Perception and Cognition

How do we see? This question has fascinated and perplexed philosophers and scientists for millennia. In visual perception, mind and world meet, when light reflected from objects enters the eyes and stimulates the nerves leading to activity in the brain near the back of the head. This neural activity yields conscious experiences of a world in three dimensions, clothed in colors, and immediately recognized as (say) ground, sky, grass, trees, and friends. The visual brain also produces nonconscious representations that interact with other brain systems for perception and cognition and that help to regulate our visually guided actions. But how does all of this really work? The answers concern the physiology, psychology, and philosophy of visual perception and cognition. Gary Hatfield's essays address fundamental questions concerning, in Part I, the psychological processes underlying spatial perception and perception of objects; in Part II, psychological theories and metaphysical controversies about color perception and qualia; and, in Part III, the history and philosophy of theories of vision, including methodological controversies surrounding introspection and involving the relations between psychology and the fields of neuroscience and cognitive science. An introductory chapter provides a unified overview; an extensive reference list rounds out the volume.

Perception and Cognition

Essays in the Philosophy of Psychology

Gary Hatfield

CLARENDON PRESS · OXFORD

OXFORD

UNIVERSITY PRESS

Great Clarendon Street, Oxford OX2 6DP

Oxford University Press is a department of the University of Oxford.
It furthers the University's objective of excellence in research, scholarship,
and education by publishing worldwide in

Oxford New York

Auckland Cape Town Dar es Salaam Hong Kong Karachi
Kuala Lumpur Madrid Melbourne Mexico City Nairobi
New Delhi Shanghai Taipei Toronto

With offices in

Argentina Austria Brazil Chile Czech Republic France Greece
Guatemala Hungary Italy Japan Poland Portugal Singapore
South Korea Switzerland Thailand Turkey Ukraine Vietnam

Oxford is a registered trademark of Oxford University Press
in the UK and in certain other countries

Published in the United States
by Oxford University Press Inc., New York

British Library Cataloguing in Publication Data

Data available

Library of Congress Cataloging in Publication Data

Hatfield, Gary C. (Gary Carl)
Perception and cognition : essays in the philosophy of psychology / Gary Hatfield.
p. cm.
Includes bibliographical references and index.
ISBN 978–0–19–922821–8 — ISBN 978–0–19–922820–1 1. Perception (Philosophy)
2. Experience. 3. Neurosciences. I. Title.
B828.45.H38 2009
121'.34—dc22
2008046063

Typeset by Laserwords Private Limited, Chennai, India
Printed in Great Britain
on acid-free paper by
CPI Antony Rowe, Chippenham, Wiltshire

ISBN 978–0–19–922820–1 (Hbk)
ISBN 978–0–19–922821–8 (Pbk.)

10 9 8 7 6 5 4 3 2 1

For
William Epstein,
teacher, collaborator, friend

Preface

These essays are about how we see. They concern the character of our visual experiences (i.e., the way things look), together with the physical, physiological, psychological, and philosophical facts and theories that explain why they look that way. They also concern how vision can guide our action and permit us to gain knowledge and information about the environment, whether through conscious visual experience or through nonconscious visual processes and representations.

To understand how we see and why things look as they do, we must pay attention to what we see. If we started a list, it would include many things: we see buildings, furniture, trees swaying in the wind, where to step, trolleys coming, friends, passersby, children playing, dogs chasing cats, drawings, paintings, photographs, movies, the moon and the stars, the sky and clouds, the rainbow, sunlight streaming in from a window, shadows on the lawn, afterimages, and stars and dots in the dark. For our purposes here, I will classify what we see according to the types of visual contents that are present in our experience or are otherwise represented in the processes of vision. That work begins in the Introduction and continues in the subsequent chapters.

In our investigations of seeing, we will consider a variety of sources of information and potential insights, including our own visual experiences, the writings of philosophers (past and present), and the work of vision scientists. Vision science, and especially the psychology of visual perception, provides the framework for much of what follows. Many of the essays are exercises in the philosophy of visual perception and cognition considered as a branch of the philosophy of science.

In the philosophy of science more generally, it is common to examine the conceptual foundations and methodologies of the various sciences and scientific theories, as in philosophy of physics (space-time, quantum theory, causation, etc.) and philosophy of biology (foundations of evolutionary theory, function, adaptation, reduction, etc.). Here I take an analogous approach to the experimental psychology of visual perception and cognition, while also considering the relevant philosophical literature in the philosophy of perception and cognitive science. The various chapters analyze notions of function, representation, and content within active perceptual and cognitive theories, and they argue the conceptual and methodological autonomy of psychology as a science distinct from the neurosciences. From these arguments and analyses, they generate results that bear on debates in philosophy of mind, pertaining to nonconceptual content in perception, the notion of representational content, the conditions of object reference, the status of qualia (qualitative visual experiences), the debates concerning representation and naive realism, and the mind–brain relation and the possibility of neurophysiological reduction.

I have been fascinated with vision for many years. In grade school, I volunteered to give a report to my second-grade health class on how we see. My presentation took weeks to prepare and involved blowing up and copying numerous figures and drawings from the *Book of Knowledge* onto large sheets of manila paper, using an opaque projector. When I finally was in front of the class, I first reviewed the basic facts of anatomy and physiology that had been deemed suitable for a children's encyclopedia, referring frequently to my drawings. I pointed out the retina, the blind spot, and the optic nerves (the optic chiasma was shown in one of the drawings). I spoke about nerve activity and the brain. Finally, I ended by paraphrasing a statement that reads in part: "Light impulses arising in the retinas of our eyes are carried over chains of cells to the optic nerve and along this nerve to the brain. We become conscious of the sensation of vision only after the impulses reach the brain. In other words, we really see with our brains" (Edds 1951, 3807–8), a passage that the author summarized as: "Once the visual impulses have reached the visual cortex, we see" (ibid., 3808). I repeated this summary phrase, but instead of "visual cortex" I probably said "back of the brain." (The article said to place one's hand over the back of one's head in order to learn the location of "the visual cortex where all light impulses are finally received.")

When I had finished, someone in the rear of the class raised his hand and asked "Yes, but how do we really see?" I reasserted the point about impulses, the back of the brain, and our then just seeing. He wasn't satisfied, and neither was I. Subsequently, I gave the presentation to the other second- and third-grade classes in the school (and to my own second-grade class again, with visitors from the local university present), but the answer to that question never got any better.

I retained an interest in seeing through junior high and high school, expressed mainly in art classes through drawing and painting. In college, I was drawn to the study of the history of art in part because that major exploited and developed visual skills. I was also delighted to learn that in psychology one could earn credit hours for studying theories of visual perception. At Wichita State University, I took an undergraduate course on the Psychology of Perception from Robert Borresen in the Fall of 1973. Borresen followed a policy of teaching alternating versions of his course: one year he would teach a "standard" version, the next year he would take the first six weeks to survey this standard material (basic material in auditory and visual perception, from physiology to social factors in perception), followed by two months' intensive study of James J. Gibson's *Senses Considered as Perceptual Systems* (1966). With hindsight, I can say that I was fortunate to hit a Gibson year. I was deeply impressed by Gibson's book, including chapter 9 on the evolution of the visual system. Few psychologists at this time were sympathetic to an evolutionary approach.

In 1974, I took my Gibsonian sympathies to the University of Wisconsin, where I pursued a joint-degree program in the history and philosophy of psychology (focusing on perception), which combined the doctoral requirements (up to and including prelims) of the Departments of History of Science, Philosophy, and Psychology. Wisconsin at that time was ideally suited to the study of the history, philosophy, and psychology of perception. In history of science, David Lindberg was completing his *Theories of Vision from al-Kindi to Kepler* (1976). Victor Hilts taught the history of social science, and Robert Stauffer the history of biology (within which he allowed paper topics in sensory physiology). In philosophy, Fred Dretske had already published *Seeing and Knowing* (1969) and was working on *Knowledge and the Flow of Information* (1981). Elliott Sober had just come to Wisconsin, with his own interests in perception and cognition (and, very soon, in the philosophy of biology). Berent Enç also was interested in the philosophy of psychology. Finally, within perceptual psychology, William Epstein, who had published *Varieties of Perceptual Learning* in 1967 amid his ongoing work on the perceptual constancies, had agreed to work with me. The faculty also included Sheldon Ebenholtz and Willard Thurlow, who were soon joined by Lola Lopes, who taught the information-processing approach. Epstein soon put me in the laboratory, and I spent most of my five years in Madison engaged in experiments in the morning, conversations in the afternoon, and reading and writing in the evening (punctuated by visits to the dozens of film societies on campus or to the Union Terrace, or sailing the waters of Lake Mendota). The final product of the joint-degree program was a dissertation on the history and philosophy of spatial perception, which, after extensive revision, became *The Natural and the Normative: Theories of Spatial Perception from Kant to Helmholtz* (1990).

Epstein was not a Gibsonian, but he was more sympathetic and tolerant than many "constructivists" (theorists who view perception as the product of psychological processes that combine various sources of information). At Wisconsin I learned to think about perceptual mechanisms and processes in psychological terms, despite Gibson's strictures (discussed in the Introduction and Part I) against such thoughts. For this reason, my position is not truly

Gibsonian. I retain from Gibson an appreciation of higher-order stimulus variables and of the importance of ecological and evolutionary considerations, but I view perception as a product of psychological processes.

The essays exhibit my ongoing attempts to understand how we see. A comprehensive Introduction (Ch. 1) sketches my view of perception in a unified manner and draws together themes from the remaining chapters, which are divided into three parts: Part I, Foundational and Theoretical Issues in Visual Perception and Cognition, which focuses on explanations in perceptual theory, primarily concerning the perception and cognition of spatial properties and material objects (Chs. 2–7); Part II, Color Perception and Qualia (Chs. 8–11); and Part III, History and Philosophy of Perceptual and Cognitive Psychology, which addresses the history of theories of perception and attention and examines methodological issues concerning introspection, psychology and neuroscience, and psychology and cognitive science (Chs. 12–16). The chapters within Parts I and II are ordered by date of publication; those in Part III, topically. Depending on their interests, readers may wish to follow a different order. Those interested primarily in the philosophy of cognitive science might begin with Chapters 2, 3, 14, and 15; those focused on the foundations of the psychology of perception, Chapters 4–6, 8, and 12–13; those examining topics in traditional philosophy of mind, Chapters 7, 10, 11, and 16. The individual chapters stand on their own. Some later chapters adapt earlier arguments and conclusions to new contexts and applications.

These chapters describe various aspects of what is known about how we see, which goes some way toward satisfying my classmate's question. A good deal is known about the structure of optical stimulation, the anatomy and physiology of the retina and brain, the psychological processes of color vision, the types of theory that may explain spatial vision, and the structure of the concepts that are applied to visual objects and that mediate object reference. At various junctures, I propose my own answers to questions in the philosophy and psychology of visual perception. The question of exactly how brain processes yield conscious seeing has not been answered by anyone, and it is not even clear what form an answer will take. But work continues toward an answer.

Of the sixteen chapters, three appear here for the first time (Chs. 1, 6, 7). The remaining thirteen have been previously published and appear with permission (the details of original publication are provided with each chapter). Four of these last have been substantially edited: Chapter 2 has been thoroughly edited for style; Chapter 3 merges two previously published papers (Hatfield 1991a, b), edited for style; Chapter 11 has been edited down and revised; and Chapter 15 has been augmented by a section, otherwise expanded, and retitled. In going over the remaining nine chapters, I corrected typos and emended minor infelicities. All of the previously published chapters are edited to conform to a uniform style of citation by author and date, and to provide internal references to other chapters as published here. Cross-references within the work are identified by the use of initial capitals: Part, Chapter, Section; the corresponding parts of other works are denoted in lower case: part (or pt.), chapter (or ch.), and section (or sec.). Finally, the few editorial insertions are placed in square brackets.

In the Introductions to Parts I–III, I describe the genesis of the previously published chapters (for a full set of personal acknowledgements, the original papers must be consulted); Chapters 1, 6, and 7 contain their own acknowledgements. Here I want to express gratitude to my teachers at Wisconsin and to students and colleagues at various universities, institutes, and centers. At Wisconsin, besides Lindberg, Epstein, Dretske, Enç, and Sober, Terry Penner both challenged and inspired with his critical acumen and intellectual purpose. Among fellow students, John Kalfayan and David Ring were close intellectual companions. In my first postdoctoral position, at Harvard, Hilary Putnam, Burton Dreben, and John Rawls were generous about discussing perception; Stephen Kosslyn sent some very good psychology students to attend my course in philosophy of psychology (including Martha Farah and Mark Gluck). During these years I was admitted to the "secret seminar" that met at Ned Block's home in Back Bay (to which I was conducted by Joseph Levine, who was also in my course in philosophy of psychology). At Johns Hopkins, Alfonso Caramazza and Howard Egeth were wonderful colleagues in psychology. When Marr's *Vision* (1982) appeared, Egeth, together with the visiting Kosslyn, taught a joint seminar on it that I attended. Our weekly lunches at the Hopkins Club turned into the Hopkins Cognitive Science Group, and led to the joint Hopkins–College Park cognitive science discussion group.

When I came to Penn in 1987, Ed Pugh (with whom I subsequently co-taught a seminar on color vision) and other members of the vision group, including Gershon Buchsbaum, Peter Sterling, and Al Laties, were welcoming. It was a special treat when Leo Hurvich and Dorothea Jameson came down from New York for a conference on the philosophy and science of color perception at the Institute for Research in Cognitive Science in 1994. The Institute itself is a constant source of stimulation. More broadly, in the late 1990s the Provost's Power of Sight interdisciplinary seminar drew together faculty across the University to read original sources in historical and contemporary visual theory and to discuss them with visitors, including A. I. Sabra, Lindberg, James Cutting, Jan Koenderink, David Summers, and John Onians. The seminar led to the founding, jointly with Renata Holod, of a Visual Studies undergraduate major at Penn. Also during this period, the Center for Interdisciplinary Research at Bielefeld twice hosted me in a stimulating environment populated by philosophers and psychologists, with the Mind and Brain Group in 1989–90 and the Perception and Evolution Group in 1995–6. More recently, Sarah Allred, who studies lightness constancy at Penn and has a background in neuroscience, has been a spirited partner in discussing the relations between psychology and neuroscience and the role of conscious experience in perception. My doctoral students with interests in sensory perception and the philosophy of psychology, and especially Larry Shapiro, Alison Simmons, and Morgan Wallhagen, brought excitement and challenges to the collaborative work that characterizes doctoral study.

Peter Momtchiloff of Oxford was both persistent and patient in bringing these essays together, and he arranged for helpful comments from an outside reader on the previously unpublished Chapters 6–7. Krisanna Scheiter did an excellent job as my research assistant. Holly Pittman posed many interesting questions and made life otherwise worthwhile.

G. H.

Contents

1

Introduction:

PHILOSOPHY AND SCIENCE OF VISUAL PERCEPTION AND COGNITION

Consider your visual experience. In that experience, mind and world meet. The world is presented to you with its shapes, colors, and textures: a green expanse with moving blobs on it; or a whitish grey ribbon with shaped volumes of color moving at great speed. The mind responds by categorizing the objects and anticipating their behavior: here is a park with people playing volleyball, and someone is about to spike the ball; there is a busy highway as you navigate your vehicle at high speed, concerned that the car on the left is weaving a bit. Form, color, and meaning are all present at once in vision, and the objects of other senses usually are experienced as located within this visual world. The world we inhabit, the one in which we live, move, and breathe, is primarily a visual world.

For this reason, vision is the most thoroughly studied of the human senses. From antiquity, the disciplines of philosophy and psychology have both given special attention to vision. Indeed, the psychology of perception is the centerpiece of psychological science. Perusing a textbook such as psychologist Stephen Palmer's *Vision Science* reveals a broad range of topics, from sensory receptors and the retinal image, to the perception of color, spatial structures, motion, and events, and on to cognitive aspects of perception including object perception, conceptualization, attention, visual memory, imagery, and consciousness. These topic areas are treated experimentally and the phenomena are subject to explicit models framed within recognized theoretical traditions. Although philosophers sometimes have disparaged the notion of *psychological science*, in this case there can be no question of the just application of the honorific "science."

Sensory perception was the first topical area within psychology to which mathematics was applied, in ancient, medieval, and early modern optical writings (Ch. 12), when the science of optics sought a complete theory of vision (Lindberg 1976). During the seventeenth century, this optical tradition was integrated into the natural philosophical tradition in psychology, which extended back to antiquity (Ch. 14). Self-consciously *experimental* psychology developed only in the latter part of the nineteenth century, primarily through the application of instruments and methods from physics and sensory physiology to the problem of describing and explaining sensory perception. These early studies included both the psychophysics of Fechner (1860/1960) and others (psychophysics correlates physical stimulus values such as intensity with experienced values) and the experimental testing of psychological theories of perception by Wundt, Helmholtz, Hering, and others. Following the consolidation of experimental psychology as a university discipline, the first edition of Robert Woodworth's *Experimental Psychology* (1938) devoted about a third of its pages to psychophysics and to sensory and perceptual psychology.

During the middle third of the twentieth century, when psychology was dominated by behaviorism, the study of perception preserved an interest in phenomenal experience and mentalistic concepts. Perception was a central player in the "cognitive revolution" that unfolded from the 1950s into the 1970s (Neisser 1967; Lindsay and Norman 1972). Other cognitive areas—which had maintained a more tenuous existence—also burgeoned, including attention, memory, problem solving, concepts, and reasoning. The subsequent development of *cognitive science*, with its early emphasis on language and computer models, introduced new explanatory styles to psychology, although these were not adopted wholesale. In physiological psychology, techniques for recording from individual neurons were applied to sensory perception from the 1940s onward. More recently, the explosion of studies using electrophysiological recording and neuroimaging offers a new source of data to experimental psychology in general.

Philosophers have studied perception since antiquity, offering *natural philosophical* explanations of how the senses work, *epistemological* analyses of the role of perception in knowledge, and *metaphysical* theories of the origin and status of sensory qualities. Early modern metaphysics and epistemology from Descartes to Kant examined the relation of sensory perception to intellectual cognition; sensory perception remained important in nineteenth-century philosophy (Hatfield 1990*b*, 1998; Yolton 1984).

Within analytic philosophy, perception was the single most prominent topic in the first half of the twentieth century. With some exceptions (e.g., Broad 1923; Hamlyn 1957), these discussions were divorced from the ongoing work in the psychology of perception and started instead from everyday examples of (presumed) perceptual knowledge. Various analyses of perceptual experience and its role in knowledge were on offer, but the primary concept that is now remembered from this rich literature is the notion of *sense data*. The concept of sense data itself, and the related notion of momentary particulars, was invoked in several distinct analyses of the metaphysics and epistemology of perception, including neutral monism, naive realism, representative realism, and critical realism (Chs. 10–11, Hatfield forthcoming-*b*). In the middle decades of the century, sense data came under attack and there was a trend toward physicalism and mind–brain identity. In the latter part of the century, the theoretical options again opened up, partly through the development of several distinct analyses of color perception and color qualia. During this period, philosophers re-engaged the psychological literature on perception.

The studies herein draw on the philosophical and psychological study of visual perception in examining three things: visual perception itself; the science of psychology as exhibited in the study of visual perception; and philosophical accounts of perception and perceptual qualities. I am investigating both a subject matter and the scientific and philosophical study of that subject matter. Accordingly, philosophical considerations inform the investigation in three ways. First, I use philosophical concepts and methods, joined with scientific concepts and methods, to address questions about visual perception. Second, I bring philosophical analysis to bear on psychology as a science, in order to contribute to the philosophy of psychology, considered as a branch of the philosophy of science (on which, see Hatfield 1995*a*). Third, I address previous philosophical theories of perception at various points (esp. Chs. 3–4, 6–7, 9–12, and 16).

In this introductory chapter, I survey the basic features of the philosophy of visual perception and cognition that guides or emerges from the remaining chapters. In setting out this framework, I introduce particular conceptions from the philosophy of psychology that underlies or results from those chapters. More particularly, in succeeding sections, I first sketch my overall picture of visual perception and cognition, and I then describe the major phenomena in visual perception, the objects of explanation in perceptual psychology, the conceptions of functional analysis that I use, the notions of content and representation in play (with replies to some objections thereto), the explanatory resources in perceptual and cognitive psychology, the sorts of evidence brought to bear, and the role of philosophy in such investigations. These sections offer a unified presentation of positions and perspectives that must depend for their support primarily on the remaining essays, although in some cases I introduce arguments for points that are not directly sustained in those essays.

1. A Picture of Visual Perception and Cognition

The external senses function to put organisms in touch with their environments, in order to guide action and build knowledge. The visual system of primates, and more particularly of humans, serves to put the organism in contact with a distal environment. It does so by processing information from the optical array as received at the retinas, from bodily musculature, and from other internal sensory systems to yield representations of various visual properties, including colors (chromatic and achromatic) and spatial structure (size, shape, texture, distance, direction, motion), represented as belonging to bounded volumes that (usually) are distributed across a landscape, or, more recently, are in an architectural setting. Color, size, shape, and texture pertain in the first instance to the surfaces of those volumes and the surrounding landscape, whereas distance, direction, and motion pertain to their locations (whether viewer-relative or object- or scene-relative). The visual system also garners information about illumination (including shadows and brightness), which is of interest in its own right and as it informs the perception of the spatial and chromatic properties of objects.

Visual systems generate such representations by responding to the information available in stimulation. I take an ecological attitude toward information: stimulus information is always information for a type of organism in an environment (Ch. 2). The physical world contains conditional regularities that allow the perceptual system to glean information concerning the spatial and chromatic properties of distal objects from the stimulus values that its receptors transduce. Such regularities concern the structures in environments and the way light is reflected from those structures and received at the eyes by a stationary or moving organism. The information registered by the transducers is processed to yield perceptual representations of the surrounding spatial layout and color properties. (See also the Note on information, below.)

Some of these representations of sensible properties become available to consciousness as the phenomenal contents of visual experience, bringing the perceiver into immediate phenomenal contact with surfaces and objects at a distance. These representations directly present a world of colored surfaces and volumes, organized into figure/ground relations, and perhaps spatially grouped according to Gestalt principles (Ch. 7.7). The entire stream of representations (conscious and nonconscious) further allows the perceiver (or the perceptual system) to interpret the scene as containing objects, some of which are recognized as objects of a known kind (a dog, a table) or as known individuals (my dog, my table)—that is, to bring objects under specific concepts. Indeed, merely to represent an object as an object is, in my view, already to bring it under a concept, viz., the concept of an object (Ch. 7). Such classifications or identifications of objects, together with any affective or emotional responses the objects invoke, may become phenomenologically present as part of the perceiver's conscious experience of the visual world. The perceiver (and/or the perceptual system) can direct attention to specific objects in or regions of the scene. Visual information (conscious and nonconscious) guides the perceiver's actions in interacting with this environment.

Many perceptual psychologists divide these phenomena of visual perception into two domains, which I describe as *sense perception* and *cognitive perception* (Chs. 2–3, 7). These names do not pertain to the character of the processes underlying perception (which are discussed below), but to types of products produced by those processes. *Sense*-perceptual products include the perception of basic features and properties of the scene: color and spatial properties. These properties are represented distally (i.e., as located in a three-dimensional world), in spatially determinate and chromatically specific ways, but without being brought under concepts. *Cognitive* perception depends on concepts, including especially object concepts, pertaining both to individually identified objects and to kinds of object. Although sense perception may guide action by representing the spatial layout, cognitive perception assigns functional significance and identities to objects. Attention can engage sense-perceptual products without presupposing their conceptualization, but it can also be sensitive to conceptualized content (Ch. 13).

I regard visual sense perception as imagistic in character. It presents determinate color qualities and spatial structures arrayed in three dimensions. Like David Marr's 2½-D sketch (1982, ch. 4), it presents surfaces at a distance in a spatially articulated manner. Going beyond Marr's sketch, these surfaces are organized into volumes that show figure/ground segregation and amodal completion. Thus, although sense perception is imagistic, it does not yield a simple copy of the environment; it represents the environment in species and subject-specific ways, which include organized spatial structures and phenomenal colors (Chs. 5–11). These statements describe the spatial and chromatic content of imagistic percepts; they make no commitments regarding the processes that yield such percepts (e.g., whether these processes are symbolic or nonsymbolic, and cognitive-conceptual or noncognitive-nonconceptual). In describing our imagistic experience as presenting three-dimensional spatial structures, I am speaking of the normal case. By adopting a special attitude, we can experience something close to a two-dimensional perspective image (the "visual field" of Gibson 1950). I return to the spatial structure of our imagistic experience in Section 4.

In describing percepts as imagistic, I do not posit "images in the head" that might be seen by a neurosurgeon who has sectioned the occipital cortex. As far as I can tell, the contents of phenomenal experience have an intentional status, in Brentano's (1874/1995, 88) original sense: such contents are not physical images or pictures (even if some visual brain processes are organized retinotopically); they are phenomenal contents (further discussed in Secs. 4–8) that exist "in the mind," without literally imparting to the relevant mental state the spatial and color properties that they make present, phenomenally (Chs. 5.4, 11.6). I reject substance dualism and maintain that these intentional states are correlated with (perhaps emergent from) neurophysiological processes. The spatial characteristics possessed by these neural processes might be relevant in explaining the spatial structure of visual experience, but they are not necessarily so; whether and how they are relevant depends on one's psychoneural linking hypotheses (Ch. 4.2.3).

Further, I do not suppose that we experience the world as a sequence of static snapshots. That description goes wrong in three ways. First, as many philosophers now attest, our everyday experience is phenomenally "of the world," and not "of something experienced as an image of the world." I agree with this phenomenological report, but I do not conclude from it that we don't have imagistic experience that mediates our perception of the visual world (and I deny that the report by itself can sustain this conclusion; see Chs. 6.6, 11.2, and 16). Second, the snapshot view supposes that our experience typically is constructed from static elements. Our experience comes closest to this when we observe a still scene without moving (in such cases the eyes and body always move slightly, but the perceived scene remains stable). Often when we see, we are moving about and our perceptual systems use the flow of optical stimulation in perceiving the stable structures in the visual world; also, we typically perceive moving objects within a larger, stable environment. Third, in many cases we are actively looking and are seeking visual information; we are not merely passive receivers (though of course we do receive information that we aren't looking for). Finally, my description of visual sense perception as imagistic initially applies to conscious experience. I also allow for pre- or nonconscious imagistic representations, but the postulation of these representations belongs with the discussion of perceptual processes (below).

The conscious experience of an adult perceiver does not present bare unconceptualized images. Overall, phenomenologically, we experience a world populated by individual objects arrayed within a scene; many of these objects are experienced as being of a certain kind (a cup, a pencil, a tree, a person). Cognitive perception pervades sense perception. The type-identities and (some) individual identities are directly present to us phenomenologically: we aren't aware, in the typical case, of "working out" what we are seeing (even if nonconscious processes in fact work to identify what's there). Further, although objects may attract our attention involuntarily, we can also choose to direct our attention here and there, making some objects perceptually and cognitively more salient than others. We may focus on some objects that we intend to approach or to act on in some manner (e.g., by grasping them).

Suppose for the moment that this distinction between types of visual perceptual products (sense perception vs. cognitive perception) can be maintained. A further question is to investigate the processes by which they are produced. Theorists have proposed various types of processes, including symbolic computational processes that already involve some (at least proto-) conceptualization; inferential processes that take a primitive description of sensory stimulation as input and yield conceptualized images as output; various types of nonsymbolic processes of information-combination (or computation); in Gestalt psychology, holistically conceived configural brain processes (Chs. 4.2.3, 5.3); with James J. Gibson, neurophysiological mechanisms that simply "resonate" (to use his metaphor) to optical information specifying distal structures (1966, chs. 12−13; 1979, 239−50).

My own view is that noncognitive (nonconceptual) processes underlie sense perception, and that cognitive (conceptual) processes are required for cognitive perception. I thus reject unconscious inference as the basic cause of sense perception, but I maintain that the processes of sense perception permit a psychologically interesting decomposition into subprocesses of information-flow and information combination or computation. To this extent, I view perceptual processes as *constructive*: they produce perceptual representations by processing information. Under normal conditions of viewing, a great deal of information is available in stimulation to guide these noncognitive processes of construction.

Perhaps because I have not cognitivized the fundamental processes underlying sense perception (by viewing them as inferences, judgments, or descriptions), I find no need to posit an underlying symbol system to carry out the processes of information combination. Subsymbolic or connectionist mechanisms suffice. (I return in Sec. 6 to the character of these processes.) Although the processes of sense perception occur in relative independence of cognitive perceptual representations, they are not totally independent. Some top-down effects occur. (These are especially manifest in the perception of ambiguous figures or in cases of impoverished stimulation, but also in other cases, as in priming effects.) In accounting for the cognitive perception of objects, I eschew both causal and descriptive theories of reference. In their stead, I posit the sense-perceptual tracking of bounded, three-dimensional volumes that are subsequently subsumed under object concepts; in cases of visual reference, such objects are the targets of cognitive acts of referring intent (Ch. 7).

Although I treat conscious phenomenal content as an object of explanation in itself and also as a factor in visually mediated behavior, I do not hold that all of the visual representations that affect behavior need be conscious or even available to consciousness. Many models of perceptual processing rightly posit nonconscious representations to account for the combination of discrete sources of stimulus information to yield conscious perception, or in order to explain behaviorally manifest discriminations that occur in the absence of reportable consciousness (as in blind sight). In my view, the study of visual perception is not only about conscious vision, it is about visual processes and capacities taken generally as they mediate action and support the acquisition of conscious or nonconscious, momentary or lasting representations of the distal environment, including beliefs and perceptual or cognitive maps.

This picture of visual perception has arisen from reflection on extant psychological and philosophical theories of perception, and it is guided by the notion that human visual capacities have evolved through natural selection and are subject to biofunctional analysis. Indeed, my take on the most basic forms of information-flow and representational content is that their ascription is mediated by a decomposition of the processes of the visual system into components that are to be "functionally described" in two senses: as components in a complex system with a division of processing labor (so, as elements in Cummins-style functional decompositions, as described in Cummins 1975); and as states in a system that is ascribed an overall function in the biological sense (Wright 1973), and whose subcomponents are to be seen as contributing to that function. Thus, if a primary function of primate (including human) visual sense perception is the representation of surfaces in space with distinctive features such as color, then the subprocesses of vision can be assigned subfunctions—and indeed can be ascribed content-bearing informational states—that serve that larger function. I thus attribute informational content to sense-perceptual processes by working downward from a functional decomposition of those processes, in relation to a biofunctional description of perceptual systems. Accordingly, representations are not individuated by their causal roles alone, but always in relation to their contribution to the (bio)function of a system.

Finally, in describing perceptual experience, I distinguish between phenomenally determinate features of visual experience and other features of that experience that are part of an overall phenomenological description. As explained in Chapter 6, in perceptual psychology a phenomenological description is one that seeks to describe experience without, as far as is possible, introducing the perspective of any particular theoretical account of perception. Anything we find present in our experience can be subject to phenomenological description. Some aspects of our experience, and especially imagistic spatial structures and specific shades of color, are more or less phenomenally determinate (or at least appear to be so). I restrict the adjective *phenomenal*, and related forms, to such phenomenally determinate features. Other aspects of experience, such as the immediate experience of something as being a dog, or as being a drawing produced by a friend of ours, have *phenomenological* presence as part of our overall experience but do not possess the determinate *phenomenality* of spatial structures and experienced color qualities. Thus, *phenomenology* is an umbrella term for a descriptive attitude toward experience and the resulting descriptions. As it relates to vision, it includes the description of phenomenally definite as well as other, conceptual aspects of experience. By contrast, the term *phenomenal* applies to determinate spatial and chromatic structures (and other determinate features of visual experience, if such there be).

So much by way of sketching my picture of perception. Figure 1.1 provides a summary overview. The subsequent sections take up aspects of this sketch, broach additional questions in the philosophy of visual perception, and address some points that are not directly taken up in subsequent chapters.

2. The Objects of Explanation in Visual Perception and Cognition

Although the study of visual perception is among the oldest fields of scientific psychology, there is no agreed-upon answer to the question of what exactly constitutes visual perception, or of what the object of explanation should be in vision science. But the available answers cluster. In considering various answers, I will focus on what Marr (1982) termed *early vision* and what I have termed sense perception, since that area receives the most extended treatment by perceptual psychologists and vision scientists.

Many investigators accept Koffka's (1935, 75) question, "Why do things look as they do?" as the central question for the psychology of visual perception. Koffka's question focuses theoretical attention on visual experience or the appearances of things. In this tradition, Irvin Rock (1975, 3) places "visual appearances" at the center of perceptual theory. Whether such appearances are "veridical" (i.e., "truthfully" reflect "the objective state of affairs") is secondary; he assigns equal evidential weight to veridical and illusory perceptions (ibid.). Nonetheless, he pursues the mechanisms underlying *perceptual constancy* as

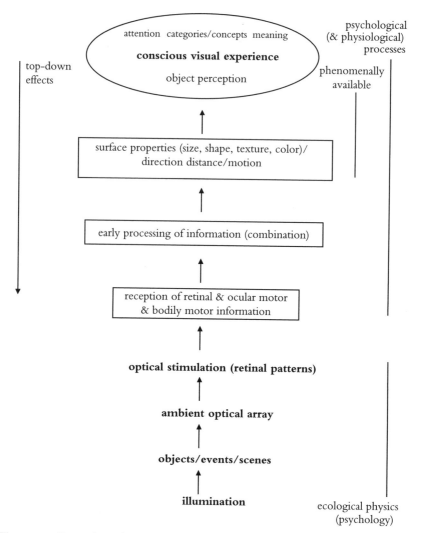

Figure 1.1. Perception: from objects to phenomenology. A chart of major causal factors, processing stages, and informational factors in the conscious perception of surfaces and objects. The diagram represents the phenomenological observation that object classification, attention, and meaning are part of our overall visual experience. See Fig. 1.2 for major response categories interacting with conscious perception.

he conceives it: the tendency of perceptual representations to remain stable (and perhaps to represent the actual sizes, shapes, and colors of objects) despite variations in the retinal image (the *proximal stimulus*). Richard Gregory (1997, ch. 1) shares Rock's focus on perceptual appearances. Each author also favors a neo-Helmholtzian explanation of perception as a process of unconscious inference and hypothesis formation. Rock (1975, 1983) is the most prominent recent theorist to contend that such inferences start from a representation of the two-dimensional retinal image (Pt. III, Intro.).

Other theorists include visual experience as part of what is to be explained, but emphasize the functional role of vision in supporting action and the acquisition of knowledge. Marr (1982) and Palmer (1999) share this general position. According to Marr (1982, 3–6), vision is the "process" of forming "representations" (both conscious and unconscious) of *what* is in the world and *where* those things are. Palmer (1999, 5) offers a formal definition of visual perception as "the process of acquiring knowledge about environmental objects and events by extracting information from the light they emit or reflect." As Palmer makes clear, the knowledge acquired may often serve in the guidance of action and behavior; it may or may not become available to consciousness as visual experience (see also Milner and Goodale 2006, and Ch. 15.2.3). Marr and Palmer both favor an information-processing approach to perceptual processes, and they each characterize these processes as inferential (Marr 1982, 44; Palmer 1999, 80).

Another group of theorists discounts the importance of visual experience as an object of explanation and focuses on perceptual mechanisms for guiding behavior and acquiring knowledge. Brian Wandell (1995, 387) regards vision, or seeing, as "a collection of inferences about the world." These inferences concern pattern, color, motion, and depth, and they are ultimately integrated into descriptions of objects and surfaces. He does not directly discount the importance of visual experience, but he largely leaves it out of his analysis of the processes of vision. His analysis concerns receptor encoding, retinal and cortical representation, and inferential processes that interpret such representations to yield the perception of color, motion, and depth. Lloyd Kaufmann (1974) sees visual perception as a constructive process, and considers the ultimate explanatory vocabulary to be physiological rather than cognitive. According to him, reports of visual experience are simply descriptive constructs of an organism who is put in a "reporting" situation (1974, 16). John Heil (1983) maintains that visual experience is inessential to visual perception, which he regards as essentially a matter of forming beliefs based on information gleaned from light. Zenon Pylyshyn (2003, 3, 133; 2007, ch. 4) discounts the importance of visual appearances as an object of explanation because he believes that the imagistic character of perception is a kind of illusion, constructed out of perceptual information that guides action and yields knowledge.

All of the authors thus far mentioned in this section distinguish the processes of sense perception from ordinary reasoning and conscious inference. In

Rock's (1983, 20) terminology, sense-perceptual processes are "insulated" from conscious conceptual knowledge. The inability of general knowledge to influence perception has long been recognized (Rock 1975, 511, 560; Ch. 4.2.1). Pylyshyn (1980) proposed that insulated perceptual systems are "cognitively impenetrable." He reasoned that if perceptual processes are cognitively penetrable (i.e., can be influenced by beliefs and goals), then the processes of perception are themselves inherently cognitive (symbolic, inferential, and conceptual). Originally, he extended such penetration quite deeply (1980, 131). Fodor (1983) countered that perceptual systems are informationally encapsulated modules within which symbol-mediated inferences occur in isolation from central cognitive systems. Theorists characterize the insulated processes differently: Rock, Marr, Gregory, and Wandell describe them as cognitive (inferential), whereas Kaufman does not. Pylyshyn (2003, ch. 2; 2007, ch. 1) now argues that early vision is largely impenetrable and so noncognitive.

Gibson (1950) took visual experience to be an important object of explanation in perceptual theory, within a theoretical context that viewed perception as guiding action and supporting the acquisition of knowledge. He rejected the traditional characterization of optical stimulation as impoverished and observed that for a moving observer there is rich information in the optical array concerning the spatial structure of the distal environment. Subsequently, he focused on the senses as mechanisms for detecting this rich stimulus information (1966, 1–2) so that an organism "can take account of its environment and cope with objective facts" (1966, 6). In his final book, he came back to questions about visual experience and approvingly paraphrased Koffka's question (Gibson 1979, 1). Throughout his writings, he is concerned with the role of visual perception in allowing organisms to navigate their environments. This involves not only detecting what is where, but also detecting change (what's happening?) and the perceiver's own motion (where am I going?). Gibson (1966, 1979) emphasizes the study of vision in ecologically valid (or normal) environments; he treats illusions as special cases that are not especially revealing of the normal processes of perception, but must be explained by deficiencies in stimulation or in physiological mechanisms (1966, ch. 14).

Gibson's emphasis on the role of perception in guiding action has been incorporated into the mainstream of perceptual theorizing (e.g., Palmer 1999). The importance of perception for guiding action has also been a theme in comparative physiological psychology of vision, in the study of the visual capacities of fish, amphibians, reptiles, and various mammals, including primates (Ingle 1967; Schneider 1967; Trevarthen 1968). This comparative work led to the postulation of "two visual systems," meaning physiologically and functionally distinct pathways of visual processing in the brain (Ungerleider and Mishkin 1982; Milner and Goodale 2006). I consider this hypothesis in Chapter 15.2.3.

Gibson (1966, 2; 1979, 251) viewed the processes underlying both the sensory and cognitive aspects of perception as noncognitive (see Ch. 2). For describing the mechanisms that "pick up" the information in stimulation, he adopted a physiological vocabulary and used the physical analogy of mechanisms that "resonate" to such information. Kaufman (1974) agrees with Gibson that *sense* perception is noncognitive; but he disagrees with Gibson's (1950, vii; 1966, ch. 13) hints that the underlying processes are unsuited to psychological study and belong instead to physiology. (Kaufman sees physiological reduction as a long-term goal, not as a prescription to avoid psychological descriptions now.) Other authors who are sympathetic to Gibson's position about the richness of optical stimulation nonetheless favor cognitively characterized processing mechanisms to pick up the information (Neisser 1976, ch. 2; Haber and Hershenson 1980, chs. 9–10).

I hold that the objects of explanation in visual perception are the visual capacities that serve to guide behavior and for the acquisition of information and knowledge about the environment. It is well established that not all of these visual capacities rely on or result in conscious visual experience. Nonetheless, consciously available visual experience is a central object of explanation in visual perception and a central explanatory factor for visually guided behavior (see also Wallhagen 2007). Koffka's question remains important for vision science, although it does not exhaustively specify its subject matter.

Explanations of the visual capacities are multifaceted. They involve explanations of visually guided behavior and of the acquisition by vision of knowledge and information. They also involve the decomposition of the visual capacities, including those that yield visual experience, into subcapacities that explain those visual capacities. The further explanation of such subcapacities may take any of several forms: physiological (as in receptor characteristics), evolutionary, cognitive-architectural (invoking connectionist or symbolist explanatory primitives), or psychological (invoking psychological explanatory primitives, such as primitive capacities for information combination). Individual investigators may choose to stop with any one type of explanation even if other types are in principle available. Some theorists hold that physiological explanations are more basic than psychological explanations, but I challenge that intuition (Ch. 15).

Although sense-perceptual capacities provide the initial focus for the psychology of vision, conceptual capacities also enter in. Gibson (1979, ch. 8) explained such capacities through his noncognitive theory of "affordances," which holds that the visual system directly detects functional properties of objects, such as "affording cutting" in the case of a knife. Most other theorists disagree, maintaining that conceptual representations must come into play when we visually recognize and identify objects. The relevant conceptual capacities are recognitional: they move from perceptual characteristics to the recognition of objects, object-kinds, and known individuals. I discuss such cognitive abilities in Chapters 2–4 and 7.

3. Functional Analysis

Functionalism entered into modern psychology in two distinct periods. At the turn of the twentieth century, the American functionalist school of psychology followed Darwin (1859, ch. 7; 1872) in viewing the mind, or the various psychological capacities, as adaptations that mediate the adjustment of an organism to its environment (O'Neil 1982, ch. 6). William James (1890) made this form of analysis prominent. The biological outlook was taken up into American behaviorism (Hatfield 2003a). Although evolutionary thinking fell under suspicion in mid twentieth-century psychology, Gibson (1966, 1979) was noteworthy for applying such thinking in perceptual psychology, and evolutionary considerations were strongly represented in comparative sensory physiology and psychology (Autrum 1979; Jacobs 1981; Trevarthen 1968).

At about the time that this sort of Darwinian functionalism in psychology was at its nadir, the philosophers Hilary Putnam (1967) and Jerry Fodor (1975) introduced a new notion of functionalism, which defined psychological states by their computational roles in mediating between inputs and outputs (stimulus and response). By focusing on the relation between input and output, this new functionalism resembled behaviorist learning theory (Ch. 3); but it differed from behaviorism in allowing mentalistic intervening variables between stimulus and response (many philosophers thought of these variables as beliefs and desires). With its focus on computational relations among internal psychological states, this new philosophical functionalism was consonant with new modes of analysis in cognitive psychology (Neisser 1967; Lindsay and Norman 1972), which decomposed perceptual and cognitive capacities into subcapacities, often represented by boxes linked together with arrows to indicate the direction of causal influence and information-flow. An analogy with computer programs was not far from the surface, and Fodor (1975) maintained that it was no analogy: he held that the routines and subroutines described in his functional analyses are literally carried out in an internal symbol system, the most basic version of which has the same fundamental status as the machine language in a standard digital computer. Psychologists themselves had mixed reactions to this particular Fodorean commitment (Ch. 14.4).

This new brand of functionalism was soon ensconced in Robert Cummins' (1975) notion of "functional analysis," which he applied to both biological and psychological systems. In a Cummins-style analysis, the ability of some entity to exhibit a capacity of theoretical interest is to be explained through a division of labor: the overarching capacity is analyzed into subcapacities that are so organized as to bring about the to-be-explained results. John Haugeland (1978) labeled the resulting explanatory style a "systematic explanation," and he observed that such explanations are typical in cognitive psychology. In this brand of functionalism as applied to psychology, representations are identified by their causal and computational roles in a system. These roles were typically described in syntactic (non-intentional) terms (e.g., Fodor 1975; 1980), although Haugeland (1978) allowed for systematic explanations involving intentionally characterized interactions that might or might not be subject to non-intentional reduction via physical instantiation.

Cummins-style analysis captured the flavor of many explanations in perceptual and cognitive psychology, which tended to chart information-flow, information-combination, and in general to decompose larger tasks into smaller ones. But it had a problem: how do we decide what the larger tasks are? Pragmatically and locally, this problem might not seem pressing: the psychologists provide the functionally characterized tasks to be analyzed, such as depth perception, color perception, object recognition, problem solving, and so on. But theoretically and philosophically, there was a problem (Hatfield 1993): how are we to understand our function-ascriptions to organic systems? Do such ascriptions simply represent our theoretical interests, or are these functions psychologically and biologically real? If some functions are real, how do we tell which ones?

Near the time that Putnam–Fodor functionalism was being incorporated into what came to be called cognitive science, philosophers of science were working on the notion of biological function (Hempel 1963; Nagel 1979; Wright 1973). This work brought the Darwinian connection between function and natural selection back onto the philosophical scene. Wright (1973) offered an intriguing answer to the question of which functions are true biological (and psychological) functions: they are the functions performed by structures and mechanisms that have been culled by natural selection because they do X. In this context, the thing that does X is in the system *in order to do X*; this description is teleological, but the teleology is cashed out by natural selection. Doing X is the function of a given structure because its doing X is responsible for its fixation in a population of organisms (or type of organism); or, in a needed adjustment to the theory, because doing X currently contributes to the fitness of the organism (Walsh 1996; Schwartz 2002).

The function of the heart is to pump blood because that is the characteristic of the heart structure that is responsible for its presence in populations or types of organisms, through the agency of natural selection. The function of the visual system is to bring animals into perceptual contact with distal objects; the function of trichromatic color vision is to make objects more discriminable by their color (let us suppose). Dysfunction (error) occurs when a system fails to perform what is properly its function. (Systems that are functioning normally can also yield nonveridical percepts: Matthen 1988.) As in Marr's (1982, ch. 1.2) "computational level"—which is actually a functional analysis in the biofunctional (teleological) sense (Ch. 3.4)—describing the tasks performed by the visual system and its subsystems is the first step in investigating those systems. The importance of an explicit *task analysis* is now widely recognized in perceptual psychology.

These two forms of functional analysis fit together nicely. The Wrightian analysis could provide an answer—or could assure the theoretician that an answer was possible—to questions about what psychological functions there are. The Cummins-style analysis indicated how the relevant capacity might be explained (through a division of labor). But there was a problem for the Wrightian (or "aetiological," meaning explanation through causal origin) type of analysis: the evolutionary process by which many biological and psychological functions have come into existence is unknown. Moreover, psychologists surely are not in the position of having to speculate about or to determine the past course of evolution in order to specify the psychological tasks that they wish to investigate and explain (Proffitt 1993). Surely they can rely on theoretical tradition, or current intuition, in deciding what the tasks or functions of the visual system and its components are.

In fact, psychological theorists often are guided by prior theory or current intuition in performing a task analysis (functional description) of the visual system and its components (Hatfield 1993; Ch. 3). But an evolutionarily guided ecological perspective is nonetheless desirable for that (Shapiro 1998). As Gibson (1966, 1979) has shown, asking questions about the conditions under which a system evolved can be heuristic in considering how the system performs its functions; for example, considering stable properties of the environment–eye relation can yield fresh insights into the sorts of stimulus variables (including texture gradients and motion flow) to which visual systems are sensitive. Ecological and evolutionary considerations are frequently invoked in the study of color vision, and genetic techniques provide new information for constraining evolutionary scenarios (Chs. 8, 9, 11, 15). And in any case, theorists can appeal to the contribution that a perceptual mechanism currently makes to fitness when describing the mechanism's biofunction (Walsh 1996). Accordingly, in invoking biofunction, theorists needn't be privy to the history of selection; they need only have a reasonable conception of how a mechanism currently contributes to the functioning of the visual system.

As set out in Chapters 2–3, 5–6, 8–11, I place heavy weight on the notion of task analysis and function-ascription in formulating descriptions of what perceptual systems do (what their functions are), and I then follow the widespread strategy of seeking to explain such capacities by positing subcapacities. There is nothing vacuous in this, if the subcapacities perform progressively less ambitious functions, until they can be discharged as functional primitives or through appeal to another mode of explanation (say, biochemical, as in the case of the visual receptors). It is through task analysis and functional decomposition that I support ascriptions of representational content to the subsystems of the visual system.

4. Content and Representations

Although the notion of *representation* did not wholly disappear from psychology during the behaviorist era (Ch. 14.3), that notion subsequently became ever more widespread in perceptual and cognitive psychology (Neisser 1967, 20, 287; Lindsay and Norman 1972, 1, 19; Haber and Hershenson 1973, 35, 159; Rock 1975, 5, 24; 1983; Palmer 1999, ch. 2.3.4). Some theorists have supposed that representations must be symbolic in nature (Fodor 1975), while others have not shared that assumption (Dretske 1981). The related notion of *content* is something of a philosopher's term of art. Recent usage of the latter term has often assumed that content is propositional in nature (e.g., Dretske 1981, 65; Heil 1983, 45; Rey 1997, 4, 19). I do not follow such usage and instead invoke the notion of nonconceptual *phenomenal content* in discussing visual representational content (see also Crane 1992b; Peacocke 1992).

As the following essays make clear, I think it is a mistake to equate representations with symbols. There surely are symbolic representations (in natural language, if nowhere else), but I doubt that all of the internal representations that are reasonably posited in perceptual and cognitive psychology are symbolic (Chs. 2–3). Further, in my version of functional analysis, representations are not defined by their causal or computational role in mediating between inputs and outputs (as in Putnam–Fodor functionalism); rather, they are assigned their content by considering what they have the function of representing. Such representations may play causal and computational roles, and those facts may be relevant to their function; but such roles alone do not yield a representation. Finally, the fact that a representational state is caused by a certain physical stimulus also does not fix its content (as in causal theories of content).

Some accounts of perceptual content first distinguish between a *representational vehicle*—a neural state, or a subject-dependent qualitative state—and its attendant representational content and then argue that the properties of the vehicle are irrelevant to the content (e.g., Dretske 1995*b*, 35–7; Tye 1991, 118). Not accidentally, such accounts deny qualia and hold that perceptual representations do nothing more than provide information about the physical properties of distal objects; on this view, there is no phenomenal content to be aware of except the distal property.

I adopt a different stance, at least for conscious contents. With noncon-scious perceptual processes of information-flow, representational content can be characterized independently of vehicle, by functional contribution. In con-trast, visual content that is carried in qualitative imagistic form cannot be characterized independently of the vehicle insofar as the vehicle has Brentanian intentional status (as phenomenal content); but it can be characterized inde-pendently of its neurophysiological realization. (This doesn't make the neural vehicle irrelevant; it simply says that the connection between phenomenal vehicle and neural vehicle is not a necessary one, so far as we know.) For imagistic percepts, the spatial structure of the vehicle itself (i.e., the spatial structure found in the phenomenal content of spatial perception) matters: the vehicle provides the spatial content. Similarly for consciously experienced col-ors: the subject's color qualia are vehicles that purvey content (normally, they purvey the colors of things). I conceive imagistic percepts as nonconceptual presenters of the spatial structures and chromatic qualities of the world—a position that rejects naive realism but is, I argue, consistent with critical direct realism (Secs. 7–8). (On introspective awareness of phenomenal content, see Chs. 5.4, 16.)

For sense perception, my ascriptions of content depend on a functional analysis of the various sense-perceptual tasks. For example, consider the (nonconscious) information provided by the outputs of the three cone types in color vision. We perceive one or another color when the visual system compares the activation of the three types of cones. The output from each cone represents, or carries informational content about, the activity of that cone (at the least). Whether such outputs also carry information about the presence of light that falls with a range of wavelengths (the range of sensitivity of that cone type)—or, better, information described by a mathematical function relating wavelength and intensity within that range—is another matter. I'm skeptical about ascribing such physically described content to the outputs of the various cones (Chs. 4, 8). In my view, such outputs may be attributed informational content because they enter into processes that have the function of producing a representation of the distal surface (Pt. II). Those processes may use cone activation to represent the presence or absence of light. Spatial mechanisms use such bottom-up information to produce representations of the spatial structure of distal surfaces, and the color system phenomenally clothes the represented surface in a specific hue. This hue represents the surface in a distinctive manner, as an illuminated surface with a color quality.

In the case of spatial perception, outputs from various small regions of the retina might represent (retinocentric) visual direction. Binocular neurons may detect disparity between like features (light–dark borders, or other features) in nearly corresponding positions on the two retinas. However, as with the cone types, I resist assigning representational or informational content to retinal mechanisms simply on the basis of a physical description of the stimuli to which they respond. Binocular neurons do not count as "disparity detectors" simply because they physically respond to disparities. Such neurons conceivably could serve other functions, such as tuning the alignment between the two eyes so as to preserve single vision (Crawford *et al.* 1993). If some disparity-responsive neurons were specialized for this function, then variation in the disparities to which they respond might simply be noise, or might serve to capture information at various grains of precision, so as to allow fine-tuning of the alignment. In all such cases, the specific content to be assigned depends on an analysis of the system that the detector mechanism serves.

Reflecting on visual perception and theories thereof leads me to maintain that, as regards sense perception (early vision), the primary representational content is spatial and chromatic. As explained in Chapter 5, I hold that the perceptual system creates a visual space. This space is not congruent with physical space but is contracted with respect to it, in such a way that visual direction is preserved (i.e., visual direction typically is congruent with physical direction) while spatial structures are represented at less than their true physical distance (in accordance with a 3-D to 3-D projective relation). Visual space contains phenomenal structures. These structures represent the physical spatial structures of objects and scenes by means of a resemblance relation. In many contexts, phenomenally present visual line segments represent physically present line segments. Sometimes, a phenomenally present trapezoid represents a physically present rectangle (Chs. 5–6), and in this case the resemblance is attenuated. If the representing structure is normally contracted for the circumstances, I count the percept as veridical.

I do not hold that these resembling structures represent the corresponding physical structures simply in virtue of resemblance. Their status as representations is set by functional analysis (as explained in Sec. 3). The fact that they resemble is a feature of their representational character; they carry information about spatial structure *by* resembling it, which can explain how visual perception is able to guide locomotion successfully. (Such resemblance is not a *necessary* feature of representation in my view, as the case of phenomenal color shows.) Further, although circular phenomenal structures do not represent a circular surface simply because they are caused by it or resemble it, visual representational types such as circles presumably have been selected during evolution or learning to represent physical circles because they resemble them (and so I favor "wide" content: Ch. 2.4). Both causation and resemblance may affect evolution and learning, but neither by itself establishes a representational or referential relation (Chs. 7, 11). Insofar as the representational characteristics of physiological structures affect their selection, then such structures are selected because of their psychological (representational) properties. Finally, I not only deny that resembling structures represent distal surfaces simply because they are caused by light reflected from those surfaces; I also deny that *sense perceptual* representations possess content that is itself of or about *individual* surfaces and objects at all. Rather, I hold that imagistic percepts represent spatial (and chromatic) properties abstractly but determinately (Ch. 7); that is, as a determinate spatial structure of a certain type, for example, a circle of certain size and viewer-relative location.

Phenomenal color qualities do not resemble the surfaces of objects, nor do they (in my view) represent the underlying physical causes of color experiences. Rather, they function to represent object surfaces (in the basic case) in a qualitatively distinctive manner. Although there are systematic relations between physically described surface-properties (spectral reflectance distributions, or SRDs) and color experience (as also mediated by contextual factors, including illumination), I do not consider the color experience to represent the SRDs—except perhaps to a well-informed theorist, and in that case the representing is mediated by theoretical knowledge. As is apparent, I endorse a version of the distinction between primary and secondary qualities (Chs. 9, 11).

In my descriptions of what visual sense experience represents, I have invoked nonpropositional and nonconceptual content. Phenomenal colors nonconceptually represent surface characteristics. A phenomenal line segment (usually) nonconceptually represents a physical line segment. It is an imagistic content. The spatial structure of the line segment as phenomenally present may guide our action, and it may also allow us to recognize the presence of a line segment through the appropriate concept. I of course also recognize conceptual and propositional content, as discussed in Chapters 2–4 and 7.

I have suggested (just now and in Sec. 2) that there are recognitional concepts. Fodor (1998) denies them. His arguments assume that a recognitional concept such as *red* not only must serve the cognitive-perceptual function of detecting instances of red, but also must explain all other cognitive abilities involving the concept *red*, including the productivity and compositionality of belief content. This objection loses force if our conceptual capacities are hierarchically layered. A recognitional concept may serve to gather instances of red in the visual world. That recognitional concept might yield the further tokening of an abstract representation of red that is not tied to present instances and that is related to other features of redness (that it is a color, that it pertains to vision). The abstract representation might itself yield the tokening of a mental word (or an English word) that enters into further computations that exhibit productivity and compositionality. As I discuss in Section 6, Fodor's argument is an instance of a widespread strategy of supporting or opposing a single-type account for all perceptual and cognitive operations, rather than allowing diversity of representational format and function.

5. Attacks on Biofunctional and Evolutionary Accounts of Representational Content

There have been some prominent objections to invoking biofunction and evolution to underwrite representational content in psychology. Fodor (2000, ch. 5) contains several, but they are easily disposed of (e.g., Ariew 2003, on Fodor's main point; Sec. 3 above on function and teleology). Lewontin (1998) offers what his editors describe as an "unremitting attack" (1998, 129) on study of the evolution of cognition. Lewontin points to problems in reconstructing the past; in using chimpanzees as a window into the last "common ancestor" between the apes and the lineage resulting in Homo; and to alleged difficulties in determining what counts as "cognition" in nonhuman species. As examples of what he is opposing, he cites two works: a sociobiological book by Charles J. Lumsden and E. O. Wilson (1981) containing identical twin studies in support of innateness, and a paper by cognitive scientists Steven Pinker and Paul Bloom (1990) on the evolution of language. Otherwise, his is entirely a "just can't" argument, which doesn't engage the specialist literature of those who think you can, including work by physiological psychologists (Donald 1991), paleoarchaeologists and paleoanthropologists (Gamble 1991; Mellars 1989;

Mithen 1990), evolutionary biologists/anthropologists (Boyd and Richerson 1985), and anthropological psychologists (resulting in Tomasello 1999), or the synthetic works in which these results are summarized (e.g., Mithen 1996). (On more recent literature, see Hatfield forthcoming-*a*.)

As regards visual perception, Fodor (unpublished, 1990) has posed an interesting objection to using evolutionary considerations in studying perception and cognition: how does an appeal to function or evolution allow us to decide which specific content should be assigned to a given structure or process? This question has famously been asked about the frog's alleged fly detector. The frog visual system and brain is such that when a fly comes in range, the frog shoots out its tongue and ingests it. The frog will also (let us say) snap up bee-bees, or paper dots, that move appropriately. So what is the detector's content: *fly*; the more generic *food*; *small black dot*; or the disjunctive *fly or bee-bee or paper dot or ...* ?

Several answers have been given. Before considering some of them, let's step back and ask how we should determine an answer. On my account, we first seek to specify the function of the frog's visual mechanism that represents the small black (or dark) dot and to learn how that representation is related to the snapping response. If the frog's visual system were such that it initially formed representations of moving items at different locations independently of a recognition and response system, then we might suppose that the content reduces to shape, color, and motion. It would still be intentional in Fodor's sense (i.e., representational): it would represent a particular shape, darkness, and motion, and be subject to misrepresentation such as misrepresenting the direction to a target, getting the size wrong, and so on. Suppose also that a subsequent ("recognitional") mechanism induces the frog to snap only at things of a specified size and direction that exhibit a characteristic motion pattern. We can now seek the function of this further mechanism that triggers snapping. Is it to detect food? To detect small black dots that move at a certain speed?

Fodor is skeptical that biofunctional and evolutionary considerations can yield any answer concerning the representational content of the frog's detector mechanism. In his view, the whole system can be treated as a causal mechanism that has been selected because it serves *to procure* flies in the usual frog environment, but not because it *represents* flies (or anything else). As Fodor (1990, 72–3) puts it (with characteristic pith): "Darwin doesn't care how you describe the intentional object of frog snaps. All that matters is how many flies the frog manages to ingest in consequence of its snapping."

There have been several responses to this sort of point. Dretske attempts to explain how the content gets into perceptual states such as the frog's by combining his notion of semantic information (Dretske 1981, ch. 3) with the idea of a biofunctionally characterized representational system (1988, 1995b). Suppose that a frog's eyes respond to characteristic motions that only flies make in the frog's normal environment. On Dretske's account of information, the semantic information that a fly is over there is present at the frog's eye if there is a stimulus variable that naturally indicates the fly's presence. Any physical structure that is present only if a fly is present possesses the "indicator content" that a fly is present (independently of whether any organisms do or can use this information). If a structure in the frog's visual system responds only if that stimulus variable is present, then it shares that indicator content. Thus far, we don't have a representation of a fly. For that, Dretske (1988, ch. 3) requires that the system has the function of using indicator content to guide behavior. If the tongue-snapping trigger has the function of inducing a snap when and only when the visual system's fly indicator fires, then the system *represents* flies; and, when it misfires, it misrepresents flies.

I don't accept Dretske's analysis because I am skeptical of his proposal that physical information directly yields semantic information which in turn furnishes the content for psychological representations (as if by osmosis). It's not that I deny that conditional relations might exist between motion-patterns and the presence of flies (physical information). It's rather that I don't see a way to ascribe semantic content of any kind to the motion-path stimulus variable short of finding a mechanism that is sensitive to that sort of motion *because* it indicates the presence of flies, or because it serves to increase the chance (on the frog's part) of eating, or serves some other function. By contrast with Dretske, I don't believe in semantic information without a system that creates it in response to physical information. For that reason, I must rely on the notion of a *function to represent* in ascribing content, without deriving the content from Dretskean indicator content. (See the Note on information.)

Shapiro (1992) provides another approach to this problem. Like Dretske, Shapiro appeals to evolutionary considerations to fix content. He argues, contrary to Fodor as quoted, that the phrase "was selected for representing things as F" is *not* transparent to coreferring expressions. Suppose that in the frog's environment, *moving black dot* and *food* are co-extensive. Shapiro holds that "selecting for" provides an intensional context that is opaque to substitution, on the grounds that only by putting "food" into the context do we capture the relevant generalizations from the ecological and ethological sciences that explain why the frog has the detector it has (such as the generalization that frogs that catch more food fare better).

I agree with Shapiro that "was selected for representing things as F" is an intensional context (on the intension/intention contrast, see Ch. 7.4). But I think it is doubly so, and that only one of the intensions gets us to food (or flies) as *representational content*. The "selecting for" part is intensional over the properties relevant to lawful (or otherwise explanatorily generalized) regularities concerning frogs and their food. Such generalities might pertain to the rate at which one or another version of the frog's detector mechanism snaps up food in a given environment. Although the intensionality of lawful or explanatory contexts is a controversial matter (see Dretske 1981, 75–7), I'm willing to live with the notion that objects fall under explanatory generalizations only under certain descriptions (e.g., "frog food," and not "my grandmother's least favorite insect"). But these descriptions apply to the behavior of the frog's detector as described from the outside: a behaviorist could use such descriptions. This instance of intensional opacity doesn't get us to the frog's representations.

To a limited extent, I agree with Fodor (1990) that selection is not content-specifying: the mere establishment through natural selection of a mechanism that successfully induces fly-snaps does not tell us what representational content to ascribe to the mechanism. In describing behavioral success, Darwin needn't determine the specific representational content. To account for the frog's snapping mechanism as it is relevant to selection, *food, moving black dot*, and *flies* all work (assuming they are ecologically co-extensive). But that's because a mechanism that had the function of representing any of those three would work equally well in the frog's environment (we are supposing). Presumably, a mechanism that had the frog snap at any movement at all wouldn't work, nor would one that had the frog snap an inch behind the fly's present position. As Shapiro (1992, 472) observes, Fodor never denies that the visual mechanism governing snapping is a *detector*. For Fodor (1990), the issue is whether selection assumes a specification of whether the detector distinguishes between *fly* and *food* (etc.). I answer: no, it doesn't, if the mechanism that is selected is in fact able to detect food in an adequate manner.

But just because behaviorism works for some purposes is no reason to stop there. There may still be a fact of the matter about what the frog is detecting, and *how* it "represents things as F" (our second intensional context). Evolutionary explanations start from the extant variability in a population and selection then accounts for the fixation of a trait in subsequent populations. If a certain frog in fact possessed a representation of *fly* and not *moving black dot*, and that representation triggered its snapping mechanisms with more successful outcomes than other detectors in the population and therefore was selected, then we have the functional specification of the detector's content as *fly*. I consider it unlikely that frogs have the conceptual resources for such a specific content. If, as seems plausible, the system can function with the minimal content *moving black dot here now*, I would rest content with that. But that does not mean that there is no intentionality or misrepresentation. Because we treat the visuomotor system as having the function of representing items so that they can be targeted and ingested, we have a basis for assigning representational content and for allocating misrepresentation. Further, if the states that account for the frog's success at fly-catching do so because they are representations, then, on the aetiological account, the function of those states is to represent.

A reader of a naturalistic bent might balk here. Dretske (1988, 1995*b*) attempts to reduce representational intentionality to the allegedly physical notion of semantic information, plus the notion of biological function. I do not attempt to reduce it to either. I treat representation and aboutness as features that arise in organisms and become subject to selection, but I don't explain how they arise. Perhaps they evolve through mutation from simpler mechanisms that causally co-vary with environmental states (see Lloyd 1989, ch. 3). Or perhaps they arise from the mutation of physically self-organizing aspects of organisms that in some way come to be directed beyond themselves (Walsh 2002). I offer no account of their emergence. I posit that it occurs, on these grounds: presumably, before life evolved there were no representational states (nor states with semantic content, since I don't allow semantic information without a user, or using mechanism), and now there are such. I treat representing states as emergent features that then undergo selection. This position is consistent with an *inclusive naturalism*, which includes unreduced intentionality in the natural world, perhaps as an emergent feature (see Ch. 10.5, and Hatfield 1990*b*, ch. 7.2; Shapiro 1997).

6. Explanatory Resources

The theorists discussed in Section 2 invoke a variety of explanatory notions for sense perception and cognitive perception. Most of those theorists see sense perception as resulting from cognitive operations that combine information via unconscious inferences. One prominent strand of such theory, inspired by the computer analogy (Fodor 1975) or by an analogy with logical reasoning (Rock 1983), regards these inferential processes as symbolic in nature. When such processes combine information that is described logically or numerically, they are called *computational* or *algorithmic* processes. A cognitive theory need not posit internal computations but might instead describe perception using the language of belief-formation (Heil 1983, ch. 7). Conversely, one can posit computations and algorithms without supposing that they are mediated by cognitive or symbolic processes (Chs. 2–3).

Theorists who view perception as resulting from an active process of information processing are typically called *constructivists*; they may further be specified as *information processing* theorists, because they hold that perceptual processes combine local information to yield global perceptual outcomes. Although a cognitive and symbolic conception of constructivist information processing is the most common, it is not required. In my picture of visual perception and cognition, the processes underlying visual sense perception are noncognitive and nonconceptual. I also hold that they are nonsymbolic. To the extent that processes of information-combination are quantitatively specifiable, they may be deemed algorithmic computations. Further, I hold that nonsymbolic processes can underlie conceptual and cognitive representations, although of course as cognitive operations break into language, symbols are needed—however, such symbols need not be primitively specified by the computational architecture, but may be derived and constructed entities (Ch. 3).

For sense perception, I derive representational content by working downward from a task analysis (Chs. 2–3, 8). A task analysis can tell us what is being represented, but it doesn't by itself reveal which subprocesses in fact carry out the task (Marr's algorithmic level). For that, we need to determine the structure of processing. For many tasks in visual sense perception, the relevant models postulate the registration of stimulus information (cone activations, microfeature detection, and registration of larger-pattern variables such as projective shape, or of higher-order stimulus variables that specify distal shape). The various sources of registered information (including ocular and bodily orientation) are then processed and combined in algorithmic processes, as in Figure 1.2. Registration already synthesizes across physiological receptors and is to that extent "constructive," as are the processes that combine and transform registered information to yield spatial and chromatic visual structures. Although sense-perceptual processes are in this way synthetic, constructive, and computational (algorithmic), they need not be regarded as inferential, cognitive, or symbolic (Chs. 2–5). Sense-perceptual processes yield representations (nonconscious and conscious) that subsequently engage the cognitive perceptual capacities and may invoke other responses. There can be top-down influence (from cognitive perception to sense perception), but in my view the sense-perceptual processes operate largely independently of cognition. As discussed in Section 2 (and Ch. 15.2.3), some registered information may be passed on to visually guided motor-control systems without entering consciousness (Fig. 1.2).

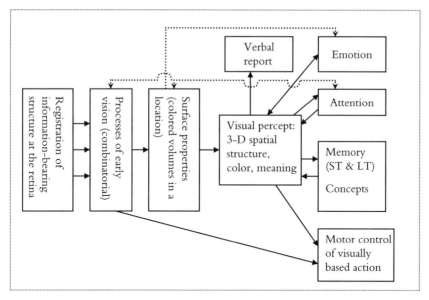

Figure 1.2. Perceptual processing stages and response categories. Response categories including concepts, attention, and emotion feed into the phenomenological content of the percept. Bodily actions such as grasping targeted objects with the hands are guided by both conscious and nonconscious visual representations (Sec. 2, and Ch. 15.2.3). Verbal reports are shown as a separate motor response to conscious visual experience. Solid lines indicate primary causal and functional relations; dotted lines indicate secondary causal and functional connections.

Different sorts of explanatory resources can be applied in explaining the processes of sense perception. In a discussion of the spatial constancies, Epstein (1973, 1977*b*) posits processes for registering, transforming, and algorithmically combining stimulus information. He does not describe the combinatorial processes as inferential or cognitive, and I take his descriptions to be compatible with my noncognitive (nonconceptual, nonsymbolic) functional algorithms (Ch. 2). Epstein (1973) treats such notions as registration, transformation, and combination as explanatory primitives. There is nothing wrong with this attitude; the viability of such primitives is tested by the empirical success of the theoretical models that employ them. But some theorists may wish to explain the basis of these capacities. Such theorists might introduce a further functional decomposition (say, of the transformational or combinatorial mechanisms), or might look to hardware (receptors) to explain stimulus registration.

More generally, a theorist might posit one or another underlying computational architecture to explain processing and combination of perceptual information. I prefer to think of sense-perceptual computations (transformations, combinations) as performed by connectionist nets (Chs. 2–3). Other theorists posit symbolic architectures, and they tend to treat the underlying processes as inferential (Fodor 1983; Marr 1982). But a symbolist need not adopt an inferential conception of sense-perceptual processes. A symbolist might hold that Epsteinian processes of stimulus registration, transformation, and combination occur in a symbol system that uses syntactically structured entities to convey nonconceptual information and to combine such information according to specified algorithms that serve as symbolically realized processing rules (see Ch. 3). I find it superfluous to use symbols in this way, for the reasons developed in Chapters 2–3.

In the literature of cognitive science there has been a great debate between symbolists and connectionists. I hope that the essays in Part I provide some antisymbolist ammunition (see also Kosslyn and Hatfield 1984; Hatfield and Epstein 1985; Epstein and Hatfield 1994). Here I would like to indicate a way in which the rhetoric employed in contemporary debates is misleading.

Sometimes authors write as if the choice between connectionism and symbolism is that between a general associationist account of the mind and a view that posits internal states with precisely specified representational contents. On this view, connectionism treats the mind as one large connectionist network, thereby eschewing any psychological division of labor among processing mechanisms. Fodor (1998, 153) puts the point this way:

What's your favorite metaphor for minds? If you're an empiricist, or an associationist, or a connectionist, you probably favor webs, networks, switchboards, or the sort of urban grid where the streets are equidistant and meet at right angles: New York's Midtown, rather than its Greenwich Village. Such images suggest a kind of mind every part of which is a lot like every other.

The mind is one big homogeneous net.

This way of characterizing the debate gives rhetorical favor to the symbolist, for it treats the division as if it were between associationists and representationalists, which can be decoded as a debate between behaviorist learning theorists and the newer information-processing psychology. Of course, associationism-connectionism (whisper: behaviorism) is supposed to lose.

Carruthers (2006, ch. 1.6) characterizes the debate in such terms, citing Gallistel (1990) in support. In fact, Gallistel contrasts general associative learning models with models that postulate internal representations, but he leaves open whether these representations are direct isomorphisms or are symbolically encoded (1990, 28–9). (On isomorphism, see Ch. 5.3.) He treats the representations in the brain as continuously varying vectors that are realized in the spatial structure of neural activity (Gallistel 1990, ch. 14). Such a system of representation is consistent with connectionism (broadly conceived). Subsequently, Gallistel and Gibbon (2002) claim to support "symbolic" models of cognition: but again the choice is between associationism and representationalism. They don't define the notion of symbol and barely mention symbols, save in their book title and preface. Their book shows that empirically successful models of conditioning attribute representations of magnitudes (including rates and statistical relations) to organisms. The only way to read Gallistel and Gibbon (2002) as providing support for symbolism is to make the unjustified slide from computation and representation to an allegedly necessary symbolic realization of computations and representations (as in Gallistel 1998). Connectionist models are of interest in part just because they offer nonsymbolic realizations of computations, representations, and rules (Chs. 2–3). They do so with an architecture of connections, activation states, activatory or inhibitory gain, modifiable thresholds of activation, and the like. Considered in the abstract, these are closer in flavor to neural properties than are symbols. However, although some connectionist models are neural wiring diagrams, most thus far are not, and so should be considered simply as connectionist computational models, whose comparative advantages must rest on other grounds than a direct match with neural reality. If, as connectionists maintain, their architectural primitives can also realize operations that are essentially symbolic (in functional or task-level description), then the need to build a primitive symbolic computational architecture into organisms is obviated. Connectionism wins on parsimony, since it can handle symbols but needn't import them where they're not needed.

I use connectionist notions as a proposed implementation for psychological models that posit as fine-grained a functional decomposition of perceptual processes as you like. In the domain of sense perception, there needn't be much associationism in such models. Many basic computational routines (for color perception, spatial direction, accommodation and convergence, and stereopsis) could turn out to be innate (hard-wired), subject only to minor environmental tuning (which might be associationist). The processing rules for such routines need not be realized symbolically; they can instead be *instantiated* connectionistically (Ch. 3.7). In the domain of cognitive perception, it seems clear that many recognitional concepts are learned. Some of this learning may be statistical and locally associationist, some may involve more structured representations (which nonetheless receive a connectionist implementation). In no case would one posit a single, large connectionist net, even to account for only the visual recognitional concepts. There is presumably a division of labor that is modeled by functional decomposition, and that ultimately must be realized in the appropriate hardware.

Finally, I treat neurophysiological structures as explanatorily relevant for psychology, but not as the ultimate bedrock of explanation. Perceptual psychology and neurophysiology exhibit an interplay, in which psychological models usually lead the way. Neurophysiological data can serve to confirm psychological models and can suggest the need for new psychological models. The basic point is that neurophysiology can be relevant for psychology without our needing to suppose that psychology can be reduced to neurophysiology (which I doubt).

7. Sources of Evidence: Visual Phenomena, Behavior, Neurophysiological Data

The sources of evidence in vision science include introspective and phenomenological reports of visual experience, whether illusory or veridical; behavioral measures in response to visual stimuli; and neurophysiological data, including invasive recording from nonhuman animals and neuroimaging of both human and nonhuman animals.

I have mentioned neurophysiological mechanisms in previous sections and I discuss neurophysiological data in Chapter 15. Behavioral data are collected in experiments in which subjects respond to various visual stimuli, sometimes of brief exposure. In analyzing such data, experimenters may consider: the stimulus variables they have manipulated, including their ecological validity; the task they set for their subjects; the theoretical models of perceptual processing they intend to test; subjects' response options (pressing a button, verbal response, selecting a matching stimulus, making a drawing); and the conditions under which subjects make a response (e.g., under instruction to respond as rapidly as possible, or only once they are sure of what they have seen). On the basis of the interactions among such factors, the experimenter qua theorist may conclude that one or another theoretical model of perceptual processing is confirmed or disconfirmed. Often, these models include the postulation of unconscious processes. Chapters 5–7 and 13–16 describe examples of data used to test or confirm theories, and Palmer (1999) describes many perceptual experiments. I want to consider more closely the status of phenomenological observations.

Psychologists of visual perception only sometimes discuss the role of phenomenological reports, which often target spatial or chromatic phenomenal qualities. Nakayama *et al.* (1995, sec. 1.1) endorse the role of phenomenological reports in vision science, as do Rock (1975, 21) and Palmer (1999, 349–50).

As mentioned in Section 2, others discount the role of phenomenological evidence and also doubt that phenomenal experience is an important object of explanation in perceptual psychology.

From the point of view of psychological science, it is important to determine to what extent phenomenological descriptions describe real features of perceptual experience. It is not that there would be nothing to study about phenomenal experience if it were discovered to be "illusory," because one could still study the reported content of the illusion. But phenomenological reports take on greater salience if there is reason to believe that they tap into genuine features of visual experience.

A notorious challenge to the reality of phenomenal experience comes from Daniel Dennett (1988, 1991). In his view, spatially articulated (imagistic) qualitative experience of spatial and chromatic features is not real. What is real are various descriptions, largely of features of the world, that exist as "multiple drafts" for perceptual judgments (1991). Our apparently coherent phenomenal experience is a fictional construct of these internal descriptions, as if we are talking to ourselves about what we see (1978). Dennett does not, to my mind, adequately address why our descriptions have the coherent fictional phenomenology they do, but he does insist that description is all we have.

Dennett's position is complex and I'll give just one example of the type of argument he sometimes offers (or once did in a talk at Penn). Visual psychologists studied *change blindness* during the 1990s. If an image is significantly altered during a saccadic eye-movement, or even if it is appropriately modified while the subject is looking at it, the subject typically does not notice the change (Palmer 1999, 538–9). The change can be large (the removal of bushes from a region of an image), but it cannot be at the unbroken point of fixation. Dennettians conclude from such data that perceivers don't really have an imagistic percept that includes the bushes (or whatever), and that they suffer from an illusion that their experience is both detailed and spatially articulated like an image (or, as I hold, like a three-dimensional imagistic structure).

This type of argument against rich, detailed phenomenal experience, although it became widespread (e.g., Blackmore *et al.* 1995), is inconclusive. The argument confounds whether the subject can report a phenomenal change with whether there was one. But theories of perception regularly distinguish what is phenomenally present from the response mechanisms that mediate an overt response. There are many contexts in which this distinction is made, but the most salient is research in attention (Ch. 13). Theorists regularly posit that there is more available in a percept than subjects can categorize and notice. The fact that a bank of bushes goes missing may alter the percept but not be noticed. Indeed, the change-blindness scenario is artificial: usually, a bank of bushes doesn't disappear all at once, but must be removed bit by bit, with each bit tracing a continuous motion trajectory as it is cut and removed. My observation that the change-blindness argument confounds perception with perceptual reporting does not decisively show that perceptual experience is spatially and chromatically detailed in an imagistic manner, but it does stay the bite of that argument.

A related issue concerns the spatial definiteness and extent of our imagistic percepts. Subjects are often surprised to find that, within a momentary fixation, the central region is clear and detailed but that the portion of the field beyond about 30° from the center is considerably less clear. This has led some theorists to suppose that, while we may have rich detailed spatial structure near the center of the visual field, we are deluded in believing that (say) a whole wall of books across the room in our study is visually present to us.

Alva Noë (2004) has responded to these concerns by noting, first, that the central portion of the visual field in fact is rich and detailed, and, second, that the books (in my example) to the left and right are "virtually present": we can move our eyes to see them, and it is part of our visuomotor skill set to know that we can attain detailed experience of them. Noë's emphasis on visuomotor skill is partly inspired by Gibson (1979). I prefer a different Gibson-inspired answer. Gibson (1979, 195) describes the momentary scene as a three-dimensional perception of the environment as seen-at-this-moment-from-this-point. Such a view is clear and detailed in the middle and fades off. But our ongoing visual experience is not a series of momentary (3-D) snapshots that we piece together; rather, as our eyes move we integrate the optical flow pattern into an awareness of a visual world that surrounds us and that, within the specious present, extends beyond the momentary vista. The surrounding books are present to our ongoing visual awareness, and not simply (as with Noë) implicit in visuomotor knowledge.

Noë (2004) and Gibson (1966, 1979) are both *physical direct realists*, so they interpret the content of this phenomenology (however described) as consisting in the books and shelves themselves, unmediated by a perceptual representation. I am a *critical direct realist*, so I interpret this phenomenology as presenting me with visual experiences as of shelves in a room with ceiling and walls, all in some sense visually present as I move my gaze about. Noë (2004, 72) points to "transparency" in favor of his view; as mentioned in Section 1, I doubt that this argument can establish his points about the metaphysics of (non) representation (see also Crane 2000).

Where does this leave us concerning the reliability of our phenomenological descriptions of a spatially and chromatically rich visual experience? In the absence of compelling reasons not to, I take such descriptions at face value.

Phenomenally, we are presented with a stable visual world that surrounds us and is immediately available for a closer look. That's phenomenology. The metaphysics of visual experience (what the real underlying basis is for such experience) is another matter.

8. Role of Philosophy

In the history and continuing development of theories of visual perception, philosophy plays several roles. In the guise of natural philosophy, it has been a source of theories and analyses. These include: the distinction between primary and secondary qualities as developed by Robert Boyle and John Locke (with foreshadowing from Descartes, as discussed in Hatfield 1986b); the notion of unconscious inference in perception, as developed by Ibn al-Haytham and subsequent theorists; an associationist theory of size and distance perception, deriving from George Berkeley (Ch. 12); and the concept of sense data from the early twentieth century. Philosophy also has been a source of methodology, in the guise of introspection and phenomenology. Philosophical analysis has examined the explanatory structures and metaphysical commitments of the various theories of vision, and philosophers currently participate in a dialogue with visual scientists concerning such structures and commitments. Philosophy examines questions that some visual scientists also propose to answer, such as "what is color?" Philosophers also venture into topics that visual scientists usually skirt, such as the status of phenomenal experience (Chs. 10–11), the mind–body problem (Chs. 10, 15), or the manner in which sense perception justifies knowledge.

Discussions of the role of perception in knowledge recently have focused on whether nonconceptual perceptual content could be epistemically relevant. John McDowell (1996) believes that nonconceptual content cannot provide a basis for epistemic justification. He reasons that if the sense perceptual states that I've described were to be assigned correctness conditions (as they certainly may be, since they present the world as being spatially and chromatically a certain way), any appeal to those conditions in epistemology would commit the "naturalistic fallacy" (1996, xiv). Like Fodor and Carruthers above, McDowell foists onto his opponents a putative one-step account of how perception supports knowledge. But as Chapter 7 describes, sense perception may initiate epistemic contact with objects, by making them salient perceptually. As we move into an epistemic context, sense-perceptual representations must be brought under concepts; the application of concepts and the assertion of conceptual content may be as epistemically norm-governed as you like, despite its engagement with nonconceptual, naturally produced phenomenal content (see also Hatfield forthcoming-c).

The status of phenomenal experience is widely discussed of late. The current trend is to try to reduce phenomenal experience to something else: it is nothing but pure informational or representational content (Dretske 1995b; Tye 1995); or it is nothing more than an unmediated awareness of the physical world itself (the new naive realism). I oppose this trend, which is partly driven by distaste for sense data or other perceptual intermediaries. As originally conceived, sense data are supposed literally to possess the qualities they appear to have: bulgy and red, for tomato-y sense data. In some versions, this claim about sense data was motivated by a type of direct realism; one which led, in one stream of thought, to neutral monism (Ch. 10), thereby reducing the material world to qualitatively characterized (e.g., bulgy, red) elements. However, neutral monism won't work if one believes, as do I, that physical things are made of atoms and molecules.

The ongoing objections to perceptual intermediaries are phenomenological and theoretical. First, on the face of it, perception doesn't *seem* to be mediated. We seem to face the world directly; we are not ordinarily aware of any need to move from mediating appearances to things in themselves. Second, there is the problem of how to fit qualitative phenomenal experiences, as states of the perceiver, into a naturalistic framework. I offer answers to these problems in Chapters 5.4, 10–11, and 16. As previously mentioned (Secs. 1, 7), I agree with the phenomenological point about phenomenally direct perception but deny that it can sustain a metaphysical conclusion about whether our perception of the world is mediated by qualitative experiences. If perception is so mediated, it is not those qualitative experiences that we *see*; rather, by means of having them, we see the world. In this regard, I am a critical direct realist, that is, a direct realist who acknowledges the need for subjectively conditioned representations and qualia. As to fitting phenomenal experience into nature, I don't believe that this is such a problem: it's already there. Some philosophers are reluctant to accept the reality of the phenomenal prior to achieving a theoretical understanding of what it is. As I see it, phenomenal experience is real, no matter what it really is.

In the best of its engagements with perceptual psychology and vision science, philosophy is neither underlaborer nor imperious judge. Rather, philosophers engage with the living inquiries of perceptual psychologists and vision scientists in addressing current issues. In so doing, philosophers may bring a perspective informed by the broader philosophical concerns of epistemology, metaphysics, and philosophy of science. They may also join perceptual psychologists in conducting empirical work and proposing phenomenological descriptions. In all of these endeavors, my own view is that philosophers should seek to participate in a discussion, rather than to criticize from the sidelines or simply to describe in clear terms what the sciences are saying (see also Hatfield 2001). Just as, on the scientific side, when theories are undergoing development there is no such thing as "just doing science" without also producing philosophy, so too, for philosophers, there is no such thing as talking in a substantive way about visual perception without engaging the science of vision, whether wittingly or not.

As philosophical and scientific discussions of visual perception continue, I believe that each party will gain from engaging the work of the other. Philosophers can contribute by raising new questions and challenging old answers. One thing is for sure. There is no danger that the mysteries of seeing will be completely solved in the near future. There isn't much that is as puzzling as is seeing itself.

Note on the Concept of Information in Perception

The notion of information was widely invoked in psychology during the 1960s and 1970s, and it is now firmly entrenched in discussions of perception and cognition in psychology, cognitive science, and philosophy. Descriptions of perception point to information in the light reflected from objects, information transduced by receptors, information processed by perceptual systems, and information contained in perceptual representations and stored and retrieved from memory. Although the word "information" is common to all these discussions, the notion of information has undergone development, and more than one concept is now in play. Thus, some sorting out is needed in order to make clear which notions of information I favor, which not, and why.

The concept of information that initially was prominent in psychological discussion of the 1950s and 1960s derived from Claude Shannon and Norbert Wiener (see Shannon 1948). Fred Attneave (1954) was among those who brought this new concept into the study of perception. Shannon and Wiener developed a mathematical theory of information as a means for measuring information transmission in communication devices. Their concept of information had nothing to do with content; it concerned only the amount of information transmitted. Technically, they defined information as negative entropy, or as the reduction of uncertainty. Their measures were widely used in perceptual investigations in the 1950s and 1960s, but this use subsequently waned because such measures did not correlate well with stimulus characteristics that perceptual psychologists found to be empirically important.

We needn't explore the technical definition of information, or chart its passing from the psychological literature (see Corcoran 1971, ch. 2; Haber and Hershenson 1973, 160), in order to understand the core idea that was ultimately retained from this notion. The Shannon–Wiener notion effectively proposes that information transmission involves the existence of conditional probabilities between two distinct entities or sets of events (Dretske 1981, chs. 1–2). Information is transmitted between A and B if the states of B exhibit a conditional relation to A. Smoke bears information that there is fire because, usually, where there is smoke there is fire. The lengths of shadows bear information concerning the time of day because they are conditionally related to the height of the sun in the sky, and the height of the sun measures time of day (relative to season). The structure of light reaching the eyes bears sufficient information to specify the layout of the distal environment if, given a certain structure at the eyes, the distal environment must have a specific spatial configuration. (This relation of specification exists only given certain assumptions, such as that the environmental structures tend to keep their shape, so that when an observer moves his eyes the changes in stimulation result from that motion and not from a simultaneous deformation of the environment.)

A second impetus toward talk of information in psychology stems from Gibson. His notion of information pertains, in the primary case, to relations of structure. There is information "in the light" because the structure of the light specifies the structure of the layout from which it was reflected (subject to some background conditions). Gibson himself at first endorsed a relation between his concept of information and the notion of conditional structural relations as derived from information theory (1966, 245), but he subsequently came to doubt that his notion of information was consistent with information theory (1979, 242–3). I agree with Neisser (1976, 60) that Gibson's notion of information is consistent with the core idea of information as conveyed by structural dependencies between objects and the stimulus array. But Gibson's specific concept differs from the generic notion derived from information theory. Gibson's notion is ecological: the structure in the light is information for an organism in an environment. Ground texture is information for distance only if the texture is comparatively homogeneous at a scale appropriate to the height of the organism that samples the optical texture generated by that ground texture (Gibson 1979, fig. 5.1).

In my view, the idea of physical or optical information available in the light should be accepted without difficulty. Theoretical questions arise in considering what is needed for a perceptual and cognitive system to respond to, register, and represent that information. These questions are raised by the tendency to view the flow of information from the world to sensory systems, or to the organism more generally, as a process of absorption. The perceptual system simply "picks up" the needed information, and the perceiver then directly perceives the distal layout. As mentioned in Sections 1–2, Gibson himself believes that there are mechanisms involved, which he describes as "resonating" to the information in stimulation, making it seem as if the information is simply absorbed. But it strikes me that there is no reception and transformation of information without mechanisms—including receptors and subsequent processing mechanisms—that register and transform the information. No information can get into or be used by the system unless the system has receptors that can register the structure of light, and no registered structures can yield the perception of a distal environment unless there are mechanisms for producing representations of the distal environment using stimulus information.

In this connection, I agree with Ralph Haber and Maurice Hershenson (1973, 159):

Since the retinal projection of the light itself cannot get "into" the organism, a representation of it, which we call information, is the content that we will describe in our theories. When this information is stored, we will want to know its relation to the information in the retinal projection of the stimulus. Is it in the same form or has it been transformed? Is it coded in some way?

Information in stimulation is one thing. Information as registered by the visual system and subsequently processed and transformed is another.

The processes that register information in the light begin at the retinas. The most basic units for human daylight vision, the cones, respond to the intensity of light within a range of wavelengths (depending on cone type). Information about the retinocentric direction of the light is associated with the cone's position in the retina and presumably is preserved in the retinotopic projection of stimulus information into the visual cortex. The retina and cortex also contain various mechanisms that compare the activation of adjacent or nearby cones. These detector mechanisms may respond to features in the light, such as light–dark boundaries, and may detect the presence of motion in a direction.

The registration of a Gibsonian higher-order stimulus variable, such as an optic flow pattern, clearly depends on comparing and integrating the outputs of such detector mechanisms across the retina. For example, Gibsonian theorists are interested in a pattern of optical expansion described by a mathematical function known as *tau* (Proffitt and Kaiser 1995). There are several applications of tau to describe flow patterns that might specify the observer's motion or the motion of objects toward the observer, including *global tau* (a global expansion of optical texture around a point specifying the observer's heading) and *local tau* (the expansion of a local area within the optic array, such as would be produced by an approaching object, e.g., a baseball). Presumably, the visual system has mechanisms to detect a local tau-pattern and mediate the perception of approaching objects. But notice that it is no good simply to have a tau-detector that tells the system that a tau-pattern is on the retina. In order to help explain how we experience approaching objects, this information must be incorporated into a perceptual representation of a solid volume approaching from a direction. Tau-detection in itself is not helpful unless the distal significance of tau enters the process (even if only in the structure of a reflex response).

As I see things, the representational significance of external physical information cannot simply be absorbed at the retina but must be generated by the receptors and subsequent processing mechanisms according to their functions to represent. Cones (or their activations) do not represent the presence of light simply because light causes them to respond; rather, because they respond to light, they have been wired into the system as light-detectors. The mechanisms that use local tau to generate representations of solid volumes approaching from a direction do not get their content by simply absorbing the information in the optic array; rather, because the structure of the array offers information about distal events, these mechanisms have been wired up to respond to that information by generating a representation of the distal motions. We must look to the properties of the visual system to understand what representation-generating mechanisms it has. I assume that the basic mechanisms have been selected in evolution because they respond to stimulus structures by generating representations that are reasonably accurate portrayals of the distal situations that produce those structures (Sec. 5). Consequently, I don't build my concept of representation from the concept of information, but I treat representational content as arising *sui generis* as the perceptual system evolves.

I thus distinguish information in the light from information registered by the system. The former exists independently of being transduced or registered, even if, in accordance with ecological optics, the classification of structural information in the light proceeds in a species or genus-specific manner. Information in the system is always, for me as for Haber and Hershenson (1973), represented information. And I see its content as contributed by the system—although presumably the system produces a specific content because, for receptor mechanisms, such content accurately represents a light-structure present at the retina, or, for subsequent mechanisms, because by integrating registered information it produces representations of the distal scene.

In this regard, my notions of information in stimulation and information in the perceptual system differs from Dretske's concept of information. Dretske's *Knowledge and the Flow of Information* includes an exposition of the mathematical theory of information, which brings out the core idea of conditional dependency (1981, chs. 1–2). Thus far, this concept of information is similar to the core idea from information theory that is shared by Gibson and myself: conditional dependence. Dretske then adds to this concept the idea of *semantic information*. He says in effect that when B bears information about A, this information exists in semantic form in B without being detected or represented by a system. He inserts semantic content into the physical state. Semantic information is what is distinctive to the Dretskean concept of information.

Dretske's extension of traditional information theory by adding semantic information is not uncontroversial (e.g., Sturdee 1997; Lombardi 2005). It is what allows him to "naturalize" representational content in his sense. He does so by supposing that a mechanism (B) in an organism that fires only when A is present would thereby instantiate the semantic information *that A* (1981, 65). This semantic information then becomes the basis (in ways described in Dretske 1981, chs. 6–7; 1988, ch. 3; and 1995b, ch. 1) for the representational content that accrues to the representations that incorporate it. In this way, semantic content (allegedly) is absorbed into representations from the information in the world.

I do not accept Dretske's postulated semantic information. Accordingly, optical structure may bear information, but that information can be extracted and rendered into semantic form only by mechanisms that bring their own representational content with them. There is no semantic content without representations and concepts. In this sense, information doesn't perform any psychological work unless there are mechanisms for registering, detecting, and processing it. Information yields representational content, but it does not do so by being absorbed. It does so when information-bearing structure is registered and transformed by mechanisms having the function to represent (Chs. 3, 11).

PART I

Foundational and Theoretical Issues in Visual Perception and Cognition

Introduction

Assuming that sensory perception has the function of representing the world in the service of action and cognition, there is much to explain. Focusing on vision, we can ask about the physical means by which objects affect the eyes as sense organs, about the physiological processes that take place in the nervous system, about the psychological processes that yield visual experience (as well as nonconscious representations), about the character of that experience itself, and about the ways vision guides action and yields knowledge and other cognitive or affective states.

Although the essays in Part I touch on all of these aspects of perception, they focus on the psychological processes in spatial perception (leaving color to Part II) and the phenomenal and cognitive upshot of those processes. In thinking about perception, questions about the relation between perception and cognition arise at several points. First, to what extent does even the most basic perception of the spatial layout in early vision, which yields a presentation of surfaces arrayed in depth (and their motion, or the perceiver's motion), already depend on cognitive processes? That is, is the bare act of seeing itself the product of cognitive operations such as inference, or does it arise through noncognitive (and nonconceptual) psychological operations? Second, to what extent is the content of visual experience itself fundamentally cognitive and conceptual? Third, how does visual perception allow conceptualized cognition of the objects around us, that is, how does cognitive perception of objects take place?

All of these issues are raised in Chapter 2, on the notions of representation and content in extant psychological theories of perception. The originally published version of the chapter was long in preparation, and it provides the framework for the subsequent chapters. The chapter ultimately descends from two papers written in graduate seminars at Wisconsin in 1976. The first of these, written for Fred Dretske in a seminar on Fodor's *Language of Thought*

(1975), discussed the role (or lack thereof) of cognitive processes in what Marr (1982) called *early vision* and what I call (following Rock 1975, 24) *sense perception* (in contrast with cognitive perception, which requires concepts). The second paper was written for Elliott Sober in a seminar on hypothesis choice. I submitted a descendant of these two papers, entitled "Perception and Cognition: Seeing Isn't Necessarily Believing," for presentation at the Seventh Annual Meeting of the Society for Philosophy and Psychology (Chicago, 1981). For the meeting, I produced a revised version, entitled "Direct Theory versus Constructivism: Contrasting Kinds of Perceptual Explanation," on which Zenon Pylyshyn commented, and which I subsequently discussed in Daniel Dennett's seminar at Tufts.

The roots of this chapter lie in my original exposure to Gibson's work (as described in the Preface) and in subsequent discussions with Epstein, Dretske, and Sober at Wisconsin. Epstein, although not a Gibsonian, appreciated Gibson's point about higher-order stimulus variables, including texture gradients and kinetic information. He believed that none of Gibson's arguments blocked an examination of the processes of perception in terms of the combination of (even higher-order) information, and he was prepared to treat such combinatorial processes in noncognitive terms (Epstein 1973, 1977*b*). Epstein and Dretske shared my interest in the role of cognitive factors in perception. The place of function in psychology was also under discussion: not merely the usual sort of Putnam–Fodor "functionalism" (input–state–output functionalism, on which see Shapiro 1994), but also psychological functions understood on analogy with biological functions. The debate between Cummins (1975) and Wright (1973) over the notion of *function* was in full swing. Cummins believed that "functional role in a system" was the more basic notion, by which he meant the causal and explanatory contribution that a system's elements make to the overall behavior of the system. By contrast, Wright held that functions should be assigned by attending to what structures and processes *do* that has been causally efficacious in the process of natural selection and so accounts for their presence in a population. I found Cummins' (1975) analysis of functional *explanation* useful, but believed that his position offered no principled means for identifying the *natural functions* that need to be explained. For that purpose, I favored Wright's aetiological approach, extended, as seemed natural, to include not only selection but current maintenance of traits (in this case, processing mechanisms and their state-types).

These factors flowed into the early versions of Chapter 2. Subsequent versions were shaped by students' responses to my Gibsonian leanings in my philosophy of psychology seminars and by discussions with Howard Egeth and Stephen Kosslyn. I drew on the ongoing revisions in Hatfield and Epstein

(1985), and in an American Psychological Association Symposium honoring Irvin Rock's work (in 1986). The essay was discussed in the joint Hopkins and Maryland-College Park Cognitive Science Seminar, and Kim Sterelny (who was visiting College Park at the time) took a copy with him back to Australia, where it circulated. I presented it to colloquia at Penn, Duke, and Maryland, and it was ultimately published in 1988.

I now find three main contributions in the essay, which are further developed in other chapters. The first is the notion that noncognitive functional algorithms serve as a *psychological* level of explanation and analysis. The question of whether psychology studies anything distinct from physiology, on the one hand, and systematized common sense ("folk psychology"), on the other, was much discussed at the time. Some questioned whether scientific psychology was possible (Davidson 1973; Grice 1974–5). Putnam (1967) and Fodor (1968, 1975) had provided "functionalist arguments" (from multiple realizability) for the autonomy of psychology, which provided hope. More interesting to me—since I knew that experimental psychology was possible, given that it was actual—was the question of the subject matter and object of explanation in psychology. Many philosophers accepted the conception that *belief* and *desire* are the core theoretical notions in psychology. These philosophers regarded the task of psychology as that of explaining behavior, and they made belief and desire do the primary explanatory work (see Ch. 3; also, Shapiro 1994). In the face of challenges to that program (Davidson 1973; P. M. Churchland 1981; P. S. Churchland 1980), philosophers debated the legitimacy of belief–desire psychology (pro: Fodor 1975; Pylyshyn 1984; contra: Stich 1983).

Philosophers arguing for the legitimacy of scientific psychology typically sought to legitimate the belief–desire version; they assimilated psychological content to the propositional attitudes and so to contents that were propositionally (or sententially) conceived. Even those who appealed to actual scientific psychology to make their cases assimilated mental contents and processes in such psychology to transitions among propositions or syntactically characterized states (Cummins 1983). Von Eckardt (1984) was an exception: she realized that although the cognitive science of Fodor (1975) and Pylyshyn (1984) focused on sentential representation, not all cognitive-style psychologists (e.g., Anderson 1978; Kosslyn 1980) followed suit. Chapter 2 begins by contrasting two styles of perceptual explanation. The first style is the cognitive constructivism of Rock (1983) and Gregory (1978), and the complementary philosophical approach of Fodor (1975), according to which even sense perception results from unconscious cognitive processes of hypothesis formation or inference. The second is the "direct theory" of Gibson (1966), according to which there are no psychologically analyzable processes underlying sense perception (rather, the processes are merely physiological). The chapter then develops a third alternative: a psychological account of perceptual processes that is noncognitive and nonconceptual—that is, that does not treat belief as the exclusive model for psychological states that are endowed with content. Ultimately, this alternative account enables a version of constructivism in perceptual psychology that views sense-perceptual states as, in the first instance, the product of noncognitive processes that modify and combine sense-perceptual content in early vision.

The second contribution is related. It pertains to the idea that function (in the biological sense) might be used to fix content ascriptions, whether noncognitive or cognitive (nonconceptual or conceptual). The chapter invokes the biofunctional notion of function in comparing an artifactual "tensional adder" to a naturally evolved system. Others in the 1980s also appealed to biological function to support ascriptions of content. They typically conceived content in propositional terms (e.g., Millikan 1984; Dretske 1981, 137, alludes to analog representations as pictorial, but his core concept of "information" is cashed out propositionally, p. 65). I believe that perception has a core of nonconceptual, imagistic content that represents things spatially (and chromatically, but that's for Part II), and that the system has evolved to provide such spatial representations. This idea is further worked out in Chapters 3, 5, and 6 (and, for color, Chs. 8−11), and also in Hatfield (1993).

A third contribution of the chapter is the discussion of connectionist implementations for noncognitive functional algorithms. Such implementations promise to carry out psychological processes that combine and transform perceptual information without doing so via the interaction of formal symbols. Kosslyn and Hatfield (1984) had already broached these topics. As Chapter 1 recounts, I like connectionist models of perceptual processes because they provide a way of thinking (albeit abstractly) about possible neural implementations of rule-bound psychological processes. This idea is further developed in the notion of rule instantiation (Ch. 3.7). My characterization of connectionist models as nonsymbolic may appear contentious, since some theorists close to connectionism in spirit remained committed to symbols (e.g., Marr 1982, ch. 7). As discussed in Hatfield and Epstein (1985, 178−83), I interpret the new connectionism as extending a theoretical stance found in the Gestalt psychologists and in more recent discussions (e.g., Attneave 1982).

Chapter 2 (as also Ch. 3) argues against symbolism in part by comparatively assessing the psychologically primitive capacities of symbolist and connectionist systems. It alludes to Fodor's (1975, ch. 2) reliance on primitive symbol-manipulating capacities in psychological systems in order to block an infinite regress of symbol-reading capacities. It argues against symbolism by offering connectionist computational architectures as an alternative, having preferable explanatory primitives. This argument of course does not assume or conclude that psychological systems have no symbolic capacities. Further, it does not prevent a theorist from seeking (as some theorists, e.g., Stich 1983, are wont to do) to define "syntactic representations" independently of their function to represent something beyond themselves (i.e., independently of my preferred approach). Without invoking a Fodorean "machine language" (Chs. 2.3, 3.1), such a theorist might describe syntactic representations by their functional roles in rule-described interactions. Such an approach is not inherently symbolist, for it does not require *primitive* symbolic operations; in effect, such purely syntactic approaches posit a *functional role syntax* in which symbols are defined only by their functional roles. Such roles might just as well be realized connectionistically.

Of the remaining chapters in Part I, all but one were written in the past nine years. Chapter 3 combines two published papers written for philosophical anthologies on connectionism (Hatfield 1991*a*, *b*). Chapter 4 arose from the Bielefeld group on Perception and Evolution. Chapter 5 was prepared for a special journal issue honoring Emanuel Leeuwenberg. The final two chapters are new (and the occasions of their discussion are noted in them).

Chapters 2–3 each treat "aboutness" or intentionality as a "stands for" relation. In this way they reflect my belief that perceptual psychology deals with the way in which perceptual systems represent actually distal things. Content is not defined merely by a representation's relations to other states internal to the system. These two chapters focus mainly on object properties (space, color) and they don't separate out object-reference from representation of spatial structure or other properties. In writing Chapter 2, I did not endorse Dretske's (1981, ch. 3) notion of semantic information (though I was sympathetic to it at the time). Subsequently, I rejected Dretske's notion (Ch. 1, Note) and held instead that representational content is wholly, not partially, parasitic on a "function to represent" (where "function" means biofunction). This position is adumbrated in Chapter 2 and further developed in Chapters 3 and 6 (as in Chs. 8–11), and I answer objections to a biofunctional account in Chapter 1.5.

Each of Chapters 2–7 takes seriously the idea of imagistic perceptual content. Chapters 4–6 go more fully into the implications of this notion. Chapter 4 observes that the phenomenal character of perceptual images is an explanandum of perceptual psychology. Chapters 5–6 explore the geometry of visual space and the notion of the spatial constancies (Ch. 6 also touches on color). Chapter 5 diagnoses the reticence among psychologists and philosophers of the 1970s and 1980s to discuss phenomenally characterized representations. Chapter 6 provides some support for the notion that visual space is subject-dependent, thereby moving against the renewed popularity of naive realism. In these chapters, the examples of the gross geometry of visual space come from static structures, mostly viewed statically: hallways, sidewalks, roads, train tracks, plates, and tables. This fact does not reflect any lack of appreciation of dynamic factors in spatial perception on my part; rather, it is a concession to the practicalities of obtaining specifiable conditions for intersubjective comparisons of the structure of phenomenal experience. For hallways, sidewalks, roadways, and the like, the phenomenal convergence of parallels as described also obtains for a moving observer. Chapter 7 discusses percepts some of which are static and some of which involve motion.

Chapters 5–6 suggest that resemblance, or a strong isomorphism, grounds the imagistic representational content of sense perception as regards spatial structures. Resemblance as a basis for perceptual representation has taken its knocks in recent decades, stemming from Goodman's (1968) arguments against the notion of resemblance in analyzing how pictures (photographs, drawings, paintings) represent. The cases are different, since picture-making and picture-interpreting include conventional elements. Nonetheless, the usual litany of objections is similar, including: the observation that resemblance is neither necessary nor sufficient for representation; the fact that resemblance is symmetrical, whereas representation is asymmetrical (the representing represents the represented, but not vice versa); the point that images may resemble one another more than they resemble their objects; and the fact that things may resemble one another in some respects but not in others (R. Schwartz 2006, ch. 9). As noted in Chapter 1, I don't take resemblance to be either a necessary or a sufficient condition for representation; the representational character of visual perception stems from the function of the visual system to represent the environment. Perception is inherently representational; the asymmetry of represented and representing is built into it. In the case of spatial properties, the representational relation is effected through resemblance, as regards topological structure from a point of view and under a 3-D to 3-D projective transformation in which line segments represent line segments, verticals and horizontals typically remain vertical and horizontal, and parallels running into depth converge (Chs. 5–6). The resemblance relation holds only in some respects, but these are well-defined within the geometry of visual space. Color perception is another matter, and I analyze it in terms of a sign relation (Chs. 5.7, 11).

Each of Chapters 2–6 invokes the separation of the sense-perceptual factors (spatial, chromatic) from cognitive-perceptual achievements that rely on concepts (such as recognition or classification), but only Chapter 7 focuses primarily on the cognitive or conceptual side. Chapter 4 examines cognitively based theories of sense perception and seeks to reveal the sophisticated concepts that must be assumed by many such accounts. Chapter 6 makes a case for the presence of conceptual (classificatory and recognitional) factors in the overall phenomenology of perception (the chapter distinguishes the concretely phenomenal from "phenomenological presence"). Chapter 7 examines a recent tendency to suppose that perceivers achieve cognitive or intentional contact (i.e., reference) to objects through a direct causal (or informational) relation. It argues that causation can't do the needed work, and supports a demonstrative or indexical account of perceptual object-reference that invokes primitive intentional capacities: intentional capacities that need not be reduced to non-intentional terms, and the explanation of which should be sought in the evolution of psychological functions (as in Chs. 5–6, 10–11).

2

Representation and Content in Some (Actual) Theories of Perception

Philosophers of psychology have examined the use and legitimacy of such notions as "representation," "content," "computation," and "inference" within a scientific psychology. While the resulting assessments have varied widely—from outright rejection of some or all of these notions (P. M. Churchland 1981; P. S. Churchland 1980; Stich 1983) to full vindication of their use (Fodor 1975; Pylyshyn 1984)—there has been agreement on the considerations deemed relevant for making an assessment. The answer to the question of whether the notion of, say, representational content may be admitted into a scientific psychology has been made to turn upon whether the notion can be squared with our "ordinary" or "folk" style of psychological explanation, with its alleged commitment to the idiom of beliefs and desires.[1] I intend to proceed the other way around, starting with experimental psychology itself and asking whether such notions as the above play a legitimate role within a particular area of contemporary theory, the psychology of perception. My conclusion is that especially the first three—representation, content, and computation—have a legitimate place in scientific theories of perception, albeit one that differs from that which a significant portion of the philosophical literature ascribes to them.

First published in *Studies in History and Philosophy of Science* 19 (1988), 175–214, copyright © 1988 by Pergamon Press. Reprinted with permission and edited for style.

[1] Fodor (1980) expresses doubts about a science of representational content. The Churchlands (1983) have suggested that the (folk) psychological notion of representation should be replaced with a neurophysiologically based notion of representation and "calibrational content" (on which, see n. 27, below).

The emphasis on "folk psychology" in philosophical arguments concerning the status of various concepts within scientific psychology is unfortunate, for it runs afoul of the ideal that the philosophy of psychology, by analogy with the philosophy of biology and the philosophy of physics, should at its core be discussing ongoing psychological theories. Especially in recent discussions of representational content, this maxim has been honored more in the breach than in the observance (Burge 1986 being an exception).[2] For while it would be interesting in itself to evaluate appeals to "folk psychology" in justifying a role for the belief–desire idiom within psychology proper, it is not at all clear that mainstream experimental psychology has adopted either the language or the conceptions of "belief–desire" psychology. To the extent that experimental psychology has proceeded in relative independence from "folk" notions, the philosophical evaluation of those notions will be less germane in assessing the notion of representational content within that body of work.[3] Put in other words, the outcome of investigations into the role of representational content in psychology is highly sensitive to what one takes psychology to be.

I therefore do not start from the relationship between experimental psychology and "folk psychology." Instead, I begin my investigation of notions such as representational content by examining their use in current psychological theories of perception (primarily, visual perception). In particular, I focus on the conflict between two broad approaches to perceptual theory: direct theory and constructivism. Both philosophers and psychologists have discussed this conflict in an attempt to resolve it on one side or the other (Fodor and Pylyshyn 1981; Turvey et al. 1981).[4] The dispute exemplifies an ongoing discussion

[2] P. S. Churchland's work, although informed about neuroscience, barely refers to experimental psychology; see the references in her 1986 book. Fodor's work in philosophy of psychology draws on his work in psycholinguistics, and his exaggerated claim (1975, ch. 1) that symbol-based computational psychology is the only game in town presumably reflects that starting point. Pylyshyn's (1984) case is more complicated, for he argues not that the *only* but that the *best* psychology will be developed through an extension of "folk" notions. I reply in Section 5.

[3] A common philosophical criticism of theories in cognitive psychology (or at least a criticism common within the walls of Harvard's Emerson Hall *c.*1980) is that, although such theories claim to operate independently of "folk" notions in virtue of possessing their own technical vocabularies, when the going gets tough the tacit "folk" connotations of ostensibly "clean" technical terms such as "interpret," "read," and "infer" do the real work, despite all disclaimers. Although such criticism is sometimes well founded, it does not obviate the present point. My claim that psychology has proceeded in relative independence from folk notions rests on successful theories in experimental psychology (examples below) that do not fail through an illicit appeal to such notions. Further, although some psychological theories (especially in social psychology) explicitly do attempt to regularize commonsense notions, these are not in the majority.

[4] Although Fodor and Pylyshyn (1981) do not describe themselves as constructivists, the shoe fits. My discussion focuses on direct theory and constructivism as competing explanatory styles in perceptual theory, not on the alleged realist and antirealist consequences of the two positions (as in Gibson 1982).

within experimental psychology over the legitimacy of fundamental notions such as information and representation. Starting from this living example, I argue for a conception of representation that is not "folk" in inspiration but that can meet the needs of the psychology of perception (and perhaps other areas of psychology).

Although the theoretical dispute between direct theorists and constructivists typically has been regarded as concerning how much and what type of information visual stimulation contains, I argue in Section 1 that the principled differences arise elsewhere. These differences stem from a disagreement over the types of explanation to be allowed in the psychology of perception. Constructivists urge that the best explanations of perception posit internal processes of hypothesis formation; indeed, Jerry Fodor and others contend that this is the *only* type of explanation available in all areas of cognitive psychology (considered as including sense perception), and that these internal processes require an internal symbol system. (In general, such symbol systems are defined by the syntactic properties of their representations; they may or may not be regarded as requiring semantic interpretation for the purposes of psychological theory.) Direct theorists, balking at the notions of hypothesis formation and internal symbols, propose a different type of explanation within perceptual psychology. According to them, perception is not mediated by cognitive operations such as hypothesis formation, and so it is not mediated by any psychological operations at all. Explanations in perceptual psychology focus on the relation between stimulus information and organismic action, in effect replacing the notion of representation with that of information, and leaving moot the character and content of internal operations. This opposition to internal psychological processes has made direct theory seem worthy of the type of scorn that is usually reserved for behaviorism.

These two conceptions of explanation in perception bring with them opposing views of the role of internal processes in the psychology of perception and of the place (or lack thereof) of representations in those processes. But implicit in some current theories of perception lies an alternative form of explanation that allows theorists to deny that perception is mediated by inference while retaining internal representations and psychological processes. I make explicit and develop this third conception of explanation in perception, which yields an alternative conception of representation. I contend that perceptual theory has open to it a kind of psychological explanation that (*a*) goes beyond mere stimulus–response correlation, (*b*) lies above the level of neurophysiology (i.e., above the level of description that is couched in the language of neural interaction), and yet (*c*) needn't invoke symbolic representations (e.g., symbol systems or a language of thought) or cognitive operations (e.g., inference or hypothesis formation), but (*d*) can nonetheless retain a workable notion of representation for use in constructing theories of perception. In order to distinguish this approach from traditional cognitive approaches and from direct theory (as I construe it below), I call it a *noncognitive psychological* approach to perceptual theory. The approach includes conceptions of representation and content that are neither "folk" nor Fodorean, and so are not cognitive in a traditional sense but are nonetheless psychological.

The availability of this third approach has radical implications for current debate in the philosophy of psychology. It shows that perceptual theorists in general and direct theorists in particular can pursue properly psychological accounts of perception without embracing the cognitive explanations of the constructivists. More generally, it indicates the existence of a type of explanation in psychology that is distinct from the current symbol-laden models, but that nonetheless provides a legitimate role for the notion of representation. The existence of psychological theories of this sort shows that belief–desire psychology is not the only type of psychology that can employ notions of representation and representational content. This result calls for a reorganization of the basic theoretic alternatives within the philosophy of psychology. "Folk psychology" no longer stands as the only alternative to eliminative materialism and the syntactic theory of mind. Scientific psychology is not in the position of either seeking a replacement for the notion of representation in physiology (as eliminative materialism demands), or of giving up the notion altogether (as in a purely syntactic theory of mind).

1. Direct Theory and Constructivism

Just as the outcome of the debate about representational content depends in part on what one takes psychology to be, so too the use of theories of perceptual psychology to adjudicate the debate is sensitive to the choice of emphasis within the field of perception itself. Possible emphases vary widely, especially if one takes traditional philosophical interests in perception into account. Philosophical discussions of perception, conditioned by concerns with epistemology, have understandably taken conceptually rich perceptual judgments about objects in the "external world" as the paradigm perceptual achievement. By contrast, psychologists of perception have tended to regard the study of the sensory discrimination of relatively simple properties such as color, shape, and size as central to their discipline. Given this diversity of emphasis, it is easy to see how investigators might form differing expectations about the type of explanation required for "perceptual" phenomena.

In order to focus discussion, let us consider the distinction that many perceptual psychologists draw between sensory and cognitive aspects of perception, or, in the terminology of David Marr, between early and late vision.[5] The study of "early vision," or sense perception proper, aims at analyzing the various sensory dimensions of perceptual experience: the perception of color, size, shape, distance, depth, and motion. Using various psychophysical techniques the investigator of sense perception seeks to answer Koffka's (1935) question, "Why do things look as they do?" The study of "late vision," or cognitive perception, concerns such achievements as recognizing, identifying, or classifying into kinds the things that we see. These achievements typically involve classifying the things we see under concepts. The difference between the two aspects of perception may be illustrated by considering how experimentalists studying one or the other might differ in their approach to the same stimulus materials. An investigation into the cognitive perception of, say, shape might focus on the names for shapes that subjects use in their perceptual judgments, and the tendency of subjects to group shapes in accordance with these names. An investigation into the sense perception of shape might focus on how well subjects discriminate various shapes under various viewing conditions. Subjects might be asked to respond in such a way that the experimenter could infer what shapes they perceived various stimuli to have, rather than what names they would give the shapes. Indeed, experimenters might seek to avoid any biases arising from the names of shapes, by presenting irregular shapes, or by using variants of a single type of shape all having the same name (e.g., all ellipses). Although there is more to say about this distinction and its justification, I introduce it here as a recognized division of labor among experimentalists who investigate the psychology of perception.

The distinction between sense perception and cognitive perception allows me to distinguish two kinds of perceptual result, or two aspects of our (phenomenally unified) experience of the world of objects and events. The distinction itself does not require an allegiance to any particular account of the processes that underlie the two kinds of end-product: separating the more sensory from the more cognitive aspects of perception does not decide

---

[5] Although philosophers of psychology and cognitive scientists are most likely to know the distinction between early and late vision as Marr formulated it (1982), esp. chs. 1–2 (he did not actually use the term "late" to complement "early"), he did not originate it. Gibson (1950, 10, 198) offered a similar distinction. Rock (1975, ch. 1, esp. pp. 2–3, 24) describes a distinction between sense perception and cognitive perception as standard within the psychology of perception.

whether cognitive operations such as inference and hypothesis formation are needed to explain either aspect. It may seem, at first glance, that recognition or identification could result only from inference, and that the sensory response to color or depth, being more biological, does not require cognitive operations. One might therefore suppose that direct theorists (who deny underlying cognitive operations) would devote themselves to the study of sense perception, and that constructivists (who emphasize cognitive processes) would limit their investigations to cognitive perception. In fact, adherents of the direct and the constructivist approaches each extend their characteristic modes of explanation to *both* kinds of perceptual result: direct theorists seek to explain object recognition without appealing to inferential or other cognitive processes, and constructivists maintain that even the perception of depth is a cognitive construction.

With these preliminaries in mind, let us examine direct theory and constructivism themselves more closely, focusing primarily on sense perception. The work of James J. Gibson (1966, 1979) and his followers (Michaels and Carello 1981; Reed 1986) exemplifies direct theory. The opposing, constructivist position comprises several lines of thought, including the neo-Helmholtzian treatment of perception as logical inference by Irvin Rock (1983) and Richard Gregory (1978), and the AI-inspired approaches of cognitive scientists such as Fodor (1975, 42–51) or Marr (1982).[6] The names given to the two approaches may be understood from their respective positions on the psychology of the perceptual process: direct theorists deny that perception is mediated by cognitive operations such as inference and hypothesis formation (hence, they say that it is "direct"), whereas constructivists affirm that it is so mediated (hence, they say that perception is "constructed" via such operations).

Standardly, the point of dispute between direct theory and constructivism is located in the amount of information available in the light reaching the eyes. And indeed, after the publication of Gibson's 1950 book, direct theorists and constructivists did clash over whether there is a sufficiently rich set of variations within optical stimulation to determine sense perception. Gibson and others maintain that the array of stimulation available to a freely moving, binocularly endowed perceiver is sufficient to specify the spatial structure of the three-dimensional visual world. The idea that optical stimulation *specifies* the distal configuration amounts to the claim that there is a one-to-one correspondence between (*a*) certain perhaps exceedingly complex variables in

---

[6] Marr places himself in the constructivist camp by characterizing perception as "the construction of a description" in an internal symbol system (1982, 343–53). Kosslyn and Hatfield (1984), 1037–41, argue that the symbolist and constructivist features of Marr's theory of vision are not essential to the theory itself.

the array of light reaching the eyes, and (*b*) the layout of the objects from which that light has been reflected. If the direct theorist is right, one could determine the spatial structure of objects reflecting light from the structure within the light alone as received at a pair of eyes. This result directly contradicts the traditional conception of optical stimulation as consisting of a static two-dimensional image that is inherently impoverished with respect to our visual achievements. On the traditional conception, internal cognitive rules (which may be acquired through experience, innate, or some of each) make up for the information lacking in the stimulus. In standard construals of the dispute (e.g., Fodor and Pylyshyn 1981; Michaels and Carello 1981, chs. 1–2, 7), constructivists rely on the traditional notion of informationally impoverished stimulation to justify positing constructive processes that mediate between stimulation and perception, whereas direct theorists, in denying the gap between stimulation and perception, also deny the need for constructive intervening processes.

If these positions on the richness of optical stimulation are taken as arguments that might establish either direct theory or constructivism, they fail. To see this, let us grant to each side its point about richness and consider what follows. Suppose that the traditional notion is correct: that optical stimulation, even under the most powerful analysis, does not specify the three-dimensional layout. Must one posit constructive processes that rely on cognitive operations in explaining perception? Not necessarily. Some scientific accounts of the intervening processes do not invoke such operations. The Gestalt psychologists, for example, accepted crucial parts of the traditional analysis of stimulation and contended that innately given physiological processes bridge the gap between stimulus information and perception (Koffka 1935, ch. 3; Köhler 1947, ch. 5). According to the notorious psychophysical postulate of Gestalt psychology, the structure of occurrent perceptual experience literally reflects the configural properties of brain states—perception of a circle, for example, results from a roughly circular brain state. In the speculative Gestalt brain physiology, the physics of ionic fields explains the configural properties of brain states. A contemporary version of this kind of explanation might eschew strong psychophysical isomorphism, but it could still propose a physiological rather than a psychological analysis of the visual process (e.g., Attneave 1982). Such a view might regard the perceptual response to stimulation as the outcome of a very complicated process of transduction—where transduction is understood as a physiological process that mediates between incoming patterns of light energy and the resulting neurophysiological activity. This view regards perception itself as the first properly psychological result of the transduction process. The well-known explanation of Mach bands in terms of lateral inhibition is an instance of this type of account (Ratliff 1965).[7]

Conversely, even if the direct theorists are right and we can in principle determine the configuration of a scene from patterns of reflected light, this does not refute a constructivist approach to explaining perception. It does, however, undercut a classical motivation of constructivism: that sound theory requires innate or learned rules of inference in order to close the gap between the two-dimensional retinal image and the ensuing perception of a three-dimensional visual world. But a thoroughly modern constructivist might well accept Gibson's point about the richness of optical stimulation and yet remain committed to constructivism. As the constructivist might put it, this option is open because the Gibsonian contention about the richness of stimulation and the constructivist account of what the organism does with this richness belong to different explanatory domains. The first is a claim about the characteristics of the patterns of light that stimulate the retinas; it pertains to geometrical optics. The second is a claim about what goes on behind the retinas; it pertains to the physiology or psychology of visual perception. A constructivist might well argue that no matter how much information is available in the optical array, it is of no consequence unless the organism can respond to it—a response that constructivists believe results from underlying cognitive operations (Fodor and Pylyshyn 1981; Pylyshyn 1984, 179–91). But the fact that an organism responds to a given pattern of stimulation cannot settle the question of whether this response is "direct" (cognitively unmediated). The answer to that question depends on how the organism is enabled to respond—a "how" question that demands an analysis of the stimulus patterns available, the transduction mechanisms for receiving that stimulation, and the subsequent processes, if any, that lead from the reception of stimulation to the occurrence of perception.

A follower of Gibson might feel that the constructivist, in treating the optics of stimulation as a fixed starting point that must be supplemented by a cognitive process to yield perception, has overlooked a crucial aspect of Gibsonian theory. And such indeed is the case. Riding in tandem with the direct theorist's claim about the richness of stimulus information is a contention about how best to conceive the relation between the stimulus array and the

---

[7] The argument of this paragraph requires only that cognitive processes *need not* be invoked to fill in an informational gap. The fact that physiological and cognitive explanations are not *in themselves* incompatible (cognitivists can allow that their posited mechanisms are physiologically realized) does not undercut the argument, which merely entails that a physiological explanation *could* be given without an attendant cognitive level of explanation, as when the processes invoked to fill the gap do not appeal to memory, to conceptual abilities, or to cognitively represented rules.

organism's perceptual response. Indeed, since constructivists can accept the claim about the richness of optical stimulation, the crux of the dispute between direct theorists and constructivists shifts to the question of how to account for the organism's ability to respond to rich stimulation. The dispute does not turn on the facts of geometrical optics *per se* but on how to conceive the relation between organism and information.

Direct theorists differ from constructivists by making the notion of information relative to specific organisms in specific environments. They deny that geometrical optics provides the appropriate analysis of optical stimulation, pursuing "ecological optics" in its stead (Gibson 1966, 1979; Turvey *et al.* 1981). In this much misunderstood portion of direct theory lies the root of the direct theorist's response to the criticisms of the thoroughly modern constructivist. According to the ecological approach, one accounts for the ability of an organism to "detect" or "pick up" the information in stimulation by supposing that the organism's visual system has evolved a sensitivity to adaptively significant variables in the optical array. The focus of Gibsonian research has often been to establish that particular types of information are available to a given organism in a given environment by showing that the organism is sensitive to the information. Direct theorists tend to treat their job as done if they have (i) discovered for a particular organism a taxonomy of the ecologically significant aspects of the organism's environment, (ii) shown how these aspects of the environment structure the ambient light that the objects reflect, and (iii) shown that the organism responds to this information in the light (rather than to some other source of information) to guide its behavior. Their point is not about rich information *per se* but about the adaptedness of visual systems to that information.

Although this approach may seem to depend on hopelessly general claims about the adaptation of organisms to their environments, in practice it can have considerable empirical specificity. The notion of rich informational content draws life not from the mere fact of successful perception but from an investigation of hitherto unknown regularities in the optical array. Although these regularities can be stated in terms of geometrical optics inasmuch as they pertain to the structure of ambient light, they are not laws of geometrical optics. They depend on contingent facts about the structure of the environment (Gibson 1966, chs. 1, 10; 1979, chs. 1–3, 14). These facts range from the general to the species-specific. An example of the first is Gibson's point about the earth below and the sky above, which entails that land-roving animals in open environments are surrounded by relatively unstructured light above and by a gradient of optical texture that becomes finer and denser toward the optical horizon below. An example of the second is that in the environment of the periwinkle or marsh snail, an occlusion of ambient light of a few degrees on the horizon is a reliable guide to a stalk of grass, a fact that is significant when the tide is coming in, and one to which the snail seems "tuned" to respond (Turvey et al. 1981, 249–50). Direct theory leads its investigators away from attempts to discuss optical information in general, toward attempts to investigate environmental regularities that are of perceptual and behavioral significance to the members of a particular species. One might label the direct theorist's project "ecological psychophysics."[8]

Describing direct theory as ecological psychophysics permits insight into why some direct theorists resist discussing the mechanisms by which organisms detect information. Psychophysics seeks to establish relationships between stimulation and perceptual response. This goal is met if a regular function between the two is found—such as would obtain between Gibsonian higher-order variables and the perception of the three-dimensional layout. For every psychophysical relationship that can be established, it might be assumed that some transduction process (though not necessarily a specialized one for each psychophysical relationship) mediates between the light impinging on the visual system and the resultant perceptual response. Direct theorists may view this transducer as just so much hardware—of interest to physiologists, but not to psychologists. So perhaps the direct theorist allows for a noncognitive account of the intervening processes in perception simply by treating a large chunk of the visual system as a transducer. On this somewhat common view of direct theory (e.g., Pylyshyn 1984, 185–6), the mechanism intervening between stimulation and perception is a physiologically complex transducer that admits of no psychologically interesting analysis. Accordingly, for direct theorists the account of perception is complete once they have discovered the relevant relation between optical information and percipient; constructivist explanations of information pickup are thereby rendered otiose.

With respect to sense perception, richness of information is not the principled core of the dispute between direct theorists and constructivists, since they might agree on geometrical optics and still disagree about the proper

---

[8] Direct theorists may find fault with calling Gibson's approach "psychophysical" because the term connotes the narrow stimulus dimensions investigated within traditional psychophysics, an approach that he rejects (e.g., 1979, 149). My use of the term "ecological psychophysics" is not inappropriate, because (1) Gibson (ibid.) does not reject the use of the term "psychophysics" outright, but proposes a particular way of understanding it, and (2) "ecological psychophysics" reflects the emphasis of direct theory on organism–environment relations and on environmentally specific regularities in explaining perception and action (Turvey et al. 1981). Moreover, I am not suggesting that direct theorists have limited their explanations to this sort of psychophysical relation; in Sec. 2, I argue that they endorse biological or neurophysiological explanations of information pickup, while forswearing *psychological* intervening processes (as they understand these).

explanation of perception. However, in turning to cognitive perception, the two approaches do in fact divide over whether object recognition can be explained by appeal to information "in the light." Sophisticated construct-ivists argue that the properties of light that the visual system can transduce are *conceptually* impoverished, as it were, with respect to our cognitive per-ceptual achievements. Fodor and Pylyshyn (1981) observe that the visual system's transducers respond to (say) brightness, color, and elementary shapes or features, but that we perceive cars and people. There is a conceptual gap between the transducible properties and the content of typical perceptual judgments, which are replete with conceptualized content. These authors argue that "nondemonstrative inferences" bridge this gap. Such inferences put more into the conclusion than was there in the premises, making possible the transition from patterns of light to conceptually rich judgments regarding one's visual surroundings. In this case, there can be no agreement between the two approaches on the availability of rich information, since the constructivist (e.g., Pylyshyn 1984, 180) denies that stimulation can carry information that matches the conceptual order of our cognitive responses (i.e., our perceptual judgments).

Direct theorists counter that even here an ecological account should be given. They do not stop at maintaining that sense perception is a matter of picking up the information in stimulation; with his theory of "affordances," Gibson (1979, ch. 8) extends this type of account to perceiving the functionally significant aspects of objects (e.g., "affording cutting" in the case of a knife). Direct theorists deny that the information detected by the visual system actually is conceptually impoverished. They maintain that the visual system "resonates" (tuning-fork style) to conceptually rich affordances. In this way, direct theory extends the thick-transducer analysis to such paradigmatically cognitive achievements as recognizing the functionally significant properties of objects. (At the limit, the whole organism may come to be regarded as a transducer for any property to which it can respond.)

Although I return briefly to explanations of cognitive perception in Section 5, for now I want to highlight the sharp distinction between direct and constructivist accounts of sense perception. Direct theorists explain sense perception in terms of the ecological psychophysics of rich optical stimulation in relation to mechanisms that have evolved to respond to such stimulation. In opposition, constructivists typically posit cognitive operations to explain the sense perception of three-dimensional spatial configurations. A typical constructivist account views sense perception as akin to problem solving or hypothesis formation, where the problem to be solved is of the following form: given current proximal stimulation, what are the sizes, distances, and shapes of the objects in my surroundings? That is, we—or our visual systems—try to infer the spatial features of the distal layout that is causing our current proximal stimulation.[9] A consequence of this view is that the phenomenal structure of our visual experience—the way things look, as opposed to what they look to be—is the result of inference or judgment.

For the ensuing discussion, I focus on the competing accounts of sense perception, and especially on the perception of spatial structure. This emphasis on sense perception comes as close as possible to finding neutral ground for the dispute, since cognitive perception may seem on the face of it to require inference or judgment in its explanation. This approach also has the advantage of directing the debate toward aspects of perception that have formed the core of experimental work within perceptual psychology.

2. Noncognitive Functional Analysis and Functional Algorithms

Even when direct theory is described as ecological psychophysics, the refusal of many direct theorists to posit internal psychological processes in explaining perception remains difficult to understand. It is true that if Gibson's psychophysical contentions are correct, so that unequivocal correlations can be established between a rich optical array and the ensuing perceptual responses, then direct theory can achieve predictive adequacy without opening the black box of the visual system. However, the ability to make predictions in this black-box manner provides no principled objection to probing the interior of the box (whether, e.g., by examining its works through measurements of physiological activity, or by inferring its internal functional organization by testing of the box's behavior under various conditions). Consider a parallel case. Under normal conditions, we can predict the behavior of a word processor from the position of the power switch, the specific program that is loaded, and the keys that a user has depressed. Even if such predictive power lies within our grasp, that fact alone provides no principled objection to our looking further in understanding the word processor. We might wish to understand more fully the normal operations of the machine—for example, why it takes so long to respond to certain commands—or to understand its behavior in abnormal circumstances—for example, why it sometimes doesn't respond to

---

[9] Charniak and McDermott (1985, 89): "Unlike many problems in AI, the vision problem may be stated with reasonable precision: Given a two-dimensional image, infer the objects that produced it, including their shapes, positions, colors, and sizes." See also Rock (1983), 11–20 and chs. 4–7.

any commands at all. Our investigations might target hardware, software, or both. The same considerations might lead us to have an interest in the internal workings of the visual system, even if Gibson's point about the richness of stimulus information is correct.

This familiar antibehaviorist argument would not, I think, have been lost on Gibson, nor has it been lost on a number of his co-theorists. It is a myth that Gibson and Gibsonians reject the postulation of *any* intervening processes in perception: they reject outright only *psychological* intervening processes. Gibson (1950, 1966) distinguished his psychological theory of information and its relation to perception from physiological analysis of the detection mechanisms that underlie information pickup. Although his chosen level of explanation has been that of ecological psychophysics, his position does not preclude an analysis of the biology of information-detection mechanisms, and indeed his co-theorists have pursued that line of investigation.[10]

We can better understand the direct theorist's resistance to positing intervening psychological processes by considering how the theoretical options typically get framed. Many theorists assume that properly psychological explanations of perception must invoke processes of inference and hypothesis formation, perhaps couched in an internal symbol system. Because direct theorists refuse to postulate intervening processes of just this cognitivist sort, it would appear that they must deny the very possibility of a psychology of intervening processes. This construal has been shared by direct theorists (Gibson 1966, 1979; Michaels and Carello 1981; but cf. Johansson *et al.* 1980) and their critics alike. Shimon Ullman (1980) criticizes direct theory for allowing only physiological

---

[10] Gibson (1950, 8) focused on psychophysically based psychological explanations rather than physiological explanations: "There are laws relating perception to physical stimulation as well as laws relating it to physiological processes. Explanation is a matter of lawfulness, although there are different levels of explanation. The level to be aimed for in the present book is a psychophysical theory, not a physiological theory." Although later avoiding the term "psychophysics" because of its unwanted connotations (see n. 8), Gibson (1966) still described two aspects of ecological explanations of perception: the discovery of "stimulus invariants" that "correspond to the permanent properties of the environment"; and the postulated "ability of the individual to detect the invariants" (1966, 3). The 1966 book focuses on stimulus invariants, but mentions possible mechanisms of detection here and there. Gibson couched such talk in the language of neurophysiology: "neural loops" "resonate" to information (1966, 5), photoreceptor output is "sent into the nervous system" (158), and "a more complex nervous system" is needed to detect higher-order stimulus information (159–60; also 251–3 and 267–71). Although such detector mechanisms are products of evolution, their use may be "tuned" through experience (1966, chs. 10, 14). Gibson (1979) simply spoke of the "process of pickup" (250), to be explicated through metaphors of "resonating, extracting, optimizing, or symmetricalizing" (246); the absence of further discussion of these mechanisms in this final book may have encouraged claims that direct theory eschews perceptual mechanisms. Nonetheless, Gibsonians have emphasized biological explanations of both perceptual mechanisms and the ecological constraints on postulating such mechanisms (Michaels and Carello 1981, chs. 4, 5); the adventuresome reader might explore Shaw and Turvey (1981) on ecosystem constraints in perceptual theory.

mediating mechanisms in explaining perception, mechanisms that cannot admit a "psychologically meaningful" decomposition in terms of subprocesses and subchannels of information flow.

I suggested earlier that this construal of the theoretical alternatives does not reflect all the available options. In order to see this, consider Ullman's use of the term "psychologically meaningful." If we assume that any psychologically meaningful analysis of perception must be formulated in terms of rules and representations as these have commonly been understood—as involving inferences over descriptions in a symbol system—then Ullman's point is correct. Any such decomposition would violate the direct theorist's aversion to cognitive accounts of perception. However, the situation changes if there is a level of analysis open to the perceptual theorist that is psychological but noninferential and nonsymbolic.

I believe that there is such a level, and that its theoretical vocabulary is couched neither in physiological terms nor in the language of cognitive operations such as inference. I call this level that of *noncognitive functional analysis* and I describe the processes of this level as *functional algorithms*.

I use the term "functional" in order to suggest that these algorithms may be discussed in abstraction from particular anatomical mechanisms or physiological processes. The term "algorithm" is drawn from existing theories of perception. It suggests a lawful relationship between stimulus input and perceptual response, but it is more specific than a mere description of an input–output relationship. For a given psychological function that is input–output determinate, there may exist several candidate algorithms for explicating the intervening process.[11]

By way of illustration, consider competing explanations of shape constancy. For this perceptual phenomenon, the overall input–output function is stable: within a (roughly) specifiable set of conditions, we perceive a given physical shape, say, a circle, as a circle, even though, owing to its slant relative to the line of sight, it projects any of a family of ellipses onto our retinas. Two competing algorithms have been proposed to account for this function (Epstein and Hatfield 1978). According to the first algorithm (A), perceived shape-at-a-slant results from combining information for the slant of an object

---

[11] The term "algorithm" may call to mind level two of Marr's three-level analysis of vision (1982, ch. 1, esp. pp. 24–7), and I think that the term as used above can be made consistent with Marr's usage. Its use here, however, is not in the first instance drawn from Marr, but from mainstream psychology of perception: e.g., Haber and Hershenson (1980), ch. 9, review a "combinatorial" or "algorithmic" approach, which they unfortunately present as conjoined with cognitivism. For accounts that permit distinguishing an algorithmic approach from cognitivism (a possibility that I develop below), see Epstein (1973, 1977a) and Ebenholtz (1977).

with retinally projected shape-information, each form of information being registered separately and processed through different channels of the visual system. According to the second algorithm (B), perceived shape results from registering a higher-order shape–slant texture gradient (a light–dark gradient of a given shape), which the visual system registers as a single stimulus variable.[12] I claim (i) that these two algorithms are to be analyzed above the level of neurophysiology, but (ii) that they need not be realized by cognitive operations using symbolic representations.

The first claim amounts pragmatically to the idea that functional algorithms can be investigated independently of neurophysiology. They lie above the level of neurophysiology because we can describe them theoretically in abstraction from any particular neurophysiological instantiation; for a given algorithm, multiple neurophysiological realizations are possible in principle.[13] My contention that the two algorithms are distinct psychological constructs is rendered concrete by the possibility that psychological experimentation can distinguish between them. They could be empirically distinguished if the expected results of disrupting visual processes in progress (say, by introducing visual noise) are different for each algorithm. We might expect that, with A, disruption at successively longer intervals from the onset of the target stimulus would yield at first pure projective shape, up to a certain threshold interval—the interval of processing time needed before the separate information channels are combined—after which full shape constancy would be obtained; whereas, for B, disruption might simply introduce random noise in the constancy response, which decreases monotonically as the interval between stimulus-onset and noise-onset increases (Epstein *et al.* 1977; Epstein and Hatfield 1978).

Even though the two algorithms can be investigated independently of neurophysiology, this does not preclude using neurophysiological and neuroanatomical results to decide which of the algorithms is realized by the visual system of a given individual or species. Although commitment to an autonomous functional level of description may block reduction, it does not imply that physiology is irrelevant to psychology. In the present example, even if both A and B could in principle be realized by distinct neurophysiological

---

[12] Some adherents of an algorithmic approach would be uncomfortable calling B an "algorithm," restricting that term to perceptual processes that combine stimulus information from at least two sources (e.g., Epstein 1973). I see the number of sources of information as distinct from the characterization (algorithmically) of the process that responds to the information.

[13] Although I accept that multiple-realizability arguments support a functional level of description, I leave open how widely the realizability extends: to only the human visual system (as actually or merely potentially multiply realizable), or to primate visual systems, or to mammalian systems, or to terrestrial animal systems but not Martians or robots, or so widely as to include the latter two.

structures, that poses no obstacle to investigating the structure of a given visual system to see which (if either) of the algorithms it instantiates. If investigation reveals that the neurophysiology instantiates A (e.g., owing to the discovery of separate channels for registering and, ultimately, combining slant- and shape-information), that is evidence that A is the appropriate functional characterization of the visual process in that individual or species. Such evidence may be available, even if different structures in fact realize the same functionally characterized process in different species, as binocular disparity is detected by functionally similar but anatomically and evolutionarily distinct structures in the visual systems of the owl and the cat (Pettigrew and Konishi 1976).[14]

My second claim, that the two algorithms need not be described in terms of cognitive operations and symbolic representations, may seem to contradict the first claim, with its commitment to a functional level of description. For it has become common for philosophers to link functionalism in psychology to the mentalistic belief–desire idiom of "folk psychology."[15] This is unfortunate because it unnecessarily confuses issues. No one would argue that functionalism with respect to genetics commits one to an "ordinary" or "folk" theory of heredity; the idea of a functional level of description draws life from the fact that genetic theory constitutes its own domain, which was for decades and still can be investigated independently of the biochemistry of DNA. Presumably, functionalism in psychology has brought with it the connotation of "folk" theory because psychology is known as the science of the mental and there is the suspicion that all mentalistic discourse depends on (so-called) ordinary conceptions. It thus might seem that psychological functionalism must be mentalistic in a traditional sense.

My alternative view asserts that the theoretical vocabulary in which theorists couch explanations of perception can be psychological without being

---

[14] Although Putnam's original articles (1975a, chs. 16, 20, 21) proposing functionalism as an argument against reductionism do not pronounce the irrelevance of physiology to psychology, later adherents of functionalism have made that assertion (e.g., Fodor 1975, 17).

[15] Stich (1983), chs. 1–2, takes functionalism and the doctrine that beliefs are sentences in the head as extensions of folk psychology; in doing so, he reflects the vision of cognitive science advanced by its leading philosophically minded proponents, Fodor and Pylyshyn. Fodor's allegiance to functionalism is clear; he typically speaks of intentional psychology rather than folk psychology, but he embraces the idea that (functional, computational) psychology should regularize and extend the kind of explanation implicit in "ordinary" attributions of belief and desire (see, e.g., Fodor 1981, 16–31). Pylyshyn (1984, ch. 1) argues that the functionally characterized internal states postulated in cognitive science must capture the generalizations implicit in "folk" explanations. By contrast, Barbara Von Eckardt (1984) cogently distinguishes the aims of folk psychology from those of cognitive psychology, appealing to the symbolist models of Stephen Kosslyn (1980, 1983) in defending Fodor and Pylyshyn from P. S. Churchland (1980).

mentalistic. This is the force of "noncognitive" in "noncognitive functional algorithms." How is such an analysis noncognitive and not traditionally mentalistic? Let us return to the example of shape constancy. Algorithm A provides a psychologically interesting decomposition of this psychological phenomenon because it analyzes the visual process in a more detailed and specific manner than does a mere psychophysical function. It commits the theorist to a specific answer to the question of *how* the visual system achieves constancy. But it does this without committing the theorist to the belief–desire idiom or to the equally mentalistic idiom of hypothesis formation, since the appropriate functional characterizations are cast in terms of "disparity detection," "registration of projective shape" (or of features of projected shapes), "motion detection," and "combination of shape and slant information." Although the notions of detection, registration, and combination may have traditionally mentalistic connotations in some contexts, these need not be operative here. For the operations described in the above terminology are to be considered as functional achievements of the visual system, not as operations performed by the cognitive agent. The theorist ascribes to a functionally characterized component of the visual system the normal function of registering projective shape; in this sense, registration is no more mentalistic than is the registration of blood-sugar level by the hypothalamus. The warrant for introducing such operations is the role they play in a functional analysis of vision; as such, we can view them as part of what is sometimes called the "subpersonal" level of description.[16] We may aptly characterize these subpersonal achievements as "psychological" because they enter into explanations of visual perception that are couched above the level of neurophysiology.

However, accepting that explanations of sense perception need not be cast in traditional mentalistic language does not by itself establish my second claim, that explanation in terms of functional algorithms is noncognitive (in all relevant senses). This is because the operative notions of "cognitive" for many cognitive scientists are not belief and desire but symbol and computation (e.g., Newell 1980). Even those cognitive scientists who see their enterprise as beginning with "folk" notions do not remain solely within the language (or conceptions) of belief and desire in formulating their theories of cognitive functions. Typically,

---

[16] Not just any psychological process can be ascribed to the subpersonal level, especially if the process is construed by analogy with the actions of cognitive agents (e.g., persons). Rock's (1983, 39) appeal to an "executive agency" treats a component of the perceptual system as a little person, but he is willing to bite the bullet. Be that as it may, there is a clear rationale for postulating functionally characterized psychological operations such as the "registration" of various stimulus dimensions, even if such operations in principle could not become available to consciousness (see Epstein 1973, 276–7). Fodor (1975, 52–3) offers a philosophical apology for postulating subpersonal psychological states.

their models comprise rule-governed operations that are defined over symbol systems (as in Fodor 1975). In the case of sense perception, this becomes the notion that the processes underlying perception comprise computations performed over descriptions of stimulation. Of course, constructivists tend to think of these computational processes as inferential, thereby making a nod in the direction of traditional mentalistic discourse. But some cognitive scientists (e.g., Kosslyn 1980, ch. 5, sec. 1.2) and some philosophical defenders of cognitive science (e.g., Von Eckardt 1984; Cummins 1983, ch. 3) observe that the notion of inference as currently understood in cognitive science is operationally defined in terms of explicit computational procedures defined within a symbol system, thereby avoiding the objection raised against the "folk" notion of inference, that it is vaguely defined and open ended. And so the question of present interest becomes: are functional algorithms cognitive in the sense of being computational and therefore symbolic?

From the point of view I am developing, there are two answers to this question. The first is "no"; the second denies that the question is properly formulated.

The case for functional algorithms without underlying symbol systems rests on providing a nonsymbolic interpretation of the processes in the visual system that compute the algorithms. Standard accounts of color vision provide an example. The perception of color is mediated by three types of cone in the retina. Each type of cone responds most strongly to a specific wavelength and responds successively less vigorously across a range of wavelengths. The rates of firing of the various types of cone together determine the perceived color. Investigators have proposed various models for combining the outputs of the three types of cone in order to account for the psychophysical laws of color vision. These models take the form of wiring diagrams, and they differ in the connections they postulate between the cones and various afferent channels: for example, in Boynton (1979, 211–12) the red–green afferent channel responds simply to the difference in input from the "red" and "green" cones, while in Kaufman (1974, 189–90) this channel takes the difference between the input from the "green" cone and the combined input of the "blue" and "red" cones. Each wiring diagram may be seen as instantiating a distinct algorithm. This shows how distinct algorithms might be instantiated by the visual system, but it would be superfluous to impute a symbol system to the visual system for describing the firing rate of each cone, or for carrying out arithmetical operations to combine these values. The combination occurs through interacting values of activation. This construal provides a nonsymbolic and noncognitive interpretation for these functional algorithms.

A constructivist of the "cognitive science" bent might accept this account of color vision but argue that it is unsuitable for extension to all of sense perception because it is too simplistic. A cognitivist could be expected to contend that perception involves the reception and processing of information in complicated ways, and that the only suitable means for modeling such information-handling is to posit an internal computational medium of some complexity (greater complexity than can be modeled via a wiring diagram, as in the color vision example). Such a constructivist might then argue: "no computation without representation, and no representation without a symbolic medium or a language of thought" (to paraphrase Fodor 1975, ch. 1 and p. 55).

In rejecting this slogan, I give my second response to the question of whether functional algorithms are computational and therefore symbolic, which is to reject the formulation of the question itself. To begin with, I deny the equation of *computational* with *symbolic*. I intend to prize apart the two notions, so that it makes sense to attribute "computations"—and even "representations"—to a visual process without thereby characterizing the process as "symbolic." But once we reject the idea that the processes of sense perception occur in a symbolic medium—replete with "descriptions" and "hypotheses"—it may no longer seem obvious that such processes should be regarded as cognitive or thought-like. Indeed, I support the view that, even though we model a perceptual system in terms of computations and representations, that is not sufficient warrant for characterizing the operations of the system as "cognitive" in the sense of involving symbolically characterized processes.

3. Nonsymbolic Computation and Representation

My contention that there are plausible notions of nonsymbolic computation and representation may perhaps best be approached indirectly by contrasting it with the standard symbolist view of cognitive processes, which was introduced into cognitive psychology and cognitive science by taking the computer metaphor very seriously. Perception and other cognitive processes are complicated, and the computer provided a powerful example of a device that could perform complicated information-handling tasks and whose operation was understood in detail. By treating the perceptual system as a computational device, investigators hoped to be able to capture its complexity in a perspicuous model.

For present purposes, it is important to see that, in taking seriously the comparison with conventional computers, psychologists would naturally be led to think that computationally characterized perceptual and cognitive processes occur in an internal symbol system.[17] In understanding the operation of the standard digital computer, it makes sense to think of the machine's internal processes as instantiating (token symbols in) a syntactically defined symbol system. The computer's internal operations are conveniently viewed as being carried out within a system of symbols that is defined by how the central processing unit (CPU) "reads" the data and instructions that it receives from other parts of the device. Sequences of on- and off-current that affect the CPU are appropriately regarded as strings of symbols, because this offers a perspicuous vocabulary within which to understand the functioning of the machine. Depending upon how the CPU has been "set," it treats a sequence of on- and off-current as an "instruction" to alter further machine states in a specified manner, or as "data" to be altered or "read" and combined with other "data" in a specified manner. These sequences of current-settings are aptly characterized as "symbols" because their effects on the machine's activity can be characterized through a "syntax" of well-formed strings of symbols and the operations performed on the syntactically characterized states are naturally likened to "reading," "writing," and "storing" strings of symbols (see Weizenbaum 1976, chs. 2–3, and Newell 1980). The plausibility of terming these internal states "symbols" does not depend on the possibility of interpreting them semantically, nor is it parasitic upon the fact that the input and output to the entire device typically is alphanumeric. We might apply the same description to the internal states of a computer driving a robotics system, whose input is received from mechanical sensors, and whose output consists in the positioning and firing of various spot-welders. In this case, the computer's internal states are viewed as symbols because this provides a good way of understanding how the system performs its tasks—for example, examining certain memory buffers reveals the programmed rules that mediate between sensor inputs and motor outputs.[18] Despite claims to the contrary, the

---

[17] The centrality of the computer metaphor in cognitive science is apparent; see Fodor (1975), esp. ch. 2, Newell (1980), and Pylyshyn (1984), ch. 3. My understanding of how deeply cognitive science depended on taking the computer metaphor literally was enhanced by conversations with Kosslyn about his and others' uses of computational models; these conversations led to Kosslyn and Hatfield (1984), in which we criticize that dependence. For a compact statement of Kosslyn's earlier view, which summarizes the working assumptions of many cognitive scientists, see his (1983), ch. 2.

[18] In general, the question of whether a given psychological or cognitive ability is a symbolic ability is distinct from whether the processes that underlie that ability occur within a symbolic medium. In the case of the spot-welder, a nonsymbolic ability (welding) is carried out by a symbolic process. Section 4 provides an example of a symbolic ability (adding) carried out by a nonsymbolic process.

appeal to an internal "interpreter" with respect to which the symbol system is defined does not lead to a regress (Fodor 1975, ch. 2, esp. pp. 65–79). There is no further interpreter within the CPU; the CPU's ability to "interpret" sequences of on- and off-current depends on the way in which it is wired (Pylyshyn 1984, ch. 4).

A typical constructivist model of perception cast in symbolist terms involves a number of elements: say, transducers, buffers, hypothesis-formation routines, and hypothesis-testing routines. The transducers take patterns of light as their input, and they yield descriptions couched in an impoverished vocabulary (of lightness and darkness, color or wavelength range, and simple features) as their output. These initial data might be held in a buffer and gone over by the hypothesis-formation routine, which contains explicit rules for positing a distal configuration as the perceptually relevant cause of the input as described. Once a hypothesis has been formed, the testing routine might check it against a wider body of data (past and now subsequent transducer outputs) and either accept the hypothesis (which is then realized as the current perceptual state) or reject it (returning control to the hypothesis-formation routine). The whole model might be programmed on a computer and tested for its adequacy by actually making it run (using simulated input from a computer tape, or input from a television camera or artificial eye).[19]

The possibility of explicitly stating rules of inference—major premises in the nondemonstrative arguments that allegedly constitute the process of perception—and testing them in a working model is both the strength and the weakness of the symbol-crunching approach. It has been the strength because it encourages explicitness of modeling; the goal of a symbolic computational account is to specify a set of operations in the language of thought that would model the relations between input and output that correspond to a particular psychological ability. In order for the model to run, the investigators must spell out its subprocesses explicitly (it is not enough just to *say* that hypotheses are produced and tested: operations must be specified for producing and testing them). It has been the weakness because of the theoretical baggage that the language of thought as a medium of inference carries with it. Because internal processing reputedly occurs in a linguistic medium, one is led to suppose that the processes should be conceived on analogy with description and inference

---

[19] Such top-down models were once the mainstay of AI and AI-inspired accounts of perception, as in Raphael (1976), ch. 7, and Haber and Hershenson (1980), chs. 14–15; see MacArthur (1982) for a review and criticism. Their popularity dwindled in the face of bottom-up accounts such as those provided by Marr (1982) and others, which are reviewed in Charniak and McDermott (1985), ch. 3, who retain top-down models for higher perceptual achievements, such as representing and recognizing scenes (sec. 3.6).

in natural language. Here it is not the "ordinary" or "folk" character of these notions that is bothersome but the fact that they direct the theorist toward taking quasi-linguistic models that appeal to internal descriptions and inferences as the only type of model available for the detailed analysis of psychological processes. Although it may seem at first blush that this theoretical direction is entirely appropriate to the distant and programmatic goal of modeling human thought in general (including language use and the ability to draw inferences), it has been downright misleading for sense perception, and it may keep researchers from seeing other viable approaches to cognitive perception.

The weight of the symbolist baggage may be compared with a different kind of computational account that allows explicitness of modeling but does not appeal to an internal symbolic medium. This type of account is provided by "massively parallel" or "connectionist" computational models (Feldman 1985b, Rumelhart and McClelland 1986b). Connectionist models are intended to have greater neural plausibility than standard symbolist models. In a connectionist computational architecture, computations are performed through the interaction of a large number of units or nodes in a network. Each node is connected to its neighbors in such a way that its state of activity can affect and can be affected by the activity of (functionally) adjacent units. "Input" occurs when a set of the nodes is activated. "Computation" occurs as they mutually interact. "Output" consists of the state of activity in the network after the nodes have been allowed to interact (perhaps achieving an equilibrium point). The connections among the nodes—both the spatial pattern of connections and the excitatory or inhibitory gain of the single connections—determine what function is being computed. By adjusting these connections, the input–output function can be altered. Given a pattern of input, these networks "settle down" to an equilibrium state much the way a soap bubble or other isoperimetric physical system achieves equilibrium at a minimum energy state. Unlike the case of the digital computer, there seems little temptation to think of the internal states of such a massively parallel device as symbols. The nodes do influence one another in a manner that can be assigned a numeric value, but nothing is to be gained by regarding the interactions between the nodes as the passing of symbols. One node does not "read" or "interpret" the activity of another node; it simply is affected by it. Such devices are nonsymbolic in that their computations do not occur in an internal symbolic medium.

Connectionist models claim to provide a more plausible account of computation-intensive processes that must be completed very rapidly. Standard symbolist models conceived on analogy with the digital computer are committed to *serial* processing (computational operations are performed one after another). In a *parallel* computational architecture, a global result is obtained through simultaneous local interactions. Fairly complex results can be achieved by adjusting the parameters of these local interactions—for example, determining three-dimensional depth from the shading in a two-dimensional image (Brown *et al.* 1982). Advocates of connectionism contend that, given the speed of actual psychological processes, parallel models are empirically more plausible than serial models.

I would like to propose a different comparative advantage for connectionist models. First, consider the elements in a symbolist account. (1) The description of the function to be performed, that is, of the psychological ability to be modeled—in this case, generating a configuration in depth from the shading in a perspective projection. (2) The specification of a specific sequence of steps, that is, of an algorithm, for generating output from input. (3) The expression of this algorithm in an internal symbol system, together with provision for "reading" and manipulating the various symbols in the algorithm. (4) The realization or hardware implementation of a control function or CPU that does this "reading" (recall that the danger of a regress of "readers" and "interpreters" is countered by appeal to the hardwiring of the CPU).

Now consider a connectionist account. Its first two elements, (1') and (2'), are identical with (1) and (2) above. There is no counterpart to (3), for the algorithm described in (2') is *directly implemented* in a computational net, rather than being described in a symbol system that has its own functional architecture. Hence, we can proceed directly to a counterpart for (4), which becomes (3'), a connectionist implementation of the algorithm. Connectionist accounts have an intrinsic advantage because they can focus directly on the questions of psychological importance: What is the precise character of the psychological ability in question? What algorithm could be used to model it? The algorithm needn't be expressed in an internal symbolic medium, whose operations require a specific functional architecture (including an internal "interpreter," etc.).[20]

---

[20] Pylyshyn trumpets item (4) as a specific advantage for symbolism, for it underlies the distinction between functional architecture and mental process that is central to the standard computational account (1984, 30−1 and ch. 4). In a related vein, he denies that massively parallel or connectionist accounts are truly computational on the grounds that the connectionist computational nets are better conceived as finite state automata rather than as universal Turing machines (1984, 71−4). Accordingly, only general purpose machines should count as computational devices, which contradicts the practice of considering special-purpose analog computers as computers and ignores the role that the notion of computation plays in psychology, which is to allow explicitness in modeling particular functionally characterized abilities (the specification of which Marr called the "computational" level of analysis!).

A symbolist sympathizer might counter that this line of reasoning neglects the advantage that symbolism offers in proposing a unified symbolic medium for modeling all psychological abilities (as on a general purpose machine). But the symbolists themselves have called into question the picture of the mind as a single computational system having one (or a few) central processors for which various subroutines must compete. The new symbolist picture emphasizes the "modularity of mind." In this picture, cognitive systems contain a number of relatively autonomous "modules" (e.g., modules for parsing sentences or for computing shape from shading) that have their own computational resources, including their own basic vocabulary and rules for processing (Fodor 1983, pt. 3). While it may be the case that the outputs of some of the modules must be intertranslatable (e.g., the results of shape perception must at least on occasion be available to speech-production systems), the internal symbol systems of the various modules need not constitute a unified language of thought. Indeed, it might seem far fetched to suppose that a unified symbolic vocabulary underlies all psychological processing, be it auditory, visual, language-motor, ambulatory-motor, etc. And so the idea of a unified symbolic medium loses its appeal.

A second symbolist response might claim connectionist models for their own by saying that connectionist systems are merely devices into which the programs have been hardwired. The symbolist claims direct implementation (which I have proposed as a special advantage of connectionism) of symbol-described programs. However, it is not clear why a device with a hardwired program should be seen as instantiating a symbol system. The device may simply be viewed as having been engineered so as to instantiate its processing rules directly in its circuits; in comparison, the symbolist conception is superfluous and obscuring. If we treat computational devices as symbol crunchers, then we are committed to an analysis of their internal operation that involves the manipulation of symbols. If we treat them simply as engineered devices (without finding it useful to regard the engineering function of any of the internal components as that of "reading" internal symbols), we lose the sense of internal symbols.[21] This may not be a large loss. For now we can turn directly to the psychologically relevant algorithms and, if it helps, to their

[21] See also Stabler (1983). The usefulness of treating an internal process as symbolic or nonsymbolic is independent of whether the cognitive ability in question involves symbols: sentence-parsing is an ability that involves manipulation of symbols at the level of the task to be performed, but which might be modeled with either symbolist or connectionist processes. Further, my argument above does not imply that all "engineered devices" are nonsymbolic; standard digital computers are engineered devices in which it *is* useful to regard the engineering function of one of the internal components as that of "reading" internal symbols. Finally, Dennett (1983) discusses "tacit" and "explicit" representation in a way that accords with my distinction between functional algorithms and symbolic representations.

implementations in neural circuitry. In so doing, we need not impoverish the psychology of internal processes.

Supposing that connectionist computational architectures provide a plausible conception of nonsymbolic computation, we have not yet shown that perceptual theory can be adequately formulated in these terms. For, although direct theorists would not agree with this terminology, an important notion in perceptual theorizing is that of *representation*: the representation of distal events by proximal stimulation, and ultimately their representation within perceptual experience. Many authors maintain that the positing of an internal symbolic medium is the best—if not the only—way to characterize the representational function from stimulus input to perceptual response. Fodor expresses this assumption as follows: "representation presupposes a medium of representation, and there is no symbolization without symbols" (1975, 55). We can safely grant the second half of this sentence. The transition between its two parts should not be so easily accepted, for it contains a prodigious leap from *representation* to *symbolization*. I have claimed that this leap need not be taken. It is time to make good on this assertion by providing a positive conception of nonsymbolic representation to go along with nonsymbolic computation.

4. Representation and Function

Although my primary aim is to offer a nonsymbolic notion of representation, I also defend the very notion of representational content in psychology. For even though symbolism was initially attractive for its seemingly easy accommodation of representations into psychology, recently the notions of representation and representational content have come under attack from within the symbolist camp. Fodor (1980) argues that there can be no scientific treatment of representational content because that would require establishing lawful relationships between (*a*) types of symbols in the language of thought and (*b*) types of environmental objects, and such laws are either nonexistent or so dependent on the as yet uncompleted sciences of physics and chemistry as to be unknowable within the next millennium. In response to these and other arguments, Stephen Stich (1983, chs. 8, 10) suggests dropping the notion of representational content from psychology in favor of purely syntactic theories, that is, theories couched wholly in terms of computational relations among syntactically characterized states of individual organisms.

I believe that a plausible alternative to a symbol-based conception of representation may be found by attending to the role that the concept of representation plays in accounts of basic psychological processes such as perception. This approach identifies representations and representational content through the functions that certain states perform in organisms and information-handling devices.[22] By way of illustration, consider a device that performs computations without an internal symbol system. Let us call this device a "tensional adder." By placing weights of known unit values (including multiples of units) into the pan of a spring scale, we use it to perform addition. "Input" consists of placing weights into the pan corresponding to the integers to be summed; "addition" occurs through the physical pressure exerted on the spring and its affect on a pointer; and "output" consists of the pointer reading on the face of the device (which, of course, is a symbolic type of output). The various weights may be said to represent numeric values, and the device as a whole may be said to compute sums, all without the benefit of an internal symbol system.[23]

I must make several points right away. First, the idea that the weights represent integers is parasitic on the notion that the device is an adder. If we had not assigned this function to the device, we might view it simply as a device for measuring weights, rather than as a crude calculator. Second, the rationale for assigning a specific representational content (say, representing the number three) to aspects of the device is parasitic on an analysis of how the device achieves addition; given that it adds by physically summing the weights, multiples of unit weights represent various integers. Third, the denial that these representations are symbolic also depends on a conception of how the adder works. Thus, I am not denying that the input–output function of the tensional adder—its global behavior—can usefully be described using

[22] I discussed this notion of representation in Kosslyn and Hatfield (1984), 1031–7. Recent "functionalist" philosophy of psychology (Fodor 1975; Putnam 1975a, chs. 16, 20, 21) emphasizes the causal or computational roles of representations in mediating between input and output (in a computer, or in an organism). My notion of representational function includes input–output relations, whether pertaining to the whole organism or to internal processes; but it also appeals to the notion of normal biological function (see notes 26, 29, and the associated text). Ruth Garrett Millikan (1984, *passim*) offers a theory of linguistic meaning that starts from the notion of biological function.

[23] Pylyshyn would not count my adder as a truly computational device (n. 20, above). In commenting on an earlier version of this chapter (at the 1981 meeting of the Society for Philosophy and Psychology in Chicago), he objected that a purely functional notion of representation is not possible; his published arguments to this effect (1984, 29 and ch. 3) suggest that only functionally characterized systems of certain types—those that employ a language-like combinatorial mechanism—can capture the generalizations of cognitive science. These arguments depend on construing the relevant generalizations as extensions of "ordinary" belief–desire ascriptions, which is part of the matter in question.

numerals and addition signs. But this says nothing about whether it is useful or advisable to understand the internal operation of the device—its mode of "carrying out" its computations—in terms of the manipulation of symbols. And indeed, unlike the case of the digital computer, in which talk of the manipulation, storage, and "interpretation" of symbols is helpful, the attribution of symbols to the internal workings of the scale seems very much beside the point.[24] Fourth and finally, analyzing aspects of the device in terms of their functional roles allows the investigator to distinguish between computationally relevant and irrelevant aspects, a distinction that symbolists capture by appeal to an internal symbol system (Ullman 1979, ch. 1; Pylyshyn 1984, ch. 3, esp. pp. 54–9). According to the symbolist, just as a theory of computation allows us to distinguish the computational aspects of a hand calculator from other mechanically necessary but informationally irrelevant aspects (such as the processes in its batteries), so too for psychological processes such as vision, the notion of a symbol system allows us to distinguish the visual information-bearing aspects of internal processes from other events in the visual system (such as cell respiration). But in the present nonsymbolic analysis, we can readily distinguish computationally relevant aspects of the device, such as the magnitudes of the weights, the tension of the spring, and the linkage between spring and pointer, from computationally irrelevant aspects, such as the color of the weights or the detail work on the pointer, by reflecting on the role (or lack thereof) that each plays in the summation process.

The first of these four points (pertaining to the adder as an artifact) may seem to undermine the applicability of the other three to the psychology of perception. For in the case of the adder, the representational content that is assigned to various aspects of the device depends on the function assigned to the device by a user or community of users. What can play a similar role in ascriptions of functions to the perceptual system? Here, theorists will assign psychological functions to the system in a manner analogous to the way they assign biological functions. One might regard the visual system as, in the first instance, a system for representing the spatial and chromatic layout and for permitting recognition of objects by means of their

---

[24] These computations do not require discrete steps for the addition operation itself (two or more weights could be placed in the pan at once), which violates the "ordinary" expectation that computation involves sequential operations. In this connection, it may be useful to regard the adder as an instance of an analog computer. Analog computers are nonsymbolic, in that they achieve their computations without an internally defined symbol system. But the notion of nonsymbolic computation developed here is wider than that of an analog computer (which it includes as an instance), for it extends to any computational system that is functionally analyzed in a perspicuous manner without appeal to an internal symbol system.

spatial and chromatic properties. We then assign representational content to various functionally characterized states of the visual system because of the contributions that those states make to these global functions, perhaps by contributing to some subfunction. Thus, in a theoretical account of shape perception, one might describe various receptor mechanisms as registering retinally projected shape; in size perception, one might posit an initial representation of projected size at an early stage, and so on. Although such purely psychological posits are sufficient for the purposes of ongoing psychological experimentation, when enough is known about the neurophysiological basis for a particular function, we can ascribe content to neural mechanisms: the firing of edge detectors in the brain would be said to represent a light–dark contrast in a specific region of the retina, the firing of other cortical cells might represent the binocular disparity between corresponding features in the two retinal images, and so on for other "feature" or "property" detectors.[25] Unlike the case of the adder, these assignments of function do not play a constitutive role in determining what the function of the system is; with the perceptual system, we are attempting to describe accurately some naturally occurring functions. In natural systems, we ascribe the functions of subprocesses in relation to the functions of the larger system; we analyze the functions of the larger system by considering environmental adaptations and by appeal to evolutionary considerations. Such analyses do not invoke the intentions of a community of users (as happens in the case of artifacts).[26]

As with the adder, appealing to function in assigning content to various processes within the visual system allows one to separate mere physical response from representation. A host of substances and structures may respond selectively to some region of the electromagnetic spectrum, but they do not all constitute representations of the presence of light. Pigmented cells in the skin change their characteristics upon exposure to sunlight. Although the resulting chemical changes may represent something to us (as when we come to know about an acquaintance's weekend trip to the beach through such epidermal changes), we do not assign to changes in pigmented human skin cells the sensory function of representing the presence of light. For

[25] The present conception of representation does not intrinsically commit one to either an analog or digital description of the content of visual states. States that represent continuously varying magnitudes—such as projective shape—in a relatively continuous manner might best be considered analog; other states, such as those that represent the presence of a discrete feature, might best be viewed as digital (see Dretske 1981, 135–41).
[26] Similarities and contrasts in function ascriptions to artifacts and to organisms have been widely discussed in the literature on functional analysis; for an overview and critical discussion, see Peter Achinstein (1983), ch. 8.

the purposes of the psychological investigation of the senses, representation is tied to function where the relevant notion of function is not mere input–output function (pigmented skin cells have that) but functional role within a system.[27]

This notion of "functional role in a system" may seem like an instance of traditional functionalism, which defines psychological states through their roles in mediating between inputs and outputs. This traditional stimulus–response version of functionalism appears adequate to the case of the adder, because we agree by stipulation that its function is to add; my analysis of the device differs from mainstream symbolist functionalism in being nonsymbolic. But an important difference arises for naturally occurring functions. Once one has assigned to the scales the function of addition, there is nothing more to investigate regarding its global function; the remaining questions pertain to how this function is performed, and the investigation can focus directly on the structure of the device. By contrast, in the case of naturally occurring functions the question of what function is being performed is an object of empirical investigation. Attempts to answer this question typically proceed by considering the relevant system in relation to its normal environment. The environmental specificity of functional role attributions comes to the fore.[28] Philosophical analyses of function statements in biology commonly recognize the inherent environmental specificity of such statements.[29] In the analysis of sensory systems the need for such recognition should be even

---

[27] This paragraph replies to Pylyshyn's (1984, 55–9) challenge to distinguish mere causal relations from representational relations without appealing to a symbolist conception of cognitive content. By contrast, the Churchlands' (1983) conception of representational content as "calibrational" (see n. 1) is either causal or merely correlative; because it does not appeal to normal function, it cannot distinguish between mere input–output function and functional role within a system. See also Pylyshyn's (1980, 164) response to Patricia Churchland.

[28] The functions ascribed to artifacts also may be environmentally conditioned (addition is a particularly fixed function); thus, physically congruent artifacts might have quite distinct functions depending on their cultural context (an object that looks like a chair to visitors from an outside culture might actually be an altar in its home culture). To the extent that ascriptions of function vary with cultural context, this variation might become the object of empirical (e.g., anthropological) investigation. However, within the home culture the functions ascribed to artifacts may depend on or be constituted through argument and evaluative judgment. For that reason, members of the culture need not accept empirical investigation into currently ascribed functions as decisive. Such cultural relativity contrasts with natural functions. (Of course, an anthropologist might, as the result of empirical investigation, describe what members of a culture consider to be the "correct" functional description at a particular time; but such descriptions are not authoritative, since they are open to immediate challenge that need not impugn their empirical accuracy.)

[29] See, e.g., Carl G. Hempel (1965) and Ernst Nagel (1979), 305–16. Biologists stress the role of environmental context in analyzing adaptations (functions produced through natural selection) and in describing natural selection itself: e.g., George C. Williams (1966), 66–71, and Ernst Mayr (1970), 5–6, 106–14.

more apparent, since the function of the senses is to sense the environment. The ability of sensory systems to carry out their functions may in fact depend on physically contingent facts about specific environments. An environmentally insulated input–output analysis is therefore inadequate for such systems.

I want to illustrate the role of environment-specific regularities in the analysis of sense perception by elaborating my previous example of shape constancy, now extended to include size as well. The algorithms underlying shape constancy described in Section 2 will work in environments in which (1) objects typically maintain a constant shape from moment to moment, and (2) the projective properties of light remain constant. The need for assumption (2) is obvious; in the absence of stable laws of optics, our sense of vision could not exist. The need for assumption (1), which pertains to contingent environmental regularities, may be less obvious. It is needed because, without it, changes in a retinally projected shape for a stationary observer might signify either the motion of a rigid object or the deformation of the object itself (as indeed happens on some occasions, e.g., with animate objects). Indeed, our visual system exploits a number of physically contingent facts about our environment; for example, that expansion of a portion of the visual field indicates the approach of an object, that deformation of the entire visual field in a certain regular manner indicates the motion of the observer, and so on.[30] These are physically contingent in the sense that one need not suppose any violations of the laws of physics in order to imagine organisms and environments for which they would not hold true. (Think of beings living in the midst of irregularly moving regions of optical media with sharply differing refractive indexes.)

The environmental specificity of function-based ascriptions of content yields an important philosophical advantage, at least for philosophers who are otherwise impressed by the environmental specificity of psychological content. Such specificity requires that the generalizations used for assigning content to various psychological states must refer to both organism and environment. This interplay among environment, function, and content distinguishes my notion of nonsymbolic representation from the traditional symbolist conception. For

---

[30] Perceptual psychologists disagree about whether the ecological regularities mentioned above are the most significant ones (and indeed whether they are correct as stated); this disagreement only emphasizes the importance of such regularities in perceptual psychology. Gibson and the ecological approach have heralded this importance, as have members of the constructivist tradition such as Brunswik (1956). Outside the ecological approach, no one has recently sustained this importance more effectively than Marr (1982); see especially his "physical assumptions," which clearly are environmentally specific (ch. 2, sec. 1).

the symbolist, the idea that something is a symbol can be separated from the question of what it represents (syntax is separable from semantics). Symbolists identify symbols by their "form," which, at least for the basic *lingua mentis*, they define relative to the control function or CPU, that is, solely in terms of the structure of an individual organism or a device. It is a separate task to relate these formally defined symbols to the world, the difficulty of which has led some symbolists to the despairing position of "methodological solipsism" (Fodor 1980). As I have mentioned, Fodor's despair stems from his belief either that there can be no scientifically respectable *laws* concerning the relations between organisms and their environments, or that such laws must await millennial developments in physics and chemistry. In maintaining that ascriptions of content in psychology must be sustained by generalizations having the status of physical or chemical laws, Fodor denies the scientific respectability of the types of environmental regularities that Gibson (1966, 1979), Egon Brunswik (1956), and Marr (1982) emphasize—although I find no argument in his writings to show that the only scientifically respectable generalizations are law statements.[31] Some direct theorists have responded to Fodor by biting the bullet, arguing that ecological laws are every bit as nomic as the laws of physics (Turvey *et al.* 1981). My argument merely requires environmental regularities that are sufficiently stable to serve in the functional analysis of the visual abilities that rely on them. From the point of view of physics (and, indeed, of biology or psychology), this stability can be a wholly contingent fact, as long as it is a fact.

Under the analysis of representation that I am proposing, the task of determining representational content is bound up with that of determining functional role: assignments of representational content are a part of the very description of the visual process (syntax and semantics—if these terms are permitted here—go hand in hand). To say that a portion of the visual system serves to detect binocular disparity, and to assign to various of its states representational contents that correspond to various values of disparity, are part and parcel of a functional analysis of depth perception. It would therefore make little sense to attempt to analyze depth perception in terms of an abstractly characterized set of computations in a symbol system, independent of any concern with the optics of binocular disparity and with the ways in which the visual system might use such disparity in the service of depth perception.

[31] Stich (1983), ch. 8, sec. 3, and Patricia Kitcher (1985), sec. 3, forcibly criticize Fodor's (1980) argument; Millikan (1986) reconceives the status and relevance of folk psychological generalizations.

Nonetheless, Stich (1983, ch. 8, sec. 3) has argued that environmental regularities of the sort I have alluded to are irrelevant to psychology, and he has done so without endorsing Fodor's (1980) demand for nomological generalizations. He appeals to an "autonomy principle," which says that psychological states supervene on the current physical states of individual organisms, independent of the organisms' histories and their relations to their environments. By way of a thought experiment, he asks us to accept that the replacement of one organism with a physically identical replica would be irrelevant from the point of view of a behavioral description of the organism (where "behavior" amounts to physical motion). The physically identical individual, which by hypothesis shares none of the history of the individual it replaces, may be expected (supposing determinism) to exhibit identical future motions. Hence, past environmental context is irrelevant to psychology (assuming that the goal of psychology is to predict physical behavior!). Granting Stich his point about the future motions of the replacement entities, he has not made his case. Environmentally specific regularities in psychology enable us to analyze the abilities or capacities of types of organisms in a relatively constant environment. As opposed to the Twin Earth examples that inspired Stich's argument (Kitcher 1985 critically examines those examples), the interests of psychology lie not in the isolated replacement of one physically identical individual with another but in how the psychological abilities of members of the same psychological type (species, or groups of species) exploit environmentally specific regularities (perhaps through evolutionary adaptation). Even for individuals, in characterizing their current physical organization psychologists are interested in the environmental circumstances that yielded aspects of that organization through learning (and not in the details of the physical organization itself). Stich's arguments do not address the kind of generalizations about the relations of organism to environment that are found in perceptual psychology (generalizations that are consistent with global supervenience of psychological properties on organism–environment contexts, but are inconsistent with narrow supervenience on individuals). His arguments do not undermine my appeal to environmentally specific regularities when I assert that functional analysis can assign nonsymbolic representational content to the visual system.

The representational content that such functional analyses ascribe will be rather coarse, in that numerous extensionally equivalent descriptions will exist for the contents so assigned. For example, we can describe the stimulus for an "edge detector" in several ways: as a luminosity boundary, as a step function in luminance, as a pattern of luminance points, and so on. What representational content should we assign to such detectors? Perhaps a content that does not discriminate among these alternative descriptions. Indeed, such coarseness of content may be a virtue rather than a fault. The representational content of edge detectors in the visual system may in fact *be* that coarse—perhaps no finer degree of content should be assigned to such detectors than arises from their role in the larger function of detecting physical edges in the visual world. Ascriptions of content will become as coarse or as fine as are the psychological functions in which they are embedded.

Although much remains to be fleshed out in this necessarily skeletal account of nonsymbolic representation, I conclude for now by pointing out that it permits an intuitively satisfying account of *mis*representation. In assigning content to a state, one wants to allow that the state could occur in the absence of what it represents, and that at least some of these occurrences will be misrepresentings, where something is represented as present when it is not. Photoreceptors in the eye respond to a host of stimuli: pressure, electric spark applied to the outside of the eyeball, stimulation by internal electrode, chemical stimulation, and so on. Visual scientists nonetheless agree (and rightly so) that the function of photoreceptor activity is to represent the presence of light, and that when such activity occurs on other occasions we have misrepresentation. Photoreceptor activity properly represents light when light has caused it to respond standardly, where "standardly" is cashed out in terms of (biologically and/or psychologically) normal functioning. Thus, we assign the content "physical edge" to those more global mechanisms of the visual system that function in such a way as to respond selectively to physical edges in the world (under normal conditions), rather than merely to local light–dark contrasts on the retina. If a cause other than the presence of a physical edge activates one of these mechanisms, this activation still has the content "physical edge" and we have misrepresentation (see also Dretske 1981, ch. 8). From the present viewpoint, the notion of misrepresentation is no more (and no less) problematic or conceptually suspect than the notions of normal and abnormal conditions relative to a functioning system—notions that may arouse suspicion when considered abstractly, but that we know how to apply in the concrete.

I hope to have demonstrated the availability of a notion of nonsymbolic representation for use in the psychology of perception. If the reader will recall the standard conceptions of *cognitive* as involving mentalistic notions such as concept and judgment or else internal processes in a symbol system, then results of this section, together with my discussions of noncognitive functional algorithms and nonsymbolic computation in Sections 2–3, make good on my promise to articulate a *noncognitive* psychology of vision. Moreover, I believe that direct theorists should find such a psychology acceptable, since it avoids cognitivism. Its acceptance by direct theorists would allow them to use a psychofunctional, rather than a neurophysiological, vocabulary when discussing the flow of information within information pickup devices. The notion of *representation* would allow them to chart the flow of information beyond the retina, and the notion *computation* would allow them to give an account of how the visual system detects higher-order stimulus information. Of course, the strongly conditioned aversion of direct theorists to the very words "computation" and "representation" may prevent them from accepting my offering. In any case, if my arguments stand, they show the plausibility of a type of theorizing that is psychological without being mentalistic in the traditional sense, while also including representations and representational content.

5. Cognitive Perception and the Limits of Cognitive Science

Suppose that the psychology of sense perception admits of nonmentalistic but nonetheless psychological explanations, and that such explanations include a notion of content. We may ask how far this style of explanation extends into other areas of psychology, including more paradigmatically cognitive achievements. At least two questions arise: (1) whether my analysis in terms of noncognitive functional algorithms will work for higher processes, and (2) whether my concept of content extends to the conceptually rich content that many recent discussions seek to explain. Both of these questions, I hasten to add, are empirical matters of a long-term sort that are judged by the success or failure of entire research programs. And although it is not the place of philosophers to forecast (or to prescribe) the outcome of empirical programs, that should not prevent us from exploring possible outcomes on the basis of what has been found to succeed (and to fail) thus far.

We may explore the first question by taking up the case of cognitive perception. Although the symbolist conception may seem the only choice for framing explanations of recognitional abilities, it is not. Take the concept of *rabbit*. Following my emphasis on perception, I want initially to consider this concept as it is manifested in an ability to separate on sight rabbits from nonrabbits (including squirrels and stuffed rabbits). If we suppose that some psychological mechanism underlies this ability, the question becomes how theorists should conceive this mechanism. Symbolists model it with internal descriptions of rabbit characteristics, whether through necessary and sufficient (or probabilistically adequate) perceptual features for recognizing rabbits, or through a representation of a prototypical rabbit together with a similarity metric to be applied to individual cases, along with notes on exceptions (see, e.g., Smith and Medin 1981, chs. 2, 7). In fact, neither necessary and sufficient conditions nor prototypes need commit a theorist to internal symbols. Necessary and sufficient conditions might be instantiated by a network of detectors for various individual rabbit (or animal) features, in such a way that when an appropriate collection of individual features are found, rabbit detection (or putative rabbit detection, as the case may be) occurs. Although the extent to which connectionist or other "wiring design" models can implement more complex cognitive achievements is as yet undetermined, investigators have implemented simple recognition networks with some success (e.g., Feldman 1985a). In any case, to the extent that object recognition can appropriately be conceived as a functional task rather than (say) as an intrinsically linguistic ability, there is no conceptual barrier to treating a nonsymbolist "functional analysis" conception of content as a serious theoretical alternative.

The main barrier to extending noncognitive functional algorithms to higher domains arises in extending the notion of content. My initial ascriptions of content depend on functional analysis, and functional analyses are environmentally specific. So far no problem. Difficulties for theory making arise, however, as contexts become more particular and more complex. For psychological functions that have a relatively fixed context—perhaps a function that has remained virtually constant during the evolution of the species (or even the genus)—functional ascriptions of content can claim wide generality. Such is surely the case with the basic regularities that underlie our sense perceptions of color and shape. The same holds true for cognitive functions that have a fixed and general context—examples might include predator recognition in the field mouse, or dam building in the beaver. Difficulties crop up with the complex content in human behaviors that are specific to context. When the biological meets the culturally conditioned, we may have less hope that the latter will offer the fixed contexts needed for developing the generalizations that support the functional analyses that underlie content ascription.

This is not to say that there can be no science of the culturally conditioned. There are two cases in which such scientific investigation is possible: when biology strongly conditions culture, and when sufficient cultural conformity exists to provide a stable context for generalization. Chomskian linguists have proposed that some aspects of the syntactic structure of language are biologically fixed, thus holding out the hope that linguists can achieve species-wide generalizations. But even if the degree of biological fixity is virtually nil, grammatical usage within a dialect or a language or a group of languages might nonetheless provide a sufficiently stable context within which to seek a general account of the psychological mechanisms underlying specific syntactic abilities. When we seek mechanisms underlying linguistic and (sophisticated) conceptual meaning, the story may be different; certainly the death of semantics as a science has been proclaimed many times in recent years (e.g., Hornstein 1984, ch. 7). Those who would raise the dead counterclaim that "situations" (or types of specific contexts) can pin down context and thereby set the stage for a general theory of meaning (Barwise and Perry 1983).[32] The success of this strategy depends on the extent to which semantic research reveals generalizations across situations. The more context-specific meaning turns out to be, the less it will make sense to pursue a general theory of meaning, or a general science of psychological content. A point can be reached at which complexity is no longer a merely pragmatic constraint, to be overcome as one's program progresses. At such a point, a switch to a qualitatively different type of analysis may be called for. Maxwell introduced his demon without supposing that the particles in a gas violate d'Alembert's equations.

The same considerations apply to the further reaches of cognitive psychology—memory, problem solving, and so forth. These are appropriate subjects for experimental science insofar as phenomena and mechanisms are shared within populations. Surely there are some shared mechanisms, such as those underlying memory. But whether these will provide deep insight into the content of memory and into the questions of central human interest, such as the selectivity of memory, is open to question. Again, whether a general theory of problem solving can be formulated depends on whether all problems have a common structure (or fit into a manageable typology), which in turn depends on what we count as a problem. If we take "problem" in its ordinary sense, the prospects for a general theory seem dim. (Think of the problem of reaching a banana from inside a cage using bamboo sticks, each of which is by itself too short; think of the problem of staying in favor at the court of Louis XIV; and now, at the court of Justinian.)

---

[32] Barwise and Perry (1983) attempt to make types of contexts (situation types) central to a theory of meaning. Others have also made context or background conditions do great service in the theory of meaning, as in Dretske's appeal to "channel conditions," that is, those conditions that must obtain for information (in his sense) to be transmitted (1981, ch. 5). Although such conditions have intuitive implications in some contexts, they stand in danger of becoming too particular to play a role in general explanations of behavior via meaning, as when information depends on intricate conventions or agreements among persons.

We may now return to a question that I set aside in the introduction: the centrality of "folk psychology" to psychology proper. Patricia Churchland (1980) and Stich (1983), reacting to the writings primarily of Fodor (1975) and Zenon Pylyshyn (1980), have portrayed the situation in contemporary cognitive science as requiring a choice between folk psychology on the one hand and either eliminative materialism or individualistic syntacticism on the other. On their view, functionalist cognitive psychology is belief–desire psychology, which, in the interest of scientific respectability, theorists should forsake for neurological explanations or, at best, for purely syntactic computational accounts.

However much folk psychological notions may be of interest and import-ance in understanding ourselves as cultural beings (and I, for one, believe that they will remain so, independently of whether they become "scien-tifically respectable"), they do not stand at the core of the experimental psychology of perception. I also deem it unlikely that such notions will be central to those aspects of higher cognitive functions that are most amen-able to experimental treatment (except, of course, in the empirical study of the folk notions themselves!). The type of functional psychology that I have described can develop representational content of a limited sort; it does so without subscribing to belief–desire psychology and without claim-ing that this functional content can replace the mentalistic notions that are central to our conceptions of ourselves within our cultural categories. This limited notion of content is at home in analyses of various repres-entational tasks, such as those in visual perception. It may be extended to higher-level cognition to the extent that researchers can discover suffi-ciently general contexts within which to formulate functional accounts of the relevant tasks.

This role for content comes at the price of acknowledging possible limitations on the scientific treatment of psychological functions. Such an admission may seem an act of despair to those who think of psychology as the science of *thought*, full stop. The conception that I have offered presents a less sweeping and grand program for cognitive science than has on occasion been proposed. But it has the virtue of being in keeping with the actual progress that experimental psychology and related disciplines have made. There is an august tradition in philosophy of setting one's sights by means of an analysis of what has made possible the success of theories or modes of knowledge that are known to work. Such a strategy need not be despairing or overly conservative, as long as it does not claim to set final or absolute limits. How far cognitive science can go is, after all, another of those long-term empirical matters. Among extant theories, I claim that in the domain of the psychology of sense perception, enough data are in to say that there can be a psychology of the internal processes of vision that is representational and computational without being either "folk" or Fodorean. This type of psychology can avoid objections that theorists have raised against the latter types of theory, without forsaking the project of formulating psychological explanations of perception.

3

Representation in Perception and Cognition

TASK ANALYSIS, PSYCHOLOGICAL FUNCTIONS, AND RULE INSTANTIATION

There is disagreement over how the notion of representation should be understood in cognitive science. Many investigators equate representations with symbols, that is, with syntactically defined elements in an internal symbol system (Fodor 1975; Pylyshyn 1984). Some urge that representation be understood wholly in terms of syntactic elements (Fodor 1980; Stich 1983, ch. 8),[1] while others implicitly adopt this position (Newell and Simon 1976; Newell 1980). This strictly syntactic symbolist view has provided a powerful tool for modeling psychological processes as governed by internal rules expressed in a symbolic medium. In particular, it interprets internal psychological processes realistically, while assuaging behaviorist scruples regarding mental processes by avoiding the traditional "stands for" notion of representation.

In recent years there have been two challenges to this orthodoxy. First, a number of philosophers have argued that "representation" should be understood in its classical sense, as denoting a "stands for" or "aboutness"

First published (without Section 7) as "Representation in Perception and Cognition: Connectionist Affordances," in W. Ramsey, D. Rumelhart, and S. Stich (eds.), *Philosophy and Connectionist Theory* (Hillsdale, NJ: Lawrence Erlbaum, 1991), 163–95, copyright © 1991 by Lawrence Erlbaum Associates; section 7 is from "Representation and Rule-Instantiation in Connectionist Systems," in Terry Horgan and John Tienson (eds.), *Connectionism and the Philosophy of Mind* (Boston: Kluwer, 1991), 90–112, copyright © 1991 by Kluwer Academic Publishers. Reprinted with permission and edited for style (and to allow two cross-references to more recent chapters).

[1] Stich opposes his "syntactic" theory of mind (1983, ch. 8) to "representational" theories of mind (chs. 7, 9) and so would not accept my description of his position. He, like most philosophers, reserves the term "representation" to describe a "stands for" relation (a usage I prefer). In parts of this chapter, I follow the more liberal use of the term as found in cognitive science, according to which there can be purely syntactic "representations."

relation between representing and represented. These philosophers include those outside the symbolist orthodoxy (Dretske 1988; Searle 1983; Ch. 2 herein) as well as those within, who maintain that symbols should be construed as referring to or representing an external world (Fodor 1987). Second, there has been a growing challenge to the orthodox symbolist view under the banner of connectionism (Rumelhart and McClelland 1986*b*; Smolensky 1988). Although this connectionist challenge is strong enough to elicit rebukes from the symbolist camp (Fodor and Pylyshyn 1988; Pinker and Prince 1988), connectionists as a group have not articulated a conception of representation to replace the symbolist view. Nonetheless, most connectionists agree on the need for a nonsymbolic notion of representation (Feldman and Ballard 1982; Hinton *et al.* 1986; Smolensky 1988; see also Kosslyn and Hatfield 1984).

In this chapter I incorporate the *stands for* (or *aboutness*) sense of representation into a general approach to cognitive science that is consonant with the connectionist challenge to orthodox symbolism. The leading idea is to marry connectionism to a particular version of functionalism, one that builds its notion of *function* on the similarity between functional analysis in biology and in psychology. This approach extends earlier work (Kosslyn and Hatfield 1984; Hatfield 1988*a* [Ch. 2 herein]) that adapted and revised Marr's (1982) tri-level approach to perception and cognition. My proposal frees Marr's analysis from an unneeded alliance with orthodox symbolism and reinterprets it through a notion of functional analysis that appeals both to "functional systems" as discussed by Cummins (1975) and Haugeland (1978) and to selection-based biological function (Wright 1973) as invoked by Millikan (1984) and Dretske (1988). Unlike these authors, however, I do not wed the notion of representation to a general analysis of behavior in terms of belief and desire. Rather, I draw a lesson from theoretical practice in the psychology of perception and cognition, in which investigators do not typically seek to explain behavior in general but to analyze the capacities that underlie behavior, such as vision, memory, learning, and linguistic capacities. According to this view, ascriptions of representational content are made not by working back from individual belief–desire ascriptions, but in framing psychological models to account for specific psychological capacities.

Because conceptions of representation in cognitive science typically are embedded in a general approach to the study of perception and cognition, an argument for the comparative plausibility of a particular conception of representation must scout these larger frameworks. I therefore first characterize the interlocking assumptions that support the orthodox symbolist approach, paying special attention to the complementarity between representation and process that those assumptions sustain. I then consider two versions of an alternative approach to representation: Dretske's (1988) and my own, and I show that my conception can underwrite a notion of rule following that is distinct from the usual symbolist accounts. Finally, I suggest that, by taking individual behaviors as its primary explanandum, cognitive science retains the influence of behaviorism just where it sought to counter it: in using ascriptions of beliefs and desires to explain behavior. Instead, I urge the merits of viewing the subject matter of experimental psychology and related portions of cognitive science as consisting in the various *psychological capacities*.

1. The Orthodox Conception of Representations as Symbols

Although the orthodox conception of representations as symbols receives lip service from many quarters, its underlying assumptions are less widely acknowledged. This is surprising, since several clear expositions of the symbolist view and of how it accounts for cognitive rules are available (Fodor 1975, ch. 1; Haugeland 1985, ch. 2; Newell 1980; Newell *et al.* 1989; Pylyshyn 1984, 1989).

As these expositions make clear, the symbolist conception of representation depends on a comparison between psychological processes and computational processes in digital computers. The comparison is not metaphorical (it is not a mere "computer metaphor"). It does not amount simply to the claim that psychological processes can be formally described in a regimented language or that such processes can be simulated on a computer. The hypothesized relation entails that psychological processes in organisms are performed by mechanisms that are functionally similar to the fundamental mechanisms of digital computers. The basic idea is that psychological processes are carried out in a *symbolic medium*. This medium is defined by the permitted interactions among strings of symbols, and it allows for the expression of specific *rules* (whose structure must be discovered empirically) to govern various psychological processes. The symbols themselves are type-individuated by their *form:* that is, by the properties that causally mediate the symbol's proper effects in interacting with processing mechanisms. The symbols and the mechanisms together define a symbol system.

Digital computers are devices in which causal interactions among physically instantiated symbols correspond (in a properly functioning machine) to the permitted transitions among syntactically characterized strings of symbols. The computer provides a well-understood example of a physically instantiated symbol system in which specialized rules (program statements) can be formulated to mediate input and output. Because symbols connote representation and talk of rules and representations has a mental flavor, and because computers are ponderable material objects, the existence of computers gives hope that the mind–body problem is not insoluble (Putnam 1967, 1975b; Fodor 1975, Introduction). The resulting symbolist view allows psychologists to respond to the rhetoric of "hollow organism" behaviorists such as Skinner (1963), who compare belief in internal mental processes to a belief in ghosts. Further, because symbol systems are language-like and are deemed to operate in a well-regimented manner, their interactions can be modeled as logical computations; symbolic models can be tested by using them to design computer programs that perform specific psychological tasks (such as object recognition).

Putnam, Fodor, and others combined the computer model with a conception of the nature of mental states known as "functionalism." In its most general formulation (Block 1980), this approach holds that the behavior of complex organisms is a function of input, output, and interactions among internal states, that is, a function among states defined by their interactions with one another and with input and output devices (such as sensory transducers and organs of motion). Stated generally, the position is distinct from Skinnerian behaviorism but remains similar to Hull's (1943) behaviorism, which permits (nonmentalistic) intervening variables, and it does not differ fundamentally from Tolman's (1936) behaviorism, which allows cognitive intervening variables. Nonetheless, the functionalist approach claims that its internal states are better suited than behaviorist intervening variables for explaining perception and cognition. Because the newly posited internal states are language-like, they might provide an appropriate medium for carrying out various cognitive tasks, including rational choice, concept learning, and object recognition. Indeed, Fodor contended that the ability to perform such tasks could be explained *only* by positing an internal language of thought (1975, ch. 1). He supported this assertion by claiming that there can be no computation without symbols (1975, 55).

Although the development of connectionist computational models under-mined Fodor's claim, the symbolic paradigm remains a powerful force in cognitive science and should be considered on its own merits before examin-ing alternatives. The reason that symbolists hypothesize internal symbol systems in target organisms is that they believe that psychological explanations of great power are thereby rendered possible. Computers are capable of carrying out complicated tasks (i.e., of performing complicated transformations between input and output) by dint of being symbol processing devices; perhaps organ-isms perform their complicated information-handling tasks according to a similar design.

The core of the symbolist approach is revealed by its response to an early objection: that the positing of an internal symbol system is the first step in an infinite regress of such systems. The charge goes like this: internal symbol systems are posited in order to explain complex information-handling abilities, such as natural-language abilities; but in positing an internal language, one must ascribe to the machinery that manipulates its symbols the ability to "read" and respond to them appropriately; but those are just the abilities that the internal symbol system was supposed to explain in the first place; hence, yet another internal symbol system must be posited to explain the abilities of this internal machinery to "read" symbols, and so on. The reply (or implicit response) to this charge varies from author to author, but the basic point is the same: some primitive abilities for "reading" and manipulating symbols must be ascribed to the organism or device. Fodor explicitly invoked the computer model (1975, 65–6): just as a computer must initially be built to respond to symbolic inputs—its central processing unit (CPU) must be hardwired to perform some primitive symbolic manipulations in "machine language," out of which its other abilities must be constructed—so too the organism comes ready-built with a primitive language of thought (a set of symbols and built-in mechanisms for manipulating them). Others simply speak of "primitive" capacities for manipulating symbols (Haugeland 1985, ch. 2; Pylyshyn 1989), or of physically instantiated symbols as having causal interactions with other symbol tokens by virtue of their physical (as opposed to formally symbolic) properties (Stich 1983, 149–51). In each case, an appeal is made to causal properties of symbols that do not depend upon their being "read" as symbols but that arise from their brute physical properties (their shapes or other structural properties) and the physical structure of the device or organism in which they are instantiated. These causal properties explain how symbol tokens interact with one another to yield transitions among symbol strings.[2]

Considering a second line of criticism reinforces the need for symbofunctionalists to impute a specific internal architecture to organisms. This objection paints the symbol-system hypothesis as vacuous by contending that, under a relevant description, *anything* can be a symbol. One could, for instance, use differently colored bricks in the side of a building to code sentences, by mapping brick colors to words and directing the receiver of the message to the bricks in a particular row; the bricks are the symbols, and a key gives

---

[2] As Stich (1983, 151) observes, an appeal to physical properties in explaining the behavior of symbol processors is compatible with the standard functionalist point that formally identical symbol systems can be multiply realized. For additional discussion of an antireductionist, functionalist psychology that can grant an explanatory role to physics or physiology, see Kitcher (1984), Kosslyn and Hatfield (1984), and Mehler *et al.* (1984).

the mapping of colors to words. One could use the same row of bricks to represent different messages by altering the key. But, the objection goes, if bricks can be symbols, and if the same brick can be now one symbol, now another, then the symbol-system hypothesis is so unconstrained as to be without content. Putnam (1988, Appendix) formalizes this objection and concludes that functionalism is either vacuous or reduces to behaviorism. He proves a theorem to show that "there is a sense in which *everything has every functional* organization" (p. xv). The theorem states that "Every ordinary open system is a realization of every abstract finite automaton" (121). The proof demarcates well-defined physical states of the system within sharp temporal boundaries, and it then defines appropriate disjunctions of such states as a sequence of machine states; subsequently, if one changes the definitions of machine states in terms of physical states, one changes the automaton that is "realized" by the sequence of physical states. Putnam acknowledges that this proof does not itself undermine "functionally characterized" systems in cognitive science, which tie the computed function to the actual states of sensory and motor processes in organisms. But he extends the original proof to show that all systems behaving "as if" they were computing a given function may be imputed that function, and then concludes that, since (in standard functionalism) possessing a given functional organization reduces to possessing a behavioral disposition, functionalism reduces to behaviorism.

In my view, Putnam's argument does not show that functionalism is vacuous, but it illustrates an important point: in symbol-system functionalism, symbols are defined in relation to a specific functional architecture for "reading" and manipulating them. In natural languages, we treat inscriptions and sound patterns as symbols (words and sentences) in a language that is relative to a linguistic community and its linguistic practices. With the brick code, individuals explicitly agree to treat certain objects or events as symbols. With artificial languages, those who create the language explicitly define the domain of legal symbols and legal operations over those symbols. In these instances, the rationale for calling something a "symbol" depends on the conventions that a group of users agree to or adhere to. In Putnam's argument, symbol systems are constrained by a merely stipulated framework of rules. Accordingly, anything can be made to seem as though it were organized as a symbol processor. By contrast, when symbol-system functionalists impute symbol systems to organisms, what counts as a symbol is not supposed to depend on convention or stipulation in any way, but is supposed to be a natural-scientific fact about how certain types of organisms are built. Although "everything" might have every functional architecture in the stipulative sense described by Putnam, the symbofunctionalist maintains that some things *naturally* have an internal organization in which some states are symbols (where "natural" is cashed out by imputing biological functions to the anatomical parts of an organism).[3]

If the symbol systems approach is not to slide into vacuity, its adherents must specify some strong constraints for deciding which internal states count as symbols and which sequences of events as the mechanisms for "reading" and "interpreting" those symbols (in the computer-science sense of "interpretation": being caused to go into the next machine state). Symbolists such as Pylyshyn, recognizing the need for such constraints, propose that functional descriptions of psychological systems should include concrete proposals about their internal computational architecture, proposals that could be tested by drawing implications for the real-time behavior of the system on specific tasks (1984, ch. 4; 1989). In a digital computer, this functional architecture is defined by the type of CPU, the clock speed, the amount of internal memory, and so on; the wiring of the CPU in particular determines the basic "symbol reading" operations of that machine, in relation to which its other symbolic abilities must be defined. In imputing an internal symbol system to an organism, the symbofunctionalist is (ideally) making a concrete proposal about the internal workings of that organism, and that proposal should include a functional decomposition of the organism's psychological systems that is empirically plausible. To the extent that this decomposition is confirmed by empirical tests that can discriminate among different computational architectures, it will make sense to be a scientific realist about symbofunctionalism. (Of course, it is still possible that arguments in the body of Putnam's 1988 book undermine symbol-system functionalisms that equate propositional attitudes with functional states. That would not undercut my rejoinder to his argument for the general vacuity of standard functionalism.)

2. The Alleged Representation–Process Complementarity

Symbol-system functionalism entails a strong representation–process complementarity: it makes no sense to speak of something as a "representation" (that is, a symbol) without specifying the processes that operate on it. The postulation of a complementarity between representation and process is a venerable

---

[3] Stabler (1987) counters arguments he attributes to Kripke (1981) (arguments similar to Putnam's) by invoking the notion of the "normal" operation of a device. I endorse his appeal to normal operations for devices and extend the argument to organisms by appealing to biological function (Ch. 2.4–5; also Kosslyn and Hatfield 1984, 1035–7).

position in cognitive science and cognitive psychology, and even investigators holding notions of representation that are distinct from the symbol-systems approach have advocated it.

Palmer (1978) and Gallistel (1990) analyze representation by drawing on measurement theory (Krantz *et al.* 1971; Suppes and Zinnes 1963). They define representational relations as holding between two domains: the represent*ing* and the represent*ed*. These relations map objects in the second domain onto those in the first, thereby establishing which objects in the representing domain stand for which objects in the represented domain. Although these theorists rely on a *stands for* relation between representations and objects, they simply stipulate (and don't explain) this relation, which is not the relation of primary interest to them. According to Palmer (1978, 266–7), the emphasis is on the *relations among objects* in the two domains: the "information" or "representational content" in the representing domain occurs in the set of relations among the objects in that domain. Once an object-mapping has been stipulated, the representational content consists in comparative relations among the objects in the representing domain.

The usual examples of this notion of representation involve the representation of some continuously varying magnitude in the represented domain by some magnitude in the representing domain. In one of Palmer's examples, the lengths of line segments in the representing domain represent the heights of rectangles in the represented domain. Any of several functions might be defined between these two magnitudes: greater length may directly represent greater height, or there could be an inverse relation between the two, or a more arbitrary mapping. Without specifying a key that determines the relevant feature of the representing objects, there is no sense in calling them "representations." With the interests of cognitive psychology in mind, Palmer thinks of the key as instantiated by the psychological processes that use the representations: "processing operations" "interpret" length as information about height. Within this framework, as Palmer contends, "one cannot discuss representation without considering process" (1978, 265).

Both the measurement-theory approach to representation and the symbol-systems approach posit a strong representation–process complementarity. This complementarity arises from similar features in each case: certain entities are treated as representations only because they are defined as representations relative to some operations for manipulating them (in the symbol-systems case) or for extracting information from them (in Palmer's case). As potential guides for theorizing about representation in naturally occurring psychological systems, the implications of the two approaches are equivalent: each defines representations in relation to the processes that operate on them.

Despite the plausibility of the representation–process complementarities scouted thus far, I contend that such complementarity does not hold for all viable notions of representation in psychology. It would therefore be a mistake to *define* representations in terms of the processes that operate over them. Psychology requires principled constraints for individuating the representational states of organisms, but these constraints need not advert to the processes operating on representations. Indeed, I maintain that the functional analysis of organisms into systems whose biological or psychological function is to represent states of the environment—the visual system is an example—sufficiently constrains the notion of representation for the purposes of empirical research, whereas exclusive use of the representation–process approach would hinder research.

I acknowledge that a complementarity between representation and process is required for some purposes. Independently of the conceptions of representation just canvassed, complementarity arises in the epistemology of ascribing representational states to an organism: an investigator cannot infer the existence of internal representations without also positing a set of processes into which the representations enter. This is the familiar point that, at present, behavior provides the primary data for ascribing psychological states to organisms. If one is to infer the presence of an internal representation on the basis of a certain behavior—say, the representation of a predator in a field mouse on the basis of the mouse's avoidance behavior—one must at the same time posit other internal representations and processes to mediate between input and output. Thus, the simple fact that a predator is in proximity and that the field mouse "behaves appropriately" does not by itself establish that it has represented and responded to the predator; besides determining how often the mouse behaves in this particular way and whether it does so in response to all approaching objects or only (or mostly) to predators, one would want to know whether the predator affected the mouse's sense organs, how sensory stimulation might have been processed to represent the presence of a predator, how this representation engaged motor mechanisms, and so on. Any ascription of internal representations made on behavioral evidence entails assumptions about internal processes.

Nonetheless, we should not conclude that what it is *to be* a representation is determined by the processes that make use of the representation. The fact that the evidence for positing representations requires imputing internal processes to an organism does not entail that those same processes supply a necessary condition on a state's being a representation. The epistemological condition on the investigation of internal representations should be distinguished from the ontological claim that internal states are representations solely in virtue of their role in mediating between input and output. I accept the epistemological point but deny the ontological one.

This distinction between the epistemology and ontology of representation may at first seem futile: surely the designation of an internal state as a representation essentially depends on the role that the state plays in mediating between inputs and outputs. This claim lies at the heart of symbofunctionalist thinking. But it is just what I deny. I hold that there are systems in some organisms (including human beings) that serve the function of representing the environment, whether individual representations in those systems enter into further processing or not. It is important to be careful here. I am not claiming that there are systems that have the function of representing states of the environment and that the representational states of such systems never affect behavior; rather, I'm making the claim that for a given token representational state to be a representation, it is not necessary that that particular state or a type-identical one *ever* enter into a process that affects behavior or even that affects other internal representations.

In my view, something can be a representation simply by virtue of its being a state of a system whose function is to represent. Accordingly, some internal states of organisms are *natural representations*; that is, they are states of an organism that have as their natural biological or psychological function to represent the environment. They may serve this function without affecting behavior. A visual percept represents the environment because it is a state of a visual system, not because it controls behavior. Of course, it might be that, for all known organisms, nothing can be a visual system unless the system as a whole contributes somehow to the control of behavior. For present purposes, I grant this condition: to be a visual system is to be capable of guiding an organism's response to its environment by extracting spatial information from ambient light. As I shall argue in contrasting my position with that of Dretske, this concession does not obviate my point.

3. Biopsychological Function and Representation

There is a growing trend toward interpreting psychological function by analogy with biological function and using this notion to ground ascriptions of content. K. V. Wilkes (1978, ch. 4) offered an early explicit interpretation of functionalism in psychology in terms of biological function. In fact, the early functionalist arguments of Putnam (1967) and Fodor (1968, ch. 3) tacitly drew upon the biological and artifactual notion of function (see Hatfield

1988*a*), while overtly emphasizing the mathematical notion of a functional relation between the inputs and outputs of real or ideal machines. The mathematical notion dominated their subsequent discussions. In recent years, Millikan (1984) and Dretske (1988) have developed accounts of content that draw on biological function, as have I (Kosslyn and Hatfield 1984; Ch. 2.4). Although these recent uses of the notion of function to ground ascriptions of content display similarities, they set out from different starting points and yield different implications. In particular, the Millikan–Dretske approach applies the notion of biological function to input–output analyses of behaving organisms; it conjoins biological function with orthodox functionalism to ascribe content to internal states mediating between input and output. By contrast, I use the notion of biological function in analyzing particular psychological systems such as the visual system; the resulting ascriptions of content arise in analyzing the system in question, not in attempting to give a theory of content for beliefs and desires in general.

Dretske's 1988 book attempts to provide a naturalistic account of meaning that could serve in explaining behavior. Dretske distinguishes between two levels of meaning. He calls the first "natural meaning" (he refers to Grice 1957) or "indication," which he equates with his earlier (1981) notion of "information" (1988, 58–9). Accordingly, many natural states are *indicators* of other natural states: tracks in the snow indicate the previous presence of the bird that made them, the width between tree rings indicates amount of yearly rainfall, and a state in an animal's nervous system may indicate the presence of food. For there to be indication in each case there must be a dependence between the indicator and the indicated, such that the indicator would not be present unless the indicated had been present (other conditions being constant). Dretske contrasts this "indicator" sense of meaning with the sort of meaning found in psychological representations such as beliefs. Beliefs differ from natural meaning in possessing a characteristic mark of intentionality: the ability to misrepresent. In defining indicators strictly in terms of dependence, Dretske rules out misindication: if the purported indicator could have been present without the indicated property or thing having been present, there is no indication. By contrast, beliefs are the sort of thing that can misrepresent, as the existence of false beliefs shows.

Dretske attempts to develop a theory of meaning appropriate to belief by building upon the indicator relation. Indicators become representations (here, beliefs or belief-like states) by virtue of their role in causing behavior. His account of representation places great weight on the role of internal states in producing behavior. In schematic terms, Dretske's account of a situation in which internal state C of organism O represents external state F is as follows:

the fact that C causes M in O (where M is an instance of O's behavior) is explained by the facts that C indicates F in O's environment and O needs or desires F. In other words, an internal state C comes to represent F when it causes appropriate behavior toward F and it causes that behavior because it indicates F. The specific causal mechanism leading from C to M is not the crucial element; Dretske is instead targeting the cause of O's being so wired that C causes M. He is asking for the cause of O's *having forged* a causal link from C to M, and not for an explanation of *how* C causes M. In his terms, he is looking for a "structuring cause" of the relation between C and M, and not the "triggering cause" of a particular instance of M (1988, 42–50, 83–7).

When the above conditions are met, Dretske says that the "intrinsic function" of C is to represent F. (He explicates intrinsic function in terms of biological function: 1988, 63–4.) Thus, a certain internal state C has the function of representing food when, in addition to indicating the presence of food, it also causes an organism, say, to approach and eat the food. In this case misrepresentation can occur because although states of type C typically indicate food, they nonetheless can occur in the absence of food (when other conditions are not constant). When they do so occur they are not indicators but, on Dretske's view, they are representations, albeit ones that misrepresent the state of affairs. Although states of type C have the function of representing food, token instances can misrepresent the presence of food because something can have a function even if it does not always successfully perform it. The function of the lens in the human eye is to promote visual acuity, even if it fails to do so in some people or for part of the lifetime of a particular person. In the case at hand, it is precisely because C's intrinsic function is to represent F that an aberrant occurrence of C has the content F.

My own view of representation places great weight on the functional analysis of an organism into systems and subsystems. The designation of an internal state of the organism as a *representation* occurs in ascribing to various systems the function of producing or modifying representations. Some states of an organism are representations by virtue of being part of a system whose function is to generate states internal to an organism that *stand for* some external state or event. Thus, we might ascribe to visual systems the function of representing distal states, and to other systems (such as pictorial memory) the function of storing and allowing access to the information contained in the representations that the visual system produces. In schematic terms: R represents D in O because the function of the system of which R is a state is to represent states of D's type, and the function of states of type R is to represent states of type D in particular. I here invoke the notion of biological or psychological function, which is the same notion of function as Dretske uses. The difference between the two approaches comes down to my insisting that some internal systems, such as the visual system, simply have the function of representing external states of affairs.[4] From this I draw the conclusion that states of such systems can *be* representations without their entering into further processing.

One might plausibly argue that, even on the symbolist view, token symbols can remain symbols without entering into further processing. Imagine a token symbol inscribed directly into a visual memory buffer that never gets cleared and is never again accessed. It remains a symbolic representation relative to the system of which it was a part, since it retains the properties that define it as a symbol: the properties that allow it to enter into the "right" relation with the CPU. Similarly, one might argue that, in Dretske's view, while states of type C must on occasion produce behavior M and must do so because they represent F, token states might be instantiated without actually causing behavior M: a given token of C might fail to produce M because O had a conflicting desire for external object H represented by internal state J which caused behavior N. In both cases, there is a sense in which an internal state can be a representation without entering into further processing: if it is a token of a type that is well defined in the usual representation–process complementarity.

Herein lies the crucial distinction between my position and that of symbolism or Dretske. A state is a representation in virtue of its relation to a CPU on the symbolist view, or in virtue of its standard behavioral upshot on the Dretskean view. In my view, whether a given type of representation enters into further processing can be irrelevant to whether its tokens count as representations; what makes them *be* representations is the fact that they are states of a system whose function is to generate representations.[5]

Suppose for a moment that the visual system in primates has the function of representing (1) the distal spatial layout, (2) changes in that layout, and (3) the motion of the organism through the layout (Gibson 1966, 156). Among the representational functions of the visual system is that of representing the precise

---

[4] Dretske admits the validity of this notion of representation but devotes only a single sentence to it (1988, 94). He focuses instead on the notion of "natural" representations that guide behavior (62–77). He avoids analyzing representations that do not guide behavior because his ultimate aim is to understand "ordinary" explanations of behavior that rely on attributions of beliefs and desires; his book is intended to vindicate naturalistic conceptions of intentional explanation (x), even if such explanations do not meet the standards of the empirical sciences (81, n. 1).

[5] Functional analysis typically treats an organism as comprising functional systems, each of which contributes to the larger system. In such analyses, the sensory systems generally might be considered as input systems, and thus as systems having the function of producing representations to be passed along for further processing. It follows that even in my view a token state R could not be a representation unless it were part of a system that regularly passed representations along for further processing. Nonetheless, it does not follow that each state-type of such a system is a representation *because* it could be passed along.

spatial configuration of distal surfaces, a function it performs well up to some limit of acuity. The possible representational states of the system range across the spatial configurations that it can represent: these form a series of possible representational states, R_1 to R_n, which is large (if, owing to limitations on acuity, not indefinitely large). I hold that we can legitimately denominate each of the states R_i as representational states even if some subset of them (*a*) never enters into further processing, and (*b*) would have no effect on behavior if it did.

Outcome (*a*) is empirically plausible: due to the well-known bottleneck effect (Sperling 1960), a large portion of any given visual spatial representation is not subject to further processing. It would not diminish their status as representations if spatial representations of a particular class of tetrahedra always happened to be part of what did not get through. Further, it also seems plausible to suppose that there are some surface layouts which, if seen, would have no effect on behavior (outcome *b*) because, for example, they happened always to occur in proximity to surfaces that were especially salient behaviorally. Thus, if tetrahedra were rarely present in the visual field and then only in the fields of hungry primates and only in proximity to food, they might pass the bottleneck but never affect behavior (assuming that their rarity keeps them from becoming "signs" of food). In each case, the status of such spatial representations *as* representations depends on the fact that they are *bona fide* states in a system whose function is to produce spatial representations. Accordingly, although the visual system may have evolved because its representations of the spatial layout helped guide adaptive behavior, the spatial content of any given perceptual representation is not determined by its past or present behavioral upshot.

This view of perceptual representation needs fleshing out so as to avoid certain kinds of objections. In particular, I need to avoid the objection that in fact only those spatial representations that guide behavior have true "content" or "meaning," and that I have mistakenly assigned content to other such representations by an improper analogy to those that do or could guide behavior. From Dretske's perspective, my alleged "representations" might be seen as superfluous states produced by a mechanism that has the function of producing states to guide behavior. From the standpoint of selectional theories in biology, they might be understood as accidental consequences of a process that was selected because it generated actual behavior-guiding representations. My "representations" would be by-products of the true behavior-guiding function of vision, just as heart sounds are a by-product of the blood-pumping function of the heart. In my view, by contrast, visual systems may well have evolved to guide behavior, but that process of evolution has yielded mechanisms whose function is to represent distal properties independently of linking any specific representation to any specific behavior. This response requires a more fully articulated functional analysis of the visual system, which I find in Marr's (1982) work.

4. Functional Analysis and Marr's Three Levels

The central feature of Marr's approach is the notion of *task analysis*: an analysis of what a given system or process is *for*. He integrated this notion into a comprehensive analysis of information-processing systems on three levels: *computation, algorithm,* and *implementation*.

Although the term "computation" brings to mind stepwise manipulation of numerical or logical arguments, Marr's first level of analysis really amounts to a functional or task analysis. This level seeks to specify what a given system is for and to describe the strategy by which it carries out its function (1982, 22–3, 25). Thus, a "computational" analysis of the auditory perceptual system might describe the kinds of information that the system extracts, the types of energy it responds to in extracting this information, and the strategies it embodies to glean information from variations in energy. Marr's second level specifies the representational system that encodes input, together with the algorithms that transform these representations during the functioning of the system. The auditory system might transduce primitive representations of pitch, amplitude, phase, and inter-ear time differences and then use a particular set of algorithms to compute the locations and characteristics of distal sound sources. The third level of analysis, the implementation, aims to describe the physical realization of the representations and algorithms from level two. In the case of natural information-handling systems, this description is in terms of neural networks; in the case of an artificial device, it might amount to a description of a real-time processor together with associated data buffers. The distinctions between the different levels should not be treated as hard and fast. In particular, the distinction between the first two levels may depend on the grain of the analysis: what is treated as an algorithm (level two) in a global description may be treated as a task-specification (level one) in a more fine-grained analysis.

Marr's task analysis of the visual system separates the relatively "pure" perceptual processes of what he terms *early vision* from subsequent visual processes such as object recognition. Accordingly, the function of early vision is to represent the spatial configuration of surfaces in the immediate environment, including the orientation and distance of such surfaces from the viewer (1982,

41–2, 268–9). Early vision is *for* representing the spatial layout. It generates accurate spatial representations that organisms may exploit on different occasions for different purposes: to guide local movement, to navigate by distant landmarks, to detect desired objects near and far, to foresee impending danger (34–6). In serving these functions, the spatial representations of early vision may be accessed by any of a number of subsequent processes, and presumably organisms would not possess visual systems if such systems did not produce representations that could be so accessed. Nonetheless, Marr's analysis confines the function of early vision to that of producing representations of distal surfaces, *simpliciter*.

This analysis of the function of early vision guides Marr's core analysis of vision (1982, chs. 2–4). He develops models of how the visual system might create accurate representations of the spatial features of objects from the patterns of light received at the retinas. Although he describes representations as elements in a symbol system (pp. 20–1), the spatial representations that his models generate are clearly intended to stand for distal surfaces (44). In explaining how the visual system constructs such representations, he imputes to the system a set of "assumptions" (which he characterizes as background knowledge) about the structure of the external world. Two such assumptions are that the visible world is composed of cohesive objects with relatively smooth surfaces, and that individual points on these surfaces have unique positions in space at any one time (112–13). He recounts how a system operating according to these assumptions might compute stereoscopic depth from binocular disparity (113–16). He provides similar analyses for shape, surface texture, and object motion. In each case, his analysis is guided by the notion that the function of early vision is to produce representations of the spatial structure of the distal layout.

Marr's theory does not by itself answer the objections posed at the end of the previous section. It is not fully obvious what the functions of the visual system are, and Marr's analysis could be wrong: early vision might have a more specialized function than that of representing properties of distal surfaces. The visual system's profuse generation of spatial representations might be an accidental by-product of its function in guiding motion for the purpose of avoiding danger and securing food, shelter, and other objects of desire. It seems more likely, however, that the production of such representations aims to yield accurate representations of the distal layout for access by further processes. From this perspective, the function of the visual system is not (or is not any longer) to produce representations for the sake of any one of these further purposes; its function just is to produce accurate representations of the distal layout.

5. Task Analysis and the Connectionist–Symbolist Debate

The *stands for* sense of representation that I have employed in previous sections does not have an exclusive affinity with Marr's task analysis approach. But as in his analysis of early vision, Marr's approach easily incorporates this notion of representation. I want now to argue that connectionist models are well suited to both the task analysis approach and the *stands for* sense of representation. Moreover, attention to Marr's three levels of analysis brings the principled differences between connectionist and symbolist approaches into relief.

The controversy between symbolists and connectionists has focused on whether connectionist models can handle aspects of human cognition such as systematicity and compositionality—aspects of cognition that symbol system models (literally) are built to handle. Symbophiliacs have maneuvered to put their connectionist foes into a no-win situation: they have argued that either connectionist models cannot handle compositionality, or that, if they can, then connectionism is not truly distinct from symbolism but amounts merely to a way of implementing traditional symbolist models (Fodor and Pylyshyn 1988). This point is often made using the terminology of rules and representations: symbolists allege that only symbol systems can model cognitive processes that involve the rule-governed manipulation of representations, and that many psychological functions, including perception, concept learning, problem solving, and language learning, require such manipulations.

These arguments misconstrue the principled differences between connectionist and symbolist models, and they disregard legitimate differences of opinion over matters that are, in the long run, empirical. First, as to the principled differences. Connectionism and symbolism differ in their conceptions of the computational machine that underlies perception and cognition. The fundamental difference is manifested in the basic or primitive operations that each approach posits. Symbol-system approaches build the ability to manipulate token symbolic representations into psychological systems as a primitive (as discussed above). Symbol systems just are systems with a primitive capacity to manipulate token symbols according to syntactic rules. Perceptual and cognitive processes instantiated by such systems can be "rule following" in a very literal sense: the rules governing psychological operations can be explicitly formulated in the internal symbol system. By contrast, the connectionist approach does not build syntactic or other language-like abilities into the basic operations it posits; rather, it starts with very simple capacities from which it constructs perceptual and cognitive abilities, including the ability to manipulate symbols. Connectionist systems compute when a pattern of activation passes among the interconnected nodes: some nodes receive input, and the states of some nodes count as output; in some systems, other nodes constitute "hidden" layers between input and output. The basic operations in connectionist systems include passing on activation when inputs to a node sum to a threshold, and altering the threshold as a result of past activity (Feldman and Ballard 1982; Rumelhart 1989). Both symbolist and connectionist systems allow for the "programming" of computations, but in different ways. Symbolist programs are conceived as rules expressed in an internal language. Connectionist models build a network that computes in virtue of its connectivity; such networks do not need to instantiate symbol-manipulation unless the specific task being computed is itself a symbolic one.

The main difference between symbolism and connectionism pertains to the built-in primitive operations in each system. Connectionism is symbol-free inasmuch as symbols are not posited among the primitive features of connectionist systems;[6] but connectionist models can provide algorithms and implementations for tasks that are symbolic under a Marr level-one description. Assuming that such models are adequate to the task (a matter still under investigation, as with symbolic models), they potentially provide an explanatory advantage over symbolist models: they would explain syntactic abilities within psychology rather than taking them as primitives that are built into the system (and so subject only to physical or physiological explanation). Connectionism makes form-based interactions among symbols—the operation of the CPU in the standard computer model—an explicit object of psychological investigation. More broadly, connectionist models need to invoke symbols only for tasks that have a symbolic task analysis, such as natural language abilities.

In the symbofunctionalist approach, all psychological processes—whether perceptual, conceptual, or linguistic—are conceived as mediated by a language of thought. Connectionist models need not construe all perception and cognition as inherently symbolic. Task analysis provides the framework for deciding what sorts of representations and processes should be posited in modeling a particular perceptual or cognitive capacity. Some tasks, such as image formation, may not require a symbolic underpinning. In fact, both symbolic and nonsymbolic models of image formation have been proposed. Kosslyn (1980, 1983) posited that his imagistic representations have a symbolic underpinning, even though they behave functionally as images. Kosslyn

---

[6] Of course, parallel computation systems can be created by linking standard digital computers together, in which case the "nodes" in this parallel network would compute via internal symbols. The connectionist models under discussion do not posit digital computational structures within nodes.

and Hatfield (1984) treat images as inherently analog, with a nonsymbolic connectionist underpinning. Psychological tasks that do not require symbolic structures can be directly realized in a connectionist net (see Ch. 2.3). To the extent that nonsymbolic task analyses occur in psychology, as might be the case in spatial representation and color perception in vision and in tasks that rely on pattern recognition (via pattern similarities), connectionist models as a whole are not "mere" implementations of symbol systems, since they cover psychological tasks that are not inherently symbolic and they do so without invoking symbols.

A second type of systematic difference between some connectionists and their symbolist foes pertains to the task analysis itself. Some connectionists believe that even apparently symbolic tasks are not truly governed by hard rules but should be regarded as probabilistic processes. According to them, hard-rule descriptions—such as those linguists give for a speaker's grammatical abilities—are idealizations; they argue that psychology should explain linguistic performance, not idealized competence (Rumelhart and McClelland 1986a). They and other connectionists contend that actual cognitive capacities such as linguistic performance should be conceived probabilistically. Smolensky (1988) has suggested that connectionist models of concepts are more realistic than traditional symbolist models precisely because they capture the context-sensitive nature and the "family resemblance" character of concepts. Accordingly, the alleged advantage of classical systems in handling hard-rule behaviors would be an illusion based on a mistaken task analysis; indeed, one might conjecture that hard-rule task analyses were projected onto many cognitive tasks by those already enamored of the symbolic paradigm. In offering probabilistic task analyses, connectionists are not claiming that their models can handle probabilistic relations and that symbolic models cannot. Rather, they are contending that a supposed advantage of symbolist models—that they are especially well suited for modeling cognition, because cognition is rule-governed and symbolist models have a built-in affinity for modeling rule-governed cognitive processes—may rest on a mistake. Which group is right is, of course, a long-term empirical matter.

Some connectionists, however, do accept the "hard rules" task analysis, and they develop connectionist models that instantiate rule-governed abilities. Shastri has attempted to model hard-rule knowledge and inference abilities connectionistically (1988). Dell (1985) marries the hard-rule approach to linguistic ability with a connectionistic model that purports to provide a better account of performance errors. Such models agree with the spirit of the task analysis in traditional approaches to rules and representations, but they claim that connectionist models provide a more powerful or empirically more plausible implementation.

Taken together, these connectionist positions hinder the slide that Fodor and others make from symbolic task analyses to the necessity of classical symbol-systems realizations for those tasks (Fodor 1987, 135, 138–9). These connectionist positions undermine the claim that all psychological operations must have symbolic underpinnings. They question whether all psychological tasks are governed by hard rules and also whether only symbolist models can effectively model those that are.

6. Connectionist Representations

In the symbolist paradigm the notion of representation is intrinsically tied to syntax (whether one is a solipsist, as in Fodor 1980, or a born-again semantic realist, as in Fodor 1987): representations are symbols defined relative to primitive processes of symbolic interaction (standardly, a central symbol processor). In connectionist models the description of a state of a system as a representation never depends solely on its being a well-defined state of the computational architecture: the designation of certain states as representations depends on their functional role in the model, which itself depends on the task that the model has been designed to compute. In symbolist models, ascriptions of specific representational structures may depend on a task analysis. Nonetheless, before symbolists even analyze a task, they have decided that the representational elements must be symbols (at the level of computational architecture).

Because the ascription of representational status to elements in a connectionist model depends on the task analysis, the way in which representations are conceived in such models may vary depending on the task in question. Thus, in connectionist models of long-term memory or stored knowledge, "representational content" is determined by the relation that a given state has to other states in memory and to representations in input and output systems. The connectionist instantiation of a particular concept might, in a given model, gain its content through its pattern of connectivity to other concepts: the concept *Quaker*, for instance, might be assigned its content because of its relation to other parts of a semantic network, including the concepts *person* and *pacifist* (Shastri 1990). It also might be assigned its content because of its relation to input systems and specifically to its role in recognizing Quakers as Quakers.[7]

---

[7] Connectionist models seem well suited to pattern-matching tasks, and thus to recognitional tasks: see Gluck and Bower (1988). Modeling actual visual recognition, though, is quite difficult (even for more tractable concepts than *Quaker*); some models purporting to address "recognition" actually

In models of perceptual abilities, connectionists confer representational status by assigning some states of a network the function of directly standing for the state of the environment (Ballard *et al.* 1983). In a model of surface perception, states of a network are ascribed a representational status because they are states whose function is to represent the distal layout (Lehky and Sejnowski 1988). In each case, the task analysis governs the ascription of representational status.

Understandably, there has been more than one conception of how connectionist networks realize representational content. Those dealing with learning or with knowledge structures have emphasized the representational function of the pattern of connectivity. Thus, in Shastri's (1988) model of knowledge storage, the pattern of connectivity (including wiring paths, excitatory or inhibitory gain, and thresholds for firing) is used to store information in propositional format (subject–predicate form) that can be queried in various ways. The pairings of subjects and predicates depends entirely on the pattern of connectivity; once the pattern is established, dynamic activation serves only in the retrieval (active representation) of the knowledge. When, as is usual at present, a model of knowledge storage is presented without a coordinated model of object recognition, the ascription of representational content depends on the relations among the representational states (as in many symbolist models: see Newell and Simon 1976, and Newell *et al.* 1989).

In models of active cognitive processes such as inference or perception, dynamic properties of nodes, such as the frequency of firing or the present pattern of activation, come to the fore. In a further elaboration of his model of knowledge storage, Shastri allows frequency of firing to represent the relation between specific objects and a predicate structure (Shastri and Ajjanagadde 1993). The predicate structure *gives* is broken down into three places: *giver*, *givee*, and *object given*, each of which is assigned a node or collection of nodes. Further collections of nodes correspond to potential individual arguments, such as *John*, *Mary*, and *Ivanhoe*. The statement "John gave Mary *Ivanhoe*" is instantiated by *John* resonating with *giver*, *Mary* with *givee*, and *Ivanhoe* with *object given*. This arrangement allows extensive background knowledge (as stored in connection weights) to be brought to bear on particular active propositions; inferences from one proposition to another that are sensitive to background knowledge are mediated by the spreading activation of the patterns of resonance. In this case, then, connectivity serves

---

model scene reconstruction, inasmuch as they show how geometric shapes might be reconstructed in representation but make no provision for sorting such shapes into kinds (Sabbah 1985). Feldman (1985a) avoids this objection.

the representational function of storing knowledge, and the pattern of activity serves the function of representing "active" knowledge and of mediating a process of inference.

In perceptual models, the pattern of activity itself typically serves the function of representation. In one model (Kienker *et al.* 1986; Sejnowski and Hinton 1989), the figure/ground relation is represented by the spatial positions and excitatory values of nodes (following the topology of "next-to-ness" defined by connectivity). Input consists of activating each node in an array to a given value; computation proceeds through a simulated annealing paradigm; and output is the state of the net in equilibrium, with perhaps two areas of similarly activated adjacent nodes, one serving as figure, the other as ground (separated by a border of "edge unit" nodes that determine which is figure and which ground). The representational content of the net is just the spatial information contained in the pattern of activation: such models do not speak to recognitional abilities, but merely to the figure/ground segregation of a spatial array. The "rules" for computing figure/ground segregation are included in the pattern of connectivity and activation. I address the status of such processing rules in connection nets in Section 7.

In this section, I have described some perceptual models in which the pattern of activation is a representation that stands for a spatial structure in the world. This pattern possesses no formal characteristics that make it a representation "in itself" (contrary to symbolist models). It is a representation of a spatial structure because it is a proper state of a system whose function is to produce such representations.

7. Rule Instantiation

Traditional "rules and representations" accounts of cognition draw a distinction between *rule described* and *rule following* systems (Fodor 1975, 74, n. 15). The usual example of a rule-*described* system is one that simply obeys natural laws, as when an object falls to earth in accordance with the law of gravity: no understanding or representation of the rule or law is imputed to the object in order to explain the fact that its motion conforms to the law. A rule-*following* system conforms to the rule or law by virtue of an explicit representation of it, as when a cook follows a new recipe: the cook's behavior accords with the steps in the recipe because the cook consults the recipe and follows its directions. I suggest that connectionist systems fit neither of these descriptions. They *instantiate* rules without being rule-following in the traditional sense. Nor are they merely rule described, as falling objects are. The rules that connectionist systems instantiate do not follow directly from universal laws of physics and chemistry but arise in tandem with the evolution or epigenesis of psychological systems of certain kinds. To mark this distinction, I use the phrase *rule instantiating* for connectionist networks that compute specific rules.

The ease with which symbolist models provide a realist interpretation for processing rules in psychology is one of their strengths: they equate processing rules with explicitly formulated statements in the internal code. Connectionists, because they give up classical computational architecture with its commitment to primitive symbolic operations, cannot generally adopt the symbolist conception of rule following (they may, of course, allow explicitly formulated rules at the task level). But, even though connectionist networks are not rule following in the way that symbolist models are, they nonetheless allow for a realist interpretation of processing rules. In connectionist models, networks are *designed* or *engineered* to instantiate a given rule, such as a rule for computing shape from shading or for pattern matching; or such networks are designed or engineered to acquire computational characteristics that enable them to perform these tasks. If connectionism is right, organisms have acquired (through evolution or learning) networks of connections that instantiate appropriate processing rules for various psychological tasks.

The term "rule" may be applied in several ways in describing connectionist networks. Generic "rules of activation" and "rules of learning" characterize the architecture of a connectionist network—for instance, the activation properties of each node—independently of the psychological rule that the network instantiates by virtue of its architecture. These "rules" of the basic architecture have a status similar to the basic "rules" of Turing machine operation: for example, the rules that govern the operation of the mechanism that allows the machine's head to be programmed. These rules need not be symbolically formulated but can be engineered into the head so that it reads a cell, writes a cell, and moves one way or the other. If the head is programmable, then it can be symbolically configured to perform these basic operations in accordance with one explicitly represented rule or another; still, the mechanisms for "reading" a cell are engineered in, and, on pain of regress, they are not symbolically formulated within the device. Similarly with connection nets: the rules of activation, rules of learning, and so on, are basic elements of the computational architecture that allow the network, in virtue of its particular pattern of connectivity and particular values of its rules of activation, to be configured in such a way that it computes one function rather than another. The function that the configured network computes is the psychological rule *instantiated* by the network.[8]

The rules instantiated by connectionist models are a diverse lot. They reflect the variety of psychological functions for which connectionist models have been proposed: computing shape from shading (Brown *et al.* 1982); separating figure from ground (Kienker *et al.* 1986); recognizing patterns (see McClelland *et al.* 1986); object recognition (Feldman 1985*a*); learning the morphology of the past tense of English verbs (Rumelhart and McClelland 1986*a*); and drawing inferences from a data base (Shastri and Ajjanagadde 1993). The connection weights and network configurations in such models variously instantiate rules of inference, knowledge structures, and rules of perceptual processing. Although the principles of network operation may be shared in these cases, the functions that the networks instantiate are diverse when described psychologically. In models of stored knowledge, the network characteristics may represent rule-structured knowledge of the world. With object recognition, connection weights instantiate conceptual representations or implicit knowledge about object characteristics. The rules that the network instantiates for computing shape from shading or for computing surface reflectance from retinal intensities do not, intuitively, seem worthy of being called "knowledge" or even "stored representations," any more than one imputes "knowledge" of the rules of color mixture to the neuronal systems that combine the outputs of the three types of light-sensitive cones in the human retina. In early vision, the rules that the network instantiates seem intuitively to be processing rules for generating visual representations rather than cognitive rules that are themselves represented.

Consider two types of connectionist model. In Shastri's model of rule-based reasoning, connection weights and node characteristics represent stored information about a domain of knowledge, say, about book ownership among a group of friends (Shastri and Ajjanagadde 1993). This information is "in" the network characteristics in this sense: solely in virtue of those characteristics, the network responds appropriately to queries about who owns which book. Now consider a model for computing shape from shading, in which connection weights instantiate rules for extracting shape by processing local differences in shading (Brown *et al.* 1982). In virtue of the weights, the network instantiates one rule for extracting shape from shading rather than another. But does the network store *knowledge* or *information* about the rules for extracting shape from shading? Intuitively, no. The "rules" of processes such as those of early vision

---

[8] One might choose to describe the engineered rules in the Turing machine head, or the generic rules of activation, as "instantiated" rules; but these would be subpsychological rules governing implementation, not psychological processing rules.

seem to be precognitive or subcognitive. Even so, the network does instantiate such rules.

The fact that various configurations of connection weights serve to instantiate a psychologically heterogeneous collection of rules does not by itself call into question the intuitive distinction between "stored knowledge" and processing rules that are subcognitively instantiated. But among theorists who emphasize the biological basis of computation there has been a tendency to elide this distinction. The distinction can be dissolved in either direction. Some authors, such as the eliminative materialist P. S. Churchland (1986, ch. 9), envision developing the vocabulary of neuroscience in such a way that this vocabulary replaces the allegedly unscientific vocabulary of "inference" or "cognitive representation," thereby dissolving the distinction in the direction of (an as yet unarticulated) neuroscientific description. Conversely, others extend the vocabulary of knowing to the lower levels, including the computations involved in deriving shape from shading. Many connectionist authors and their relatives describe the processes of early vision in terms of testing hypotheses or making inferences based on assumptions (e.g., Hinton and Sejnowski 1986; Marr 1982, 17, 159). They would thus dissolve the distinction between cognitive and subcognitive processes by extending cognitive descriptions to early visual processing.

The implications that connectionist models hold for maintaining a division between neurophysiology and psychology are worth considering. Connectionist models are touted as being more biologically plausible than symbolist models, because connectionist networks share some qualities with neural networks. All the same, the relation between connectionist networks and actual neurons is not clear; indeed, connectionist nodes might be realized by populations of neurons rather than single neurons. Still, the sense in which connectionist models constitute psychology rather than (idealized) physiology requires explication.

Advocates of symbolism draw the line between psychology and physiology far upstream. Fodor and Pylyshyn characterize any nonsymbolic processes in early vision as physiological "transduction" between stimulation and symbol. Ullman (1980) argues that Gibsonian accounts of vision are not psychology but physiology, contending that, in rejecting cognitive characterizations of the processes of early vision, Gibsonian direct theorists reject a "psychologically interesting" decomposition of early visual processes (an implication that some direct theorists would accept). But, as I discussed in Chapter 2, connectionist models afford a means for interjecting psychologically interesting descriptions of processes without conceiving them in symbolist or cognitive terms. Connectionists can describe the computation of shape from shading, or of depth in stereopsis, in the vocabulary of registering and algorithmically combining information in a computationally complex manner. By sustaining a conception of precognitive psychological processes along with nonsymbolic computation and rule instantiation, connectionist models remove any *a priori* theoretical motivation for characterizing the processes of early vision as cognitive and inferential. The dividing line between psychology and physiology then turns on the type of functional description. The functions of early vision, including the processes that yield perceptual representations of color, size, shape, and motion, fall on the side of psychology, as a systematic comparison of physiological and psychological concepts might reveal (Hatfield 1991*a*, sec. 4 [and Chs. 14–15 herein]).

8. The Subject Matter and Object of Explanation of Psychology

I have attempted to show how the *stands for* notion of representation fits nicely with a task-analysis approach to cognition in combination with a connectionist approach to psychological processes. The paradigmatic example in my discussions of representation and task analysis has been early vision, although the work of Shastri and Smolensky addresses higher cognitive functions within a connectionist framework. It might be argued that these examples do not establish that an account of representational content based on biological function as paired with a connectionist theory of computation is of general interest, because they do not demonstrate that the partners in this marriage (either jointly or singly) can handle the full-scale, intentionally characterized content of beliefs and desires: the kind of content that has been at the center of attention in the philosophy of psychology and the philosophy of mind. And surely (the argument might go), no theory of representation that cannot handle that content deserves a second look in the philosophy of psychology.

The force of this criticism crucially depends on what one takes psychology to be, and especially on conceptions of the object of explanation in psychology. By my lights, recent philosophical literature characterizes the object of explanation in psychology in a distorted manner. Most writers assume that the object of explanation in psychology is behavior, and that this object is to be explained by ascribing beliefs and desires to the behaving organism (Davidson 1973). The most popular program has been to understand beliefs and desires computationally (Fodor 1975, 1987; Pylyshyn 1984): behavior is explained by the computational relations among states that are at once syntactic (structured using symbols) and semantic (possessed of propositional content), and toward which an organism may stand in any of a variety of computational relations (which amount to attitudinal relations, including desires and other motivational attitudes). In attempting to construct scientific explanations of behavior by imputing beliefs and desires, problems arise pertaining to the standards for ascribing content to fellow organisms on the basis of outward appearances. The whole project seems in danger of devolving into a kind of hermeneutics of behavior (or worse), in which self-understanding leads the way to the allegedly "scientific" understanding of others (Stich 1983, ch. 7). In the hope of avoiding hermeneutics, some philosophers propose drastic measures: keeping the computational structure and bracketing the semantic content (Stich 1983, ch. 8), or eliminating the semantic content and substituting connectionist or some other neurally inspired computational structure for the symbolic version (Churchland 1986, ch. 10).

Despite these variations in explanans, the explanandum has been held constant: behavior. This emphasis was apparent in the symbofunctionalist program, which sought to explain outputs in relation to inputs by positing an intervening computational structure. It remains apparent in the syntactic and eliminativist approaches. Aetiology helps explain this fact. In the philosophy of psychology, symbofunctionalism arose as a response to behaviorism (Fodor 1968, ch. 2; 1975, Introduction). One way of understanding the explanandum of the symbofunctionalists is to see it as simply that of the behaviorist, now under a richer description: a description that distinguishes mere movements from intentionally described behavior. (This is a distinction that, according to their critics, behaviorists themselves relied on tacitly, despite Skinnerian or Hullian rejections of intentional or goal-oriented descriptions of behavior.) Thus, the symbofunctionalists and their kin simply negated the behaviorist proscription on appealing to mentalistic internal processes to explain behavior, and began freely positing computationally or propositionally characterized internal states to mediate between S and R (Cummins 1983, ch. 2; Dretske 1988; Fodor 1975, ch. 1; Haugeland 1978; 1985, ch. 3). Adherents of the syntactic and eliminativist approaches, having agreed with behaviorists such as Quine (1960, secs. 5, 45; 1974, ch. 1) that mentalism is hopeless, return to an austere descriptive vocabulary but continue to be liberal in positing internal states, now syntactically or neurally conceived (an updated Hullian behaviorism).

Although virtually all psychologists remain convinced that behavior is the primary source of *evidence* for evaluating psychological theories, the literature divides over the subject matter and explanatory goal of psychology. The simplest division is between those who define psychology as the "science of behavior" and those who define it as the "science of mind" (Gleitman 1986, 1). This traditional division does not mark the divide between behaviorism and cognitive psychology, for from the time of Tolman (1936) some of those who conceived of psychology as the science of behavior allowed for mentalistic intervening variables such as goals, hypotheses, and cognitive maps (see Schnaitter 1986). Moreover, among those who consider psychology to be the science of mind or of cognition there is disagreement about the object of explanation. Some authors, while regarding mental processes as the object of study, consider the explanatory goal to be that of discovering and explaining the mapping between input and output, or between S and R (Palmer and Kimchi 1986). For others, it is the psychological capacities themselves that form the subject matter and the object of explanation in psychology (Chomsky 1980, ch. 1; Massaro 1989, ch. 1), capacities such as language learning, spatial perception, mental imagery, verbal memory, and so on. The explanatory goal is to understand what the capacities are and how they are performed. Behavior becomes simply one (even if the most important) source of evidence for the existence and operation of the capacities in question.

The literature in philosophy of psychology rarely discusses the need to discover and characterize the psychological capacities. Symbofunctionalists typically assume some general description of the capacity to be explained—usually, "to behave rationally" or "sensibly"—and focus on explaining such behavior by imputing internal computational states (Fodor 1987, ch. 1; Pylyshyn 1984, ch. 2; 1989, 57). Even philosophers who tout "functional analysis" describe the goal of functional explanation as "intentionally interpretable" (viz. rational) behavior in general (Haugeland 1978). Explanation may proceed by analyzing the organism into functional subsystems, but the object of functional analysis has nonetheless remained intentionally interpretable behavior (but see Cummins 1983, ch. 3.5; Fodor 1983, pts. 2–3).

Marr (1982) again provides an exception to this approach. With his emphasis on task analysis, he renders primary the question of what tasks need to be explained. That is, Marr does not assume that the explananda in psychology are obvious: part of the investigator's job is to discover the right description of what a particular system in a given type of organism *does* (in the sense of "to do" that ascribes a function to the doing). Marr's 1982 book seeks to describe and understand vision itself as a complex information-processing ability. His project to discover the "computations" that vision performs translates, in the terminology I am using, as the project of understanding what vision is *for* and how the visual system performs its *functions*. "Understanding" involves constructing an explicit and detailed model of how the visual system, or some subsystem of it, performs a specific task. This involves both understanding the rationale for the task (Why would it make sense for an organism such as this to have a system performing this task?) and the means for carrying it out (What algorithms does the organism's visual system compute and with what neural structures?).[9] Behavior is one sort of evidence used in answering these questions; other evidence includes the investigator's own visual experience (or that of the reader of the investigator's work) and measurements of neurophysiological activity under various conditions of stimulation. But for Marr it is not behavior that is to be explained: behavior serves as the evidence for or against the hypotheses about the existence and structure of various cognitive capacities. It is those capacities that are to be explained (by positing and confirming hypotheses about algorithms and implementations).

Marr did not invent the information-processing approach, and he is not its only recent champion: it has been recognized as a general approach within psychology itself for some time. But the information-processing approach usually has remained neobehaviorist in conception. Neisser's (1967) influential textbook presented cognitive psychology as the study of the transformation of information as it made its way inward from the senses: the approach remained fundamentally S–R. Neisser and his followers acknowledged that in practice the investigator is reduced to using behavior as evidence for positing various internal mechanisms taken one at a time: mechanisms for pattern recognition, figural synthesis, visual memory, speech perception, and so on. But the goal remained that of putting these models together to form a comprehensive explanation of human behavior (Neisser 1967, 4–8; Palmer and Kimchi 1986, 38–9; Schnaitter 1986, 309).

Other adherents of the information-processing approach characterize the subject matter and the explanandum of psychology as the psychological processes themselves, rather than the behavior they mediate. Massaro (1989) in particular has articulated this conception. While Massaro speaks of psychological processes as mediating between stimulus and response, he rejects the idea that the goal of psychology is the explanation and prediction of the stimulus–response relation. He contends instead that psychology should investigate the "form of psychological behavior," by which he means the form of the psychological processes themselves (1989, 42). As he puts it, the goal of the information-processing approach "is to understand what the psychological processes do and how they do it" (20). In practice, this means restricting the goal of explanation to particular domains of human performance (such as speech recognition), or rather, to the psychological processes that give rise to

---

[9] Marr's "computational" level is much more than a simple mapping theory describing the relation between input and output, as Palmer and Kimchi (1986, 44, n. 3) have it.

such performance.[10] These processes are to be explained by being analyzed into simpler and simpler processes (18–19). Massaro does not specify a stopping place in this process of decomposition, but other authors speak of reaching a set of primitive operations that may remain unexplained (Palmer and Kimchi 1986, 49–50), just as gravitational force remained unexplained in Newtonian mechanics but nonetheless served to explain a variety of phenomena.

Assume that psychological capacities (e.g., perceptual, motor, and cognitive) are the subject matter of psychology. Does psychology, so conceived, stand a better chance of meeting the standards of natural science than does the belief–desire psychology that Quine and Stich reject? Indeed, does this conception of psychology's subject matter obviate the need for belief–desire ascriptions within psychology? Aren't such ascriptions still required to interpret the behavior that serves as evidence in testing hypotheses about psychological capacities?

It may seem that, in the end, the psychological-capacities approach doesn't avoid the problems of belief–desire psychology but merely camouflages them. The approach (as I am developing it) is, on the face of it, more modest than belief–desire psychology, because it doesn't pretend to explain naturally occurring behavior in all its complexity, taking instead a more circumscribed set of phenomena as its object. In this way, it is like classical mechanics, which did not attempt to explain the behavior of objects bouncing about in the world (e.g., the precise path of a falling leaf), but developed certain fundamental laws or principles that describe objects under laboratory conditions well, that apply to distant planets and stars, and that allow explanatory insight into uncontrolled objects (leaves do, after all, *fall*). But in psychology, it might be argued, restricting the object of explanation to psychological capacities does *not* avoid the complexities of belief-ascription, because the relevant evidence remains behavior, and if this behavior is to provide evidence about *psychological* capacities, it must be subsumed under a mentalistic description. Which, assuming this means a belief–desire description, returns us to square one. Accordingly, if behavioral evidence collected under experimental conditions is to count for or against a proposed analysis of a given psychological capacity, the experimenters must ascribe a host of beliefs and desires to each subject, including beliefs about what is expected of him or her during the experiment along with the desire to cooperate (to keep the list short).

---

[10] Massaro (1989) sometimes switches between describing psychology as the science of mental life (his official definition, p. 5) and as the science of behavior (p. 17, where he describes psychologists as "students of human behavior"). But the thrust of his book is to treat psychology as the science of the mental processes, focusing on the processes themselves as opposed to the observed stimulus–response couplings that provide evidence about those processes (see p. 13, mid; p. 15, top; p. 18, mid; p. 20, mid).

The premise of this objection is surely true: psychological experimentation typically does require investigators to rely on the background knowledge of their subjects and, often, on their desire to cooperate, and so it requires (often tacitly) interpreting the behavior of those subjects in light of a supposed body of such beliefs and desires. Does this mean that psychology requires a theory of beliefs and desires—or at least a set of clear criteria for attributing beliefs and desires—in order to interpret the behavior of subjects in an experimental situation? Does granting this premise entail that the psychological-capacities approach itself falls prey to the putative vagaries of belief–desire psychology? I don't see that it does, because I don't see that a psychological theory—or even a set of explicit criteria—is required in order to interpret behavior by imputing background beliefs.

Consider an experiment in perceptual psychology, in which the investigators wish to determine the extent to which the duration of processing time influences the perceived shapes of objects. The investigators choose as their stimuli a set of ellipses that they rotate about their vertical axes so that the ellipses all project circles onto the retina. Suppose that they construe their *subject matter* as the mechanisms underlying shape constancy (i.e., underlying the tendency to perceive a rotated ellipse as an ellipse, despite its retinal projection as a circle). Suppose further that they are trying to decide between two hypotheses: that shape and slant information are registered and processed together (in the form of a single representation of shape-at-a-slant); and that shape and slant are registered separately and combined at a later stage of processing. They anticipate that shortening or lengthening the allowed processing time will let them distinguish between these two hypotheses as follows. If shape and slant are processed together, then as they allow processing time to increase, perceived shape will move regularly from projected shape (a circle) to actual shape, and perceived slant will go from no slant to actual slant. However, if shape and slant are processed separately and *then* combined, perceived shape and slant will vary independently for a certain interval of processing time (the interval prior to combination), after which perfect constancy will result. Subjects observe the ellipses one at a time for varying durations; after each trial they indicate the shape they perceived by selecting the one most similar to it on a page of drawings. Now imagine that the results show that perceived shape and perceived slant vary independently of one another during the first 300 milliseconds of processing time, after which subjects achieve perfect constancy.[11]

---

[11] This paragraph contains a counterfactual description of experiments reported by Epstein *et al.* (1977) and Epstein and Hatfield (1978). In those experiments, processing time was controlled by

The investigators conducting such an experiment must assume that their subjects understand the experimental task and undertake it in good faith. They must attribute many background beliefs to their subjects in accordance with the first assumption, beliefs containing such concepts as *shape, slant, similarity*, and *the "look" of a thing*. If, in reporting their experimental findings, the investigators were required to demonstrate that the subjects possessed the requisite concepts and beliefs, they would face a formidable obstacle: they would need to produce a convincing account of the relation between observed behavior and possession of the relevant concepts and beliefs. But why make such stringent demands? The evidence that the subjects understood the task is that they were able to perform it; the evidence that they were serious and attentive comes from the high degree of uniformity that their behavior exhibited, both across trials for a given subject and among subjects (let us say). Of course, their attention may have wandered on occasion, and they might have adopted various cognitive strategies for guessing at the shape, leading them to report a different shape than the one the object appeared to have. Although these factors would influence the data, such worries are not new within experimental psychology. A factor such as wandering attention might occur randomly in this type of experiment and would wash out under statistical analysis. And if investigators suspect that subjects are adopting strategies for guessing, they might introduce special instructions to control the subjects' attitudes (Carlson 1977); or they might analyze the subjects' observed performances using signal-detection theory to control for response-biases that might arise from subjects' choosing different response criteria (Swets *et al.* 1961). In general, the best evidence for the plausibility of the tacit assumptions that investigators use to interpret subjects' behavior is the finding that the dependent variable (the reports of perceived shape in the example above) is under the control of the independent variables (actual shape and viewing time) in the experiment.[12] Ideally, the only other sources of variation in the dependent variable are random. The cleaner the data in a given experiment, the more likely that these assumptions were plausible.

When reading Quinean discussions of the unscientific character of psychology, one is struck by the idealized manner in which the physical sciences are described (making psychology look poor in comparison). The objectivity

backward masking, and the stimuli were more complex (for reasons of experimental design) than those I describe here. The envisioned results are also counterfactual; the actual results supported the shape–slant invariance hypothesis but did not discriminate between the hypotheses I discuss above. The point of my thought experiment is to illustrate results that would discriminate.

[12] The decision-theoretic idealizations underlying signal-detection theory were justified in this manner (Swets *et al.* 1961, 311); in many perception experiments, the results are sufficiently reliable that signal detection need not be applied (as these authors recognized, p. 337).

of physics is assured because the evidence for its posits are observation statements subject to the high standard of community-wide assent and because the
indeterminacy of posit relative to evidence is settled through the application of
scientific method (which Quine characterizes using behaviorist learning theory, 1960, secs. 5–6; 1974, secs. 1, 9–11). In contrast, psychology's (alleged)
practice of using beliefs to explain behavior seems murky and messy (1960, 221;
1974, 36). But can we understand the pursuit of physics without our attributing
to investigators some background beliefs that they bring to experimental situations? Could physics be pursued unless physicists ascribed background beliefs
and desires to one another? I think not. The interpretation of an experiment
in physics may depend on a wide range of background beliefs and knowledge,
from very general beliefs such as that no finding can violate the conservation
of energy, to specific knowledge about the principles underlying the use of a
particular instrument or technique (as in the use of x-ray crystallography to map
microstructures). Moreover, physics is a highly social practice. It depends on
communicating results among investigators within a group and between groups
in widely different locations, and on interpreting reports of results that others
similarly circulate. This entire interchange implicitly relies on investigators'
attributing background beliefs to one another.

Quineans might rejoin that background beliefs about instrumentation are
not imputed to other human beings, but are used by each physicist to
interpret the experimental situation directly. In the case of beliefs ascribed to
other investigators, the Quinean might assert that the language and practice
of physics are sufficiently precise to render the vagaries of interpretation of
no practical consequence.[13] By contrast, belief-ascriptions condition the very
object of investigation in psychology.

And so we reach the heart of the matter. If the subject matter of psychology
is not beliefs and desires but psychological capacities, then psychologists
should be permitted to engage in the same ordinary interpretive practices in
understanding the performance of their subjects as physicists are permitted in
understanding one another.

Suppose that a physicist and a psychologist are both realists about theoretical
entities and let us compare their respective experimental situations. The
physicist uses her background knowledge to interpret the bearing of a complex
set of data on the existence and character of a microstate. She uses her
background knowledge to narrow the class of events that she measures in

---

[13] Quineans, of course, issue a promissory note to cash out talk of "background beliefs" in terms of
behaviorist learning theory, which they believe will ultimately be reduced to physiological mechanisms.
Physicists' understanding of one another, they assure us, will ultimately be dealt with in the same terms.
In each case, we should wish them luck.

the experimental situation, and she relies on common background beliefs in interpreting the reported observations of other investigators who perform similar experiments. The psychologist uses his background knowledge to understand the relation between the behavior that he observes and the perceptual or cognitive structures that he hypothesizes. In particular, he uses his background knowledge to narrow the conditions in which the behavior of his subjects occurs so that the behavioral outcomes bear on specific questions about the character of (say) perceptual processing. The psychologist must ascribe background beliefs to his subjects, but the language and practice of experimental studies of perception are typically sufficiently precise to render the vagaries of interpretation of no practical consequence. The beliefs that psychologists ascribe to their subjects do not constitute the objects of their investigations (except perhaps in social psychology). Instead, psychologists tacitly assume such beliefs when they interpret their subjects' behavior as indicating their perceptual states. If asked how she knows that subjects are responding on the basis of their perceptual experience rather than simply guessing or engaging in some other task, the psychologist can point to the unbroken regularity with which subjects perform under experimental conditions and the coherence of the responses under theoretical interpretation.

Even if this response to the "camouflage" objection has succeeded, someone might object that the example used in vindicating realism about psychological capacities—the psychology of shape perception—cannot be extended to many properly cognitive domains. It is a genuine question how far the techniques of experimental psychology can go in investigating phenomena that are cognitive in the traditional mentalistic sense of the term. This would, in fact, seem to be an empirical matter. Beyond perceptual psychology, a great many results already bear on the mechanisms underlying visual imagery, memory encoding, word recognition, and so on. The study of visual imagery uses some techniques similar to perceptual studies, but there the object of study is not under the immediate control of an external stimulus. Nonetheless, Kosslyn (1980) has collected remarkably clean data concerning our imagistic capacities, and further studies of imagery impairment in brain-damaged patients have tested for hypothesized functional structures in the imagery system—for example, the relative autonomy of capacities for generating, copying, and describing images (Farah 1984). Caramazza and his coworkers study brain-damaged patients to learn about linguistic abilities, such as the capacity to spell words upon hearing them spoken or to recognize words that are spelled (Caramazza et al. 1987). Other investigators measure reaction time and error rates in order to decompose memory or recognitional abilities into relevant subfunctions (Massaro 1989, chs. 7–9, 16–17). If an investigator improperly claims to have produced a general model of "reading" when what is meant is only grapheme-to-phoneme translation (a type of claim that Caramazza *et al.* avoid), our disappointment in this exaggerated claim should not prevent us from appreciating the genuine contribution that a model of grapheme-to-phoneme translation makes toward understanding the psychological capacities that underlie reading. In any event, the only way to decide whether a science of psychological capacities can fruitfully be pursued is to examine, one by one, the proposed models of such capacities and their relations to the supporting data.

9. Coda on Function-Based Accounts of Content

Fodor (unpublished) has objected to using ascriptions of function as a basis for assigning representational content by arguing that function-ascriptions are too weak to support assignments of full-blown propositional content. In particular, he urges, contrary to Dretske and others, that function-based accounts of content cannot solve the "disjunction problem," which relates to the possibility of error. As Dretske (1988, 64–70) acknowledges, in order to capture intentionality, ascriptions of representational content must go beyond a mere causal or indicator relation between representation and represented, because those relations make a representation be "about" whatever *in fact* causes it. Human beings can get things wrong: we can represent a fly as being present when there is really only a moving black dot that causes our fly-representation to engage. We can produce the content *fly* even though only a moving black dot is present. Taking aim at function-based accounts that appeal to evolution in grounding representational content, Fodor claims that, even for the frog's storied bug detector, evolution could never provide a basis for attributing one content or the other, because selection doesn't care under what description frogs eat flies (*moving black dot* or *fly*), as long as they eat enough of them. He believes that an evolution-based functional description of the frog's perceptual mechanisms cannot discriminate between their representing flies or black dots, from which he concludes that functional descriptions cannot support fine-grained ascriptions of content.

As far as I now know, biologically based functional description may or may not be able to provide a basis for analyzing intentionality of such fine grain: the matter is under dispute. But such descriptions can capture weaker ascriptions of content: they can serve as the basis for ascribing to states of the frog's visual system the content *target fly/ moving dot*, or some such coarse-grained content. Furthermore, such content can provide the basis for an account of error, inasmuch as the system is in error when its function is to represent targets but it fires when no target is present. A Fodorean might counter that the frog's eye is really a fly-or-moving-black-dot-or-nothing detector, and that selection cares only that the detector put the tongue in action so as to catch flies sufficiently often. This counter in effect dismisses function-ascriptions that distinguish between the normal function of a system and misfunction, thereby diluting the notion of the function of a system into being whatever the system happens in fact to do.

My tendency is to believe that function-ascription, with its minimal degree of intensionality, is too deeply entrenched in the practice of biology and psychology to be dismissed so easily. Among the functions of the frog's visual system is to represent small moving things as being there when they are, and not to represent them as being there when they aren't. Until a strong case is made that such ascriptions are fundamentally wrongheaded, they remain legitimate objects of philosophical analysis. Fodor's intuitions about "what selection can do" are rendered problematic by the very fact that they call such ascriptions of function into question. Functional analysis may or may not be able to handle full-scale intentionality; but it seems a promising route toward understanding more modest representational achievements. [See also Ch. 1.5.]

By using functional analysis to ascribe content, we allow a task analysis to guide our way in imputing representations. Whether we must construe such representations as symbolic depends on the task being analyzed: linguistic abilities require symbolic representations in their level-one descriptions, but spatial perception does not. Connectionist models allow theorists to explain some representational tasks without appealing to an internal symbol system; they also afford the possibility of explaining syntactic abilities that symbolic models merely assume. Connectionist models form a nice package with the task-analysis approach. Together, they offer a framework for pursuing theories of the psychological capacities that is far more plausible than that offered by orthodox symbolism.

4

Perception as Unconscious Inference

Consider for a moment the spatial and chromatic dimensions of your visual experience. Suppose that as you gaze about the room you see a table, some books, and papers. Ignore for now the fact that you immediately recognize these objects to be a table with books and papers on it. Concentrate on how the table looks to you: its top spreads out in front of you, stopping at edges beyond which lies unfilled space, leading to more or less distant chairs, shelves, or expanses of floor. The books and paper on the table top create shaped visual boundaries between areas of different color, within which there may be further variation of color or visual texture. Propelled by a slight breeze, a sheet of paper slides across the table, and you experience its smooth motion before it floats out of sight.

The aspects of visual perception to which I've drawn your attention are objects of study in contemporary perceptual psychology, which considers the perception of size, shape, distance, motion, and color. These phenomenal aspects of vision are sometimes contrasted with other, more typically cognitive aspects of perception, including our recognition that the objects in front of us include the table, books, and paper, our seeing that the table is old and well crafted, and our identifying the sheets of paper as the draft of an article in progress. All of these elements of our visual experience, whether characterized here as phenomenal or cognitive,[1] seem to arise effortlessly as we direct our

First published in Dieter Heyer and Rainer Mausfeld (eds.), *Perception and the Physical World: Psychological and Philosophical Issue in Perception* (New York: John Wiley, 2002), 115–43, copyright © 2002 by John Wiley & Sons. Reprinted with permission.

[1] In using "phenomenal" and "cognitive" as contrastive qualifiers of "perception" and related terms, I do not mean to imply that our recognition of the table as a table is not a part of our visual experience, or is not as phenomenally immediate as the experience of the shape or color of the table. I need contrastive terms that signal the seemingly noncognitive aspect of shape or color perception (here distinguished from shape or color recognition, classification, and identification), as opposed to

gaze here and there. Yet we know that the cognitive aspects must depend on previously attained knowledge. We are not born recognizing books and tables, but we learn to categorize these artifacts and to determine at a glance that a table is an old one of good quality. What about the phenomenal aspects?

A persistent theme in the history of visual theory has been that the phenomenal aspects of visual perception are produced by inferences or judgments, which are unnoticed or unconscious. The persistence of this theme is interesting because, unlike our capacity to recognize a book or to identify something as the draft we have been working on, simply having a phenomenal experience of surfaces arranged in space and varying in color does not obviously require prior knowledge (even though describing such experience does). Nor does such experience seem on the face of it to be the product of reasoning or inference, such as we might employ in reasoning from the fact that our friend's books lie open on the table to the conclusion that she is about. Nonetheless, from ancient times theorists have accounted for visual perception of the size, shape, distance, motion, and (sometimes) color of objects in terms of judgment and inference.

Hermann Helmholtz (1867/1910) provided the paradigm modern statement of the theory that visual perception is mediated by unconscious inferences. His name is frequently invoked by recent advocates of the theory (Barlow 1990a; Gregory 1997, 5; Hochberg 1981; Rock 1983, 16; Wandell 1995, 7, 336). Helmholtz maintained that perception draws on the same cognitive mechanisms as do ordinary reasoning and scientific inference (1910, 3: 28–9), and some theorists make similar comparisons (Barlow 1974; Gregory 1997, 9–13). Others in the twentieth century have argued that perception is not literally inferential but is "like inference" or "ratiomorphic" (Brunswik 1956, 141–6), while still others postulate special-purpose inferential mechanisms in perception, isolated from ordinary reasoning and knowledge (Gregory 1974, 205, 210; Nakayama et al. 1995, 2; Rock 1983, ch. 11).

decidedly cognitive achievements such as object recognition or identification. For a statement of the distinction between perceptual and cognitive aspects of vision, see Rock (1975, ch. 1, esp. p. 24). On the distinction from a computational and neurophysiological perspective, see Arbib and Hanson (1987, esp. pp. 4–5). For a philosophical statement of the contrast, see Dretske (1995a, esp. pp. 332–5). The present contrast concerns aspects of perceptual experience itself, and does not describe the processes that produce these aspects, which may themselves be cognitive or noncognitive. In this chapter I focus on cognitive theories of the processes that produce the phenomenal aspects of experience, though I will mention noncognitive theories as well. I am not concerned with epistemological aspects of the theories; on epistemological aspects of inferential theories, see R. Schwartz (1994, 104–10). Finally, other characterizations of the objects of study in contemporary visual perceptual psychology can be substituted for the traditional list given above (size, shape, etc.), including: the spatial and chromatic layout and changes within it, or the spatial and chromatic structure of surfaces and its changes.

In this chapter I examine past and recent theories of unconscious inference. Most theorists have ascribed inferences to perception literally, not analogically, and I focus on the literal approach. I examine three problems faced by such theories if their commitment to unconscious inferences is taken seriously. Two problems concern the cognitive resources that must be available to the visual system (or a more central system) to support the inferences in question. The third problem focuses on how the conclusions of inferences are supposed to explain the phenomenal aspects of visual experience, the looks of things. Finally, in comparing past and recent responses to these problems, I provide an assessment of the current prospects for inferential theories.

1.   Unconscious Inferences in Theories of Perception

The idea that unnoticed judgments underlie perception has been in the literature of visual science at least since the *Optics* of Ptolemy (*c*.160; see Ptolemy 1989/1996). In the past millennium, Alhazen (*c*.1030; 1989), Helmholtz (1867/1910), and Rock (1983) have offered explicit versions of the theory that perception results from unconscious inferences, in the form of (respectively) syllogisms, inductive inferences, and deductions in predicate logic. I will sometimes apply the term "unconscious inference" to all such theories, despite the fact that this technical term was introduced by Helmholtz (in a German equivalent), and despite variations in theorists' characterizations of such inferences, which are noted as needed. To give some sense of the range of theories, I begin by briefly examining two areas: size and distance perception, and color constancy.

1.1.   *Perception of size at a distance*

Prior to the development of new conceptions of optical information by Gibson (1966) and their extension by Marr (1982), theories of the perception of size relied on a common analysis of the stimulus for vision. One element of this analysis was contributed by Euclid (fourth century BC/1945), who equated apparent size with the visual angle subtended at the eye. Five centuries later, Ptolemy argued that the perception of an object's size depends on both visual angle and perception or knowledge of the object's distance (1989/1996, 2.56). Surviving versions of his work illustrate the problem as in Figure 4.1. The eye at E sees objects AB and GD under the same visual angle. If size were determined by visual angle alone, the two objects would appear to have the same size. But, Ptolemy says, when the difference in distance is detectable,

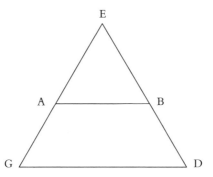

Figure 4.1. Perception of size at a distance as analyzed by Ptolemy (*c*.160).

such objects do not appear to be of the same size, but are seen with their real sizes (if our apprehension of the distance is accurate). Ptolemy was an extramission theorist who held that the crystalline humor (now known as the lens) is the sensitive element in the eye; he argued that the eye sends something out into the air, which allows the eye to feel the length of visual rays such as EA or EG (ibid., 2.26). Leaving aside the direct apprehension of distance, his position on the relation between visual angle and distance in size perception was accepted by subsequent authors, whether extramissionists or intromissionists, and whether they believed that the crystalline or the retina is the sensitive element. Indeed, the geometrical analysis of the perception of size-at-a-distance was unaffected by Kepler's discovery that the lens causes inverted images to be formed on the retinas (see Chapter 12).

Ptolemy only briefly alluded to the judgments he posited for combining visual angle and distance in size perception. Nearly a millennium later (*c*.1030), Alhazen (Ibn al-Haytham) offered an extended analysis of such judgments (Alhazen 1989). According to Alhazen, through "pure sensation" the sense of sight perceives only light and color (1989, 2.3.25). Alhazen was an intromission theorist, who held that the eye receives and transmits into the brain a cross-section of the visual pyramid, which constitutes a two-dimensional, point-for-point ordered record of the field of view (1.6.22–32). In receiving this cross-section, the sense of sight also registers the direction from which the light and color comes (2.3.97), and so has available the visual angle subtended by an object. The faculty of judgment then combines visual angle and distance information, through an "inference and judgment" that has become habitual, rapid, and unnoticed, to yield a perception of the size of an object that takes distance into account (2.3.145–8).

Although the Euclidean equation of apparent size with visual angle was sometimes rehearsed in subsequent literature (e.g., Chambers 1738, vol. 1,

"Apparent magnitude"; R. Smith 1738, 1:31–2), Alhazen's view that size perception depends on rapid, unnoticed judgments that combine perceived distance with visual angle became standard doctrine. The judgmental account of size perception was repeated in diverse works, including those of Descartes (1637/1984–5, pt. 6), Rohault (1735, 1:254), Porterfield (1759, 2:377–80), Le Cat (1767, 2:441–84, esp. 471–84), and Gehler (1787–96, 2:537–42). Berkeley (1709) rejected the judgmental account, arguing that the perceptual processes leading to size and distance perception are mediated by association, not by judgment or inference. Helmholtz combined aspects of the judgmental and associative accounts by proposing that size perception results from unconscious inference while giving an associative analysis of the process of inference itself (1867/1910, 3:24, 236–7, 242, 434, 439). More recently, neo-Helmholtzians have used the language of inference without association (Gregory 1997; Rock 1983), and so in fact are in the tradition of Ptolemy and Alhazen. Others have developed a subjectivist probabilistic analysis of perceptual inference (Bennett et al. 1989).

1.2. Color constancy

The tendency of observers to perceive objects as having a constant size at various distances despite variations in the visual angle they subtend at the eye was dubbed "size constancy" in the twentieth century. A similar constancy occurs in the case of color. We typically see objects as having the same color (e.g., as being the same shade of blue) under varying conditions of illumination (e.g., in sunlight and under artificial lighting). There is, within limits, constancy of perceived color under variations in the intensity and color of the ambient light.

Alhazen produced an early description of color constancy. He observed that light reflected by an object is modified by the color of the object. As he put it, the quality of the light and of the object are "mingled" in the light that reaches the eye. Through a cognitive act, the perceiver is able to separate light and color:

from perceiving the variations of lights falling upon visible objects, and from perceiving that objects are sometimes luminous and sometimes not, the faculty of judgment perceives that the colors in these objects are not the same as the lights that supervene upon them. Then, as this notion is repeated, it is established in the soul, as a universal, that colors in colored objects are not the same as their lights. (1989, 2.3.48)

Alhazen indicated that through experience the faculty of judgment learns the characteristics of various forms of illumination (1989, 2.3.50). He presumably held that it then is able to separate the color of the object from the quality of the illumination.

Unlike size and shape constancy, color constancy did not become standard fare in the early modern literature and was prominently discussed starting only in the nineteenth century.[2] Twentieth-century theorists have been fascinated by color constancy and achromatic brightness constancy, and some hold that the fundamental task of color perception is to extract information about the reflectance properties of objects from the light reaching the eyes. Specifically, many investigators formulate the task of the visual system in color constancy as that of recovering the spectral reflectance distribution of surfaces. A spectral reflectance distribution describes the percentage of ambient light of differing wavelengths reflected by a surface. It thus gives a precise physical description of the property of objects that gives them color: the disposition to absorb and reflect differing amounts of light as a function of wavelength. If we represent this distribution by R, let I stand for the spectral composition of the illuminant and L for that of the light reaching the eyes, then $L = I * R$. The problem for the visual system is to disambiguate I and R, which requires additional information or background assumptions.

Maloney and Wandell formulate the problem of color constancy as that of "estimating the surface reflectance functions of objects in a scene with incomplete knowledge of the spectral power distribution of the ambient light" (1986, 29). They show that approximate color constancy is possible if the visual system uses the fact that many natural surfaces can be modeled as linear combinations of a comparatively small number of surface coefficients (spectral reflectance functions), and if the range of ambient light is also describable as a linear combination of a small number of basis functions (spectral compositions). That is, they suggest that the visual system makes limiting assumptions about the composition of natural illuminants and the shapes of surface reflection functions, which allow it to make nearly accurate estimates of distal surface reflectance distributions on the basis of the incoming light. On this view, the goal of color constancy is to generate a physical description of the spectrophotometric properties of distal surfaces. In a recent theoretical survey of linear models and other computational approaches to color constancy, Hurlbert (1998) endorsed this conception of the aim of color constancy, arguing that since "spectral reflectance is an invariant property of surfaces," it is therefore "plausible, if not perfectly logical, to assume that color constancy results from the attempt to recover spectral reflectance in the more general pursuit of object recognition" (1998, 283).

---

[2] Phenomenal color constancy was mentioned by Thomas Young (1807, 1:456), using the example of white paper under varying intensities and colors of illumination. It was brought into prominence by Helmholtz (1867/1910, 2:110, 243–4) and Ewald Hering (1875a, 335–8; 1905–20, 13–17), who discussed the constancy of object colors in addition to white.

2. Problems for Unconscious Inference Theories

In order to count as a psychological or perceptual *theory*, a description of visual perception as involving unconscious inferences must do more than simply compare perceptual processes to the making of inferences. It must do such things as the following: describe the premises of such inferences, say how the premises come to be instantiated, account for the process of inference from premises to conclusions, describe the conclusions, and say how arrival at the conclusion constitutes or explains perception.

My own reflections on theories of unconscious perceptual inference indicate that they face (at least) three challenging problems. First, since they attribute unconscious inferences to the perceptual system, they must account for the cognitive resources needed to carry them out. Are the unconscious inferences posited to explain size perception and color constancy carried out by the same cognitive mechanisms that account for conscious and deliberate inferences, or does the visual system have its own inferential machinery? In either case, what is the structure of the posited mechanisms? This is the *cognitive machinery problem*. Second, how shall we describe the content of the premises and conclusions? For instance, in size perception it might be that the premises include values for visual angle and perceived distance, along with a representation of the algorithm relating the two. Or in color constancy, the conclusion might describe a spectral reflectance distribution. But shall we literally attribute concepts of visual angle and wavelength to the visual system? This is the *sophisticated content problem*. Third, to be fully explanatory, unconscious inference theories of perception must explain how the conclusion of an inference about size and distance leads to the experience of an object as having a certain size and being at a certain distance, or how a conclusion about a spectral reflectance distribution yields the experience of a specific hue. In other words, the theories need to explain how the conclusion to an inference, perhaps conceived linguistically, can be or can cause visual experience, with its imagistic quality.[3] This is the *phenomenal experience problem*.

2.1. Cognitive machinery

Inferential theories typically posit an early sensory representation that differs from ordinary perception in its portrayal of various properties of objects. This

---

[3] Dennett (1991, ch. 12) would contest this way of posing the third problem, since he denies the reality of imagistic phenomenal experience; but a theorist who subscribed to his views would still be faced with the problem of explaining how an inferential conclusion can *seem* to be the experience of a specific hue, or whatever.

original sensory representation, or sensation, might represent the shape of an object as a two-dimensional projection, so that a circle tilted away from the observer would be represented as an ellipse. Judgment or inference would then be called upon to mediate the change in representation from sensation to perception—in this case, to the perception of the true (circular) shape. The means for carrying out such inferences need to be specified, and the long history of inferential theories has seen various conceptions of the psychological processes thought to be involved.[4]

Although Ptolemy assigned a role to judgment in the apprehension of size, he provided little analysis of such judgments, simply referring them to a "governing faculty" or "discerning power" (1989/1996, 2.22–3, 76). Alhazen, by contrast, carefully analyzed the role of judgment in perception (1989, 2.3.1–42). He contended that any perceptual act beyond the passive apprehension of light and color requires judgment or inference. Such acts include recognition of color categories (as opposed to mere sensations of color), perception of similarity or dissimilarity between objects, and perception of distance. Further, the judgments or inferences in question typically require comparison with previous instances (in the case of acts of recognition), or depend on previous learning (as when the known size of an object is used together with visual angle to judge distance). But since on his view the senses themselves do not judge, compare, or learn from previous instances (1989, 2.3.17–25), the faculty of judgment must enter into perception.

Judgmental theories are faced with the fact that if perception relies on judgments, the judgments go unnoticed. In providing an explanation of this fact, Alhazen gave his fullest description of the judgments themselves. He began by contrasting the unnoticed judgments of perception with the visual theorist's careful and deliberate judgment that perception is judgmental (1989,

---

[4] My formulation of the cognitive machinery problem is distinct from *a priori* arguments that conclude, on conceptual grounds, that unconscious inference theories must be false, as when Ludwig (1996) argues that the very concept of an unconscious inference is incoherent. Among Ludwig's other arguments, only one overlaps with my three problems. He requires (1996, 38–9) that the concepts expressed in perceptual inferences be attributed to perceivers (my sophisticated content problem), and argues that the visual system could not have them (on conceptual grounds), and that children and animals do not have them (a commonsense empirical argument). None of my three problems are purely conceptual or *a priori*; the first two concern the empirical plausibility of needed explanatory apparatus, and the third concerns the explanatory adequacy of theories as developed thus far. The question of the attribution of subpersonal cognitive states has generated discussion (see Davies 1995). On this score I agree with Fodor (1975, 52–3). Although there are various moral, legal, and cultural reasons for wanting, in many contexts, to use the language of "inference" and "belief" to describe only acts of (whole) persons, for the purposes of psychological theory there are not adequate grounds *a priori* to preclude ascriptions of cognitive states to subsystems of persons, including the psychological mechanisms underlying vision. There may of course be theoretical or empirical grounds for such a preclusion.

2.3.26, 30, 36). The former judgments are rapid and habitual, the latter slow and reflective. In ordinary acts of perceiving, we do not usually undertake the slow and reflective act of determining that, say, the perception of size requires a judgment. We therefore remain unaware that a rapid and habitual judgment has occurred. Alhazen nonetheless argued that unnoticed perceptual judgments are carried out by the same "faculty of judgment" involved in all judgments, including conscious ones. He further contended that perceptual judgments are equivalent to syllogistic inferences (1989, 2.3.27–42). This identification of the process of perception with logical inference required further explanation, since perception is on the face of it not linguistic, whereas syllogisms apparently are.

Alhazen explained away this apparent dissimilarity between perception and inference by arguing that ordinary syllogistic inferences need not be properly linguistic, either. He contended that syllogistic inferences of the sort that can be expressed by a verbal syllogism need not be and typically are not actually produced in explicit linguistic form. He compared the rapid inferences of perception to cases in which we reach a conclusion rapidly, without consciously entertaining any logical steps. In one of his examples, upon hearing someone exclaim "How effective this sword is!" the listener immediately understands that the sword is sharp. She does so on the basis of the universal premise "Every effective sword is sharp." But the conclusion is achieved "without the need for words or for repeating and ordering the premisses, or the need for repeating and ordering the words" (1989, 2.3.28). As Alhazen explained, neither in perception nor in the sword example (where one premise is given verbally) does the faculty of judgment need to formulate an explicit syllogism using words in order for it to carry out an inference. Rather, from the moment it understands the content of the particular premise, given that it remembers the content of the universal, it immediately understands the conclusion (1989, 2.3.29). Alhazen would seem to suggest that in both sorts of case the faculty of judgment operates from a nonlinguistic grasp of the content of premises and conclusions. Accordingly, he could claim that the same judgmental capacity as underlies our rapid understanding of everyday events serves as the cognitive machinery for perception. This capacity carries out its operations by grasping content directly, and does not require linguistic form.

Five centuries later the philosopher and mathematician René Descartes, who wrote in an optical tradition continuous with Alhazen, appealed to unnoticed processes of reasoning in explaining size, shape, and distance perception.[5] In

---

[5] Descartes also gave a purely psychophysical account of distance perception, according to which the brain states that control accommodation and convergence directly cause a corresponding idea of distance (Descartes 1664/1972, 94; 1637/1984–5, 1:170; see Hatfield 1992b, 357).

his *Dioptrics*, Descartes explained that the size of objects is judged "by the knowledge or opinion we have of their distance, compared with the size of the images they imprint on the back of the eye—and not simply by the size of these images" (1984–5, 1:172). In the sixth set of Replies to Objections to the *Meditations*, he explained that these judgments, though rapid and habitual, are made "in exactly the same way as those we make now" (1641/1984–5, 2:295). Descartes held that sensation yields an image whose elements vary (at least) in size, shape, and color. As infants, we gain habits for judging the size, shape, distance, and color of distant objects on the basis of such images. Apprehension of shapes, size, and color in the images, as well as other relevant information (such as eye position), provide the content of the minor premises of our perceptual inferences. The major premises are rules such as the one relating size, visual angle, and distance. Through repetition the transition from visual angle and distance information to the experience of an object's size becomes habitual and so is no longer recognized as being judgmentally based. Nonetheless, Descartes affirmed that both the unnoticed judgments of perception and the reflective judgments of the mature thinker are carried out by the same cognitive mechanism, which he described as the faculty of intellect.

The fact that Descartes and Alhazen (and many others) proffered a faculty analysis of mind has been seen as an embarrassment. Such analyses were later ridiculed in the manner of Molière's famous jest in which a doctor says that opium makes people sleepy because it has a dormitive virtue (Molière 1673/1965, 143). Such jokes, and the easy dismissal of faculty psychology, fail to distinguish two potential aims of faculty theories, only one of which is sometimes laughable. Molière's joke plays on the idea that a physician has sought to *explain* how opium puts people to sleep by appealing to its dormitive virtue, rather than simply to *describe* its power to do so. Now it may well be that some of those ascribing "faculties" or "powers" to things understood this to be an inherently explanatory act, as it may be in some circumstances (see Hutchison 1991). But in other cases talk of powers is descriptive and taxonomic, and amounts to a nontrivial parsing of the real capacities of things. In the case of Alhazen's and Descartes' appeal to the intellectual faculty, Molière's joke would apply to them only if they tried to explain how the mind reasons by saying it has a faculty of reason. Instead, I see their efforts as part of an attempt to analyze the mind into a set of primitive capacities that are then used to explain particular abilities. So, in the case of size perception, a seemingly pure sensory ability is explained by appealing to an interaction between the capacity for rational inference and the passive reception of sensory information. The mind's capacity for rational inference is invoked to explain how sensations are transformed or supplanted to yield perceptions of shape. The judgmental capacity itself is not explained.

One might expect that since Descartes argued that the same intellectual faculty is involved in perception and other reasoning he would hold that perceptual judgments are subject to modification and correction in relation to consciously entertained knowledge. But he (in effect) admitted the opposite. In the familiar illusion of the straight stick that appears bent when half submerged in water, Descartes held that the appearance results from unnoticed judgments (habits of judging visual position) learned in childhood (1641/1984–5, 2:295–6). When an adult suffers the illusion, the intellect operates by habit, without forming a new judgment for the occasion. At the same time, the intellect is able, by reflecting on its tactual experience, to know that the stick is really straight. Descartes wrote with full appreciation of the fact that this judgment does not affect the appearance of the stick. In general, the unnoticed judgments he posited to explain perception were not open to conscious revision. Later, Immanuel Kant drew explicit attention to the fact that the moon illusion is impervious to knowledge, presumably because the judgments that underlie it are habitual and unnoticed and so not open to scrutiny or correction (Kant 1787/1998, 384, 386; see Hatfield 1990b, 105–6).

Berkeley introduced a new position into the psychology of visual perception when he sought to replace the accepted judgmental account of the processes underlying perception with an associational account. Motivated in part by a desire to support his immaterialist metaphysics (Atherton 1990, ch. 12), Berkeley rethought visual theory from the ground up, focusing on the psychology of vision. He began from a point that was shared by intromission theorists, that distance is not "immediately sensed" (as Ptolemy, an extramissionist, had held), but must be perceived via other cues or sources of information, whether contained in the optical pattern or received collaterally (as in feelings from the ocular musculature). In Berkeley's terms, since distance is not directly perceived, it must be perceived "by means of some other idea" (1709, §11). From there, he mounted a frontal assault on the widely shared theory that distance is perceived via "lines and angles," as when distance is allegedly perceived by reasoning using the angle-side-angle relation of a triangle and the perceived convergence of the eyes, or using the known size of the object together with perceived visual angle. Berkeley's argument unfolded in two steps. First, he maintained that "no idea which is not itself perceived can be the means for perceiving any other idea" (1709, §10). Second, he denied that we are ever aware of "lines and angles" in visual perception: "In vain shall all the mathematicians in the world tell me that I perceive certain lines and angles which introduce into my mind the various ideas of distance so long as I myself am conscious of no such thing" (1709, §12). He explained the perception of distance by means of several cues, including: (1) the interposition of numerous objects between the viewer and the target object (1709, §3; 1733, §62), (2) faintness of the target (1709, §3; 1733, §62), (3) visible magnitude in relation to known size (1733, §62), (4) height in visual field (objects further off are typically higher in the field of vision but below the horizon, 1733, §62), and (5) the muscular sensation accompanying the rotation of the eyes during convergence (1709, §16; 1733, §66).

Counterparts to each of these five cues were in the optical literature. Berkeley departed from previous accounts in contending that in none of the cases is there a "rational" or "necessary" connection between cue and perceived distance. The various factors listed in (1) to (5) serve, in his view, as so many arbitrary visual signs, whose meanings with respect to tactually perceived distance must be learned. For example, for angle-side-angle reasoning in distance perception he substituted an acquired association between ocular muscle feelings and tactually perceived distance (1709, §§12–20). Such associations, or connections of "suggestion," are formed between two ideas that regularly co-occur. They are not the result of a cognitive connection judged to exist between the perceived contents of the ideas, but arise solely from repeated co-occurrence. But, Berkeley argued, connections made through blind habit are distinct from (content-sensitive) inferences (1733, §42). His process of habitual connection or suggestion is equivalent to what became more widely known as the association of ideas.

Berkeley is the originator of the associationist account of distance perception. He also made famous the position that we "learn to see" objects in depth at a distance. In the 150 years after he wrote, various judgmental or associationist accounts of perception were proposed. Some authors took the analysis of perceptual experience into sensational ingredients even further than Berkeley, and attempted to show how spatial representations could be derived from aspatial or punctiform elementary sensations via association (Steinbuch 1811) or via a combination of reasoning and association (Brown 1824, lecs. 22–4, 28–9). Others adopted the radical analysis of spatial perception into aspatial elements, but posited innate laws of sensibility (distinct from judgment and inference) to govern the construction of spatial representations (Tourtual 1827). In each case, the authors supposed that each nerve fiber in the optic nerve produces a single sensation, varying only in quality and intensity. Meanwhile, the textbooks repeated the older account that size perception starts from an innately given two-dimensional representation and proceeds via unnoticed judgments (see Hatfield 1990b, ch. 4).

In the latter half of the nineteenth century, Helmholtz formulated the classical statement of the theory that spatial perception results from unconscious inferences. The primary statement of the theory occurred in section 26 of his *Handbuch der physiologischen Optik* (1867/1910). Helmholtz combined the associative and inferential accounts by giving an associational account of inference. He compared the inferences of perception to syllogisms in which the major premise has been established inductively. He adopted the radical punctiform analysis of visual sensation. In his account, stimulation of any given retinal nerve fiber initially yields a sensation that varies in only three ways: hue, intensity, and "local sign." A local sign is a qualitative marker peculiar to each nerve fiber (Helmholtz 1867/1910, 3:130, 435–6). These signs originally carry no spatial meaning, but through coordination with bodily motion and sensations of touch (which are assumed to have spatial meaning) the observer acquires the ability (unconsciously) to localize sensations on the basis of local signs. For example, the observer might acquire a universal premise that light hitting the right side of the retina comes from the left (3:24). Helmholtz described the process of learning the spatial meaning of local signs in terms of active testing, and compared it to hypothesis testing in science. But in both cases he conceived the psychological processes that yield inductive conclusions from testing as associative. In the case of learning the meaning of local signs via touch, Helmholtz maintained that "while in these cases no actual conscious inference is present, yet the essential and original office of an inference has been performed" (3:24).[6] The inference is achieved "simply, of course, by the unconscious processes of the association of ideas going on in the dark background of our memory" (ibid.). In this way, Helmholtz assimilated inference to association.[7]

The most explicit recent analysis of unconscious inferences in perception is due to Irvin Rock (1983). Rock identified four sorts of cognitive operations at work in perception: (1) unconscious description, in the case of form perception (1983, ch. 3); (2) problem solving and inference to the best explanation, in the case of stimulus ambiguity or stimulus features that would yield

---

[6] The translations are mine. The third German edition of 1910 reprinted the text of the first edition of 1867 and added a great deal of useful apparatus and commentary by the editors, and it was translated by J. P. C. Southall as Helmholtz 1924–5. Southall conveniently provided the corresponding page numbers for the third German edition at the top of each page, which makes it easy to coordinate my citations of the German with his translation. Southall's translation, while useful for many purposes, is misleading on numerous occasions, especially concerning Helmholtz's psychological theory.

[7] Helmholtz (1910, 3:23) cited John Stuart Mill in support of his associationist account of inductive inference, and in fact in his *Logic* of 1843 Mill endorsed an associational account; but in the 1851 edition he qualified this endorsement (Mill 1974, 664). For additional problems with Helmholtz's associative account of inference, see Hatfield (1990b, 204–8).

unexplained coincidences if interpreted literally (1983, chs. 4–7); (3) relational determination of percepts, such as those involved in perceiving lightness and relational motion through the interpretation of relational stimulus information in accordance with certain assumptions (1983, ch. 8); and (4) deductive inference from a universal major premise and an unconsciously given minor premise, used to explain the constancies (1983, ch. 9). All four operations posit unnoticed cognitive acts. The first operation is not inferential but merely descriptive; it illustrates Rock's view that the cognitive operations of perception are based upon internal descriptions in an (unknown) language of thought (1983, 99). Rock's formulations are cautious: he says perception is "like" problem solving and deductive inference (1983, 1, 100, 239, 272, 341). But his account is not merely ratiomorphic. In the end, he held that perception does involve unconscious reasoning, including both inductive formation of rules (1983, 310–11) and deductive inference from rules. The cognitive machinery for such inferences operates in a linguistic medium and follows the rules of predicate logic (1983, 99, 272–3). The rules governing perceptual inference may be either learned or innate—Rock (1983, 312–16) rejected Helmholtz's emphasis on learning.

Rock's cautious formulations reflect the fact that he recognized a sharp divide between the processes of perception and the processes that underlie conscious describing, problem solving, rule-based calculations, and deductive inference. Some separation of this kind is demanded by the fact known to Descartes, Kant, and others: that the perceptual process often is impervious to knowledge, as when visual illusions persist despite being detected. It is a seeming paradox for cognitive accounts of perceptual processing that perception is isolated from and inflexible in the face of other cognitive factors, such as the conscious knowledge that the lines are the same length in the Mueller-Lyer illusion (Rock 1983, 336–7). Rock responded by proposing a strict separation between ordinary cognition and the cognitive processes underlying perception. He separated the knowledge relevant to perception into two divisions: immediate stimulus-based information, and unconscious descriptions, concepts, and rules (1983, 302). The unconscious processes typically take into account only such information about a particular stimulus as is available in current stimulation; he called this the condition of "stimulus support" (1983, 303). Achromatic color illusions, such as the Gelb effect—in which a black circle appears white if it alone is illuminated by a spotlight in an otherwise dark room—disappear when a white contrast paper is moved into the light, but reappear as soon as the stimulus support provided by the white paper is removed. Apparently the perceptual system is caught up in the moment! Rock further postulated that the concepts and rules used in the unconscious cognitive operations of perception are isolated from central cognitive processes of description, categorization, and hypothesis formation (1983, 306, 310, 313, 315). He in effect posited a special-purpose domain of concepts, rules, and reasoning to support the processes of perception.

Rock supported his comparisons of perception to problem solving and inference with an extensive program of empirical research. Others, pursuing general theories of mind in the fields of artificial intelligence and cognitive science, have used perception as an example of a mental process that fits their general model. Such theoreticians have of necessity been explicit about the cognitive machinery. They have sought to provide an explanation of the cognitive capacities that were used as explanatory primitives by earlier theorists.

Fodor (1975) was an early and articulate advocate of the theory that the mind is importantly similar to a general purpose digital computer and that its cognitive operations are carried out in an internal language of thought. He compared the language of thought to the machine language in a computer (1975, 65–8). Just as a computer is "built to use" its machine language, and so need not acquire it, the brain comes with its own built-in language. This language then serves as the medium in which perceptual hypotheses are framed and tested. Although I agree with Crane (1992b, 148) that it remains an open question whether one absolutely must posit an internal language in order to account for the inferential abilities of humans and other cognitive agents, Fodor's posit of a language of thought does provide a powerful model for unconscious inferences. In this model, the inferential machinery of perception is a full-scale language, with syntactically based inference rules for drawing conclusions from premises.

Fodor (1983) took into account the same fact that we have found in Rock (1983), that perceptual inferences are relatively insulated from the consciously available knowledge of the perceiver. Largely in response to this fact, Fodor adopted the position that perceptual processes take place in cognitively insulated modules. Although Fodor (1983) did not describe precise structures for his innate machine language, he gave no reason to suppose that the language of thought of the various perceptual modules is the same as that of other cognitive modules. Theory would dictate that the output of such modules must be usable by subsequent processes. But there is no necessity for the postulated linguistic medium that underlies the processes of shape perception to have precise analogues of the shape vocabulary of the central cognitive processes of shape identification. The modularity thesis and its counterpart in Rock (1983) undermine the assumption that perceptual inferences are one with ordinary thought.

Acceptance of the modularity thesis forsakes the (perhaps implausible) parsimony of traditional inferential accounts. From Alhazen (*c*.1030/1989) to Helmholtz (1867/1910), theorists had posited a unity between the mechanisms underlying perception and those underlying thought more generally. The notion of cognitively isolated (Rock 1983) or insulated (Fodor 1983) modules replaces this simple unity with distinct cognitive mechanisms and processes for the postulated inferences of perception and the inferences of conscious thought. This separation of processes places a new burden on contemporary inferential theories, for now they must account for the cognitive resources employed in perception independently of the general cognitive resources of perceivers.

2.2. *Sophisticated content*

Theorists who posit that perception occurs via inferences from sensory premises to perceptual conclusion take on a commitment to the psychological reality of the premises and conclusions. This in turn requires a commitment that the visual system, governing agency, faculty of judgment, or the intellect has the resources to think the premises and conclusions. If perceptual processes are indeed unnoticed judgments, then the cognitive faculty that carries them out must be able to comprehend the content of such judgments. In more modern terms, if unconscious processes are posited that involve descriptions, then the perceptual system or its auxiliary must have the conceptual resources to express the content found in the descriptions.[8]

Early theorists recognized the need for supplying conceptual resources to the visual system by bringing the faculty of judgment or the intellect into perception. Thus, when Alhazen argued that one and the same intellectual faculty operates in everyday cognition and in the unnoticed judgments of perception, he presumably assumed that the faculty has the same conceptual resources available in both cases. Alhazen held that over the course of a lifetime,

---

[8] As is explained at the end of this section, I am assuming that genuine inferences are couched in representations that express their content in such a way that it is available to the subsystem performing the inference. Systems that merely transform and transmit information without sensitivity to its content, such as a computer keyboard system (which transforms physical pressure into internal symbols, and may do so conditionally, as with the "shift" key), do not count as performing inferences. By contrast, in a conceptual encoding, having a concept requires its being connected to other concepts (Crane 1992*b*, 142–9; E. E. Smith 1995). Philosophers have of course been interested in the question of how there could be systems in which conceptual content is expressed (e.g., Dretske 1988). Further, it has been thought that inferential operations might take place solely in virtue of the syntax of internal inscriptions; but even in such cases, the syntactic entities will have to be related to other syntactic entities in sufficiently complex ways for us to treat some of them as predicates corresponding to concepts (Fodor 1975, ch. 2).

we learn to recognize instantaneously all of the visible properties of things, without being aware of the acts of recognition or judgment involved (2.3.42). He thus believed that the perceiver's full range of concepts is available for perception.

Descartes also maintained that sensory perception relies on habitual judgments of the intellect. Because he attributed innate ideas to the perceiver, one would expect him also to believe that the intellect has all its concepts available for perceptual inference. Nonetheless, he recognized a *de facto* limitation on the conceptual vocabulary expressed in unnoticed perceptual judgments. He suggested that we are unable to revise our habitual judgment, formed in childhood, that objects contain something "wholly resembling" the color we experience (1644/1984–5, 1.70–2). Because the childhood judgments have become frozen as unnoticed habits, we are unable to use the concepts of the true physics, discovered through mature intellectual reflection, to revise our early judgments about resemblance. As befits the infantile formation of unnoticed perceptual judgments, their conceptual content is restricted by comparison with the sophisticated concepts of the metaphysician and natural philosopher.

By contrast, Berkeley's associationist account avoided any need for the unnoticed processes of perception to use sophisticated conceptual content, because the processes he described make no use of conceptualized content of any sort. In his account of size perception, visual ideas corresponding to visual angle give rise to perceptions of size as a result of acquired associations among visible magnitudes (visual angle), visual cues for distance, and tactual perceptions of distance. The elements to be associated are related to one another as arbitrary signs. In his view, there is no intelligible connection between cues such as ocular muscle feelings and tactual distance. The mind does not perceive distance because it understands that certain muscle feelings result from accommodations of the lens that vary with distance; rather, the perceiver is simply trained by experience to associate specific muscle feelings with specific tactual distances.

Berkeley contrasted his account with Descartes', in which a perceiver might make use of intelligible relations among ideas, as in angle-side-angle reasoning about distance.[9] He challenged the proposal that perceivers make use of geometrical lines and angles in everyday perception by asserting that most people do not possess the requisite notions. He denied that lines and

[9] Although Descartes provided a purely psychophysical (and so noncognitive) account of distance perception via convergence, in some cases he attributed unnoticed geometrical reasoning to the perceiver, as in the perception of distance from known size and visual angle (see Hatfield 1992b, 357).

angles are "ever thought of by those unskillful in optics" (1709, §12). Ordinary perceivers therefore cannot bring the technical concepts of optics to bear in unconscious or unnoticed descriptions of the objects of vision. He further argued that since perceivers (whether geometrically sophisticated or not) are not conscious of reasoning from lines and angles, they do not reason from them. On the face of it this argument seems weak, for Berkeley himself posited unnoticed processes of suggestion (or association). But he might argue that it is plausible for at least some noncognitive habits to remain unnoticed throughout both their formation and operation, while sophisticated geometrical inferences could not. Some noncognitive motor habits are surely formed without our even knowing we have them (e.g., habits of gait). By contrast, we are all familiar with the ways in which we at first have to pay attention to new cognitive tasks, before they become habitual. But the adherents of unconscious inference posit inferential acts of which we seem never to have been aware. Hence Berkeley might be proposing that the sort of sophisticated mathematical reasoning ascribed by the "natural geometry" argument is not the sort of thing that could become habitual if it had not first been part of a conscious reasoning process. By contrast, his unnoticed processes are habits formed through blind acts of association, which serve to connect ideas to one another simply as a result of their temporal co-occurrence.

Early nineteenth-century theorists, such as Steinbuch (1811) and Tourtual (1827), developed extensive analyses of visual perception that described its initial content as phenomenal and unconceptualized. They described the sensational elements of visual perception as unspatialized punctiform sensations varying in hue and intensity, and then gave a detailed account of how psychological operations create spatial representations from this nonspatial sensory core (see Hatfield 1990b, ch. 4). Both theorists posited noncognitive operations, distinct from judgment and intellect, that order sensations by quality and intensity. Steinbuch posited learned associations among muscle sensations, built up slowly, starting *in utero*, to create a mapping from retinal fibers to two-dimensional representation (allegedly) on the basis solely of phenomenal similarity and temporal contiguity.[10] Tourtual posited innate laws of sensibility, also operating on the qualitative character of elemental sensations. In each case, there was no question of sophisticated conceptual content doing the ordering, since the operations were conceived as preconceptual.

---

[10] Although Alhazen (1989, 2.13.22) treated similarity as something to be detected intellectually, the associationist tradition in the nineteenth century posited laws as operating blindly over one-dimensional similarities (as among sensations within a single modality, or along a single dimension within a modality, such as hue).

We have seen that Helmholtz also posited aspatial elemental sensations, but that he characterized the transformative processes as at once associational and inferential. His contention that unconscious inferences could be explained psychologically as resulting from associational processes meant that his analysis of the psychology of perception could focus on the phenomenal character of sensations, since association operates on phenomenally characterized sensations. His description of the resultant perceptual images as the conclusions of inferences introduced a certain tension into his account, because of the apparent difference between perceptual images and the linguistic conclusions of logical inferences. But Helmholtz held that there is "only a superficial difference between the inferences of logicians and those inductive inferences whose results we recognize in the intuitions of the outer world we attain through our sensations." (By "intuition" he means a perceptual image.) He continued: "The chief difference is that the former are capable of expression in words, while the latter are not, because instead of words they deal only with sensations and memory images of sensations" (1896, 1:358; 1995, 198). So the content of perceptual premises and conclusions are sensations and images.[11] What about the major premises, the universal rules for localizing sensations in space? These are associations among sensations, forged through relations of contiguity and resemblance. They operate over the phenomenal properties of sensations, including, for vision, punctiform sensations varying in hue, intensity, and local sign, and feelings of innervation of the ocular (and bodily) musculature. Helmholtz's associationist account of unconscious inference allowed him to restrict the content and operation of perceptual inferences to the phenomenal properties of sensations and phenomenal relations among sensations, operated upon by conceptually blind laws of association. There is no need to attribute sophisticated content to Helmholtzian perceptual inferences.

In the twentieth century, appeal to laws of association operating over aspatial sensations characterized by phenomenal qualities has fallen out of

[11] Helmholtz believed that an image can contain the content of a judgment: "it is clearly possible, using the sensible images of memory instead of words, to produce the same kind of combination which, when expressed in words, would be called a proposition or judgment" (1896, 1:358; 1995, 199). Indeed, Helmholtz considered concepts of objects to be resolvable into a series of images of the objects, comprising both perspectival and cross-sectional images (1882–95, 3:545; 1894/1971, 507). As Fodor (1975, 174–84) has observed, any theory that attempts to equate propositions with images faces problems of ambiguity. For example, does a picture of a man walking on a slope and facing upwards express the content that he is walking up, or walking down backwards? If propositional content is to be expressed, one cannot avoid introducing an active mental element of grasping or connecting the "relevant" aspects of an image with other images. The continuation of the passage quoted in this note suggests that Helmholtz was sensitive to this point and believed that associative connections would suffice.

favor.[12] The most developed of today's inferential accounts posit underlying language-like representations to mediate the inferential connections. As we have seen, theorists such as Rock (1983) and Fodor (1983) posit special cognitive subsystems for perception. This allows them to restrict the range of concepts attributed to the subsystem. Rock's isolated cognitive domain requires only a comparatively modest conceptual vocabulary for describing sensory aspects of objects, such as form and other spatial characteristics. His problem-solving and inference-formation operations work on these perceptual features. A typical Rockian inference might combine information about the egocentric tilt of a line with information about head-tilt to yield a perception of real-world orientation, or combine visual angle and distance information to yield a perception of size (Rock 1983, 273–4). The descriptive vocabulary here is impoverished relative to general cognition, focusing as it does on spatial properties in egocentric and environmental frames of reference (1983, 331–2). Fodor's (1983, 86–97) point about the conceptually "shallow" outputs of perceptual modules provides a more general framework for attributing special-purpose, modest conceptual vocabularies to the visual system.

Other computational accounts of vision strain the bounds of plausibility in ascribing perceptual inferences with sophisticated content. Difficulties arise especially for certain computational models of color constancy. We have seen that Maloney and Wandell describe the task of the visual system in color constancy as that of "estimating the surface reflectance functions of objects in a scene with incomplete knowledge of the spectral power distribution of the ambient light" (1986, 29). If one takes these authors at their word, they attribute a rich conceptual vocabulary to the visual system, including sophisticated physical concepts such as surface reflective function (spectral reflectance distribution). It seems implausible to attribute such content to encapsulated processes of early vision. The human species came upon these physical concepts only late in its development, after the time of Newton. But human ancestors developed trichromatic color vision hundreds of thousands of years earlier (Goldsmith 1990). So the mechanisms and processes that yield our trichromatic color vision, whether viewed as occurring in a language of thought or via nonlinguistic processing mechanisms, could not have had

---

[12] Connectionism is often regarded as carrying on the associationist tradition (Quinlan 1991, 2–3). Further, some connectionist models provide a noncognitive basis for detecting similarities among patterns (Quinlan 1991, 49–56). The patterns are matched via the activation of patterns of input nodes, not by unreduced phenomenal qualities of hue and intensity. Still, in cases in which the input nodes are feature detectors, these accounts bear an analogy to a dephenomenalized Helmholtzian account, with the important exception that they probably are not aptly characterized as inferential accounts (on which, more below).

access to sophisticated physical concepts. And if they are encapsulated, as seems certain, then these processes still would not have access to such concepts (even if the perceiver has "central system" knowledge of physics). Consequently, the output of the color system does not conceptually encode such notions.

There is an alternative way of construing the statements of Maloney and Wandell (1986), which would make sense of their saying that the visual system contains information about spectral reflectance distributions, but which would cut against inclusion of their color constancy model in the family of "unconscious inference" theories. The mathematical notion of information, developed by Shannon (1948) and others and brought into perceptual theory in the 1950s by Attneave (1954), provides a way of describing the information contained in a signal (or a perceptual state) without needing to attribute knowledge of or access to that information to the containing system. Dretske (1981) further developed this notion of information for use in describing perceptual content. On this way of viewing things, if perception of a particular hue is strictly correlated (under appropriate environmental background or "channel" conditions) with a particular reflectance distribution in the stimulus, then perception of that hue carries the information that the reflectance distribution is present (but see Ch. 8 [and Ch. 1, Note]). It can do so without the perceiver even knowing what a reflectance distribution is—for, as Dretske explains (1981, ch. 9), this notion of information is distinct from conceptual meaning. But if so, then any supposition that the visual system "estimates" the physical properties of the distal stimulus from its "knowledge" of retinal values is thereby undercut. Inference and estimation are cognitive acts. Our best philosophical and psychological accounts of such acts suggest that they occur through operations over premises that encode knowledge conceptually (Crane 1992b, 142–9; E. E. Smith 1995). But the color constancy models mentioned above make no provision for that sort of cognitive act. Hence, they would appear to be better classed as cases of the metaphorical application of an inferential model to perception. The computational aspects of color vision would then be understood as cases of informational combination and transformation via noncognitive mechanisms.

2.3. Phenomenal experience

The aim of much visual theory has been to explain the contents of phenomenal experience, the "way things look." This has been the case in central areas of perceptual theory, such as the perception of spatial and chromatic aspects of things. To meet this explanatory aim an unconscious inference theory of perception must provide some explanation of how inferences yield phenomenal experience. A complete explanation of the production of phenomenal experience would presuppose a solution to the mind–body problem. It would require explaining how perceptual processes in the brain produce phenomenal experience, which is a difficult problem. But less ambitious explanatory agendas are available. One might, for instance, posit psychophysical linking propositions (Teller and Pugh 1983), or psychoneural linking hypotheses (Hatfield and Pugh, unpublished), to bridge the gap between the brain states and experience, without thereby seeking to explain the ontology of such links. Similarly, one might treat the conclusions of inferences as a certain kind of data array (Marr 1982, ch. 4; Tye 1991, ch. 5), and use the representational content of the data array to explain imagistic experience.

Alhazen sought to explain the looks of things, as is apparent in his distinction between size as a function of visual angle and (phenomenally) perceived size. I think he would have had little problem explaining the looks of things via judgment, since on his view the judgments of perception are not linguistic and they operate directly on phenomenally given materials. He was, however, not explicit on how inferences operate on sensations to produce the ultimate looks of things. Two possibilities suggest themselves: inferences operate either to transform the representation of spatial properties in sensation into a representation of perceived spatial properties, or inferences operate to create a new representation exhibiting the perceived properties. Leaving aside metaphysical difficulties about the status of phenomenal experience itself—which are common to all theories and remain unresolved—no special problem of phenomenal experience arises for Alhazen.

As we have seen in the previous section, perceptual theory from Descartes to Helmholtz retained phenomenally defined theoretical primitives. Descartes followed Alhazen and the optical tradition in conceiving the premises of perceptual inferences as graspings of phenomenally given sensations, and the conclusions of such inferences as phenomenal experiences. The associationist tradition developed a finer analysis of the processes by which the spatial representations of perceptual experience are constructed from sensory elements. Aspatial sensory elements are conjoined associatively to yield phenomenal representations of a three-dimensional visual world. Although Helmholtz adopted an inferential account of perception, he offered a phenomenalist account of the conclusions of perceptual inferences. Since he considered the conclusions of such inferences to be images, he left no gap between conclusion and experience.

The notion that perceptual psychology attempts to explain the "looks of things" was fundamental to the work of the Gestalt psychologists (Köhler 1929, ch. 1; Koffka 1935, ch. 1 and pp. 73–6), who used a principle of spatial isomorphism to explain how brain states are related to experience. They argued that experience of voluminous shaped regions is produced by (or identical with) three-dimensional isomorphically shaped areas in the brain, so that the experience of a sphere is caused by a spherical region of brain activity. Although the Gestaltists' brain theory has been rejected, many investigators hold that phenomenal experience is a primary explanatory object for perceptual theory (Cutting 1986, p. 4, ch. 15; Gibson 1971, 4; Goldstein 1996, 15, 29; Natsoulas 1991), though some disagree (for instance Kaufman 1974, 16). Despite this explanatory goal, no detailed explanations of how the processes posited in perceptual theory yield the phenomenal aspects of sense perception are yet extant. The strategy of Helmholtz and his predecessors, of maintaining that perceptual experience is constructed from phenomenally characterized sensations, is no longer accepted. But no generally accepted model of how brain events are related to phenomenal experience has arisen to replace the one-fiber, one-sensation doctrine. Explaining phenomenal experience itself remains an unrealized goal of modern perceptual (and cognitive) theory.

Some proposals have been made. Wandell offered the intriguing suggestion that phenomenal color, or color appearance, "is a mental explanation of why an object causes relatively more absorptions in one cone type than another object" (1995, 289). Although providing a detailed theory of how information about surface reflectance might be recovered (1995, ch. 9), he does not offer anything further on the problem of how an estimation of a surface reflectance's relative effect on a cone type yields the experience of color.

Others have suggested that percepts are generated from early representations in the processing stream via cognitive, language-mediated processes. In his 1975 book, Fodor conjectured that perceptual processes are initially carried out as operations on sentence-like objects, with images subsequently being constructed from symbolic descriptions. He speculated that this construction might be likened to a "digital to analog" conversion (1975, 193, n. 26), but said nothing further about how this might occur.

Rock (1975, ch. 11) was acutely aware of the need for and difficulty of explaining perceptual experience. He considered percepts themselves to be "analogic, picturelike, and concrete" (1983, 52), by contrast with descriptions of percepts framed in the language of thought. He clearly stated (1983, 272) that the outcome of perceptual inference "is a percept rather than a conclusion" (by which he meant a linguistically expressed conclusion). But he did not say how such percepts are generated from the unconscious descriptions found in perceptual inferences.

Michael Tye (1995, ch. 5) has most fully elaborated a conception of how a language-like symbolist view of perceptual and imagistic representations might explain phenomenal experience. Drawing on Marr (1982, ch. 4), he proposed that imagistic representations be conceived as symbol-filled arrays. Such arrays are formed from a matrix of cells that represent distal surface locations in two dimensions. The individual cells (matrix units) are addressed by the relative positions they represent, corresponding to columns and rows. The physical locations of the cells in the brain is irrelevant on Tye's view; rather, the arrays are treated as having imagistic content in part because the processes operating over them treat the cells with numerically adjacent column and row addresses as if they were adjacent (1995, 94). Further imagistic content is provided by symbols within the cells, which represent the depth, color, intensity, and surface texture of a distal point (small area). Full image content arises only when the arrays are associated with a sentential interpretation, such as "this represents a pig." Our imagistic experience arises from the fact that we have symbolic representations of spatial, chromatic, and categorial aspects of things, which we access by symbol-reading processes that treat the areas represented in cells which have contiguous addresses as being distally contiguous. An image is constituted by thousands of words, containing labels for spatial location attached to descriptions of depth and color. The matrix arrays are not analog, but they do represent spatial relations of small areas that may be treated as forming a continuous surface.

Tye's view has the advantage that it can draw on ongoing work seeking to explain the production of the symbol-filled array, including Marr's (1982) explanations of the production of the "2½-D sketch" (which was a model for Tye's symbol-filled array). But there remains a question of why Tye believes the postulated symbol-filled array explains phenomenal experience. It is the array's representational or informational content that does the work for Tye (1991, 136, 142), and not any relation to neural states or to nonsymbolic mental states. Specifically, Tye posits that phenomenal experience arises when we have symbolic-matrix representations of distal states that are ready to be taken up cognitively (e.g., brought under description). As a description of the role that phenomenal experience itself might play in perception and cognition, in providing representations for further cognitive response, this strikes me as a good description. But Tye intends it to explain our (apparent) phenomenal experience itself. In the case of color vision, he says that phenomenal blue simply arises when we have symbolic states that represent distal blue things (1991, 133; 1995, 145−7). He rejects sensations, qualia, or other mental items that might present phenomenal blue (1991, ch. 7). The phenomenal blue, he explains, is not in the head, but is on the surfaces of things. He is aware that the property possessed by some distal things, which makes them blue, is the physical property of having a spectral reflectance distribution that falls within a certain class of such distributions. It is his view that a nonconceptual representation of this property in the visual system at a stage ready for conceptual description just is the perception of the distal blue surface in a phenomenally blue manner (1995, 137–43). No further explanation of the phenomenal content is given.

Kosslyn (1995) surveyed the literature on visual imagery and proposed that there are two sorts of symbolic systems in the head: propositional and depictive. Propositional representations consist of discrete symbols of various classes (signifying entities, relations, properties, and logical relations), with rules for combining them. The spatial relations among the symbols have only an arbitrary significance. Property-symbols may always be written to the right of the entity symbols to which they apply, but this does not mean that they are on the right hand side of the entity! By contrast, spatial relations of symbols in the depictive style of representation have that sort of nonarbitrary spatial meaning. The depictive style of representation involves only two classes of symbols, points (small punctiform areas) and empty spaces. The combination rules are merely that the symbols must be put in spatial relation to one another, and any relation is allowed (Kosslyn 1995, 280–2).

It is misleading for Kosslyn to label the points that compose his depictive representations "symbols," since no operations are defined which respond to the points based on variation in their form, as happens in classical symbol-processing models (Fodor 1975, ch. 2; Pylyshyn 1984, ch. 3). Indeed, Kosslyn seems to assume that noncognitive processes yield the depictive structure of the basic parts of images. At the least, his mature theory is not discernibly committed to positing cognitive or inferential processes to generate the spatial relations internal to image parts.[13] Interpretive processes operate over spatial relations found in the image, which is composed of points in spatial arrangement (Kosslyn 1995, 273–5). The images are spatially concrete. The potentially continuously varying spatial relations among points give them their content. Because continuous variation in spatial relations is permitted, the medium is analog.

Originally, Kosslyn (1983, 23) understood the spatial relations found in images to be a functional space consisting of paths of access among address labels for represented points as read by processing mechanisms (a conception similar to Tye's symbol-filled array). Neuroscientific findings led him to suggest that these functional relations may indeed be realized by real spatial relations in the cerebral cortex (Kosslyn 1995, 290–2). Although Kosslyn does not explicitly say so, he appears to suggest that the spatial relations experienced in images

---

[13] To put the point in Kosslyn's technical vocabulary, there is no discernible commitment that the operations by which compressed images (1994, 118–19) are used to reconstruct depictive representations are cognitive, though of course the decompression process may be initiated cognitively.

result from isomorphic spatial relations in the brain, presumably in accordance with a linking proposition (Teller and Pugh 1983). This proposal is similar to the Gestalt psychologists' earlier postulation of a spatial isomorphism between brain events and the structure of perceptual experience (Köhler 1929, 61–6, 142–7; Koffka 1935, 56–67; see also Scheerer 1994). An extension of Kosslyn's theory in this direction would yield a noncognitive principle of explanation for the spatial structure in phenomenal experience via spatially isomorphic patterns of activity in the brain. If we treat linking propositions as hypothesized laws of nature, then the existence of spatially organized phenomenal experience is explained as the lawful product of the spatial properties of activity in certain areas of the brain.

Stepping back, it would seem that the most promising route for inferential theories to explain the spatial structure of perception is the postulation of language-like inferential processes that produce analog or depictive representations. If we give due regard to Rock's and Fodor's point about encapsulation, then these inferential processes would take place in a conceptually impoverished vocabulary, perhaps limited to spatial and chromatic properties and focusing on the production of a representation of the spatially articulated surfaces of objects via a symbol-filled array.

At present there is no worked-out account of how an encapsulated inferential process would produce either a genuinely analog representation or one of Marr's arrays. Moreover, there are rival accounts of processing mechanisms that could yield analog representations without relying on a language-like or inferential medium. Historically, the Gestalt theory of self-organizing dynamical systems in the brain provided a noncognitive basis for generating perceptual results (Hatfield and Epstein 1985, 178–9). In more recent times, connectionist models provide a conception of perceptual processing in which perceptual information can be combined in regular ways to yield analog representations, without positing cognitive operations such as inference (Chs. 2–3). To the extent that these rival accounts provide a means for modeling the production of analog representations, they go further than inferential accounts in addressing the production of the spatial structure of phenomenal experience.

3. Conclusion

Highly articulated theories of unconscious inference in perception have been extant for a thousand years (since Alhazen c.1030), and have been widespread for nearly four hundred years (following Descartes 1637). The structure of the theories has varied, as can be seen by reviewing their various theoretical primitives, that is, what is taken as given as opposed to what needs an explanation. Prior to the nineteenth century, the inferential machinery required to make unconscious inferences was taken as a given: it was the intellect, or the faculty of judgment. Subsequently, various proposals were made to explain this machinery: via association in the case of Helmholtz, via an unconscious language of thought in the case of Fodor and Rock. Prior to the latter twentieth century, it was assumed that the same concepts are employed in unconscious inferences and conscious thought. In recent decades, the fact that perception is often impervious to consciously entertained knowledge has led investigators to posit a separate, encapsulated domain of perceptual processing, which must then be supplied with its own cognitive resources. Finally, prior to the twentieth century the primitive elements posited in perceptual theories were sensations with phenomenal properties. Processes were then posited to augment or transform those properties, for example, by ordering the sensations spatially. In the twentieth century such sensational primitives have been rejected. For contemporary unconscious inference theories, the problem then arises of explaining how linguistic inferential processes can yield the phenomenal aspects of perceptual experience.

The literature of artificial intelligence and computational accounts of vision is replete with talk of "descriptions" and "inferences." In some cases, such as Marr (1982, 342–4), the approach has been allied with a Fodorean conception of symbolic computation. But in many cases no real support is given for such talk. It is as if causal transitions among information-bearing states of a system that occur according to rules and that lead to appropriate outcomes should be counted as inferences on the face of it, without supplying cognitive machinery or making provision to explain the conceptual content found in the inferences. As we found with the work on color constancy discussed above, such discussions are best classed as metaphorical uses of the concepts of inference and description. They are not inferential theories of perception, but theories of information transformation in perception.[14] The problem with taking these

[14] It is possible to read this literature as implicitly proposing that all inference should be treated as information transformation, without worrying about the system's sensitivity to the content of the information. More generally, it seems clear that Horace Barlow (1974, 1990a) adopts the attitude that mechanisms of information transformation, from the bacterium to the human, are best treated as lying on a continuum, with no in-principle dividing line separating the processes and marking off what I have called concept-mediated inferences from the "inferences" of the bacterium. This line of thought is of great interest. At the same time, without further articulation and defense of its claims about continuity, it slips too easily into panmentalism; for it equates thought content with information transformations of any kind, and so does not account for the internal structure of conceptual thought (see Dretske 1981) that distinguishes cognitive beings from computer keyboards.

positions as literal inference theories is that they make no provision for the cognitive resources that would be needed to sustain unconscious inferences.

Literal theories of perceptual inference that do posit cognitive resources, in the manner of Fodor (1983) and Rock (1983), have the opposite problem. They need to defend their invocation of cognitive apparatus to carry out rule-based transformations on information-bearing states in perception. Recall that our discussion has been limited to the phenomenal aspects of sense perception, that is, to the generation of imagistic perceptual representations. Rock argues that the outcomes of perception are clever enough to require truly intelligent (or at least genuinely cognitive) mechanisms in their production. The question of whether "smart mechanisms" must simply be engineered smartly (or evolved "smartly"), or must contain genuinely cognitive apparatus, is of great interest (Runeson 1977). More generally, it would be interesting to contemplate similarities and differences among the various processes by which sensory information is encoded, perceptions are formed and brought under concepts, words are applied to perceptions, and meanings of words are altered on empirical (inductive) grounds (Barlow 1974, 132). But for present purposes it will be enough to consider briefly an alternative means for conceiving perceptual processes noncognitively.

One of the reasons that unconscious inference models are attractive is that perception is mental and involves transformations of information in accordance with rules. It has seemed reasonable or even necessary that the rules would be represented and applied by a cognitive apparatus. But the development of connectionist computational architectures provides a means of conceiving of rules for information transformation that are instantiated in neural nets, without being cognitively represented and accessed. Connectionist models can treat information processing in perception as the outcome of stimulus driven inputs to nodes in a connectionist net and the subsequent settling down of that net (or one downstream) into a stable state. Spatial information might be carried in such nets by adjacency relations within a retinotopic projection (Bienenstock and Doursat 1991). By organizing a pyramid of nets that respond to the spatial properties of represented images at many different scales, local computations can respond to global features of images in a reasonable number of steps (Rosenfeld 1990). Within the connectionist framework it is possible to think of networks of nodes as instantiating processing rules (Ch. 3 and Hatfield 1991a) without representing those rules in explicit symbolic form or operating upon them via language-like inferential apparatus. Because such nets process information in accordance with rules without the necessity that the stimulus be described internally in a conceptual vocabulary (however modest), such models are noncognitive (see Ch. 2). For basic sensory processes, evolutionary engineering presumably has shaped the instantiated rules. Marr's (1982) theory of early vision, long a bastion of symbolist and inferential conceptions of psychological processes, admits of a nonsymbolic, noncognitive connectionist interpretation (Ch. 3; Kosslyn and Hatfield 1984).

Noncognitive models of sense perception face (counterparts to) only two of the three problems discussed herein. As the complement of the cognitive machinery problem, they must provide computational machinery to explain transformations among perceptual representations. As the complement to the phenomenal experience problem, they must explain how the phenomenal aspects of sensory perception arise from noncognitive processes and operations. They are not faced with the sophisticated content problem in relation to sense perception, since they do not posit cognitive operations that represent conceptual content (sophisticated or no) in their explanations. Connectionist versions of noncognitive theories do, of course, face the problem of sophisticated content in framing explanations of cognitive achievements such as object recognition. They will in that case need to provide their own models of conceptual content and object recognition (on which, see Quinlan 1991, 120–31).

The previous hegemony of inferential models of the psychological processes underlying sense perception (by contrast with cognitive or meaningful perception) has fallen subject to challenge (Epstein 1993; Kanizsa 1979, ch. 1; 1985; Ch. 2). The fate of inferential models will be decided in the longer course of empirical research and theoretical assessment. It is clear that the mere presence of specified processing rules or of "clever" perceptual outcomes cannot support the theory that sense perception results from inference, to the exclusion of noncognitive theories. Although seeing usually leads to believing, it remains an open question whether simple seeing results from belief-like inferences. The slow movement of theory is towards thinking that it does not.

5

Representation and Constraints

THE INVERSE PROBLEM AND THE STRUCTURE OF VISUAL SPACE

1. Introduction

At an ecologically relevant scale, the physical world is spatially three-dimensional, and human beings (along with other animals) perceive a world in three dimensions when light appropriately affects the eyes. The light obeys known laws of transmission, which form a set of constraints (C) on the proximal stimulus patterns (S_p) that light reflected from surfaces of objects (distal stimuli, S_d) can present to the visual system. Perceptual psychologists have investigated the processes (P) that take those patterns (or aspects of them) as input and yield perceptual representations (R) as output. Various proposals have been made about the relations among objects O, environmental constraints C, processes P, and perceptual representations R (along with the use of such representations to guide action). These proposals constitute the theories or subtheories of visual perception.

Various questions can be posed about the perceptual situation. In psychophysics, one asks how the properties of S_d are represented R. In information-processing psychology, one seeks to characterize the processes (IP) that mediate between the proximal stimulus S_p and R. Theorists such as Gibson (1950) and Shepard (1984, 1994) have proposed that the existence of constraints C can provide a clue to the structure of representations R; Shepard would add that attention to C can point the way to a proper characterization of the task or end-goal as well as the structure of IP. Nonetheless, it may be useful to describe perceptual outcomes independently of a specific process mode. Leeuwenberg's structural information theory is one example (Leeuwenberg 1969; Helm 2000), and geometrical descriptions of visual space may provide another.

As a philosopher engaged by contemporary visual theories, my intention is to step back and pose some questions about the assumptions underlying the notion of environmental constraints and attendant conceptions of the representational task of perception. Taking a cue from Kubovy and Epstein (2001), I will examine the extent to which environmental constraints as discussed by Shepard (1984, 1994) can be said actually to have been "internalized" by the visual system. Taking a further cue from Buffart and Leeuwenberg (1978), I will ultimately frame this question in terms of the relation between representations R and distal stimuli S_d in spatial perception. My aim is to describe some general features of this relation, drawing on the experimental literature and my own observations. In so doing, I will challenge the widely held assumption that the global structure of visual space, or of the object structures presented in visual space, is (isotropically) Euclidean. I will also query a methodological premise about the relations among R, P, S_p, and S_d: that R is the result of solving an "inverse problem" of inferring the correct spatial structure of S_d from the proximal stimulus S_p along with various internal "principles" or "assumptions" about environmental structure and optical constraints (e.g., Palmer 1999, 23–4; Proffitt and Kaiser 1998, 177–82). This premise suggests that processes IP should be investigated under the assumption that they have the task of generating a complete and physically correct solution to the inverse problem.

Throughout the chapter I discuss various relations between perceptual representations and physical stimuli. In these discussions I assume a realist perspective on the physical world: that it has the spatial properties ordinarily assigned to it in physical descriptions (at least at the mid-sized scale pertaining to perception), that light has properties of wavelength and frequency, and so on. The arguments I make do not require this realist perspective (they could be recast in other frameworks),[1] but adopting it makes for convenient exposition. I also discuss the phenomenal aspects of visual experience, and seek

[1] The argument of this chapter can be recast within any framework that accepts that phenomenal experience is found in (at least) human perception. Beyond that, ontological commitments may vary. The arguments of the chapter are, for instance, compatible with a phenomenalist perspective such as that of Ernst Mach, William James, and Bertrand Russell (see Ch. 10), according to which primary reality consists of phenomenally characterized entities (Mach's elements, Russell's momentary particulars), and the physical word is, in Russell's terms, a logical construction from such entities. Questions about the representationality of spatial perception would be recast in terms of relations between (a) the spatial structures found in phenomenal experience, and (b) those posited through logical construction. Such questions can also be recast in a physicalist framework such as Dennett's (1988), which privileges physical description and treats the phenomenal as a logical (or intentional) construction. In either case, questions about the relations between phenomenal and physical spatial structure remain empirical.

to characterize the sort of representational relation that might exist between spatial structures presented in visual experience and the spatial properties of physical objects. I do not assume a particular notion of that representational relation in advance, but introduce various notions as needed. In the meantime, in discussing the work of specific authors I employ the term "representation" according to each author's usage.

2. The Internalization of Environmental Constraints

In a series of articles, Shepard (1981, 1984, 1994) argued that many aspects of visual perception can be explained if the visual system is thought of as *internalizing* environmental regularities. He described these regularities as *constraints* on perception, or rather on successful perception and action. They are stable physical regularities that have been found in the environments of various species, perhaps for eons. Examples include the 24-hour diurnal cycle of day and night, and the laws of geometrical or ecological optics (including that light is transmitted rectilinearly, and that the surfaces from which light is reflected typically belong to coherent, persisting objects). Shepard maintains that these regularities may be internalized by the perceptual system as constraints on the domain of acceptable visual representations. They would act as principles of perceptual processing, perhaps embodying sufficient information to reduce or negate the underdetermination of the distal scene by proximal stimulation.

In a careful examination of Shepard's (1994) notion of constraints, Kubovy and Epstein (2001) propose some terminological clarifications. They focus on Shepard's proposal that various principles of kinematic geometry governing the displacement of objects in three-dimensional space have been internalized. Using an apparent-motion paradigm, Shepard (1984, 1994) showed that apparent motion "solutions" to various stroboscopically produced stimuli seem to embody the constraints of kinematic geometry on the displacement (including rotation and translation) of objects in physical space. Kubovy and Epstein distinguish three factors: constraints as physical regularities in the extraorganismic (or extracerebral) physical world; the internal representation of such constraints in the processes of perception, through rule following or rule instantiation (Hatfield 1991a; Kubovy and Epstein 2001; Ch. 3.7); and the internalization of such constraints through evolutionary selection. In their view, environmental constraints can set conditions on the successful operation of a visual system, and perceptual systems may as a matter of fact meet those conditions; but this fact does not entail that the constraints are represented or instantiated in the internal processes, and so does not require that the contraints have been internalized through evolution. (In this case, they leave aside questions of why the perceptual system operates in accordance with environmental regularities; it just does.) They correctly portray Shepard as endorsing the contrasting view that a counterpart to environmental regularities (the principles of kinematic geometry) is both (1) internal, and (2) the result of internalization. Kubovy and Epstein (2001) argue that Shepard (1994) has not made an adequate case for these two points. They suggest that his findings could be accounted for if kinematic geometry were seen simply as a descriptive model used by the investigators to describe aspects of motion perception.

This distinction between environmental regularities and their representation is helpful as far as it goes. However, it needs to be supplemented in at least two ways. First, if (e.g.,) kinematic geometry provides a useful "descriptive model" for aspects of motion perception, it is reasonable to ask what relation the descriptions of this model bear to the aspects of perception they describe. Candidate answers would include a mere relationship of analogy, or direct description (to some degree of accuracy) of aspects of perceptual structure (in this case, aspects of perceived shape and motion). If kinematic geometry provides a direct description of perceptual structures, then it can still be asked how such structures are generated in perception and why the perceptual system should exhibit precisely those structures in its representation of distal events. This question raises the second point, which is to ask what relation the perceptual structures themselves bear to their extraorganismic counterparts (physical objects moving in the world).

Kubovy and Epstein (2001, 621) use the term *homomorphism* to describe the relation between model and perception, and between perception and world. They do not define this term, but it is frequently used in vision science (e.g., Palmer 1999, 77–8). This term, and the earlier term *isomorphism*, can describe a variety of relations between theory (or model) and perceptual structures, and between perceptual structures and distal stimuli. Finer distinctions among these relations will allow more specific answers to our questions about theory–perception and perception–environment relations.

3. Representation and Isomorphism

The original notion of perceptual isomorphism is due especially to the Gestalt psychologist Wolfgang Köhler (1947; see Scheerer 1994). He proposed, as an empirical thesis, that during perception the shape of a spatial structure in the world causes brain events exhibiting similar shape ("isomorphism" means *same shape*), which yield a phenomenal presentation in experience of that shape (as seen from a point of view). There is thus a threefold realization of the given spatial structure: in the extraorganismic world, in the pattern of brain events, and in the spatial structure present in perceptual experience.

The notion of isomorphism in perceptual and cognitive representation was further developed by Shepard (1975, 1981). Focusing on representation–environment relations, he distinguished three sorts of isomorphisms: first-order concrete, first-order abstract, and second-order. First-order isomorphisms involve concrete or abstract sameness of structure between two domains—in this case, between distal stimuli in perception and either brain events or functionally defined mental representations. In Shepard's terms, Köhler and the Gestalt psychologists posited a concrete first-order spatial isomorphism between brain events and distal stimuli. He sought instead to characterize abstract first-order structural isomorphisms and second-order functional isomorphisms among representational elements. In the abstract first-order case, the representational elements would not "resemble" (in shape perception, *have the same shape as*) the distal stimulus. Rather, various brain events or representational elements would first be put in one-to-one correspondence with the elements of the stimulus; in the usual case, this would be done in virtue of the fact that the internal elements or events are in regular, causally mediated correlation with the stimulus elements. Isomorphism now enters to describe the relations among the internal and external elements; the relations among internal elements are found to correspond (abstractly) to the relations among the external elements. The isomorphism is abstract because it consists in correspondences among logically or mathematically describable relations among elements, but does not posit an identity in the type of relation (see Ch. 3.2). Second-order isomorphism is then defined in terms of the relation that first-order structures bear to further processing. A second-order isomorphism occurs if brain or representational structures exhibiting a first-order isomorphism yield similar results in further cognitive processing or the production of behavior.

Consider the example of a square (Shepard 1975, 1981). A concrete first-order isomorphism would result if a square in the world gave rise, during visual perception, to a square pattern of activity in the visual cortex. Shepard (1981) follows Skinner (1963) in suggesting that the squareness of the brain process would not by itself be explanatory, because it would not explain further cognitive or behavioral responses. But he contends that the fact that some elements in the head were isomorphic to the distal rather than proximal stimulus would constitute a beginning for explanation. In order to fill out the explanation, an abstract first-order isomorphism (Shepard 1981, 291) would suffice, and does not require literal sameness of shape but merely sameness of abstract structural relations. Thus, there might occur in the head four brain events that are deemed to be representational elements corresponding to the four corners of the square, and which stand in relation to one another internally in a way that represents external relations of next-to-ness and the like, without their needing to be literally next to one another. The next-to-ness relation might be represented in the brain by a specific neural-connectivity relation, and on the representational level by formal or logical relations among the representational elements corresponding to the four corners.

The notion of representation is here employed in connection with three different relations: (1) causal correlation (the representation is regularly produced by the external object); (2) abstract structure (the relations among internal elements in some way mirror the relations among external elements); and (3) functional role (representational structures enter into and guide further perceptual processing, to similar effect). The relation of causal correlation, which establishes the initial representational relation, does not depend on the notion of isomorphism. In Shepard's proposal, isomorphism is needed to describe the abstract correspondence between the relations among internal and external elements. This sort of abstract first-order isomorphism is what is now more typically called a *homomorphism*[2] (Palmer 1999, 77), as in the usage of Kubovy and Epstein (2001).

4. Accommodating the Phenomenal

In alluding to the spatial structures found in visual perception, I have been tacitly relying on a phenomenalist perspective. Thus, in mentioning a perceptual experience that presents a square, I have supposed that readers will understand what I am saying because they have experienced phenomenally present squares, and find it reasonable to describe this experienced structure using the term "square." This methodological attitude, which allows descriptions of direct experience into the ambit of perceptual research, was highly touted by the

---

[2] The change in terminology avoids the historical connotation of the prefix "iso" in the Gestalt notion, as signaling genuine sameness or identity of kind of relations within structures, by replacing it with the prefix "homo," which is intended to connote mere abstract similarity or alikeness of relation. In model theory an *isomorphism* implies identity of structure, whereas a *homomorphism* merely entails similarity of structure in some respects (Hodges 1997, 5).

Gestalt psychologists (Köhler 1947, ch. 1; Koffka 1935, ch. 2). In the period after 1950, the notion became suspect, especially outside the community of psychologists of perception. As I wish to build on the methodological advice of the Gestaltists, these suspicions must be addressed.

Conveniently, Shepard (1975, 1981) can be taken as a representative theorist who voiced concerns that were shared by others. Although proclaiming himself a friend of phenomenology and introspection, philosophical reservations about objectivity precluded him from including phenomenal structures in the domain of scientific investigation. Having excluded the phenomenal, he defined representational relations and first and second-order isomorphisms in terms of the physical or functional properties of brain events. When mentioning spatial representations (such as that of a square), he did not intend to describe phenomenal structures; he limited scientific discourse to functional relations among representations in the brain that could themselves be related to external physical objects (as in Place 1956, and Smart 1959). By including second-order functional relations, he could abstract away from concrete descriptions of brain activity, to a functional (and, in his terms, "mental") level of analysis of psychological processes and their behavioral upshot. In line with the philosophical functionalism of the 1970s and 1980s (e.g., Fodor 1975), he conceived psychological investigation as directed toward the inferred structure of internal processes, functionally conceived. Phenomenal reports were to be regarded merely as instances of observable behavior.

Many psychologists and philosophers have expressed skepticism about the usefulness of describing the features of phenomenal experience, or about its very existence (Dennett 1988). Shepard (1981, 280–1) offered a diagnosis for such skepticism when he described phenomenal experience as a "mental" entity that is "nonphysical," hence inaccessible to objective study. He offered two bases for this last conclusion, one ontological, one epistemological. Ontologically, visual experience presents a shape at a distance, and so on. And yet no one now believes that in the brain there is a physical event with a precisely corresponding shape, or a representation that varies in distance to some part of the brain precisely in accordance with perceived distance. It seemed to Shepard (1981, 280) and others that if brain states are not shaped in conformity with phenomenal content, then phenomenally experienced shape would have to be reckoned as "nonphysical." Shepard therefore restricted his discourse to abstract, functional descriptions of representational states in the brain, so as to avoid the (alleged) need to posit nonphysical entities (as in mind–body dualism or dualistic epiphenomenalism). On this way of viewing things, a materialistic psychologist who wanted to embrace phenomenal shapes would be forced to posit a neural image in the head (the physical image-in-the-head view disparaged in Shepard and Chipman 1970)—a most unfashionable position.

This dilemma for the materialistic psychologist is based on an overly narrow conception of mind–body relations. On a broader conception, it is conceivable for a materialist to accept phenomenal structures into a materialistic framework. Such a materialist might posit that brain states have additional properties besides those presently explicable via physics and chemistry, such as the property of realizing conscious mental states with various spatially articulated phenomenal contents. This position (or a close relative) could be developed as a form of materialistic emergentism or materialistic property dualism (or as a dual-aspect monism)—none of which posit a separate substantial, nonphysical mind, and so none of which lead to Cartesian dualism.[3] Accordingly, brain events that are not literally square might nonetheless realize the phenomenal experience of a square, which presents a squarely structured region.

The properties of brain events that serve to realize the conscious presentation of visual qualities, such as shapes or colors, are not at present known. But if, as seems reasonable to suppose, phenomenal experience is realized by brain events of some kind or other, then phenomenal contents such as color and shape can be realized by the brain without the brain itself taking on the shapes and colors found in phenomenal experience. Those shapes and colors have the status of *intentional content*—content that is present in a mental representation, but in such a way that the represented properties do not literally pertain to the brain state that realizes the representation (nor to some other ghostly entity such as a state of a soul).[4] A phenomenal square can be present in consciousness without requiring that anything physically square be present in the brain, or that a substantial square patch occur in a separate mental substance.

[3] According to materialistic emergentism, the ability of the brain to realize conscious, phenomenal experience is an as yet unexplained emergent property arising from the combination of physical and chemical properties found in the brain. According to materialistic property dualism (or perhaps n-alism), material things have, in addition to the properties now described by physics and chemistry, other properties, including mental properties. According to dual-aspect monism, the single basic stuff of the universe (not itself characterized as material) has both mental and physical properties. For a review of these positions, see Crane (2001, ch. 2); on the need to move beyond simplistic materialism, see G. Strawson (1994).

[4] This notion of *intentional content* invokes Brentano (1874/1995). It accepts that a square spatial structure can be present in phenomenal experience without the brain (or some state of the soul) literally being square, and without the phenomenal content being wholly reducible to its relation to physical squares. It is distinct from the "intentionalism" of Dretske (1995b) and Tye (1995), and applies the term "content" with a broader meaning than do they, who (along with others) equate content with informational content. Here, whatever is phenomenally present may count as phenomenal content.

The metaphysical accounts of the mind–body relation that permit phenomenal content without requiring either brain images or dualism have not been definitively established. But neither have the competing versions of materialism, including those that would exclude phenomenal content. Hence, current philosophical thinking on the mind–body problem does not require denying phenomenally spatial objects in subjective experience. In my view, it would be a strategic error for psychology to require a definitive solution to the mind–body problem before permitting serious discussion of the properties of phenomenal experience. Those psychologists who posit a phenomenal domain (see next section) should be allowed to proceed with their investigations independently of predicted solutions to the mind–body problem. If such theorists would like to proceed consistently with the assumption of materialism (or, less contentiously, with a denial of substance dualism), they should know that various extant philosophical proposals regard phenomenal contents as realized by or emergent from brain activity (Crane 2001; G. Strawson 1994).

Shepard (1981) also raised an epistemological problem for phenomenal experience, the alleged privacy of each person's experience (the privacy of other minds). This led him to conclude that in any case phenomenal experience lies outside the domain of scientific investigation. In support, he referred to philosophical discussions of privacy and subjectivity. But this conclusion also is not forced by current philosophy. The assumption that one person's experience is like another's (beyond detectable abnormalities, such as color blindness) can be based on the notion of biological sameness of kind (Flanagan 1992, ch. 5). Further, on the assumption of a lawful universe, one might posit psychophysiological laws relating brain states to phenomenal experience (Chalmers 1996, ch. 6). In principle, as a matter of natural law things might be such that visual cortexes of the same biological kind produce color experience of similar kind under similar stimulation.

This excursus into metaphysics and epistemology is intended to loosen the grip of mid twentieth-century philosophy of mind, which retained vestiges of narrow behaviorism and physicalism even in Fodorean functionalism (see Ch. 14). The long-standing suspicion of phenomenal experience has abated in philosophy. Short of definitive word on the mind–body problem, psychologists might ask themselves why they should be unwilling to infer from the character of their own experience to that of other human beings. If they will make that inference, then in addition to inferring similarity of functional process from similarity in behavioral response, they should not hesitate to infer similarity of phenomenal experience under similar stimulus conditions.

5. Phenomenality and Representation

Some contemporary theorists take phenomenal experience as an object of explanation in perceptual psychology (e.g., Buffart and Leeuwenberg 1978; Hershenson 1999; Indow 1991; Palmer 1999; Rock 1975; 1983, 32, 52). The Gestalt psychologist Kurt Koffka (1935) posed as a central problem for perceptual theory the question "Why do things look as they do?" Rock (1975) and Palmer (1999), among others, refer to this question in formulating the tasks of perceptual theory. They interpret the question as Koffka intended—as a question about the visual experience of perceivers, and thus as requesting an explanation for the characteristics of visual experience itself.

Perceptual theorists who define phenomenal experience as an object of explanation regularly distinguish between the *physical properties* of objects and the *phenomenal presentation* (or *representation*) of those properties.[5] As a matter of physical description, objects may reflect light differently depending on its wavelength, may have a shape, be at a specific distance from the perceiver, in a particular direction, and so on. In visual experience, objects appear with phenomenal color, have a phenomenal shape, appear to be at a distance, in a direction, and so on. The phenomenal presentation of objects depends subjectively on the perceiver, while the object's physical properties may depend on the object alone (as with spectral reflectance properties) or on its physical relation to the environment or the perceiver's body. Phenomenal colors (reds, greens, etc.) are thus distinguished from their physical basis in objects, phenomenal shapes can be distinguished from the physical shapes of things, and so on.[6] All the same, we use similar terms to describe physical properties and their phenomenal counterparts; thus, we talk both of the squareness of the physical object, and of the phenomenally present square.

A distinction between phenomenal presentations and corresponding object properties permits questions to be posed about the relations between them. In particular, it allows discussion of whether, and how, phenomenal presentations of colors, shapes, and so on *represent* distal objects. Assuming that a primary

[5] I prefer the term "presentation" for describing the contents of phenomenal experience themselves, and here I use the term "representation" to pose questions about the information-carrying or representational relation between presented contents and distal objects.

[6] Several popular philosophical theories of representation, preserving the antiphenomenalist bias of functionalism, deny any such distinction (Dretske 1995b, ch. 3; Tye 1995, chs. 4–5). They take the content of perceptual representations to be exhaustively analyzable into the physical properties of distal objects (perhaps together with functional facts about the organism).

function of perception is to represent the distal environment, it is plausible to consider at least some phenomenal presentations to be representations. Such representations fall within the immediately available content of visual experience, including phenomenally presented colors, shapes, sizes, and distances of things (this list is not exhaustive). Although earlier theorists held that the "real" phenomenally immediate experience is of a two-dimensional image, those visual theorists who adopt phenomenalist descriptions today typically take immediate experience to be as of a world in three dimensions. Various spatial and chromatic aspects of visual experience can then be taken to represent the corresponding physical object properties.

Although phenomenal representations are tacitly endorsed by the theorists mentioned above—or explicitly acknowledged, as in Rock (1975)—the manner in which they represent typically is not discussed. The primary models of representation remain causal correspondence and (abstract) homomorphism (Palmer 1999, 77). However, allowing representation via phenomenal spatial structures would permit a different kind of representational relation to be considered, that of *resemblance*. This opportunity can be clarified by contrast with standard causal and homomorphic accounts.

When representations are assigned their referents through causal correlation, they serve essentially as referring signs. As such, the alignment of elemental signs with their referents can be arbitrary. In Shepard's (1981, 290) terms, such signs are "unanalyzable" or "unitary." A homogeneous color is an unanalyzable or a unitary sign for a (class of) physical reflectance properties. In a spatial structure, the representation as a whole is analyzable into subparts, but Shepard emphasizes that the representational relation is not one of resemblance or concrete first-order isomorphism; perceptual representations of a square do not relate to distal squares by presenting the same structure (a square structure or its close relative). Rather, representational elements gain the referring relation through causal correspondence, and structural properties (such as squareness) are represented through abstract first-order isomorphisms and second-order functional isomorphisms (Shepard 1981). Here again, the representing elements can be arbitrarily related to their referents, as signs. The elements and relations in the representing world need not resemble the elements and relations in the represented world (Palmer 1999, 77–8).

Now consider the relations between phenomenal presentations and represented objects or properties. We may agree with Rock (1975, 4–5) and other theorists that phenomenal color does not resemble the corresponding surface property that causes us to see color. With phenomenal color, the representational relation plausibly might depend on causal correspondence (but see Chs. 10–11). In the case of spatial properties, however, resemblance can again enter the picture.[7] Phenomenally presented spatial structures exhibit objects with a shape, at a distance, in a direction, with or without a motion, and so on. Those are (phenomenally) spatially articulated presentational contents. The represented domain (of physical objects) includes objects that have a physical shape, are at a distance, in a physically defined direction, are moving or not, and so on. The types of phenomenally presented properties (various phenomenal spatial properties) exhibit homogenous kinds of structure by comparison with the represented properties (physical spatial properties), even if those structures are not realized in the same manner (intentionally in the one case, physically in the other).

6. Phenomenal Representation, Internalization, and Constraints

With the concept of phenomenal spatial structure in place, we can consider more fully the relations among representations, constraints, and internalization. In the process, we can fill out the scheme of organism–environment and representation–environment relations.

Let us consider various ways in which environmental conditions, regularities, or universals might be internalized. We will begin with the general notion of internalization, and move on to cases of homomorphism and resemblance.

One sort of internalization would result from a literal incorporation of physical and chemical properties of the environment into the organism. Organisms are of course constructed from naturally occurring chemical elements, some of which conjoin to form organic molecules not otherwise found in nature. In the process of evolution, some features of the inorganic chemical environment were internalized. Many marine invertebrates show concentrations of common

---

[7] The notion of resemblance long provided a philosophically attractive means of accounting for the representational relation between the spatial properties of material objects and the spatial aspects of phenomenal experience. It fell out of favor in the 1950s and 1960s, with the rise of a simple version of the materialistic identity theory (e.g., Place 1956, Smart 1959). It was widely assumed that to take phenomenal spatial structure seriously, one would need to posit concretely isomorphic shaped structures in the brain (Shepard and Chipman 1970). Further, Nelson Goodman (1968), relying on "new look" psychology of perception and radical empiricism, mounted an apparently convincing challenge to the notion of resemblance itself as applied to pictorial representations, including the spatial aspect of perception. Recent philosophers (Hopkins 1998) are rehabilitating the notion of resemblance as applied to spatial perception and pictures or images, emphasizing especially outline shape (from a point of view). Herein, I apply resemblance to the perception–object relation, as with 3-D surface-shape perceived from a point of view, under the characteristic contraction of visual space (Sec. 7).

ions such as sodium, magnesium, calcium, potassium, chlorine, and sulfate in their bodily fluids that are very close to those of sea water (Schmidt-Nielsen 1990, ch. 8). Even amphibians and mammals show relative concentrations of sodium, potassium, and calcium ions very close to the relative concentrations of sea water (Loewy and Siekevitz 1969, 87). Here, presumably, sea water was literally internalized from the ambient environment of early living cells, and some aspects of the internalized environment have been retained throughout the course of evolution.

This is not the sort of internalization that Shepard and his critics have been concerned with. They have been concerned with internalized regularities that show up as processing rules that internally constrain the structure of representations. However, comparing such cases with the literal internalization of ionic concentrations may help us to differentiate various relations obtaining between environmental regularities and an internalized counterpart.

Shepard's favorite example of internalization is the diurnal cycle (Shepard 1984, 1994). Keeping in mind internalized ion concentrations, we may ask if this is a case of internalized representation, or simply the internalization of a physical regularity by mimicking or re-instantiating it. Organisms have internal processes that show a 24-hour cycle, which can cause them to exhibit waking and sleeping behavior on a 24-hour schedule even under unvarying ambient light (as in an enclosed laboratory with constant lighting). Such animals have an internal physicochemical process that cycles diurnally. Does this internal process *represent* the diurnal time cycle, or simply *correspond* to it physically? The answer is not obvious. There are clear cases of internal states that do serve as representations (many states of the perceptual and cognitive systems, or so I am assuming for present purposes). In the diurnal regulation of behavior, however, the basis for choosing between saying a system *represents* the 24-hour cycle or merely *mimics* that cycle is not clear. Presumably, further investigation would proceed by examining, species by species, the role that diurnally cycling internal states play in the regulation behavior, the extent to which such states engage with systems that are paradigmatically psychological, and so on.

The notion of internalized environmental regularities can suggest a variety of representation–environment relations even in perceptual and cognitive cases. The most complete form of internalization would be for the perceiver to produce an internal model of the three-dimensional environment, down to its physical and chemical details. Clearly, perceptual systems do not make accessible such complete representations, whether via phenomenal structures or abstract homomorphisms. Rather, perception represents only some features of the environment.

Which features of the environment does perception represent, and how does it do so? This question concerns the function or task of perception,[8] and its manner of realization in specific cases (here, in human visual perception). A common assumption of many recent theorists is that perception aims at *veridicality*; that is, it aims to form representations that present the properties of the environment truthfully, so as to guide behavior (Palmer 1999, 6, 24; Rock 1975, 3, 274). The notion of *truth* here is not that of the proposition or judgment, but of accurately conforming to a standard, as when wood is planed *true*.

Granting this description of the aim of perception, the manner of accomplishment can vary greatly. Consider the sense of taste. Recent work suggests that taste receptors are responsive to the shapes of molecules, not to their specific chemical composition (Lindemann 2001). Shall we say that experienced tastes represent molecule shapes, or that they merely partition gustatory stimuli into contrast classes? In the latter case, a specific phenomenal taste could represent each class as an arbitrary sign; it would not need to be ascribed the function of conveying information about molecular shape. Accordingly, the function of taste would not be to detect specific chemical structures, but to establish regular gustatory contrasts among naturally occurring ingestants. The existence of relevantly different soluble substances would constrain the possibilities of taste, but not so as to tempt one to say that such constraints were internalized as process rules or as specific representational content.

For vision, even assuming veridicality as the primary aim, conceptions vary concerning which environmental features are to be represented and in what manner. According to one prominent conception, the task of visual perception is to accomplish an *inverse inference* from the ambient light received at the eyes to the various physical properties that have structured the light (making use of auxiliary principles or assumptions to reduce or eliminate the ambiguity of the proximal stimulus S_p). Accordingly, the features of the world that perception is presumed to represent are the precise physical features that structure light. Some theories of color perception propose that its task is to specify a spectral reflectance distribution (Palmer 1999, ch. 3; Shepard 1994). This is to conceive color vision by analogy with a physical instrument. Such theories suggest that color vision aims to represent the unique spectral reflectance distribution seen on a given occasion. To the extent that the visual system does not provide such representations (as happens with metamerism, where different distributions can

---

[8] The notion of *function* invoked here is to be distinguished from Fodorean functionalism. The latter concerned input–output relations (whether for processing units postulated within a system, or between stimulus and response). The former notion builds on the concept of biological function and the related notion of task analysis; see Hatfield (1991*a*), Shapiro (1994), and Chapters 2–3.

look the same under a given illuminant), it fails to achieve its representational goal (for discussion, see Ch. 8).

A second way of asking what is represented in vision (and how it is represented) refines Koffka's (1935) classical question. Asking why things look as they do invites consideration of the phenomenal. We can refine the question by asking a prior one: "How do things look?" This more basic question also concerns the phenomenal. In responding to his question, Koffka rejected the answer that things look as they do because they are as they are. Phenomenally speaking, perception groups things, it enhances figure/ground relations, and it represents reflectances with phenomenal colors. These are ways things look. By comparing them with a physical description of how things are, we can make progress toward understanding how things are represented in visual experience.

How do things look? Typically, we see surfaces spatially arrayed and imbued with color. Surface colors exhibit considerable perceptual constancy, though not perfectly. Not only does metamerism occur, but a single colored surface that retains "the same" color across changes in illumination does not remain phenomenally unchanged (Mausfeld 1998). If we do not regard color perception as having the function of fully decoupling reflectance from illumination and so solving the inverse problem, these facts need not signal perceptual failure. We might instead see color perception as having the function of yielding comparatively stable distinctions of objects from one another by their differing reflectance properties. The existence of classes of objects that differ in reflectance properties would still be necessary for color vision, and to that extent would serve as an environmental constraint. But perfect inverse inference to the exact spectrophotometric properties of objects would not be required as output. Nor would one need to think of vision as having internalized the photic regularities of natural illuminants (as in Shepard 1994); it would be enough for the visual system to have hit upon representational processes and mechanisms that permitted a stable division of naturally occurring objects by reflectance groupings (Ch. 8; Thompson 1995). For this, the various models that achieve less than perfect constancy would well suffice (Mausfeld 1998).

How do things look spatially? One answer can be generated from the supposition, held by some theorists (e.g., Epstein 1995; Shepard 1994, 16), that spatial perception successfully solves the inverse problem, and so infers back to the three-dimensional (nearly) Euclidean objects of the ambient physical environment. This conception of the outcome of spatial perception, as presenting a phenomenally Euclidean world (under full-cue conditions), has frequently been expressed (Gibson 1950, 12; Heelan 1983, 27–8; Palmer 1999, 23; Toye

1986, 91; Wagner 1985, 493). But does it match visual phenomenology? Do things actually appear with their Euclidean structure?

This question can be approached via size constancy. Descriptions of size constancy typically say that despite the fact that retinal image size (or visual angle) varies with distance for a given object, "perceived size is not affected by distance" (Gordon 1997, 11; also R. Schwartz 1994, 59). This makes it sound as if, when size constancy obtains, the same physical thing at different distances *looks exactly the same* as regards size, as if the inverse problem had been perfectly solved. Data show that perceivers, when asked to attend to true size, match perceived test stimuli at a distance to standards close at hand much more nearly according to true (physical) size than retinal image size. At the same time, some theorists who are very familiar with these results are troubled by the fact that, phenomenally, objects of the same physical size take up less of the visual field with increased distance. As Rock (1975, 38–9) observed, even under conditions of constancy, the same physical thing, when farther away, exhibits a smaller phenomenal extensity, or takes up less of the visual field.[9]

Consider further that when looking down a street of constant physical width, or a straight hallway, or railroad tracks, the curb, the walls, and the rails phenomenally converge. They take up less of the horizontal visual field farther away. Also, an area of flat ground takes up less of the field farther away than a physically equal area nearer to the observer. By comparison with physical measurements, there is contraction along the dimension stretching away from the observer (see Toye 1986; Wagner 1985). At the same time, the edges of the street, the walls of the hall, and the rails do not seem themselves to be approaching one another, nor do they appear to shrink physically; for near to middle distances, constancy prevails. Nonetheless, phenomenally the scene is not an accurate Euclidean portrayal of the physical structures, since parallels converge and surfaces contract with distance. The phenomenal world is not unproblematically Euclidean. Solving the inverse problem cannot be the whole story in spatial vision. If it were, there would be no spatial contraction and no phenomenal convergence under conditions of constancy.

---

[9] Rock (1975) made this observation under conditions of constancy, as opposed to conditions in which observers have been asked to adopt a special attitude, such as the "painter's attitude." He explained the point about visual extensity as follows: "The reader can appreciate what is meant here by noting that when he holds a finger a few inches from his eye, it looms large, filling almost the entire visual field, despite the fact that it still appears to be the size of a finger. By contrast, a finger (perhaps someone else's) viewed at a distance, is sensed as filling only a small sector of the field, although its size is perceived to be the same as when it was viewed nearby" (Rock 1975, 37–8). In this description, extensity pertains to visual angle and Rock does not equate it with the phenomenology of imagining the features of objects projected in perspective onto a plane in front of the observer. Yet in a nearby passage, he does equate extensity with projective size (see n. 15 below, and Ch. 6.2).

7. Visual Space

Some theorists regard visual experience as presenting a *visual space* (French 1987; Heelan 1983; Hershenson 1999; Indow 1991, 1995; Luneburg 1947; Suppes 1977). Consonant with our phenomenal approach, we will assume the existence of such a space and examine more closely its relation to physical space. I will take visual space to be defined by the spatial structures that are presented phenomenally, including the experience of empty volume between bounding surfaces. Such phenomenal structures are found in everyday perceptions of ground and sky or walls and furniture. Physical space includes the spatial structure of the ground and of atmospheric processes that yield the illusion of a domed sky, and that of the walls and furniture.

Considerable psychological work has been done on particular aspects of this relation, especially for distance, size, and shape perception. However, as Indow (1991) observes, the question of the relation of physical space to visual space overall has only rarely been examined. Haber (1986) notes that there have been few studies of the perception of an entire spatial layout, as opposed to imagining or remembering a layout (but see Toye 1986; Wagner 1985). By far the most intensive work in this area has concerned the geometry of visual space, although discussion of point of view in early vision (Marr 1982) is also pertinent.

One way to think about the relation between visual space and physical space is to ask whether visual space has a metric structure and, if so, how that structure is related to physical space. Buffart and Leeuwenberg (1978, 4) posed the question as follows:

It is attractive to imagine visual space as metric space.... If one regards visual space as metric space, one must investigate whether and to what extent objects in the physical space determine these metrics. The fact that there are stimuli that are perceived differently from their physical existence gives rise to considering visual space as non-Euclidean space.

The question of what metric structure visual space itself has, if any, might in principle be distinct from a question about the relation between visual space and physical objects. Neither question need in itself make assumptions about the use or instantiation of geometrical formalisms in the perceptual process. Rather, these questions are usually seen as seeking the geometrical structures that correctly describe phenomenal spatial structures.

Investigations of the metric of visual space have focused on the relation between visual space and physical space. In an early study, Luneburg (1947) concluded that visual space is a non-Euclidean hyperbolic space of constant negative curvature. Luneberg relied on earlier experiments in which subjects arranged black cords against a white ground (Hillebrand 1902), or arranged small test lights in an otherwise dark alley (Blumenfeld 1913). The subjects sought to achieve either phenomenally parallel rows or equidistant receding intervals. From the reported findings, Luneburg (1947) inferred a hyperbolic metric. Subsequent research has given him some support, though it is now questioned whether one should expect to find a single metric exhibited by structures in visual space (Indow 1991, 1995). It may be that different metrics apply at different distances or for differing tasks, or when the environment is not reduced to a few lights against the dark. A recent finding suggests that, while there may be no consistent metric to visual space, it internally satisfies the weaker constraints of affine geometrical structure (Todd *et al.* 2001).

In considering the relation between physical objects (or whole visual scenes) and visual space, Indow (1991, 450) has emphasized that when human beings view whole scenes, their visual space "is dynamic, not a solid empty container into which various percepts are put without affecting its contours and intrinsic structure." From observations taken in natural environments, investigators have concluded that there is no single metric relating physical space to visual space (Indow 1991; Koenderink *et al.* 2000).

I wish to step back from the question of a precise metrical structure, and examine some general features of visual space in human perception. It will be helpful to do this from two perspectives. First, we can ask what we would expect about the general structure of visual space if the inverse problem were successfully solved and the results presented in phenomenal experience. Second, we can ask what picture arises if we pursue further Rock's (1975) comments about extensity and our own observations pertaining to visual space.

Human visual perception takes place from a point of view. Supposing that the world itself is (very close to) a three-dimensional Euclidean structure, a veridical *visual* representation of that world nonetheless has a point of view. While there may be "object-centered" representations at later stages of visual cognition (Marr 1982), the primary visual spatial representation, as in Marr's "2½-D sketch," has the characteristic that only the parts of objects that face the viewer are directly seen.

Accepting that point-of-view is intrinsic to specifically visual representation, we may still ask whether the spatial structure found in full-cue spatial perception is three-dimensionally Euclidean, or not. Let us investigate the properties we should expect to find in a phenomenal perceptual representation of a scene if the inverse problem were successfully solved and Euclidean structure were recovered fully.

Consider the view looking straight down a closed alley with physically parallel walls. Assume the viewer is located at one end of the alley, midway between the side walls. From this point of view, the facing walls of the alley would be seen, not the sides away from the viewer. With the perceiver fixating the horizontal center of the end wall at eye-height, all other positions on the visible portions of the end and side walls would be seen at an angle from the straight-ahead. Since, by hypothesis, the inverse problem has been solved and the results brought into phenomenal experience, each position would be phenomenally represented at its exact distance from the viewer, in full conformity with the physical Euclidean structure of the alley (Fig. 5.1). Further, the width and height of the alley would be represented with absolute constancy. The segment CD would therefore appear exactly the same size as the segment AB, and the heights of columns attached to the walls and rising vertically from A and B would appear to be the same, and so on.

Although some descriptions of size constancy suggest that the inverse problem is fully solved (Epstein 1995; Kubovy and Epstein 2001), the implications (drawn in the previous paragraph) do not match phenomenal descriptions of visual experience. Perhaps we can develop a description that takes into account both varying extensity and the tendency toward constancy.

Let us continue with perception of an alley. It will be best if the reader looks down an actual hallway. The sides of the walls facing the viewer are seen, and the various positions along the walls are phenomenally present under a specific angle; indeed, let us assume it is the same angle as in the previous case, so that visual direction matches physical direction.[10] We must now take into account the fact that, phenomenally, the parallel lines running away from the observer converge in the visual field. If we assume a constant phenomenal convergence in a projective transformation from one three-dimensional structure to another, we can generate Figure 5.2. It shows the visual space (phenomenal space) of an observer O in dotted lines, by contrast with the physical space that reflects light into the perceiver's eyes (the alley structure itself). The phenomenal structure as described here is intended to capture common aspects of phenomenal experience in viewing a closed alley, though in a simplified and idealized way. Phenomenal segment CD now takes up less extent than segment AB, and the columns at C and D would take up correspondingly less extent vertically. The

---

[10] For the situations represented in Figs. 5.1 and 5.2, let us assume a cyclopean viewpoint, so that the angles are defined from a point between the two eyes (Hershenson 1999, ch. 2). Then, to assume that the points in the alley are seen under the same angle in both cases is just to assume that phenomenal visual direction is accurate in relation to physical direction, even if (as in Fig. 5.2) phenomenal distance contracts with respect to physical distance.

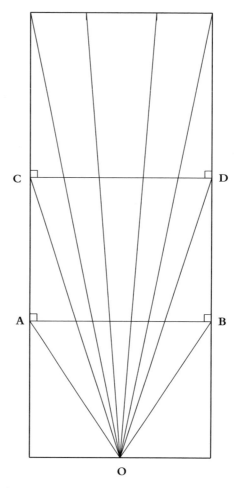

Figure 5.1. Physical and visual space with the inverse problem fully and correctly solved. A top view of observer (O) looking down an alley with physically parallel sides, showing lines of sight at eye level. The structure presented in visual space is congruent with the structure in physical space.

physical structure is represented in an ever more phenomenally contracted manner, in proportion to physical distance.[11]

---

[11] Fig. 5.2 presents a generic representation of the gross structure of a particular visual space. It simplifies by assuming that the projection is from one Euclidean structure to another (from an isotropic, infinite Euclidean space to a finite model of a visual space); empirically, it might well be that a non-Euclidean model would better fit this visual space, but I believe that a finite Euclidean model captures the gross structure. To get some sense of the contraction, preliminary observations were taken in a hallway 1.5 m wide. Two observers, while standing in the center of the hallway, aligned

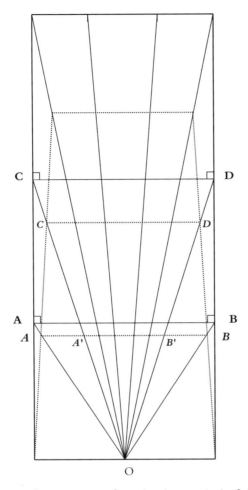

Figure 5.2. Phenomenal space as a transformation (contraction) of physical space. The physical space, observer, and lines of sight are as in Fig. 5.1. Visual space is now represented by dotted lines, showing the phenomenal convergence of the sides of the alley and the contraction of distance. Phenomenal visual direction is assumed to match physical direction.

Observation suggests that the gross structure of this phenomenal space is a projective transformation of physical space. In a projective transformation, line segments map to line segments (preserving straightness), and junctions and

a comparison stimulus placed directly in front of them just below eye level to match the perceived convergence of the left wall at 1.5 to 2 m in front of them, and again at 3.5 to 4 m; the mean value for two observations from each of two observers was 9° and 8°. Fig. 5.2, which is merely illustrative, shows each side wall converging at an angle of 5°.

between-ness relations are preserved.[12] For planes perpendicular to the line of sight, the plane in visual space is (in gross structure) related to a corresponding plane in physical space by a transformation known as a *similarity*. In this transformation, affine relations are preserved, hence, parallels map to parallels, and in addition shape is preserved; only size is different, and is here contracted in the phenomenal structure in relation to its physical counterpart. For planes along the line of sight (the floor and walls), the relation is merely projective (parallels are not conserved).

Two further points may clarify this phenomenal description and its graphic representation. First, the phenomenology represented in Figure 5.2 is not of a two-dimensional or flat scene such as might result from taking the painter's attitude. Perceiving the alley as if projected onto a plane a few feet in front of the observer would be an instance of the painter's attitude. It yields a dramatically different spatial structure. For instance, the angles between a vertical line on the wall (not shown) and the line where wall and floor meet at A and B would be much more acute than when the base lines of the alley are experienced as receding in depth (as in Fig. 5.2).[13] The phenomenology of Figure 5.2 is of three-dimensional depth.[14] Locations on the walls are seen at a distance, even though they are not phenomenally presented at the precise inverse or actual physical distance. Distances are contracted, but present. Perceived size does not reduce to visual angle; distance conditions it. Extensity alone does not determine phenomenally presented size; CD is phenomenally larger than would be $A'B'$, even though $A'B'$ would take up the same visual extent.[15]

[12] The projective relation here is a mathematical relation between geometrical descriptions of physical space and phenomenal space; although the relation between the two spaces is causally mediated by an optical projection into the observer's eyes, the present projective relation pertains exclusively to the two spaces as given structures, not to their causal relation. On projective geometry, see Yaglom (1962–75).

[13] In preliminary observations in the hallway described in n. 11, observers set a caliper to match (1) the perceived angle at which the floor-wall junction recedes from a vertical door frame 2.8 m in front of the observation post, and then (2) to match the angle for the same junction when imaginatively projected onto a plane at arm's length in front of them (they were allowed to close one eye if they wanted). In four observations, the mean value in the first condition was 85°, in the second condition, 29°.

[14] French (1987) argues that even if our experience includes the surface of the 2½-D sketch (varying in depth), a two-dimensional topology is adequate to describe such a surface. (Helmholtz 1924–5, 3:159, made a similar point.) From this, he concludes that visual space is "really" two-dimensional. However, even in describing the surface present in the 2½-D sketch, it is convenient to use a three-dimensional space in which the surface is embedded. More importantly, if distance from the perceiver is taken to be a part of phenomenal experience (and hence as an aspect of phenomenal space as presented in experience), as I have taken it here, then three dimensions are required for describing visual space.

[15] The present description thus differs from Rock's (1975) theoretical description of extensity. Rock equated perceived extensity with visual angle, and hence with "projective size, analytic size, or visual-field size" (Rock 1975, 39, note). But Fig. 5.2 represents phenomenal size in accordance with

Second, this description need not imply a lack of constancy, on two counts. First, according to the relational (or proportionality) hypothesis for size constancy (reviewed in Rock 1975, ch. 2, and Palmer 1999, ch. 7), constancy arises from the constant proportion objects bear to one another when viewed together at various distances. These proportions remain constant because all objects undergo the same contraction. If I observe a man and his dog, the dog remains knee-high whether I observe the pair at 5 m or at 20 m. These objective proportions are preserved even though phenomenal space is contracted. Second, constancy judgments may be attained despite phenomenal contraction if part of what underlies such judgments is a further cognitive act, which uses phenomenally perceived layout to infer Euclidean size. Indow (1991) calls this the "Euclidean mapping," and he assumes that it goes on even if phenomenal space is non-Euclidean (or is projectively contracted). In the situation in Figure 5.2, perceivers might treat the phenomenally contracted spatial structure as a representation of a physically Euclidean structure. In *personal space* (Cutting and Vishton 1995), the effects of contraction are nonexistent or negligible (in the central portion of the visual field). Those sizes might be taken as standard sizes. The phenomenally contracted spatial structures with which more distant objects are presented would then be used to judge (or might tacitly be associated with) isotropic Euclidean physical structure. This might occur through conscious learning, unconscious association or judgment, or innately. The relation between phenomenal spatial structure and perceivers' judgments of spatial properties is complex (Carlson 1977), and this Euclidean mapping has been little investigated.

The precise geometry of visual space remains unknown, and it may not have a homogeneous metric structure. Still, a phenomenological description of the sort associated with Figure 5.2 illustrates how visual space can present us with objects in depth (preserving various objective proportions, and various nonmetric relations), without phenomenally presenting an isotropic Euclidean space. This sort of description is consistent with the notion that structures in visual space *resemble* (but are not congruent with) physical space; so are the more specific investigations of geometrical transformations between physical and visual space (e.g., Koenderink *et al.* 2002; Todd *et al.* 2001). This resemblance relation rests on the projective relations described above between structures in visual and those in physical space (such as lines, angles, and surfaces). It can sustain a notion of veridicality in which information about physical spatial structure is phenomenally presented by a resembling spatial structure.

---

both visual angle and (contracted) distance. Hence, things seen at different distances under the same angle vary in phenomenal size, as remarked above.

8. Representation and the Tasks of Visual Perception

Visual perception allows sighted organisms to interact effectively with their environments. To serve that function perception must represent the environment with some degree of accuracy. Need it represent the environment "as it is"? That depends on the notion of accuracy or veridicality in play. Clearly, full and accurate representation of the physical, chemical, or biological properties of the environment is not required, nor does perceptual representation even remotely approach such completeness. Otherwise, knowledge of nature would be easier to attain.

In Section 5, I distinguished two sorts of relations between perceptual representation and the represented environment: a sign relation, and a relation of resemblance. In principle, it would be possible for the perceptual system to rely exclusively on a sign relation in carrying out its task. That is, perception might simply generate regular correspondences between types of environmental state and arbitrarily selected states of the organism. The organism would be well served if certain representational signs were realized in it *if and only if* certain biologically salient states of affairs obtained in the world. A flower of a certain reflectance property would induce one internal state, a shadow pattern with a certain rate of increase in its size would induce another; these might then guide behavior (e.g., approach or avoidance).

Color is a good candidate for a sign–representational relation. Objects differentially reflect light of various wavelengths, but they appear phenomenally red, green, yellow, blue, and so on. These phenomenal colors do not resemble a spectral reflectance property, but they might serve as signs for various classes of reflectances.

Reflecting on this relationship, we might say that the world appears colored because we experience it that way. That is, the property presented as phenomenal color is not an intrinsic or basic physical property (as it was thought to be in Aristotelian physics). Phenomenal color has intentional or phenomenal existence as a sign for properties of physical surfaces. We see the world as colored because of the phenomenal properties of the vehicle that represents it to us, phenomenal color experience. [See also Ch. 11.]

It would in principle also be possible for spatial relations to be represented entirely through sign relations. An arbitrarily complex homomorphism of elements and relations could represent arbitrarily complex spatial structures. Thus, triplets of numbers can represent locations in three-dimensional space. If these triplets are encoded as numerals (or sequences of neural spikes, or what have you), the spatial properties of the representational vehicle are irrelevant to their representing function. No resemblance relation would be needed. (Edelman 1998 develops Shepard's second-order isomorphism along such lines.)

However, there are grounds for positing a resemblance relation in human spatial perception between the represented domain (Euclidean three-dimensional physical space from a point of view) and the representing domain (a contracted projective transformation, with or without homogeneous metric). Physical spatial structures are represented by phenomenal spatial structures. Unlike a mere sign relation, both the representing and the represented domains exhibit spatial structure; the representing domain represents physical spatial structures via transformed but similar phenomenal spatial structures. It did not have to be that way, but it is. Why so? I am tempted to say that we see the world as spatial because it is that way. Assuming that the world actually has spatial structure, we may presume that human representational capacities have been shaped to present that structure via phenomenal visual space. Although philosophical skeptics or idealists might contend that space is no more "really" a property of the world than phenomenal color, and hence that we merely think the world is spatial because we experience it that way, a touch of realism about the physical world suggests the opposite.

During the mid twentieth century, talk of phenomenal or visual space was nearly banned from psychology and philosophy. The arguments that Shepard (1981) reviewed, as examined in Section 4, offer some insight into this curious phenomenon. In those days, it seemed as if a simple materialism might suffice for thinking about the mind–body problem. All the same, some perceptual psychologists continued to think and write about phenomenal experience (Rock 1975), and some theorists distinguished between (phenomenally defined) visual space and physical space (Buffart and Leeuwenberg 1978; Luneburg 1947), a distinction much invoked of late (Hershenson 1999; Indow 1991; Koenderink et al. 2000, 2002; Todd et al. 2001). More recent discussions in philosophy of mind (e.g., Chalmers 1996; G. Strawson 1994) suggest that the considerations summarized by Shepard (1981) were less constraining on perceptual theory than he imagined. Perceptual theorizing is constrained not only by regularities in the environment (and possibly their internal representation). It is also constrained by philosophical presuppositions. In both domains, continuing research can reveal new features of constraints and create a new environment for theorizing.

6

On Perceptual Constancy

Human perception normally occurs through stimulation of nerve endings that leads to brain activity and conscious perception.[1] For example, vision normally occurs when light reflected from objects stimulates the receptor cells in the retina. Phenomenologically speaking, the content of the visual perception corresponds more closely to distant objects than to the patterns of light on the retina. When we are observing a rectangular table while standing at one end, it projects a trapezoidal shape onto the retina, yet our experience of the shape of the tabletop tends toward that of a rectangle in depth. As we walk along the sidewalk, the features of the objects around us sweep across the retina (expanding outward from our fixation point), and yet we do not perceive the world as expanding outward or as moving; rather, we perceive ourselves as moving through a stable world.

These and other phenomena are instances of what is called "perceptual constancy." From the times of Ptolemy, Ibn al-Haytham, and Descartes (see Epstein 1977*a*, and Ch. 12), theorists have noted and discussed the phenomena of *constancy* with respect to size, shape, and color (though without using that

Previous versions of this chapter (which is first published here) were presented at the Riken Brain Science Institute, Tokyo (August 2004); the Center for Cognitive Sciences, University of Minnesota (October 2005); the Philosophy Department, CUNY Graduate Center (February 2006); the Philosophy Department, Ohio State University (April 2006); and the Institute of Philosophy, University of London (October 2006). I am grateful to audience members for their comments and criticisms and to Mark Wagner, Carl Granrud, and an anonymous referee for the Oxford University Press for written comments.

[1] Some forms of perceptual response, broadly construed, may not involve consciousness, such as blind sight (Weiskrantz 1986) and preconscious responses that determine "perceptual set" (e.g., facilitating or interfering in tasks involving color naming following subliminal presentation of consistent or inconsistent color words, Marcel 1983). Further, the question of what counts as "conscious" (attended content? phenomenally present content? conceptualized content?) is an intricate matter that evokes differing answers depending on one's theoretical perspective. At this point, I am simply signaling my intent to focus on "conscious perception," leaving until later any further qualifications.

specific term). These phenomenal observations resulted in various theoretical proposals about the kinds of mental or psychological processes that underlie the tendency toward constancy. Ibn al-Haytham and Descartes (see Ch. 4) each proposed that unconscious processes combine received information to yield perceptions of size and of shape that differ from proximal stimulation (visual angle and projective shape). They, and many subsequent theorists, did not explicitly address the extent to which human vision actually achieves constancy (to use the modern term).

More recently, theorists have proposed (or assumed) that the aim or function of perception is to achieve full constancy with respect to several physical aspects of visual objects. In the case of shape and color, complete constancy entails that a rectangular table would "look rectangular" whenever its surface is viewed from a sufficiently high elevation for perceivers to see it well, or that a colored object would present the same specific shade of color to perceivers under a wide range of illumination (morning and afternoon sunlight, indirect sunlight, even artificial illumination). According to this conception, a perceptual outcome that does not attain full constancy should be regarded as a failure to achieve the functional target of perception.

In accordance with this conception of the function of perception, theorists have postulated underlying processes in which the visual system combines or analyzes information so as to yield constancy. In the case of the table, this might involve combining the projective shape of the table with information about its slant so as to yield a representation (and a phenomenal experience) of the table as rectangular. For colored objects, this might involve decoupling the illumination falling upon an object from the reflective properties of the object's surface, and representing (and phenomenally experiencing a shade of color corresponding to) those reflective properties. For objects of the same size at different distances, it would involve combining the objects' various projective sizes (as recorded at the retina) with information about the distance of each object so as to yield a representation (and a phenomenal experience) of the true size of each object: all are of equal size.

My purpose in this chapter is to reconsider the notion of perceptual constancy from the ground up. This will involve distinguishing the *phenomenology* of perceptual constancy and stability from a *functional characterization* of perception as aiming at full constancy. Once these are distinguished, we can attend to the phenomenology of constancy itself, and ask to what extent human perceivers attain constancy, as usually defined. In discussing the phenomenology,[2]

---

[2] In philosophy, the term "phenomenology" properly refers to the phenomenological movement (of Brentano, Husserl, and Heidegger), which sought to philosophize by starting from descriptions

I distinguish *phenomenal presentations* of spatial features and color properties from *categorizations, conceptualizations,* and *judgments* that underlie verbal or other responses to those presentations. In making this distinction, I do not assume that visual experiences of colors and shapes normally occur without our categorizing or conceptualizing those colors and shapes; rather, I simply distinguish the phenomenal presentation of colors and shapes from the perceiver's categorizing them. Although phenomenal presentation and categorization commonly co-occur, they are distinct aspects of experience.[3]

The chapter begins by reviewing several standard descriptions of constancy from the psychological literature, which have also been incorporated into philosophical discussions. I then present laboratory findings and my own phenomenological descriptions by way of showing that, although perception "tends toward" constancy, human perceivers do not usually attain full constancy for either spatial or chromatic properties—a fact that many investigators acknowledge. Using examples that I believe to be uncontroversial, I catalogue some ways that color perception falls short of full constancy. I then turn to spatial perception. Here, I find that the phenomenology has been systematically misdescribed, and I offer a more adequate description of the phenomenology of everyday spatial perception.

My greatest quarrel with previous theory concerns the functional aim of the constancies. I argue not only that perception does not achieve full constancy but that we should not characterize it as aiming for full constancy. Rather, perception seeks a stability of representation suitable for guiding our actions and which can also, as needed, enable us to classify and re-identify objects by phenomenally presented properties such as shape, size, or color.

---

of experience that were devoid of the terminology of any particular metaphysical or epistemological theory. Phenomenologists took a "neutral" or "descriptive" attitude toward the content of conscious experience. I am here employing the term in the same spirit with respect to descriptions of perceptual experience; in this usage, the term carries the connotation that the descriptions are free of commitment to a particular theory regarding the representational content or function of perception. Theorists in the Gestalt psychological tradition (philosophers and psychologists alike) used the term this way, including Köhler (1947, 3–5), Koffka (1935, 73), and Gurwitsch (1964, 5); this *psychological* phenomenology differed from *philosophical* phenomenology in that it did not invoke a methodological or theoretical suspension of belief in the existence of perceptual objects and of the world of physics (see Gurwitsch 1964, 163–4). As described here (and in Ch. 1.1), I distinguish the phenomenological method of description (and its results) from the *phenomenality* or *determinate phenomenal character* of spatial structures and colors in perceptual experience.

[3] This distinction does not assume that perceptual content is inherently nonconceptual, for it is consistent with a view that allows modularized conceptualizing processes to produce color and shape representations that central processes then categorize (as in Rock 1983 and Fodor 1983, although Rock doesn't use the term "modular"). In fact, however, I believe that bare perceptions of color and shape arise from nonconceptual processes and possess nonconceptual content. In my view, however, that does not make them nonintentional (nonrepresentational): see Chs. 1–3, 5, 9, 11.

Further, I argue that theorists should not confuse these classifications with the qualitative character of phenomenal experience. My arguments underscore the need to distinguish phenomenal representation (better, "presentation") from conceptual categorization, and to distinguish perceptual presentations from subsequent processes that are involved in responding to them.[4]

1. Descriptions and Theories of Constancy

The constancies attracted considerable attention in perceptual psychology throughout the twentieth century. From early on, two ways of describing the constancies appeared in the literature: as bare facts about the comparative stability of perceptual experience, and as tendencies of perception to represent the "real" or "true" properties of objects.

The first conception of constancy highlights the tendency of perceived qualities to remain stable or constant despite large variations in the proximal stimulus (for vision, the retinal image). Irvin Rock explained the term "constancy" by noting the following "general fact" about the "phenomenal world": "perceived qualities such as color, size, and the like tend to remain *constant* despite the fact that the proximal stimulus, for example, the retinal image of objects, is continually changing" (Rock 1975, 10; see also Shebilske and Peters 1995, 227). Here, constancy is defined by contrasting *phenomenal stability* with proximal *stimulus variation*. There is no implication that these stably perceived qualities accurately represent the properties of the objects (their colors, sizes, shapes, etc.) that cause the proximal stimuli and, ultimately, the resulting perceptions.

In the second usage, constancies yield stable perception of the objective properties of things despite proximal variation. Robert Woodworth, having noted the "radical" changes in the retinal image as we move about, proposed that "in spite of the visual flux the objects seem to remain in the same places. In short, what we perceive is the objective situation" (1938, 595). Perceptual constancy is not a matter of mere stability; rather, it is the stable perception of

---

[4] Nothing in what I've just said entails that categorization or conceptualization plays no top-down role in the production of perceptual representations. That is an empirical matter. My conceptual distinction between these two aspects of the overall process of reaching a perceptual judgment permits questions about the specific relations between perception and categorization to be posed, without assuming a particular answer to those questions. Of course, it wouldn't make sense to draw the distinction unless one assumed that perception is not *wholly* top down, but this assumption (that there is *some* receptor-driven contribution) is not controversial. Finally, as in Ch. 5 (n. 5), I use "presentation" for phenomenal contents themselves, and "representation" for their actual or putative relations to objects and their properties.

things *as they are* (that is, with the sizes, shapes, colors, etc., that they have). (See also Gibson 1950, 23.)

The second conception is the more theoretically ambitious, for it suggests not only a fact about perceptual experience but a functional context in which to understand the fact: perception aims to represent things as they are, with respect at least to properties such as size, shape, and color. Accordingly, a given perception of these properties must achieve full constancy in order to be fully successful. Otherwise, it has failed to meet its functional aim.

Perceptual theorists disagree over whether perception typically achieves full constancy. James J. Gibson (1950), in drawing his distinction between the "visual field" and the "visual world," concluded that full constancy is normally attained. The *visual field* has the properties of a two-dimensional projection in "linear perspective": parallel lines converge, as when we look down "a highway" or "railroad tracks" (p. 35), and shapes present a "projective" aspect (circles at a slant appear elliptical). In the phenomenal *visual world*, by contrast, objects "remain constant in size, whatever their distance" (33). Similarly, the shape of an object in three-dimensions (its "depth shape") "remains constant from whatever direction it is viewed," while the "projective shape" varies with viewing angle (34). Gibson maintained that such constancy occurs in what are typically called "full cue" conditions, in which the light is good and the observer is free to use both eyes and to move about in a normal environment. Other theorists who assert that full constancy of shape and size usually occurs in such conditions, at least within certain limits on distance or on object-slant, include the psychologists Rock (1975, 38–9) and Stephen Palmer (1999, 23–4) and the philosophers Patrick Heelan (1983, 27–8) and Robert Schwartz (1994, 59).

The experimental literature on the constancies paints a more varied picture, in which perceptual experience may not exactly match either objective or projective properties. From the classical articles of Robert Thouless (1931, 1932) onwards, investigators have acknowledged that, even in full cue conditions, the perception of size and of shape may exhibit "underconstancy": reported phenomenal size is near to but less than real size, and reported phenomenal shape is nearer to real shape than to projective shape. In describing these findings, Thouless explicitly distinguished projective shape and real shape, as stimulus properties, from apparent or perceived shape, as present in visual experience. Theoretically, apparent or perceived shape might match either the projective or the real shape, or even a different (but related) shape. He presented his subjects with square and circular stimuli, which he rotated about a major axis so that they were viewed at one or another degree of slant; the square projected any of several compressed diamond shapes and the circle projected various ellipses. He asked subjects to match the shape that they perceived to a series of standards (or to draw what they saw). Typically, subjects reported a shape closer to real shape than to projective shape. Thouless (1931, 344) called this "phenomenal regression to the 'real' object," and he found it for size, shape, chromatic color, and achromatic (white/black/grey) color. Other authors subsequently reformulated Thouless' phrase as "phenomenal regression *toward* the real object" (Woodworth 1938, 597). The finding of underconstancy has been partially replicated for both shape (e.g., Epstein *et al.* 1977) and size (Epstein 1963; Granrud 2004, 79; Wagner 2006, 130). Many investigations have found that children exhibit more underconstancy for size than do adults, who often exhibit good constancy or even overconstancy (Granrud 2004, 75−6).

The literature further establishes that the way in which the experimenter explains the perceptual task to subjects greatly affects the outcome. Depending on what instructions subjects are given, or what questions they are asked, their perceptual reports differ systematically (Carlson 1977). The early literature did not explicitly control such factors and some ambiguity resulted. Woodworth and Schossberg (1954, 485) noted such ambiguity in the use of the term "perceived size," with authors variously using that term to describe "judged size" relative to a standard (subjects point to a matching standard); "apparent or phenomenal size" (a report of experience, as in Thouless); or "estimated size" (a guess in terms of feet or meters).

In fact, matters are even more complicated. For tasks involving shape, experimenters may variously ask subjects to judge or estimate or report the real shape of things, relying on their perceptions; to describe the phenomenal or apparent shape, leaving aside their guesses about real shape; or even to judge or report the projective shape (the shape that the object would project onto a two-dimensional plane at right angles to the line of sight). Several investigators have studied the effects of such varied instructions on subjects' responses. Reviewing this literature, V. R. Carlson (1977) distinguished "projective," "apparent," and "objective" instructions. The first type asks subjects to assess the projective shape; the second, to report neutrally (without cognitive "correction") how the shape looks; and the third, to report the real shape they believe the object to have. Overall, projective instructions yield close to projective results, apparent instructions yield underconstancy or perfect constancy, and objective instructions yield constancy or overconstancy (the size is overestimated, the shape is overcorrected). Similar effects of apparent and objective instructions have been found for achromatic color constancy (Hurvich and Jameson 1966, 102−3) and for color matching (Arend *et al.* 1991). Under apparent instructions, subjects are asked to describe the phenomenal properties of perceptual presentations; under objective instructions, they seek to describe the properties that they judge the object to have.

I want to consider various descriptions of the aim of constancy, postponing my examination of the phenomenology of constancy until Section 2. Where theorists explicitly address the aim of constancy, they almost universally agree that the perceiver, or the perceiver's perceptual system, aims at full constancy. The precise theoretical description of this aim has varied. In the earlier literature, theorists spoke of achieving phenomenal presentations that represent an object with the properties that it has: its veridical or objective size, shape, position, or color. Here, we should understand veridical size, shape, and position phenomenally: they are properties of objects as they appear and as those properties might be objectively determined using household measuring instruments (ruler, plumb bob); the terms do not refer to the microphysical properties that underlie the spatial extension of an object and the object's rigidity (Thouless 1932, 1, n. 1). Color also was understood as a phenomenal property: the objective color of an object's surface is the one that it phenomenally presents under "normal" or "common" viewing conditions; objective color typically was not defined through the physical reflectivities that underlie it (Hering 1905–20/1964, 3, 14; Thouless 1932, 1, n. 1; Woodworth and Schlossberg 1954, 429–30, 433).

Although some investigators continue to understand the constancies of size, shape, and color in phenomenal terms, others have adopted a physicalist attitude toward the problem of constancy. This attitude is most clearly present in formulations of perceptual constancy as seeking to solve an "inverse problem": that of inferring back from the proximal stimulus to its physical cause. For perception of surface color, this becomes the task of recovering the spectral reflectance distribution (SRD) of an object's surface. An SRD is a physical description of the reflectance properties of a surface for each wavelength in the range of visible light (see Fig. 8.1); specifically, it graphs the percentage of light that the surface reflects (and so, the complement of what it absorbs) for each wavelength. The task of recovering SRDs is difficult because the light reaching the eye is a product of the SRD and the ambient illumination (which can differ in its spectral properties, even in natural conditions, as in the spectral differences between midday light and early morning or late afternoon light). Investigators who endorse this task analysis have developed sophisticated theories of how the visual system might use information about (or assumptions about) ambient illumination to discount that illumination's contribution to the light reaching the eye. In that way, the visual system might determine (or approximate) the value of the SRD (Maloney and Wandell 1986; Hurlbert 1998). Here, the aim of constancy is to produce a mental representation of the physical properties of surfaces.

Some investigators also cast the spatial constancies as inverse problems. This builds upon the usual description of spatial vision as a problem of solving the "inherent ambiguity" of the visual stimulus by "inferring back" to the structural features (size, shape, position, orientation) of the objects. However, as William Epstein (1995, 11–12) has observed, in describing the spatial constancies as inverse problems, one need not endorse the traditional view of the retinal image as a two-dimensional static pattern: one is permitted to acknowledge the additional sources of information that arise from motion, texture gradients, stereopsis, and the like. Even if the information sources are rich, the visual system must still recover the distal structures by using this information (together with processing rules and/or assumptions). In any event, unlike the case of color constancy, the inverse-inference approach to spatial constancies does not portray the visual system as inferring back to microphysical reflectance properties, but rather to macrolevel geometrical structures. Nonetheless, to the extent that the description of these structures is formalized in one of the known physically possible geometries (Euclidean or non-Euclidean), we may describe the resulting formulation of the inverse problem as *physicalist*. The physicalism in this case guides the selection of candidate geometries for describing the gross structure of perceptual space.

2. A Closer Look at the Phenomenology of Constancy

Before considering more closely the various *models* of color constancy and the spatial constancies (in subsequent sections), we must carefully attend to the *phenomenology* of the constancies. In this effort, I rely primarily on my own phenomenological observations, which I describe for the reader so that he or she can confirm them; but I also refer to published reports and laboratory results.

Simple phenomenological reflection reveals that constancy is not perfect, for color or for spatial properties. Let us consider each in turn, paying close attention to the phenomenal prediction that would match full constancy, and comparing it with ordinary experience.

If color constancy were perfect, uniformly painted walls would appear in an absolutely uniform manner: we would discount the effects of illumination, shadow, reflected light from adjacent colored surfaces, and the like, in order to retrieve either the color as it appears in standard conditions (in the earlier definition of constancy) or the SRD of the pigment (in a more recent conception). We patently do not achieve such constancy, as most investigators readily concede. Perceived color typically does move toward constancy and away from hues corresponding to retinally projected patches of light; but we do not experience full constancy. At the same time, we do not typically form false beliefs about the pigmentation of uniformly painted walls. While the effects of varying illumination and shadow are readily apparent to us phenomenally, these effects do not make us complain to the painter that the pigmentation is not uniform (as if the painter had used several cans of paint that didn't match). We readily judge that the paint is uniform (similar to Carlson's "objective" instructions). Still, the phenomenal appearance exhibits the differing illumination, and so constancy is not perfect (see also Jameson and Hurvich 1989 and Mausfeld 2003).[5]

Deviations from full spatial constancy, while frequently noted, have proven more difficult to describe and conceptualize. Recall Gibson's (1950, ch. 3) distinction between the visual field and the visual world. The visual field has the properties of a perspective projection, in which train tracks converge and objects appear with their projective shapes, whereas in the visual world, the tracks do not converge and a slanted circle appears as a circle in depth. Gibson (1950, 35) intended these as mutually exclusive phenomenal structures,

---

[5] Some recent philosophical works address breakdowns in color constancy and the effects of instructions on the experience of constancy. The authors accommodate these facts to their own theories of the metaphysics of color or of color experience. Hilbert (2005) contends that physicalism about surface colors can be defended against the failure of full constancy by assuming that the visual system is also representing the physical characteristics of illuminants and shading, so that a shaded area of a white surface might look similar to a more brightly illuminated grey surface, and the mottling of a uniformly pigmented surface would be produced by the visual system's representing physical variations in the illuminant. Noë (2004, ch. 4) holds that we use our knowledge of changes in "apparent color" under varying lighting conditions in order to perceive the "invariant" "actual color" of a thing (p. 127). Cohen (2008) counters that full color constancy *does not* require that a uniformly pigmented surface appear uniform under mottled illumination but consists in the fact that observers can infer what the surface would look like under ideally uniform illumination (an ability that I assimilate to a judgment made under "objective" instructions), which is an apparent revival of a "memory color" interpretation once commonly discussed in the psychological literature (e.g., Woodworth 1938, 597). By contrast, Mausfeld (2003) contends that color perception is not about retrieving an invariant physical property or an ideal appearance, but involves both (1) representing surfaces in comparatively (but not invariantly) distinctive ways and (2) perceiving facts about illumination. I appeal to the failure of full color constancy and to the effects of instructions in supporting my biopsychological account of color perception (presented in 1992 in what is here Ch. 8 and further developed in Hatfield 1999 and Chs. 9–11). As recounted in Sec. 3, I maintain with Mausfeld that colors are not simple, determinate properties of things, but I differ from Mausfeld in considering the functions of color perception in an evolutionary and comparative context.

and he averred that we experience the visual field only under reduced cue conditions or by adopting a special attitude. Rock (1975, 37–9), by contrast, contended that aspects of both geometries are simultaneously present in phenomenal experience. He appealed to artist's perspective in describing the appearance of converging railway tracks or of people farther away as appearing in some sense smaller, which he labels "perceived extensity" as opposed to "objective" perception (Rock 1975, 38). Rock later characterized this visual extensity as a "proximal mode" representation that mirrors the retinal image (1977, 339–49; 1983, 254–65). He explained the phenomenal convergence of railway tracks during the experience of constancy as involving simultaneous access to both objective properties and the proximal-mode representation.

These positions offer us two alternatives: full constancy or a two-dimensional perspective projection. Accordingly, if we find that the train tracks (or the sidewalk, the roadway, or a hallway we look down) exhibit phenomenal convergence, we should believe we are accessing such a projection. If we find ourselves perceiving that the train tracks (and the other pathways) do not show phenomenal convergence, we should think of ourselves as experiencing them with full constancy, while perhaps (in Rock's view) simultaneously accessing the perspective properties.[6]

I contend that these phenomenological alternatives are incomplete. As descriptive tools, I find that they are inadequate in two respects. First, I believe that the typical gross structure of visual experience matches *neither* full constancy *nor* a perspective projection; rather, it has some qualitative features of the latter (convergence of parallels within experience) but it is metrically closer to the former (tendency toward constancy). Second, I hold that our ability to respond to true, objective, or physical sizes and shapes arises from judgmental or recognitional abilities that are psychologically distinct from the visual appearances themselves but are phenomenologically integrated into our occurrent experience. In the remainder of this section I will present

---

[6] Some philosophers, following the standard psychological literature mentioned here, also offer these two options, e.g., Peacocke (1983, 12, 19–24), who follows Rock (1977) in holding that both aspects are simultaneously present in perception. Lowe (1992) contends that "visual experience" is isomorphic to the two-dimensional retinal image (a perspective projection), and that we apply tacit knowledge of geometrical transformations to come to know three-dimensional objects. Noë (2004, 83–4, 166–7) holds that through "apparent shape" (a linear perspective projection, as in Gibson's visual field or Rock's extensity) we at the same time experience the objective shape (by having sensorimotor knowledge of how the perspective shape can change as we shift our viewpoint). I offer an alternative phenomenology, in which perceptual experience typically deviates from full constancy in the direction of but in a markedly different manner than Rock's described extensity (or proximal mode representation).

phenomenological descriptions to support the first point, putting off until Section 4 my arguments for the second point.

In my experience, the train tracks (roadway, sidewalk, hallway) always give an appearance of converging lines in normal perception. These lines, however, do not appear to converge in the way in which a perspective projection would. If I were experiencing a perspective projection as I look down a hallway, the lines formed where the walls meet the floor would appear to be on a two-dimensional surface and would rapidly converge as they ran up the picture plane. That is not how the hallway looks when it presents an apparent convergence. Instead, the hallway appears to be a three-dimensional structure that phenomenally contracts with greater distance. The contraction does not at all fool me, and I readily judge that the hallway does not become narrower as it proceeds away from me (similar to the reports of subjects under "objective" instructions). Similarly, people sitting in the back of a room in which I am lecturing exhibit less visual extent than those in the front. They do not have the appearance that would coincide with a retinal projection, in which they would diminish in area as the square of the distance: someone at eight yards would occupy one-sixteenth the area of someone at two yards. Rather, I see them as having a size-at-a-distance, which is noticeably diminished in visual extent (they fall under a smaller visual angle) but is not equivalent to a perspective projection (experienced as in a plane near the observer).

The phenomenology of size and distance perception is usually misdescribed because this third descriptive alternative, of a contracted three-dimensional space, has largely been ignored. As a result, the contracted space has not been distinguished from a perspective projection, and so has not been available as a description of a perceived space that exhibits contraction and diminution of phenomenal size while also remaining closer to full constancy than to projective values. Such a description accommodates the phenomenology of converging lines in a manner distinct from both Gibson's visual field and Rock's proximal-mode extensity.

Part of the reason that the phenomenological divergence from full constancy has not been prominent in the literature is that scientific as well as philosophical investigators have not appreciated the phenomenological implications of full constancy. Some of these implications have been well described, especially for size constancy: with full constancy, objects of the same size should appear with exactly the same size despite being at different distances. (Again, "appear" here does not mean simply that we can *tell*—that is, judge—that they are the same size from how they look.) But researchers do not as readily acknowledge the implications of full constancy for hallways and railway tracks: two five-foot lengths of track should, with full constancy, occupy as much phenomenal extension in depth when viewed at two yards as when viewed at ten yards. With full constancy, we should see a hallway with no phenomenal convergence whatsoever; the distant and the near portions of the hallway should take up equal portions of my three-dimensional phenomenal space.[7] But appearances are normally otherwise, or so I claim: with distance from the observer, three-dimensional space phenomenally contracts.

This contraction is uniform, or nearly so. That explains why the railway tracks (and the lines where the walls meet the floor in a hallway) appear straight (even while converging). The contraction is greatest in the depth dimension, but it occurs to a lesser degree in the horizontal and vertical dimensions, so that visual direction is preserved (see Fig. 6.4, below).[8] Visual direction is also preserved with full constancy, and it can be preserved in a perspective projection onto a plane. But a perspective projection is two-dimensional, and my contracted phenomenal space is three-dimensional. My contracted visual space and a visual space of full constancy are two different versions of three-dimensional transformations of physical space into visual space (the full-constancy transformation yielding total congruity).

---

[7] The reader who has trouble visualizing this scenario should examine Fig. 5.1 and compare it to 5.2 (or attend to the outer, solid lines in Fig. 6.4 below as "full constancy," and compare that to the dotted lines). Note that a five-foot length seen at two yards would be seen under a larger angle than would the same length at ten yards, but that both would have the same extension-in-depth. A reader may object that the experience I describe here is precluded by the fact that our seeing of the hallway is from a point of view, so that the contraction is a direct product of the geometry of the lines of sight in the hallway. I invite that reader to study Fig. 5.1 and to note that it portrays a visual space in which (1) visual direction is preserved, but (2) full constancy (no convergence) is obtained. Sections of the hallway farther away are seen under smaller angles, but the lines between the side walls and the floor do not converge, because true or physical distance is phenomenally present. I thus decouple visual angle from perceived (two-dimensional) extensity.

[8] In preserving visual direction, my contracted space differs from that of other proposed contractions, such as Wagner's (2006) affine and vector contractions, which occur only in the dimension running away from the perceiver, not in the height and width of the plane perpendicular to the principal line of sight. My contraction is greatest along the depth dimension, but it also occurs in the horizontal and vertical dimensions (as in Fig. 5.2 and Fig. 6.4). It is similar to the description of phenomenal size provided by Aage Slomann (1968), who also criticizes the standard view of size constancy. In Gogel's (1990) scheme, my proposed phenomenology for typical viewing conditions would be represented as follows: perception of direction is accurate (or nearly so, for foveal and near peripheral vision); distance is systematically contracted; and perceiver's motion is accurate as to direction. Another way of describing my contracted space says that it projects physical three-dimensional structures into visual space along the lines of sight toward the observer, but only part way (whereas the usual perspective projection goes into a two-dimensional surface). Of course, the perceptual system mediates these "projections" from physical to visual space. In effect, I am comparing the physical structure that anchors Wagner's (2006, 132–6) stimulus transformation (from object structure to retinal pattern) with the product of his "inverse transformation" (from registered proximal values to perceptually represented spatial structure). His notion of *inverse transformation* allows a variety of relations between proximal values and perceptual structure, even though, like inverse-problem theorists (Epstein 1995; Palmer 1999, 23), Wagner himself (2006, 134) assumes that full constancy is the aim.

This contraction does not explain the elliptical aspect of dinner plates: that is a matter to be explained in terms of visual direction and visual angle. The width of the dinner plate in front of the person across from us has a greater visual extent than does its depth, front to back (from where we sit), simply as a matter of visual direction. Because the plate is slanted in depth relative to our principal line of sight, the two side points diverge more in visual direction than do the front and back points, and so the angular extent is wider from side to side than from front to back, which might account for the reported phenomenal extensity and sense of ellipticity if the observer attended to visual angle while ignoring phenomenal depth. Nonetheless, the shape may appear as a tilted circle in three dimensions (there is no experienced frontoparallel ellipse, except under a visual-field attitude). The compressed angularity from front to back does not result from a planar perspective projection, nor does it depend on the spatial contraction that I've described. A similar projective transformation of visual direction would occur for a slanted circle under full constancy of size and distance. Under my phenomenal contraction, a dinner plate at a slant is only slightly diminished in its more distant hemicircle. Consequently, phenomenal shape constancy for relatively small objects seen at moderate slants should be close to full, whereas size constancy—under apparent as opposed to objective instructions—should deviate from full constancy at a regular rate with distance. (I discuss phenomenal shape for larger objects in Section 4.)

How, then, do I account for the fact that, under objective instructions, perceivers achieve full constancy? I propose that our contracted spatial experience enables us to recognize or judge the real, objective physical shapes and sizes with some accuracy. Further, the products of such judgments or acts of recognition are phenomenologically present in our experience, in the same way that its being the case that we are experiencing a table or seeing a meadow is phenomenologically present, despite the fact that recognizing something as a table or as a meadow is a conceptual achievement that results from learning. I call this the *phenomenological presence of the conceptual*. I distinguish what is phenomenologically present in consciousness (including the products of recognition, classification, and judgment) from what is presented in a phenomenally concrete manner—in vision, spatial and chromatic properties, such as colored surfaces with a shape at a location. Visual consciousness includes the concretely phenomenal and also other, more abstract, content (Chs. 1, 7). In labeling acts of recognition "conceptual," I assume that some basic concepts are functions among the varying appearances of an individual, that is, that some concepts are recognitional.

For the moment, I will simply assume that my phenomenological observations are basically correct as descriptions of the gross structure of our experiences of colors, shapes, sizes, and distances. I want next to consider how reflection on these observations might affect our conceptions of color constancy and the spatial constancies.

3. Color Constancy and the Functions of Color Vision

What are the functions of color vision? What is color vision *for*? In posing these questions, I mean to be asking about the biological and psychological functions of color vision, not about the personal or cultural values that any of us may place on colors and our experiences of them. I am asking a question that might be answered by considering the biological evolution of color vision. For the human case, we can approach this question by considering the advantages of trichromacy over dichromacy from the standpoint of natural selection.

Color vision occurs when an animal's nervous system enables it to respond to differences in the spectral composition of the light that reaches the eyes. In surface-perceivers such as mammals, color perception makes surfaces appear differently colored. Color vision requires at least two types of photoreceptor that are sensitive to different ranges of the electromagnetic spectrum (within what is termed the "visible" range). These photoreceptors are characterized by their maximal sensitivity to a specific wavelength, with diminishing sensitivity to surrounding wavelengths (as in Fig. 6.1).

Most mammals are *dichromats*, which means that they have only two cone types: one type that is sensitive in the short-wavelength portion of the spectrum (short-wavelength-sensitive, or SWS, cones), and one in the middle portion (at or near the middle-wavelength-sensitive, or MWS, cone type shown in Fig. 6.1). In dichromatic color vision, the nervous system compares the relative activation of these distinct cone types. The experienced hue varies according to whether only one of the two receptor types fires, or each type fires to some degree, or only the other type fires. Dichromats lack the third cone type that is characteristic of *trichromats*, such as human beings and some other primates. A trichromatic visual system compares the activation of three cone types, including a new cone type in the long-wavelength portion of the spectrum (a long-wavelength-sensitive, or LWS, cone type, as in Fig. 6.1). Trichromacy arose when the MWS cone type bifurcated to yield two cone types with somewhat differing sensitivities: the MWS and LWS cone types. In the current human population, the MWS

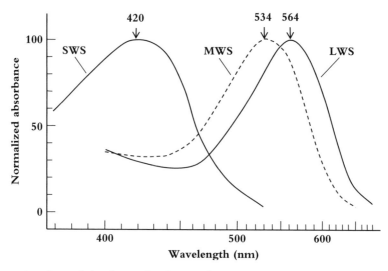

Figure 6.1. Spectral absorbance distributions for cones in a normal human trichromat. The absorbances are normalized in relation to the maximum absorption for each cone type. Although the MWS and LWS cones are more sensitive than the SWS cones, that difference is not shown here. Typical dichromats (including most mammals) have two cone types. The point of maximum sensitivity for dichromatic photoreceptors varies from species to species (see Jacobs 1993), and usually (but not always) includes a SWS cone paired with a cone near the range from the MWS to LWS cones. These curves are after Bowmaker and Dartnall (1980, fig. 2).

and LWS cones each show a small polymorphism in their peak sensitivity of about 5–7 nm (Neitz et al. 1993). Presumably, in the course of evolution, a larger polymorphism allowed two distinct cone types to arise in the middle-to long-wavelength end of the spectrum (separate MWS and LWS cones), which yielded trichromatic color vision once the nervous system changed so that it could compare the outputs of three cone types (SWS and the now distinct MWS and LWS cone types). Trichromacy yielded greater discrimination in the spectral region in which we now see green, yellow, orange, and red.

According to one hypothesis, other mammalian dichromats have blue–yellow color vision. When trichromacy arose, a green–red color system was added. Since the late nineteenth century, the dominant explanation for the evolution of the new, trichromatic sensitivities has been the fruit-discrimination hypothesis. What appear to trichromats as green leaves and yellow, orange, or red fruit would have differed only in brightness to dichromats (or leaves and fruit would have shown minor variation in shade within a single hue). For trichromats, the yellow, orange, or red fruit stands out phenomenally from green foliage (Mollon, 1989). Recent discussions suggest that other heightened discriminations may also have been involved (Vogel *et al.* 2007).

I will assume that the fruit-detection hypothesis, or an extension of it, is true. The question is how to describe the selection pressure that yielded the fixation of trichromacy. Responses to this question in turn depend on how we conceive the function or task of color vision.

Let us consider two different analyses. According to one, which inverse-inference physicalists favor, the task of color vision is to recover the SRDs of distal surfaces. Trichromacy is an advance over dichromacy because tri-chromats approach the full recovery of unique SRDs more closely. They get closer, but not all the way there: as the phenomenon of metamerism shows (see Ch. 8), the human trichromatic system is incapable of fully recovering unique SRDs. Accordingly, if one equates object colors with SRDs, objects have colors that trichromats are unable to detect under ecologically normal illumination (see Hilbert 1987, 91). (This failure is distinct from the failure to fully discount variations in illumination as described in Sec. 2.) Because this analysis regards recovery of physical SRDs to be the functional target of color vision, I call it the *physical instrument* conception of color vision (Ch. 8).

According to a second conception, a function of color vision is to increase discriminability of objects based on hue rather than brightness. For this purpose, resolution of unique SRDs is not needed. The selective advantage of trichromacy would be explained if trichromacy makes things more usefully discriminable by hue. On the fruit hypothesis, the ready discriminability of yellow, orange, and red from green explains the advantage. We may call this the *perceptual systems* conception of color vision.[9] According to it, selection works on receptors and neural mechanisms that yield phenomenal experiences of color—or color qualia—so as to present us with a world in phenomenal colors that enhance discriminability. The precise hues assigned to ranges of physical stimuli, and indeed the range of hues itself, are presumably to be explained through accidental variation in the brain tissue that produces hue-experience, with such tissues then being selected during the subsequent evolutionary

---

[9] As in Ch. 8, I label the second conception a "perceptual systems" approach, to indicate its affinity with the ecological approach of Gibson—despite the fact that Gibson's own few remarks on color vision (1950, 168; 1966, 183; 1979, 30–1) are closer to a physical instrument conception (and, in my view, thereby favor classical physics over Gibsonian ecological physics). This second conception is consonant with the "sign discrimination" analysis of the epistemic function of phenomenal color content in Ch. 11. Of course, either a perceptual-systems or sign-discrimination view could come to hold that what color represents in objects is in fact a unique SRD; but neither starts with a prejudice in favor of physicalistic descriptions, and neither is likely to arrive at such a description for color (or other sensory attributes).

process.[10] In order to achieve enhanced discriminability, color vision need neither recover unique SRDs nor achieve full phenomenal constancy.

This approach can encompass other functions of color vision that do not require full constancy. In considering the evolution of color vision, Jacobs (1981, ch. 6; 1993) describes the comparative advantages of color vision for object detection, object recognition, and object-property signaling. The first works when a trichromatic primate perceives red or yellow fruit as standing out from its surroundings, or perceives an individual piece of fruit as a unified object despite dappled lighting or despite a fragmented view (as when illumination is broken by the leaves of a tree or an object is seen through a leafy bower). The second involves recognizing the fruit to be of a given type by its color (and, presumably, by its shape as well); and the third might involve detecting a degree of ripeness.

None of these tasks requires full constancy. Fruit will be more discriminable to perceivers if, under natural variation in illumination, it looks some shade of red (but not necessarily always the same shade) by comparison with whatever shade of green for the leaves that surround it. Similarly for the other tasks. The fruit can be detected as red, or as ripe, if it appears with a relatively stable range of reddish hues. It need not exhibit exactly the same shade under changes in illumination.

On the perceptual-systems view, when color vision does not achieve full constancy, it is not failing its task, because achieving full constancy is not its function. We should judge the performance of color vision in terms of discriminability, recognizability, and property signaling. Color vision may fall short. But the judgment that it does fall short will not be based on the fact of metamerism or on the fact that perception does not attain full constancy. As Dorothea Jameson and Leo Hurvich (1989, 2–3) have observed, perception of shadows and other aspects of illumination that are phenomenally present may be advantageous because they provide information about lighting conditions, time of day, or even about the weather. Indeed, Rainer Mausfeld (2003) shows that color scientists in the 1920s and 1930s prominently discussed the perception of illumination as part of the phenomenology of color perception, and they demonstrated such perception through laboratory findings. Perceiving the illumination may be another function of color vision.

---

[10] No theory of color experience can, at present, explain why we experience the phenomenal hues that we experience: that would require a solution to the mind–body problem. Here (and in Ch. 11) I simply assume that the receptors and brain tissue that yield phenomenal experience of hues arise through mutation or otherwise exhibit variations that are subject to selection. A deeper explanation of the qualitative character of those hues requires further work (some progress might be made by considering signal properties, such as red for ripeness and for sexual readiness).

Finally, the perceptual-systems view of color vision may explain how perceivers can recognize objects by identifying their stable colors, without implying that object colors should be equated with a precise shade. Here, the proper standard of "same object color" will not be a precise match in phenomenal hue (of a certain saturation and brightness). This view frees us to modify the concept of "same physical color" so that it allows for a variation in phenomenal appearance under differing conditions of illumination and in relation to adjacent colors or other aspects of the perceptual context. Accordingly, to qualify as a particular instance of red, it would suffice to appear within a certain range of red hues under normal variations in illumination (Ch. 9). This relaxed standard of what counts as a determinate object color (see also Hatfield 1999 and Mausfeld 2003) goes a long way toward removing objections to color objectivity that subjectivists such as C. L. Hardin (1988) have posed.

4. Size and Shape Constancy and the Geometry of Visual Space

In Section 2, I argued that the phenomenology of size constancy has been misdescribed. I challenged the belief of some investigators that full phenomenal constancy obtains at least for moderate distances. In the case of shape constancy, I maintain that phenomenal constancy is expected for small objects under my contracted visual space, and that this contraction explains apparent deviations from full constancy for larger objects (such as table tops). I am also challenging the widely held theoretical tenet that full phenomenal constancy is or should be the *aim* of size perception, and it is to that question—of whether full phenomenal size constancy *should* obtain—that I now turn.

According to inverse-inference theories, the visual system seeks to infer back to the actual three-dimensional structure of physical objects. At the scale of human spatial perception, this structure is Euclidean. Figure 6.2 shows the implications of inferring back. Objects O_1 and O_2 would be phenomenally identical in size. Similarly, in Figure 5.1, the actual location of the walls of a hallway would be presented to us phenomenally; there would be no phenomenal convergence.

The conception that full phenomenal constancy is and should be the target of size constancy rests upon the physicalist assumption that perception aims phenomenally to present physical sizes "as they are." Accordingly, such a presentation would be required or·would at least be selectively preferred for successful spatial behavior.

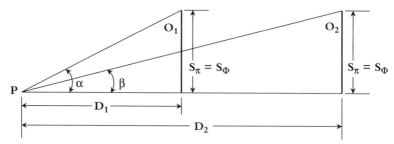

Figure 6.2. Representation of full phenomenal constancy for two objects, O_1 and O_2, of the same size at different distances (D_1 and D_2) from the perceiver. Because the objects are at different distances, the perceiver, P, sees the objects under different angles; the nearer object (O_1) is seen under a larger angle (α). The perceiver who achieves full phenomenal constancy would nonetheless phenomenally experience the actual physical size in each case, and so would find the objects to be phenomenally the same in size. In that case, where S_Φ is phenomenal size and S_π is physical size, $S_\Phi = S_\pi$.

It strikes me that full phenomenal size constancy would not be adaptive, if only because it would give equal representational weight to the near and the far. But surely it is better to give greater phenomenal weight to what is near, while still preserving adequate information about the size, shape, and direction of what is far. As James Cutting and Peter Vishton (1995) have argued, human perceptual space is focused on near and moderate distances. As I have observed (and as readers can observe), at even moderate distances objects diminish somewhat in phenomenal extent. Things within reaching distance are represented so that sight and touch exhibit strong and precise agreement (see Sec. 5). With distance, the phenomenal extent of objects falls off. The exact structure of this contracted visual space is an empirical matter. As with color qualia, its exact properties presumably could be explained by considering the evolution of spatial representation.

The apparent desirability of full phenomenal constancy has rested on the assumption that it would be needed for effective object cognition and for guiding action. But a phenomenally contracted space also allows accurate judgments and effective action. How can this be? There are two factors to consider. First, the posited contraction affects all spatial structures in it: the trains are phenomenally smaller down where the tracks have converged. If you see a man and his dog, the dog is knee-high whether the man is at ten paces or twenty paces. In general, human perceivers see objects in contexts that provide proportional size information (Rock and Ebenholtz 1959; Palmer 1999, 319–20); perceivers may also derive proportional size information from the amount of surrounding optical texture that an object occludes (Gibson 1950, ch. 9). Second, we have lived with the phenomenal contraction all our lives, so we are used to it. People in the back of the room occupy the phenomenal space that we expect people of their size to occupy at that distance (I here adapt A. A. Blank's position, as reported in Grünbaum 1973, 156). In that sense, their diminished size is neither an error nor an illusion (any more than metameric matches are errors in color vision). Spatial structures normally exhibit such phenomenal diminution, and these phenomenal presentations nonetheless enable perceivers to perform recognitional or judgmental operations.

Under conditions of contracted appearances, then, we might well expect accurate judgments of physical size. Indeed, some theoreticians have suggested that "full constancy" size judgments are in fact just that: judgments of actual size rather than accurate descriptions of appearances. Carl Granrud (2004), in particular, has argued that, for both adults and children, apparent size diminishes with distance. However, between the ages of 5 and 10, children typically learn to correct for this apparent diminution. More specifically, he reports that both adults and children enjoy full phenomenal size constancy for things up close (to 3 meters); there is underconstancy for near distances (5 or 6.1 meters, in his experiments); and, for adults and children who are savvy to the effects of distance, there is full constancy or slight overconstancy at a far distance (61 meters). Upon investigating the role of perceptual knowledge in developmental changes with respect to size perception at far distances, Granrud found that children who have learned to reason about the effects of distance on apparent size show slight underconstancy at near distances (5 or 6.1 meters). For far distances, they exhibit underconstancy under instructions to report "apparent size" (as do adults), but they exhibit full constancy or overconstancy under instructions to report "objective size." By contrast, children who did not show they could reason about the effects of distance exhibit no difference between apparent and objective instructions. Granrud (2004) proposes that "adults and children have the same perceptual experience" (p. 78) of apparent size diminishing with distance, and that "far-distance size constancy results from a cognitive judgment and is not a feature of perception" (p. 89), by which he means that it is not a feature of the phenomenal spatial structure of perceptual experience but is an added cognitive result.

Granrud (2004, 78) believes that phenomenal size perception diminishes with distance "due to poor depth cue information"; poor information causes physical distance to be under perceived, which, in accordance with the size-distance invariance hypothesis, yields a perception of size that is diminished with respect to physical size. Several investigators in the twentieth century proposed that poor depth information is not required for diminishing phenomenal size to occur. They maintained that visual space is structured so that, even in full cue conditions (such as Granrud employed), the entire visual space contracts with distance, yielding diminished phenomenal size with increasing distance (again, in accordance with the size-distance invariance hypothesis). This hypothesis was initially studied in Germany by Franz Hillebrand (1902). He directed subjects, under full cue conditions, to arrange black cords on a white tabletop so that they appeared to form parallel line segments that departed from two points of fixed separation at the distant end; he also asked subjects to adjust a curtain of threads suspended from above so as to produce phenomenally parallel walls. He found that, in order for the cords to appear parallel, subjects set them to diverge as they ran from near to far (and that the wall of threads also diverged and was slightly curved). Subsequently, Walter Blumenfeld (1913) asked subjects to adjust individual lights in an otherwise dark alley so that they formed either phenomenally parallel lines from far to near (the "parallel alley"), or equidistant horizontal intervals at various distances (the "distance alley"). Blumenfeld found that, under these reduced-cue conditions, the parallel-appearing lights diverged even more than had Hillebrand's cords. Neither experimenter supposed that their findings supported a non-Euclidean geometry for visual space; each inferred a phenomenal contraction.

In the 1940s, the mathematician Rudolf K. Luneburg, working at the Dartmouth Eye Institute, reinterpreted these results in accordance with non-Euclidean geometry: he proposed that visual space is a hyperbolic space of constant curvature. His argument depended, in part, on the difference that Blumenfeld had found between the parallel and distance alleys. Subsequently, Tarow Indow investigated these same findings, collecting further data under parallel and distance conditions (Indow *et al.* 1962). Figure 6.3 plots his primary data. In the experiment, the farthest points (Q) were fixed and the subject set lights to be parallel (filled circles) or to yield equidistant pairs (open circles). With some reservations, Indow (1982) concluded that his findings are consistent with Luneburg's conclusion that visual space is a non-Euclidean space of constant negative curvature. Luneburg (1947, 39) explained the desirability that the space be of constant curvature on the grounds that such spaces meet the conditions usually associated with *physical possibility*: that objects can freely rotate and move in space without altering their shapes. He added that only spaces of constant curvature permit true size constancy. Indow (1991) reaffirmed the desirability of constant curvature, while also expressing caution about empirical fit. From other data, he concluded that planes perpendicular to the line of sight are Euclidean in structure, so that any

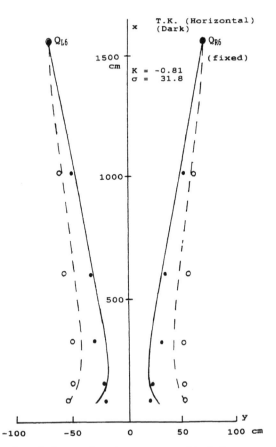

Figure 6.3. Data from Indow *et al.* 1962, as presented in Indow 1995 (fig. 1.2). The filled circles are the parallel condition; the open circles, the distance condition. Although Indow (1995) has fit a curved line to the parallel condition, which is consistent with a hyperbolic non-Euclidean space, the data points line up as straight lines, which is consistent with a 3-D to 3-D transformation that yields a contracted Euclidean space. Copyright © 1995 by Lawrence Erlbaum and reprinted with permission.

curvature of visual space would be in the depth dimension (relative to the viewer).

Let us reconsider Indow's empirical finding. First, consider the parallel condition. Although Indow has drawn a curved line (in Fig. 6.3), consistent with the hypothesis of a non-Euclidean space of negative curvature, the dots in fact fall very near to a straight line. This finding is consistent with a contracted three-dimensional Euclidean structure. If phenomenally parallel lines expand physically from near to far, then physically parallel lines would contract near to far. The distance alley exhibits a slight curve, more on the left than on the right. However, the procedure of setting lights to be equidistant differs from that of setting lights to be phenomenally parallel. These two tasks are different, but Indow assumes that they both yield measurements of the positions of the lights in a common visual space. However, the difference between the phenomenally parallel and the distance alleys may be due either to task differences or to phenomenal differences (or to both). Indow's conclusion that the geometry of visual space is non-Euclidean requires the second interpretation, whereas my contracted three-dimensional space is consistent with the first.

Indow is one of a few recent investigators who have empirically studied the global structure of visual space. Mark Wagner, who has also done extensive empirical work in the area, provides the most thorough discussion of the theoretical alternatives (Wagner 2006). Wagner is skeptical that visual space would actually meet the axioms that define a consistent physical space, including free mobility of objects without distortion. He reviewed literature that shows deviations from Euclidean structure (e.g., Koenderink et al. 2000) while producing no single constant metric, and also showing dynamic effects on judgments of size and orientation that depend on the presence or absence of stimuli besides the target object (Thorndyke 1981; Schoumans et al. 2002; see also Indow 1991, 450). Wagner favors the position that there is no single metric for visual space but that multiple metrics may arise depending on the visual task, and that variable metrics may apply to a single phenomenal experience. He thus concludes that "no single geometry can fully encompass human visual experience" (2006, 223; see also Suppes 1977). All the same, he proposes as a general fact about human visual experience that it contracts with respect to physical space in the depth dimension, that is, the direction running away from the observer (Wagner 2006, ch. 7).

I agree with Wagner that no single geometrical structure describes the relation of human visual experience to physical spatial structures. This is true even if only for the following reason: if the visual field experience of the artist fully transforms into a phenomenal experience of objects as projected onto a two-dimensional plane (Gibson's "visual field"), the result differs from ordinary three-dimensional experience. I also agree with Wagner (and others, see Wagner 2006, ch. 3) that it is unreasonable to suppose (as did Luneburg 1947) that visual space must conform to axioms that also characterize a physically possible space (understood to include free mobility). From the Ames demonstration in which a rotating trapezoid appears to be a rectangular window that waggles back and forth (Ames 1961), we know that phenomenal spatial structure can violate physical constraints. In the demonstration, a solid rod placed in the rotating window appears to make a complete rotation while the window appears to change direction and waggle back; the rod appears to pass through the solid window frame (Gregory 1997, 188).

Wagner proposes a contracted space in the depth dimension only (defined as perpendicular to a vertical plane that might transect the midpoints of the observer's eyes). By contrast, I have proposed a contraction with respect to physical distance along all lines of sight. The contraction is such that visual direction is preserved (at least for foveal and near peripheral vision). Direction can be preserved only if height and width are also compressed.[11] As shown in Figure 6.4, the compression is greater in the depth dimension than in height and width.[12]

My proposal is that, under full cue conditions, the gross structure of visual space exhibits a contraction as I have described it. I have left the degree of contraction unspecified, even though, of necessity, Figure 6.4 shows a specific degree. From my own phenomenal experience, I would guess that the contraction is uniform or nearly so, but its precise structure is an empirical matter. Further, it is quite possible that there are distortions near the edges of objects under some conditions, or that there are slight bends (even variable slight bends) as one proceeds outward in depth (or from near into far peripheral vision). Such deviations again are a matter for empirical investigation. They do not detract from the general phenomenal fact of a direction-preserving contraction.

This contraction of phenomenal space can explain the apparent convergence of train tracks, walks, roadways, and hallways without supposing that, during normal vision, we phenomenally access a proximal mode representation of the retinal image. In a true perspective projection of a hallway, perhaps observed from midway between the walls and looking down the long axis (as in Fig. 6.5), the angle made by the junction of a doorjamb, as a physically (and phenomenally) vertical line, and the line formed by the juncture of floor and wall, is quite acute (about 37° in Fig. 6.5). But in our phenomenal experience of the hallway in three dimensions, with the line formed where floor and

---

[11] In Gogel's (1990) scheme (n. 8), visual direction is (nearly) accurate in the following three cases: full phenomenal constancy; my contracted space; and a perspective projection. The three cases are in the same family of projective transformations (which allows many 3-D structures between the two extremes). For full phenomenal constancy, distance would be presented at the physical distance; for my contracted space, distance would be systematically contracted, as in Fig. 6.4; for a perspective projection, distance along each line of sight would be contracted onto a plane near the observer.

[12] Fig. 6.4, which is adapted from Fig. 5.2, shows a greater compression than Fig. 5.2. Its compression is closer to the empirical results reported in Ch. 5, n. 11 (for angle of apparent convergence), and it is also closer to the empirical values for compression discussed by Wagner (2006, ch. 7).

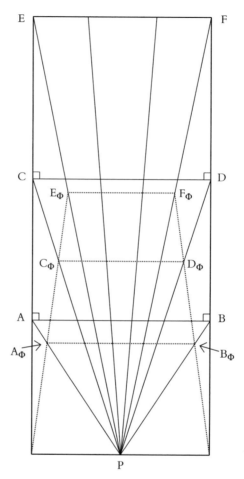

Figure 6.4. Phenomenal visual space as a transformation (contraction) with respect to physical space. A top view of a perceiver P looking down an alley with physically parallel sides. The view shows the lines of sight at eye level. If full phenomenal constancy obtained, the perceiver would experience points A–F in their physical locations (A–F). In a contracted phenomenal space, which the dotted lines represents, the sides of the alley converge, the distant end is phenomenally nearer, and physical points A–F are presented phenomenally at A_Φ–F_Φ. Note that in this contracted space, visual direction is preserved; further, perceivers encounter equal lengths (such as AB and CD) under decreasing visual angle with distance, a fact that obtains both under full phenomenal constancy and in the contracted visual space that I propose. In the contracted space illustrated here, the sides of the walls converge at an angle of 8° relative to physical space (see Ch. 5, n. 11).

wall meet running away from us in depth, the same angle has been measured at between 80° and 85° (Ch. 5, n. 11). The same angle presumably characterizes the convergence of the walls of the hallway. This phenomenal convergence occurs in depth. The phenomenally experienced hallway, with converging sides, is a three-dimensional structure. It thereby deviates radically from Gibson's two-dimensional visual field and Rock's proximal-mode two-dimensional image, but it also differs from Gibson's and Rock's uncontracted Euclidean visual world.

My proposed contracted space doesn't exhibit free mobility and so does not meet the usual conditions on a physically possible space. Objects diminish phenomenally with distance. Since direction to physical locations is preserved for any given scene, we have basic information for navigating this space successfully. Further, in accordance with Granrud's proposals, we are readily able to judge true physical size and shape. As I see it, the results of such judgments may become phenomenologically present to us not as phenomenally concrete spatial structures but as cognitive information that permeates our experience of such spatial structures, just as the fact that something is a book or a table also is typically present in our total phenomenological experience of a scene. This is what I have labeled the phenomenological presence of the conceptual.

Finally, this contracted space also affects phenomenally presented shape. For relatively small shapes, such as a dinner plate that is slanted with respect to the line of sight, the contraction has little effect. For larger objects, such as a rectangular table, the phenomenal contraction is quite evident. Descriptions of this contraction often assimilate it to a planar perspective projection. My view, to repeat, is that we experience tabletops as running away from us in depth. The tabletop has a three-dimensional phenomenal structure that contracts away from full phenomenal constancy; it is, however, closer in phenomenal shape to constancy (rectangularity) than it is to a true perspective image. Again, I do not regard this contraction as being either an error or an illusion. It is the normal mode in which we experience physically rectangular shapes that are at an angle to the line of sight. As with size, we are readily able to judge the physically rectangular shape from the trapezoid that is presented phenomenally in depth.

5. Spatial Vision and the Guidance of Action

A primary function of visual spatial perception is to guide actions. After Wagner (2006, 177) reviewed a substantial body of literature indicating that

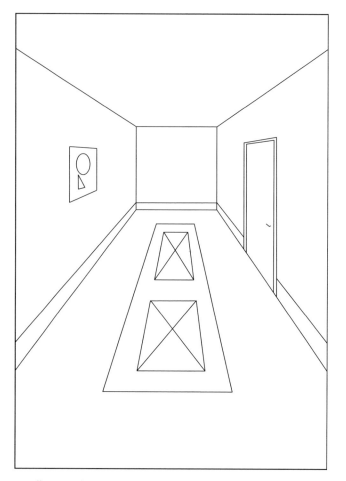

Figure 6.5. Hallway with picture, rug, and doorway. In a two-dimensional perspective projection, a right angle formed by the floor and the upright doorjamb may project as an acute angle. In this figure, the angle between the doorjamb and the line formed by the juncture of the floor and wall is 37°. Phenomenally, the angle formed in depth when perceivers observe a real hallway and experience it in three dimensions is between 80° and 85°. The hallway as normally perceived runs away in depth, unlike a perspective image, which takes the three-dimensional structure into a two-dimensional plane.

structures in visual space deviate from structures in physical space, he rightly asked: "Given that our perceptual world is so distorted, how can we survive?" He offers a variety of answers: many tasks do not require accurate distance perception; we may learn to judge size and shape from "distorted" visual experience; in a regularly contracted space, the geodesic (shortest path) is the same as in standard Euclidean space (2006, 177–81). Further, he cites studies showing that, for tasks such as way-finding and catching a fly ball, perceivers do not require and most likely do not employ metric information about distance. Instead, perceivers are sensitive to information in optic flow that represents relations among visual directions (Todd 1981; McBeath *et al.* 1996).

I am sympathetic to many of Wagner's conclusions, but I would modify and supplement them. First, instead of describing visual space as variously "distorted" in relation to physical space, I say that visual space is variously *transformed* from physical space. To call it "distorted" suggests that perceptual space *should* phenomenally present the physical Euclidean structure. The operative dimension of "shouldness" here, as Wagner intuits, is adaptive guidance of interaction with the world. But if a contracted visual space can nonetheless guide action and can also support reasonably accurate judgments of size, distance, and shape, it meets this "should."

Beyond the factors that Wagner notes to explain how a transformed visual space could guide successful action, I would add that, for the range of near vision, any contraction or other transformation is not great (the precise structure of personal space is an empirical matter). Further, visual direction is conserved (or nearly so) in my contracted space. Reaching requires coordination between the visual and tactual systems. For direction or metric distance in the ambit of personal space (about one meter in front of the perceiver), few problems would arise. Further, studies with distorting lenses suggest that the visual and tactual systems constantly seek agreement between their represented spaces (reviewed in Rock 1975, 174–80). In these studies, reaching behavior readapts to a visual world that is truly distorted. This suggests that in the normal case touch and slightly transformed vision would stay in harmony.

In addition, the worlds of tactual and visual experience have a common basis in the physical world. As we move through the world, things that were presented as phenomenally smaller loom larger, in that they occupy a larger visual angle. This is true on any plausible transformation scheme (perspective, contracted 3-D, or full phenomenal constancy). It is also true that, on any transformation scheme, the stable properties of the objective world anchor the series of transformations that we expect. The transformation scheme that I have described yields contracted but regular phenomenal constancy (i.e., stable phenomenal underconstancy). A series of regularly contracted three-dimensional vistas should enable us to recognize the stable physical properties of things, for example, the rectangularity of the table.

Finally, relying on my own phenomenal experience, I propose that, for ordinary uses of vision in full cue conditions, the gross structure of contracted visual space is relatively stable and that the metric of contraction is close to constant, subject to dynamic interactions or local bending. If so, this general regularity in visual space could help explain how our judgments of objective size and shape reach something close to full constancy (corresponding to experimental subjects who receive "objective" instructions).

But if phenomenal spatial structure is stable, how do I account for the reports in the literature of overconstancy and full constancy with respect to size perception? To explain the overconstancy judgments, I follow Walter Gogel (1990) and Granrud (2004) in pointing to cognitive overcorrection. Individuals know that objects farther away take up less phenomenal extent (as determined by visual direction); when told to give the "real size," they overcorrect. I would apply this explanatory strategy on a case-by-case basis to the various experiments on size and shape constancy, seeking to sort out cognitive or judgmental factors from reports of phenomenal structure.

6. Theories of Vision and the Reality of Visual Qualities

Perceptual constancy—to whatever degree, and whether apparent or object-ive—is the result of physiological processes that we must characterize psychologically if they are to enter into explanations of perception (see Chs. 14–15). In this chapter, I have proposed that phenomenal constancy of size, shape, and color is only partial, and that cognitive processes of recognition and judgment underlie responses that attain objective constancy. These acts of recognition and judgment—of things as red or blue, round or square, at a distance and in an orientation—depend on concepts, and they may involve inferences. I hold that the results of these conceptual acts are phenomeno-logically present in visual experience, as when we see a dog and its doghood is part of our overall experience.

What psychological processes underlie phenomenal constancy, or the pro-duction of phenomenally concrete visual experiences of things of a size, shape, and color at a distance? Such concrete experiences constitute the pictorial aspects of vision: experiences of sizes and shapes at a distance, of a shade of color, etc. The psychology of vision offers several types of explanations for these sense-perceptual aspects of vision, including Gestalt, Gibsonian, and con-structivist theories (Ch. 2). The Gestaltists (Koffka 1935, Köhler 1947) found the ultimate explanation of size and shape constancy in brain patterns that respond to invariant features in the stimulation that objects produce, yielding phenomenal constancy. Gibson (1950, 1966) developed a fuller analysis of such higher-order stimulus variables, and he proposed that the brain resonates to such information. Even if most theorists today accept Gibson's point about rich stimulus information, they believe that psychologically interesting processes must be responsible for detecting and responding to this information (see Ch. 2). They differ on the characteristics of those processes: whether they are inferential and therefore cognitive in nature (and then modular or not), or whether they arise from combining information in rule-instantiating mechanisms (Ch. 3.7; also Epstein 1995, 16).

Within the philosophy of perception, there is disagreement over whether phenomenal experience is conceptual or includes nonconceptual elements. This is in part a disagreement over whether imagistic or pictorially structured experience actually exists (Dennett 1988). Even without considering phenomena-denying phenophobes, disagreement remains concerning the content of visual experience: whether it is conceptual all the way down, or has *sui generis* phenomenal characteristics. Some hold that nonconceptual content would not be representational, whereas others (including myself, Chs. 1–2, 8–11) maintain that it can represent (see Crane 1992*b* and Peacocke 1992 for discussion).

These theories and disagreements are largely orthogonal to my investigation of the phenomenal structure of visual experience, chromatic and spatial. Whether perception results from brain resonance, noncognitive combining of information, modularized perceptual hypotheses, or unconscious cognitive inferences, the phenomenology might still be just as I have described it. A disagreement on phenomenology needn't reflect a disagreement about what underlies perceptual experience. As to philosophical theories of perceptual experience, even the phenophobe allows that it *seems as if* we have visual experience, and so one can ask what phenomenal structure it *seems to have*. More generally, in debates over whether the fine-grainedness of color experience can be accommodated on a conceptualist theory of visual experience, both sides admit that phenomenal color includes a rich range of shades (McDowell 1996, 56–60). Hence, adherence to any one of these positions regarding the psychological processes underlying perception or the nature of visual experience need not, in principle, disincline anyone toward my view, nor will holding my view push anyone into a particular camp (without other inducements).

Some theoretical positions are inconsistent with my adherence to color qualia and to a visual space distinct from physical space: the direct realism of Gibson (1966, 1979) and the related naive realism (Campbell 2002, ch. 6) and pure representational theories (Dretske 1995*b*, chs. 1–3; Tye 2000, chs. 3–4) of recent philosophy. Gibsonian and naive realism privilege physical properties and physical descriptions of the world. They hold that we simply perceive the world as it is, period. Other theorists, who posit representations to underlie visual experience, hold that, in veridical perception, the representational content of our experience just is the physical properties that are in front of us, which are available to us "transparently" (without any subjective intermediary); in illusions or hallucinations, we perceive content that is as if such physical properties were present.[13]

These positions typically adopt the view that phenomenal constancy is or should be complete: that color experience should track SRDs, that spatial experience should present an uncontracted Euclidean world.[14] Physical properties could then exhaust perceptual contents. In accordance with my phenomenal descriptions, I hold that visual experience presents the world in a way that is systematically related to but not congruent with physical structure. Color experience is systematically related to SRDs, but it does not represent that physical property. Rather, it presents various classes of surfaces as chromatically distinctive and so discriminable, but the classes do not have physical kinds (single SRDs) as their bases: from a physical point of view, the classes are disjunctive collections of SRDs. Spatial experience preserves directions and other features (such as straight lines), but it compresses space in the horizontal-vertical planes as they recede in distance, and even more so in depth along the lines of sight. Visual space exists in the phenomenal content of visual experience. It is world presenting (it presents the world from a point of view) in a *subjectively conditioned manner*, as opposed to a manner that is constituted

[13] There is an apparent tension between naive realism and physicalism: shouldn't the naive realist be more naive? In fact, earlier physicalist treatments of color in the philosophical literature were naive: they assumed that there is one physical property corresponding to each perceived shade (so, ignoring metamerism and context effects), as if light reflected from surfaces were from a narrow band of the spectrum (as opposed to the usual broadband SRDs of typical surfaces). By contrast, Dretske (1995*b*) imputes sophisticated representational content to the perceiver's visual system at a subpersonal level (in a way that is dependent on a causal or informational account of such content). Bill Brewer (2007) wants to develop a naive realism in which object properties themselves provide the content for perception (in ways that may be unknown to us). The color appearances of objects are to be explained wholly by object properties and lighting conditions, among other factors, thereby implausibly removing all subjective contribution to context effects and ignoring metamers, or perhaps saying that metameric surfaces are "physically similar" in an unspecified way—and a way that I claim *cannot* be specified except in relation to the perceiving subject (see Ch. 11.3).

[14] Some transparency theorists attempt to accommodate phenomena such as the allegedly elliptical "look" of the plate oblique to the line of sight by invoking objective physical "appearances" that obey the laws of pictorial perspective (e.g., Noë 2004, 83). They are caught in the old phenomenology and are attempting to explain an appearance that is, on my view, the artificial product of taking a special point of view. My contracted visual space is contracted in a way that can't be explained simply by pointing to physical facts; an explanation of its specific structure would need to account for the subject's special properties as a perceiver (which presumably result from a specific evolutionary history).

by the objective physical structure, or simply represents that structure. Our visual experience allows us to see the world, and thus to see it directly. We do not see our visual experience, even if that experience presents the world in a subjectively conditioned manner. Acceptance of subjective conditions to perception is consistent with a critical direct realism (see Chs. 1 and 11).

7. Conclusions

The phenomena of perceptual constancy have been noted for nearly two thousand years (for shape) and one thousand years (for color). In the twentieth century, two main conceptions of the constancies prevailed: as tendencies toward phenomenal stability, and as tendencies toward representing objects with the stable properties they have. The second conception has two versions: a tendency toward presenting colors as they appear under standard conditions and presenting gross physical shapes as they are; or, a tendency toward recovering the physically described SRDs of surfaces and the flat Euclidean structure (or other physically possible structure) of a scene's spatial properties. The second conception is an instance of physicalistic attitudes that were prevalent in many philosophical circles during the latter half of the twentieth century.

The conception that constancy seeks to recover object properties as they are is often allied with the view that the task of the perceptual system is to solve an "inverse problem": from proximal stimulation, the system aims to recover the actual properties of objects, usually under a physical description. I have argued, on phenomenological grounds, that perceptual systems typically do not yield full phenomenal constancy: color vision does not fully discount illumination and other contextual factors; metamerism occurs within the range of natural illuminants; size and shape constancy are not complete (although phenomenal sizes and shapes are normally nearer to objective sizes and shapes than to projective ones). Those who favor the inverse-problem approach would explain this circumstance as marking a failure of the visual system to achieve its targeted outcome.

I have argued that we should instead change our conception of the task of the perceptual system. We should not see it as seeking to present the world as it is physically, but rather as seeking phenomenal stability and regularity of appearance that are sufficient to serve discriminatory and recognitional tasks. Perceptual systems aim for phenomenal stability that allows perceivers to visually discriminate surfaces by hue, size, and shape and to recognize surface properties by generic hue groups and by size and shape, in part so perceivers can conceptualize and identify (or re-identify) objects by color, size, and shape. In this view, it is not an error or an illusion that uniformly painted walls vary in appearance because of contextual factors, that metameric surface colors are indistinguishable in daylight, that objects become phenomenally smaller with distance, or that rectangular objects appear trapezoidally in depth. Rather, these are normal appearances that are consistent with construing the function of the perceptual system as being to present the world in a way that can guide action and cognition. These representations may even be more serviceable than would be full phenomenal constancy: it might be better not to fully discount illumination, because phenomenal information about illumination may carry valuable information about local conditions; and it might be better to give greater phenomenal representation to nearer objects than to more distant objects, which entails that things are phenomenally smaller at greater distance and that shapes, when slanted to the line of sight, are compressed with distance.

As regards spatial perception in particular, I have proposed that visual space is contracted in a way that preserves visual direction. This contraction is greater in the depth dimension than in the horizontal and vertical dimensions. I propose that, in its gross structure, the contraction is constant over distance, although it may show dynamic effects near object boundaries, or exhibit small amounts of bending.

I distinguish phenomenal structures from judgments of physical size and shape and of stable hue category, and I contend that the results of such judgments are present phenomenologically in our overall perceptual experience. I recommend that the experimental literature be interpreted in a way that distinguishes the task of judging physical properties from that of providing phenomenal reports of spatial and chromatic appearances.

My phenomenological results and my reinterpretation of the task of constancy are orthogonal to many of the debates concerning the psychological processes underlying visual perception and to philosophical interpretations of visual experience. One can be constructivist or Gibsonian and still incorporate my claims about task analysis, while making suitable adjustments to one's overall position. One can be conceptualist or nonconceptualist about phenomenal content while accepting my results.

There are two exceptions. These results tell against the rampant naive realism and the pure representational theories of recent philosophy of perception. Naive realism says that the physical world itself constitutes the content of perceptual experience; pure representational theories hold that perceptual experience is constituted by informational content that represents the physical properties of objects. If my proposals about the constancies are correct, the world is presented to us through chromatic experience that collapses over physical descriptions of surface reflectance, and in a visual space that is systematically transformed from physical spatial structure. This spatial transformation cannot be predicted just by knowing the properties of the retinal image or the geometry of visual stimulation: it is not generated from an in-some-way-more-refined physicalist description. The ultimate explanation of our chromatic experience and of the normal geometry of visual space would come from deciphering the evolutionary processes that selected brain structures that yielded these specific phenomenal representations.

Perception presents the world with stability and constancy by comparison with the variation in proximal stimulation. It does so by yielding spatial and color experience that is closer to the physical spatial structure and color appearances in standard conditions than are retinal spatial forms and color patches. Although the structure of phenomenal experience deviates from full phenomenal constancy, it does so in such a way that visual experience can guide action and cognition. The structure of experience does not track physical properties physicalistically conceived, but it tracks object properties well enough to provide an adequate guide for navigation and to support ordinary cognitive tasks. Why expect it to do something else, when what it does do serves these purposes so well?

7

Getting Objects for Free (or Not)

THE PHILOSOPHY AND PSYCHOLOGY
OF OBJECT PERCEPTION

As adult human beings, we perceive objects effortlessly. We not only see the objects, in the sense that they are present in our visual fields, but we perceive them *as* objects. That is, we perceive them to be persisting, cohesive, unitary, individual things, many of which may be expected to retain their properties for weeks, months, years, or even millennia.

What does it take to perceive an object? This is a tricky question. If we construe it merely as asking what it takes to perceive something that is in fact an object,[1] we get a quick answer. Perceiving objects is easy, especially for humans and other surface-perceivers. We perceive things that are in fact objects merely in virtue of their being represented as discrete spatial structures in our field of vision. In the central cases, this means that a thing is perceptually represented as a segregated volume bounded by a surface. Anyone who visually represents as a segregated region what is in fact an object *sees* that object.

In asking what it takes to perceive an object we can, however, be asking for more. We may be asking what it takes to perceptually represent something *as* an object, or to be in a cognitive and perceptual state that has the representational

An earlier version of this chapter was presented in May 2003, in Paris at a joint colloquium of the Equipe Rationalites contemporaines, Department of Philosophy, University of Paris–Sorbonne (Paris IV), the Institut Jean Nicod, and the Department of Cognitive Studies of the Ecole normale supérieure; subsequent versions were presented to the Fourth International Conference on Cognitive Science, Sydney, Australia, July 2003, and the Philosophy Colloquium, University of Goias, Brazil, September 2003. I am indebted to the audience on each occasion for critical discussion, as also to an anonymous referee of the press for written comments.

[1] For the purposes of this chapter, I assume that middle-sized material objects exist as coherent, discrete entities. For those who disagree, I hope that my account of preconceptual perceptual segregation (Sec. 7) provides a common starting point from which various metaphysical theories about objects might proceed, each in its own way.

content *object*. To see something as an object, we need to have the concept of an object: of a persisting, spatially segregated individual entity. It is not enough merely to see something that is an object; we must be in a position to expect that it retains its identity over time, that we could (in principle) track its location in space, that we might encounter it (the same object) again on a later occasion, and so on.

In perceiving objects, often we do not merely perceive them as objects, but we perceive them to be objects of a particular type (this is especially true of objects we attend to). This sort of perception requires additional conceptual resources. To see something *as* a K, where K is a particular type of object (a table, a cup, a dog), we must possess the relevant concept (of *table*, *cup*, or *dog*). That involves more than simply seeing the thing over there to be a discrete thing; seeing something *as* a K classifies it as a particular type of thing. Sometimes, we do even more than that. We perceive the thing to be a known individual: my copy of *Gravity's Rainbow*, my friend David, my neighbor's car. Here we require more than conceptualizing the thing as an individual thing, or as an individual of a particular type; we conceptualize it as a previously known individual. That is to say, we *recognize* it.

The contrasts among these four notions can be illustrated by thinking of a perceiver who sees a particular object, say, my neighbor's cherry pitter. If we know that a perceiver with good eyesight is looking at the cherry pitter attentively under good conditions of observation, we can be reasonably sure that:

(1) He sees the cherry pitter.

(We can call this "simple seeing," or Dretske's (1969) "seeing$_n$.") But we need to know about his conceptual capabilities and background knowledge in order to distinguish the following cases:

(2) He perceives it as an object.
(3) He perceives it as a cherry pitter.
(4) He perceives it as my neighbor's cherry pitter.

In these cases, three relevant concepts are in play. A normal human perceiver who does not know what cherry pitters are might still perceive something that is a cherry pitter as a coherent thing, as an object of some (otherwise unknown) sort (as in (2)). If the perceiver is to perceive the thing as a cherry pitter, to represent it as being a cherry pitter, he or she must possess the concept of a cherry pitter (as in (3)). And a still more specialized conceptualization would be needed to see it as my neighbor's cherry pitter (as in (4)). All three conceptualizations classify the thing as an individual: as distinct from other objects and other cherry pitters, and as potentially reidentifiable (if only by its shape and location). But only (4) requires the ability to recognize it as the specific individual it is.

If we ask about object perception as involved in cases (2) through (4), the bar is raised. In order to ascribe *object content* to a perceptual act, we need to be able to ascribe to the perceptual and cognitive system the representation of the thing as a persisting individual entity. And in order to ascribe *object-kind content*, we need to be able to ascribe the ability to represent the thing as being of a particular kind. Finally, to allow *recognition* of an individual as a specific individual, we need to ascribe the conceptual resources involved in specifying a known individual.

In the past thirty years, object perception has been much discussed by philosophers (albeit usually as subsidiary to object reference in a belief context). They have devoted special attention to what it takes to make cognitive contact with an object in such a way that a subject's perceptions and thoughts are "of" or "about" the object. That is, they have asked how organisms make representational or referential contact with individual objects. Among naturalistic philosophers of mind, Tyler Burge (1977), Kent Bach (1982, 1987), François Recanati (1993), Fred Dretske (1995b), and others have sought to find a naturalistic relation that could effect contact. On their view, to perceive an object is just for the object to be in the right sort of relation (usually, a causal relation) to the perceptual system. In Dretske's (1995b, 25) terms, a referential relation—reference *de re*, "of the thing," as it is called—can be established merely by an object's being in a causal relation with the perceptual system; Burge (1977, 346) speaks of a *de re* "aboutness" relation, and Bach of a *de re* "representational" or "of-ness" relation, each established causally.[2] These authors rely on a relation between perceiver and object as in case (1), specifically arguing that the sorts of conceptualizations required in cases (2) to (4) should not enter into the most basic aboutness-fixing relation.

---

[2] The terminological differences here noted arise because Dretske (1995b, 25) and Recanati (1993, 98, 104) describe the relation between perceptions and object as a *referential* relation, whereas the other authors reserve the term "reference" for beliefs and linguistic acts (on which, see n. 3). In my discussion up through Section 6, I sometimes speak of *de re* referents of percepts (and pictures) as do Dretske and Recanati, while also glossing the relation as one of "aboutness" or "of-ness" in deference to Bach and Burge. From Section 7 onward, in perceptual cases I restrict the term "reference" to instances of mentally intending to single out an object. Finally, as do the authors I discuss, I may consider the aboutness relation as obtaining between distal objects and percepts or other states of the subject's visual system; while the personal/subpersonal distinction is important in many contexts, my discussions in this chapter concern how persons (or other organisms) can achieve a representational "of-ness" relation to objects through the operation of their perceptual and cognitive systems to create representations that may be subpersonal.

In my view, this makes object perception too easy. It has object perception arise as merely a result of *de facto* object seeing (of the "simple" sort, seeing$_n$). As I see it, this is to give the perceptual system its objects for free. I have nothing against free things. But when there's work to be done, it needs to be done. And I think there is work to be done here.

Psychologists are sensitive to questions about what it takes to perceive an object, and they have explored such questions with special attention to infant perception and cognition (Spelke 1990; Carey and Xu 2001). In investigating the structure and development of the concept of an object, or *object concept*, they have made proposals about what it might take to represent individual objects as objects. To that extent, they have raised the bar. But with respect to perceiving individual objects as individuals (as in (2) above), they have again tended to take their objects, or at least their individuals, for free.

My aim is to raise the bar yet further. In much of the work on infant psychology, object perception is equated with infant achievements that amount to perceiving something as a bounded, connected, cohesive, occludable, (perhaps) movable, (short-term) trackable volume. I believe that perceptually representing objects as individual objects requires more extensive resources than are needed for tracking volumes. For perception of a bounded, trackable volume to occur, the bounded area need not be individuated as a particular object but can be treated simply as a spatially coherent region. Such regions are occurrently countable, but their presence in perception does not yet require or imply an object concept, and it certainly does not entail a specific individual as content. To perceive objects in a cognitively pertinent manner, one must perceive them as individuals, which requires the relevant background conceptual capacities—at a minimum, those needed for (2), above. Further, the ability to refer to objects (or to enjoy perceptual states that establish or yield reference) requires this same background. Getting object content into a perceptual state, then, involves perceiving things *as* objects. Or so I will argue.

In developing my account of object perception, I start by considering the familiar example of photographing identical twins. Then I consider some causal theories of direct reference, or of reference or aboutness *de re*, and their motivation. I offer reasons that such theories don't suffice to account for aboutness fixation, and I also provide a way of thinking about what's right in such theories. I continue by critically developing some resources for thinking about object perception from the literature on tropes (or abstract particulars) and from the psychological literature. Finally, I sketch what is required for a successful account of object perception and perceptual reference-fixing.

1. Twins

Fred and Bill are identical twins. Today they are dressed identically, in blue jeans and t-shirts, and they have just gotten identical haircuts. There are no (readily visible) distinguishing marks for telling them apart. Fred's girlfriend, Amy, wants to take his picture. As a joke, Bill stands in for the photo, and Amy unknowingly photographs Bill, not Fred. The picture comes out looking fine. It looks just like Bill, and it looks just like Fred. If Fred had in fact stood in the same spot for the photo, it would have looked just the same (or any minute differences would have been undistinguishing). Nonetheless, we rightly believe that, unless Amy has a secret thing for Bill, she would be unhappy if someone told her the truth. She might well say: "I wanted a picture of Fred, but I got a picture of Bill." Even though the picture looks exactly as it would have looked with Fred in place, Amy refuses to think her picture is of Fred when she learns of the trick. To her, it is a picture of Bill, because he was the one standing in front of the camera when she took the picture.

As fellow picture-takers, most or all of us will agree that Amy's picture is of Bill, not Fred. I take such agreement for granted. What I want to know is *why* the picture is of Bill, not Fred. What makes it be the case that, even though the picture would have looked just the same no matter which twin stood there, the picture nonetheless is *of* the person who stood in front of the camera? Let us call this a question about the *referent* of the picture,[3] the object that the picture is a picture *of*—as opposed to the question of whom the picture *looks like*, since it looks like Fred as well as like Bill.

I extend the same question to perceptual states. When Amy looks at Bill to line up her photograph, she sees a young man before her dressed in blue jeans and t-shirt, with closely cut hair and a smooth face. I intend these phrases to describe the imagistic character of her experience of the young man at that

---

[3] Dretske (1995*b*) and Recanati (1993, 104) use the terms "referent" and "reference" to describe a two-place relation between an image (or a perceptual state) and the thing to which it refers. Earlier, Kaplan (1969, 225–6) spoke of a causal relation establishing which object a picture (or a perception) is *of*, by contrast with the picture's (or perception's) "descriptive content" (its resemblance to things); this "of-ness" relation is also two-place. As explained in n. 2, for now I follow Dretske and Recanati in using "referent" and its cognates as they do. This usage treats *mental reference* and *image reference* as distinct from the two-place relation of linguistic reference (between word and object), which, as Bach (1987, 39–40) suggests, may be parasitic on the four-place relation of speaker's reference, involving speaker, audience, term, and object. I return below (n. 23) to the question of whether mental reference to an object is a two-place or a higher-place relation. In Sec. 2, I argue that the of-ness relation for photographs is a three-place relation among objects, photos, and conventions of photography (or the attitudes that realize those conventions).

moment. I will call this imagistic aspect of her visual experience the "percept" for short. It corresponds to some aspects of her perceptual state that she wants to capture in the photo. (But not to others: percepts may include motion that is perceived clearly, whereas motion causes blur in photos.) As she takes the photo, she believes that her visual experience is presenting her with Fred, not Bill. Is the imagistic aspect of her perceptual state, her percept, a portrayal of Bill, of Fred, of both, or neither? Do percepts have referents of the sort that I have been willing to assign to the photo?

Depending on the context, we might answer these questions in various ways. I am particularly interested in asking whether there are any (non-intentional) natural facts, facts that rely simply on (non-intentional) natural properties, laws, or regularities, that make it the case that Bill is the referent of Amy's picture, or of her percept. Significant numbers of philosophers in the Anglo-American tradition maintain that there are such facts, and that such facts fix the referents of both pictures and (at least some) perceptual states. These philosophers, who include Dretske (1995b), Burge (1977), Recanati (1993), and Gareth Evans (1982), agree that in many ordinary contexts the referent of pictures and percepts—the object the picture or percept is "of," *de re*—is fixed by the object in the world that is in causal (or, perhaps, informational) contact with the photograph or the perceptual system. (These causally determined facts of reference subsequently enter, in various ways, into these authors' accounts of linguistic expressions, which topic is not our focus here.)

It is my thesis that, although there may be contexts in which we wish to speak of the causal fixation of reference, there are no non-intentional natural facts that *by themselves* serve to fix the referents of pictures or percepts. For photographs, I recognize that we typically do allow non-intentional natural facts about which objects are in front of the camera to fix the referent, but I maintain that we do so as a matter of convention. (That is, we really do *allow* such relational facts to play this role.) Our practice of photography, our intentions in designing and using cameras, play an essential role here, and the facts about which twin reflected the light entering the camera cannot by themselves fill that role. I also contend that, in the case of percepts, a natural relation of the sort envisioned by Dretske and others is not enough to *fix* a referent (even if it may be *relevant* to fixing the referent). More is required. Finding out what more is needed entails examining the notion of object perception and situating it in relation to other biopsychological capacities in perception.

2. Causal and Conventional Accounts of Photographic Reference

Many philosophers would agree that we should account for Amy's distress by invoking a causal relationship between Bill and the picture. The picture is of Bill because he's the one whose body and clothing actually reflected the light that altered the film in the camera. Even though light reflected from Fred would have caused the film to react in the same way, the fact that it was light from Bill that actually struck the film settles the matter. For photographs, the referent is fixed by causation.[4] As Evans puts it, for "information storage" devices, such as cameras, "we can say that the product of such a mechanism is *of* the objects that were the input to the mechanism when the product was produced" (1982, 125).[5]

Let's consider more closely whether the fact that Bill causally affects the film, independent of the human practice of taking photographs, actually establishes a referential (or aboutness) relation between the photograph and Bill. Consider for a moment what an ordinary, old-fashioned photograph is. The camera contains film that reacts to the intensity and wavelength of light. It also has a lens system, which focuses the light coming from surfaces in front of the camera onto the film in such a way that there is an ordered correspondence between small regions on the surfaces of things outside the camera and small regions on the film. This system operates as an enhanced camera obscura, to produce an image on the film that differentially affects the film, depending on the intensity and character (for color photos) of the light (as well as on lens characteristics, aperture size, and length of exposure).

So far, we have film reacting to light. Does the bare fact that Bill served as "input" mean that the altered film is now "of" Bill (*de re*)? I think not.

---

[4] According to such a theory, reference is fixed by which object is in the "right relation" to the film (or the sensor array, if we go digital). Many causal factors contribute to taking the photo: the presence of light, the facts that the lens cover is off, that the shutter is working, that the camera is pointed at Bill rather than at the sky or ground, and so on. Supposing the picture is taken out of doors, we can ask what makes it be a picture of Bill, when the sun is also causally responsible for the light that enters the camera. The sun sends out parallel rays of streaming light. Bill's body reflects and structures those rays, in such a way that a pattern is formed on the film that otherwise wouldn't have formed there unless Bill (or, as it might happen, Fred) was in front of the camera. This is what is meant by "the right" causal relation. Considerable work could be expended just in spelling out this relation. But we won't pause here.

[5] Although Evans accepts the "photograph model" for determining the objects (or, as he elsewhere says (1982, 139), the "target") of photographs and (nonconceptual) perceptions (1982, 78, 122–5), he of course does not accept it in the analysis of singular thoughts (or in his analysis of understanding singular referring terms); in these latter cases, he requires a second factor, a "mode of identification" (e.g., 1982, 138–9).

To suppose so would be to allow that a mere physical relation of causation is adequate by itself to establish a type of representational relation, in this case, a relation of reference. But if that were so, relations of reference would be everywhere. If the sun's light warms a stone, by virtue of this causal relation the heat of the stone would refer to the sun. In a game of billiards, if the cue ball moves another ball, the second ball's motion would refer to the cue ball. Relations of reference would be too easy.

In the case of the photograph, a further context allows us to account for our shared intuition that Amy's picture is of Bill, not Fred. It is the context of our attitude toward the camera as a designed and manufactured device that enters into our practice of taking pictures. Photographs are ways of recording the appearance of people, objects, and scenes. We treat them as records of how things looked, or of how things were arranged at a certain moment in an event. If, in a sentimental context, we view a photograph as a record of how our loved one looked, we want it actually to have been he or she in front of the camera. For most people, a double won't do. Amy wants it to have been *her Fred* in front of the camera, even though the picture would look the same with either twin. It is an embedded feature of our practice of picture-taking that photos are *of* the things in front of the camera. Such attitudes mediate (even if unreflectively) the fact that the occurrent relation between object and film fixes the object of the resulting picture.

In the ordinary practice of taking photos, the causal facts need not enter into determining whom the picture is of. A person needn't understand or be aware of the causal facts in order to use a camera. And those who use cameras know, by experience, that you (usually) get a picture of the scene at which the camera is pointed (they know this from relations of resemblance or visual similarity between the objects photographed and the resulting photos). Causal mechanisms, of course, underlie the fact that photographs give us pictures of recognizable scenes. But in order to participate in the practice of taking pictures, we needn't reflect on those mechanisms or even be aware of them. Nonetheless, we might still react as did Amy if we learned that a person other than our own special friend was in front of the camera when we took his or her photo.

All the same, philosophical sophisticates may prefer the facts of causation as the proper analysis of photographic reference. But my conventionalist account can easily accommodate this preference for causation. We believe that the person, scene, or thing that reflects the light is the object (referent) of the photograph. This belief about how *de re* reference is fixed may determine the referent of the photograph more precisely. In the conventionalist account, these causal facts are part of our understanding that cameras are devices for recording patterns of light to yield pictures. We insist that, for a photo to be a genuine record of a scene, the pattern of light and color in the photograph must have been produced by light reflected from the surfaces and structures in that scene. Accidental or contrived look-alikes will not do. Conceptually, then, the natural processes of light reflection and the like are implicated in determining the referents of photos for philosophical sophisticates. But an understanding of the mechanisms of making a photograph mediates the role of these natural processes.

As philosophers, we might appeal to the facts of causation to settle the matter of what the picture is "really" of when the canons of ordinary practice are not sufficiently specific, as might happen when conditions are abnormal. To illustrate this point, consider a case in which the camera produces a photograph by nonstandard causal means. Suppose that earlier exposure to X-rays accidentally produces a pattern on the film that matches the picture-taker's view of a cloud formation in a grey sky at a later moment. At that moment, the camera's owner believes he takes a picture of the sky, but the shutter sticks. When the film is developed, the picture looks like the clouds as he remembers them. But, we would say, the causal situation determines that the picture is not in fact of the clouds, independent of whether the picture-taker, or anyone else, actually knows this causal history. It is a record of an X-ray pattern. (Whether it is a conventional photograph of that pattern, or another kind of record, is another matter.) Facts about causality, mediated by our understanding of photo-making, enable us to decide what the picture is *of* in such cases. But those facts don't do so by themselves; their effect is mediated through our concepts and understanding.

3. Percepts and *de re* Reference

Now let us consider the case of perception itself. For present purposes, I want to focus on what I earlier called the percept. Among other things, our eyes and visual systems enable us to see the shapes, sizes, colors, distances, and motions of surfaces and volumes. They do this in part by generating imagistic visual experience that presents shapes, sizes, colors, distances, and motions phenomenally, or by way of appearance. The current visual representation of these dimensions of a scene is what I call the percept.[6] Percepts may change

---

[6] Some authors question whether we have coherent, imagistic percepts. I don't find their arguments convincing (see Ch. 1), but if you are convinced, that fact needn't affect the discussion here: just suppose that I am talking about the coherent experience that we merely seem to have (or its fragmentary basis),

from moment to moment. Further, percepts themselves are not like static snapshots: they may include motion. Within a given perceptual moment, we typically experience the presentation of surfaces and volumes with shape, size, and color, at a distance, and in motion or stationary.

In preparing to analyze perceptual experiences (my "percepts"), Dretske (1995b) draws a distinction between the *referent* and the *content* of a picture. The content of the picture includes the *properties* that it represents, and these properties make it be the kind of picture it is. Dretske (1995b, 23–4) frames this distinction by contrasting black-horse pictures and pictures *of* a black horse (see also Goodman 1968, 21–6). A black-horse picture portrays something black in color and with a horse shape. Because the picture presents the content black-horse, Dretske classifies it as a black-horse picture. He has no interest in using the horse-content (expressed most obviously in the horse-shape) to fix reference. Within the content of the picture, he focuses on the representation of properties such as shape, motion, and color (e.g., 1995b, 29); for him, such representations are nonconceptual. In Dretske's (1995b) terms, this nonconceptual content derives from "indicator content," that is, from relations providing *natural information* that exist independent of perceivers (see Ch. 1, Note). Indicator content becomes perceptual content when it attains the biological function of representing the properties it indicates. The perceptual system evolves to exploit environmental regularities in such a way that, typically, if there is a red and round thing in the environment, then redness and roundness are represented nonconceptually in the percept. We can think of such content in terms of the imagistic representational features of percepts.[7]

Dretske's position accords with that of David Kaplan (1969, 226), Evans (1982, 125), Bach (1982, 47), Recanati (1993, 104, 112–13), and others in holding that a contextual or causal relation makes the image (in this case, a perceptual image) be *of* a particular object. If one is looking at a particular black horse, the causal relation between the horse itself and the resulting percept renders that percept into a percept *of* that black horse. This relation holds independent of horse-content (i.e., picture content); so, it holds even if the horse appears brown, or is disguised as a camel, and so on.[8]

---

and then that I am discussing the place of such experience in object perception. Even if perception is merely fragmentary, we nonetheless perceive object properties such as shape, size, and motion.

[7] Not everyone accepts Dretske's indicator content (in fact, I don't, as explained in Chs. 1, 11). More importantly, not everyone accepts nonconceptual imagistic content (which I do; Chs. 1–2). Those who don't accept such content should see the issue here as being about whether causation alone fixes perceptual content of whatever sort.

[8] For economy, I henceforth speak only of a causal relation, not bothering to mention that Dretske allows the possibility of other "contextual" relations, including an informational relation as detailed in

According to this distinction, Amy's photograph might have the *content* of being "Bill or Fred," or "one of the twins." That's the *kind* of picture it is. The properties of shape and color it presents don't specify its content as being either Bill or Fred, since they look the same. Hence, it is a Bill-or-Fred-picture. But its referent is Bill. And the same would go for Amy's percept as she was lining up the shot. It is a Bill-or-Fred-percept in content, but the referent is Bill. The content does not determine the referent. That is determined by the causal or contextual relation that Bill is the one whose body and clothing structured the light that was reflected into Amy's eyes.

Causal theorists (e.g., Dretske 1995b, 34; Evans 1982, 268) generally concede (and rightly so) that content *might* suffice to fix reference, perhaps in conjunction with additional conceptual capacities and background knowledge. Most human beings are not identical twins. If Amy were dating John, who has no twin, she wouldn't face the current problem. Suppose that John has no double; then, in ordinary circumstances, she could tell that she was looking at John from the content of her percept, by attending to the size, shape, and color of his body and face. Her ability to do this would presumably rely on more than the mere imagistic experience of John. She would need to recognize, from the image, that it portrayed a unique individual. In principle, the imagistic or nonconceptual content could in some cases provide all the information needed in order for recognitional abilities to come into play.

Given that content might provide adequate grounds for fixing reference in many cases, we may ask why Dretske and Evans make *de re* fixation of reference basic. I think the answer is similar for both philosophers. They each view basic sense perception as having an essentially nonconceptual core: its imagistic aspect. They also realize that, although such nonconceptual content may be adequate for presenting properties such as shape or color, that content is not sufficiently sophisticated to specify individual things. Perhaps if content were to be used to specify individuals, it would have to be conceptual content. But, for reasons I broach further on, neither Dretske nor Evans would like to appeal to conceptual content to fix individual reference in the primary instance. (They, as many others, also would not want to rely exclusively on definite descriptions to fix reference in the linguistic case.) They would like to find a simple, natural relation that serves as the basis for fixing the referent of the nonconceptual, imagistic core of perception. They choose a causal relation, one that can be described in the naturalistic vocabulary of physical objects

Dretske 1981. Evans (1973, 1982) explicates what he calls an informational relation in terms of causality. Further, for pictures and percepts, Evans (1982, 125) speaks of the object they are *of* (as do Bach and Burge, n. 2), rather than speaking of reference; I continue to employ Dretske's referential terminology for now.

and their relations to physical sense organs. They hope that the referential contact that causal relations provide in sense perception can then ground more sophisticated cognitive contact with the world.

Because Dretske and Evans rely on a natural causal relation to fix imagistic reference, we must ask whether they are subject to my earlier objection: that causation by itself is not enough for reference, since otherwise the heat of a stone would refer to the sun. They respond to this worry and with similar strategies, by first conceding that the causal relation is not by itself *adequate* to fix reference. The causal relation is *necessary* for fixing reference, but it can do so only in relation to a system of the appropriate type. What type? In Evans' case, an "informational system" (1982, 122–9) and in Dretske's case a "representational system" (1995b, ch. 1). The stone's warmth doesn't represent the sun, but Amy's perceptual image represents Bill, because of the kinds of things the stone and Amy's perceptual system are. The stone is not a natural representational system, but Amy's perceptual system is. Although Dretske (1995b) gives an extensive analysis of what it takes to be a representational system, he provides no explanation for reference fixation other than the causal relation. The imagistic representational system does not yield the specific content "of Bill," which would fix the referent. The causal relation fixes the referent, and the content portrays Bill as lean and tall. Once Dretske has a (nonconceptual) representational system in place, the causal relation suffices to fix reference.

I think Dretske and Evans are right that the type of system involved is crucial in allowing a causal relation to fix reference (in cases where it does). But thus far, they have simply redescribed the facts: causal relations can fix reference for the right kind of system. Such a statement is also true of my conventionalist account of photographic reference: causal relations can fix reference in the right context of photographic practice.

Dretske, Evans, and others are here trying to get something for nothing, or to "get objects for free."[9] They contend that a causal relation can *import*

[9] Another sense in which some authors may try to have their objects for free arises in considering whether "object" is a natural kind, or indeed whether individual material objects exist as individuals independent of human (or other cognitive) conceptualizations. Some philosophers hold that middle-sized objects exist only insofar as they are "carved out" by human concepts (e.g., by the conditions of application for sortal terms, as in Thomasson 2007, ch. 10; see Ayers 2005 for a counterposition). The individuation of some objects (such as human-made artifacts) surely is mind-dependent, that is, depends on the relations such objects bear to maker's intentions or other culturally instilled attitudes (see Searle 1995; Heil 2005). The issues are complex, for even if some objects are individuated only in relation to perceivers, they may still constitute natural kinds if some perceivers possess an object concept innately (or inevitably acquire the concept through innate mechanisms). Further, some objects might constitute natural kinds because they enter into scientific theories (Elder 1996). Any objects that exist

object reference into informational or representational systems. On their view, a system can obtain a referential or aboutness relation to objects without the system itself contributing content adequate to specify the individual as an object (even if merely as a unique individual that is otherwise unknown). The object carries its own individual identity in its very existence, and it imparts that identity to the representational system through the causal relation alone. The object's identity enters into the representational system's aboutness relations, its intentional relations to the world, simply through the causal relation.

Although I acknowledge that a causal relation *can be* relevant to fixing reference in some cases, I deny that causation alone can suffice to fix reference for perceptual systems. Background conceptual resources must also be brought to bear. Further, although these resources may depend on certain causal relations being in place, we do not need to conceptualize these causal relations in order to fix reference. But we do need the concept of a material object, or of a unique individual. This concept need not act "descriptively," and it can suffice without appeal to causal factors. In order to support this proposal, I first consider more closely what it is to see objects, and I then consider how perceptual and cognitive systems might establish cognitive contact with and achieve reference to objects that are seen.

4. Non-Epistemic Seeing and Observer Knowledge

Dretske (1969) is famous for the notion of non-epistemic seeing, or seeing$_n$. Non-epistemic seeing occurs when something is present in our visual field as a discriminable feature or region, independent of whether we know what it is, think anything about it, or have the concepts needed to describe it. If I am the grandson of the civil engineer who built the Eleventh Street Bridge in Wichita, Kansas, then it is true of anyone who is looking at me that they see, non-epistemically, the grandson of that civil engineer. It is also true of other sighted animals that can see well enough to discriminate me from my surroundings that they see that grandson. Non-epistemic seeing does not require recognition, identification, or conceptualization, which is what Dretske hopes is also the case for *de re* perceptual reference. Hence, we should consider how non-epistemic seeing relates to perception *de re*.

as individuals only relative to a conceptualization are bad news for standard *de re* theories, since those theories take objects to have natural identity independent of conceptualization, which identity provides the (externalist) singular referential content for perception and thought. My position can bypass such considerations, for I describe a perceptual basis for object segregation (Sec. 7), which can serve as a starting point for one's favorite further account of object metaphysics.

Dretske (1969) originally articulated the notion of non-epistemic seeing in terms of intensional and extensional contexts within sentences that describe perceivers and what they perceive. Some philosophers hold that "sees" is always intensional: that it shows the same sensitivity to conceptualization or mode of description as other cognitive verbs, such as "believes" or "wants." A clear case of an intensional context is:

(5) Susan saw that some spies were in the neighborhood.

For Susan to do this successfully, that is, for the sentence to be true, she must have the concept of *spy*, and she must have come to know, by visual means, that some spies were present. Suppose, now, that the spies work in a circus as their cover. From this fact,

(6) The spies work as circus performers,

together with (5), it does *not* follow that:

(7) Susan saw that some circus performers were in the neighborhood.

This doesn't follow, even though the spies are in fact circus performers, because intensional contexts do not permit substitution of co-referring terms.

We need not explore further the various analyses of intensional contexts. For our purposes it is important to understand the kind of *extensional* reading of "sees" that Dretske (1969) sought to legitimate. Dretske agreed with the usual intensional readings of (5) and (7). But he contended that other uses of "sees" are extensional.

The most basic case is the seeing relation itself: that someone sees something. This relation is ambiguous. If someone says:

(8) Susan saw the spies in the neighborhood,

one could conceivably argue that this is another way of expressing (5) above, and so does not allow the sort of substitution that was rejected in (7). But one might also argue that (8) can express

(9) Some spies were in the neighborhood, and Susan saw those people.

Here, it is intended only that Susan saw some people who as it happens were spies. It is not intended that Susan knew that they were spies, or even what a spy is. Hence, if these spies are circus performers, from (6) and (9) one can legitimately infer

(10) Some circus performers were in the neighborhood, and Susan saw those people.

Again, there is no implication that Susan knew that the people she saw were circus performers. But, in this extensional and non-epistemic sense of "sees," Susan saw them, and co-referring terms are substitutable while preserving the truth of the sentence.

The intuition is that Susan non-epistemically sees whatever is phenomenally present in her field of vision, independent of whether she recognizes what the thing she sees is, or believes anything at all about it. If we now take the further step of supposing that non-epistemic seeing fixes reference, then the object of Susan's perception can be described as a spy, even if she doesn't have the concept *spy*. Suppose that Susan sees a short skinny fellow, who is a spy. Letting the causal relation fix reference, we might get:

(11) Of the person who is a spy, Susan saw that he is short and skinny.

Which we might choose to write as:

(11') Susan saw of the person who is a spy that he is short and skinny.

These sentences report whom Susan saw, and what she saw about him, without implying that she knew that he was a spy.[10] At the same time, according to Dretske's (1995b) and Evans' (1982) ways of thinking, Susan's perceptual state is "of" a spy, because of causal *de re* reference fixing.

I don't dispute that sentences such as (9) through (11) can be useful in various contexts. For purposes of factual reporting, they are perfectly appropriate. We might want to know whom or what Susan saw, independent of what she herself knows. For instance, suppose Susan's boyfriend David has another girlfriend, Elaine, whom Susan neither knows (has never met) nor knows about. Susan's friends might find it interesting to learn that Susan saw Elaine in a shop, despite the fact that Susan had no idea who Elaine is. They might say:

(12) Susan actually saw Elaine the other day.

In this case, one of Susan's friends tells another whom Susan saw. When (12) is used in this reporting way, the sentence is consistent with Susan's *not* knowing who Elaine is.

Sentences such as (9) to (12) do describe objective facts about whom Susan sees. But that does not in itself imply that these sentences report the referential object of Susan's perceptual state. Indeed, as Dretske (1969) originally described it, the relation of seeing$_n$ is wholly non-epistemic. In his original theory (1969,

[10] I follow common philosophical usage in treating "seeing that" as intensional and "seeing of" as extensional. I don't deny that other usages are possible; but since I am not arguing from the particulars of linguistic usage, such possibilities (as described by Bach 1982, 129–32, for belief contexts) don't worry me.

chs. 2–3), the fact that Susan sees someone who is a spy tells us nothing about Susan's representational state. Seeing$_n$ was a necessary but not a sufficient condition for Susan's having a visual epistemic or representational relation to an object. In Dretske's (1995b) new theory, it remains true that Susan must know about spies and must apply that knowledge in order for (5) to be true; but (9) to (12) serve to establish a (non-epistemic) intentional representational relation.[11] In accepting a causal account of reference fixation, Dretske in effect accepted that non-epistemic seeing can fix the object of perception *de re* (assuming that systems that can see are representational systems in his sense: 1995b, 30). We still want to know why (or whether) we should accept this view of reference fixation, a question I defer to Section 6. In the meantime, I continue to use "see$_n$" in its original, non-epistemic (nonconceptual and non-intentional) sense.

I grant that sentences (9) through (12) *can* fix a referent for a human cognizer in certain cases, which I consider to be uncontroversial: for observers who have the relevant background knowledge to assert them. Here, the knowledge possessed by the observers who have identified whom Susan saw mediates proper reference. They refer to Elaine when reporting Susan's non-epistemic visual state. In cases of third-party perceptual reporting, the desire to convey the *de facto* object of Susan's perceptual state to other parties leads us to countenance a reference relation that is beyond Susan's own knowledge, and perhaps (if Susan doesn't know what a spy is) beyond her conceptual ability. Those who are in the know can say truly that Susan saw the spies or saw the other girlfriend. But they can say this precisely because they *are* in the know.

This reporting sense of "sees" may also be used in scientific contexts to report facts about what an organism sees. Suppose that Susan is a subject in a color perception experiment in which she is asked to discriminate color patches created by combining lights of various wavelengths. The experimenters might describe what Susan sees as:

(13) Susan saw lights of RST and XYZ wavelengths.

If Susan is unable to discriminate the two sets of wavelengths, the experimenters might say:

(14) Susan did not visually discriminate lights RST and XYZ.

---

[11] Although Dretske (1995b, 11) still regards conceptualized knowledge as required for Susan to *know* (or even *believe*) that she sees spies, he adds a layer of intentionality below knowledge and belief, building on Dretske (1981); at this lower level, a causal relation establishes the intentional object of perception (1995b, ch. 1, secs. 3–5).

The experimenters use this language independent of whether Susan herself has ever heard of wavelengths or the spectrum. They use sentences such as (13) and (14) to report what Susan in fact saw, without implying that she even knew that light can be described in these ways. The scientists consider the fact that the light was of a certain spectral composition to be relevant in describing what Susan was in fact looking at during the experiment. This scientific use can extend to contexts in which observers evaluate what an organism can and cannot see$_n$. Some organisms may be unable to see$_n$ objects at distances beyond 20 meters, because objects beyond that distance fail to produce a discrete spatial structure in the visual experience or the spatial representational system of those organisms. Organisms that are not surface-perceivers but react only to local features without integrating them into segregated units may be unable to see$_n$ objects at all (Marr 1982, 32–4).

The sentences used in the ordinary and in the scientific cases do not, in the absence of further theory, attribute to Susan (or to other subjects) an intentional or referential relation to an object or type of stimulus. Nonetheless, the sentences could easily be read as attributing such relations because many sentences that are used with the "reporting" sense of "sees" can be ambiguous. We might naturally conclude from

(15) Susan saw Elaine

that Susan was in cognitive contact with Elaine. But in order to draw that conclusion, we would need to know whether (15) was used to describe Susan's cognitive state, or simply to report a fact about whom she saw$_n$. If Susan's friend asserted (15), and if one of Elaine's friends overheard it, she might easily conclude that Susan was privy to Elaine's identity in all relevant respects. But that would be a mistake, if, in asserting (15), Susan's friend only intended to report an interesting fact.

In my view, a background practice of describing what perceivers have in fact seen plays a role in the reporting uses of "sees" similar to that of photographic practices in deciding the referent of a photograph. Our attitudes toward photography lead us to accept that a causal or a spatial relation to the camera fixes the reference of the photograph. In the reporting cases, our interest in knowing some facts about what Susan has seen allows us to describe her perceptual state as being of a spy, or of Elaine, or of light of a certain composition, but only in a derivative sense that relies on outside knowledge and may be neutral with respect to the intentional object of Susan's percept. In none of the sentences (9) to (14) does this relation provide a basis for imputing the referential relation to Susan, or to her representational (in this case, her visual) system. That would be to allow the representational system to get its referents for free, or by charging them to someone else's outside knowledge.

5. *De re* Reference in the Round

Dretske's and Evans' appeals to a causal relation to fix perceptual reference are embedded in a larger movement in philosophy, rooted in analyses of singular terms (such as proper names), which refer to individuals, and in a related analysis of how terms refer to natural kinds ("gold" or "water"). In the 1970s, the view was widely held (e.g., Kripke 1972; Evans 1973; Burge 1977) that a speaker's or thinker's ability to think about or refer to individuals does not depend fundamentally upon descriptions of the sort found in Russell's theory of descriptions. Indeed, it was held that a speaker's or thinker's ability to refer to individuals does not even depend on the speaker's possessing concepts that pertain specifically to the individual. Singular reference, for thought and language, was to be understood as founded on an indexical relation to a present object (in the fundamental case). Among others, Evans (1973, 1982) invoked a causal relation to fix the indexed (or demonstrated) object; Burge (1977) invoked a causal notion for fundamental cases of what he termed belief *de re*.[12]

One reason for turning away from descriptions in accounts of reference arose when philosophers of science considered what happens to theoretical terms as a scientific theory changes. Suppose that the ability to refer to theoretical entities such as electrons were to depend wholly on the descriptions that scientists give of them (as charged particles possessing certain properties). Since electrons are submicroscopic, these descriptions would depend on physical theory. As the theory of electrons changes, the description changes. If description fixes reference, then, as description changes, the purported referent changes. This conclusion was thought to entail that, as physics developed throughout the twentieth century, it couldn't have been talking about the same things (i.e., electrons) all along. Rather, the earlier theories were talking about things that didn't exist at all, and the later theories are in danger of being in the same

---

[12] As Evans (1982, 78–9) has observed, some discussions of the "new theories" of direct reference and singular terms in the 1970s confuse two distinct theories: the theory that the causal history of the use of a name (as discussed in Kripke 1972 and Putnam 1973*a*) is what allows a name to refer successfully at the present time, and the theory that a present causal relation establishes reference in individual acts of referring. Putnam (1973*a*, 204) disavows the latter, even while speaking loosely in a manner that might suggest it (203). I am focusing on authors who proposed that a present causal (or informational) relation fixes a present instance of *de re* reference.

position, assuming that the theoretical description of electrons will continue to develop.

Against this descriptivist theory, some philosophers maintained that scientists had been talking about and referring to electrons all along (Shapere 1969; Putnam 1973*a*). The descriptions changed as the scientists learned more about electrons. But the referent remained the same. How so? Because, according to these philosophers, reference was originally fixed by the scientists' relations to the electrons themselves when they introduced the term "electron" in a baptismal act (one that, according to Putnam 1973*a*, must include sufficiently accurate descriptive knowledge to enable the scientists to focus on a physical magnitude or entity being baptized). The thing in the world ultimately fixes the referent (Putnam 1973*b*). This is what happens with the referents of indexicals such as "here" or "now," which, in basic cases, refer to the area around here, wherever that is, or to the present time, whenever that is. Within the philosophy of language and the philosophy of mind, corresponding analyses that emphasized indexical or demonstrative fixation of reference were on offer for direct reference (Kaplan 1989*a*) and for proper names as singular terms (Burge 1973).

I do not dispute that scientists and others have the ability to refer to things under a *de re* attitude. As mature users of language, scientists who are visiting a particle accelerator can intend to refer to the particles in the accelerated stream, whatever they may be. Suppose that five visiting scientists enter a control room, rightly believing that a stream of particles has been created in the accelerator. For whatever reason, the host scientists are unsure of what the particles are. Suppose that some of the visitors believe that the particles are baryons and some of them believe that they are mesons. In fact, the particles are tachyons, a type of particle that not one visitor actually believes to exist. Nonetheless, it may be true that each and every one of them wants to know what the properties of the particles are, no matter what the particles turn out to be. We can, then, attribute to them the desire to understand "that stuff," whatever it is. The object of their desire to understand is in fact the stream of tachyons. At the least, the stuff in the world fixes the referent as the stream of particles, owing to the *de re* referring attitude that the visiting scientists share. (Whether the visitors are thereby already referring in an intentional manner to the tachyons, or merely to subatomic particles of an as yet undetermined type, depends on how much of an externalist one is about linguistic meaning—a topic that needn't detain us here.)

In this example of *de re* reference, the thinker or mature language user is already in place. In allowing the scientists to refer *de re* to the particle stream, we know that we can rely on their intentions to refer to "whatever the thing is." The scientists' ability to refer with intent plays a similar role here to that assigned to convention in my analysis of Amy's photograph, or to the observer's knowledge in perceptual reports (as scouted in Sec. 4).[13] However, these cases do not get us the account that we need: an account of the most basic perceptual, cognitive, and representational relations involved in directly seeing an object. These relations are prior to third-person observer's knowledge or to the sophisticated attitudes of a mature language user. They are what sustain the perceptual contact through which mature thought can develop.

6. Causally Based Perceptual Relations in Perceptually Mediated Thoughts

Because perception plays the fundamental role in establishing basic contact with objects, the question of what is needed to establish *perceptual reference* (see n. 2) entered this literature. Kaplan (1969) developed a photographic model of what an image, including a perceptual image, is "of"—a position like the one that I rejected in Section 2. Evans (1982, 122–5) accepted the photographic model for photographs and percepts (as nonconceptual). Kaplan and Evans each found the photographic model to be incomplete as an analysis of perceptually mediated thoughts about objects, which they took to involve both perceptual and conceptual aspects (in Kaplan 1969, the conceptual elements function descriptively; in Evans 1982, not).

Many of the philosophers who invoke *de re* perceptual relations in fixing object reference embrace some version of what Evans (1982, 138) described as a two-factor theory for perceptually mediated thoughts and beliefs about objects. In two-factor theories, causally based perceptual relations join with conceptual elements. In Evans' account (1982, 138–9), a causally based "informational relation" serves as a condition for perceptually mediated thought to achieve successful reference to an object. This perceptual element must be joined with conceptual content (1982, 178) that takes the object to be an object of

---

[13] I separate two aspects of reference *de re*: reference *de re* itself *and* the means by which the *de re* referent is fixed. As regards the first aspect, some philosophers advocate that some words or expressions refer directly to singular things (individuals) in an unadorned manner, by which they mean that the reference is not mediated by a description of the (purported) referent that would pick it out through its properties (as with the usual understanding of a description such as "the present king of France"). Regarding the second aspect, some philosophers have argued that such direct referential relations are fixed by causal relations alone. I am not opposing the first point, although I am not focusing on linguistic cases but primarily on *de re* reference fixation in perception and cognition. I am disputing the second point, and I offer an alternative account in the perceptual case of what *de re* reference amounts to and how it is fixed.

some sort or other (if only a "material body"). Of course, since Evans was not at base a descriptivist, the conceptual element need not be adequate to single out the object descriptively: the perceptual context, with its causal or informational relation, yields individual reference. But this conceptual take on the object gives content to the thought about the object to which the thinker is perceptually related.

In subsequent literature, Bach (1982, 1987) and Recanati (1993, 99–103) described the perceptual factor as a "mode of presentation."[14] For the most basic case of perceptual belief, Bach (1987, 18–22) described this mode as a "percept" and as a way of being "appeared to," which then serves as a mental indexical that enters into a belief about the object that is being perceived. The belief supplies the conceptual element. Let us consider these two factors one at a time, beginning with perception.

Advocates of *de re* reference (here represented by Bach 1987) developed sophisticated accounts of singular perception partly to deal with so-called "Frege cases." Suppose that someone purports to establish that two objects he has seen are in fact the same. If reference to individuals is simply fixed *de re*, then the subject would be asserting a tautology, *a* is *a*; for the causal relation would ensure that in both cases he was referring to the same individual. But, as the famous case of Venus as "morning star" and as "evening star" makes clear, we can nontautologically assert that individual things we perceive on separate occasions are the same thing. In another case, suppose that a perceiver attributes inconsistent properties to the same object. In observing one long train while intermittently gazing out a window, the perceiver may mistakenly assume that she has seen two trains, one composed of only red boxcars and the other of only blue boxcars. If reference were fixed simply by her causal relation to the train, we would be forced to ascribe to her an inconsistent belief about the one train: that it is red and not-red (in this case, blue). But, as the example already makes clear, she is not guilty of a purely logical contradiction; her problem is an empirical one: she failed to detect that there is only one train. If *de re* reference is fixed under a specific mode of presentation or "appearance" (A) of a given individual, then in the case of Venus we have the individual under A_1 being the same as the individual under A_2, which does not assert a tautology. In the train case, we have the same individual under A_1 as P and

---

[14] Bach (1987, 41–5) and Recanati (1993, 98–101) reject some features of Evans' (1982) position (e.g., Evans asserts that when the appropriate causal relation is lacking, as in hallucination, the perception-based thought lacks content, whereas Bach ascribes content to such thoughts but not truth value). My positive comparison of the three positions pertains to their accepting the two factors, a nonconceptual perceptual factor and a conceptual factor, in analyzing perception-based thoughts about objects.

under A_2 as not-P, which is not a logical contradiction. Of course, in the second case the subject mistakenly believes that the individual under A_1 is not the same as the individual under A_2. In an unadorned causal *de re* account, she refers to the same train in the same way both times (and contradicts herself). That account does not capture the fact that her problem is not logical but empirical: she has failed to note that the train under A_1 is the same as the train under A_2.

As in the cases of Venus and the train, the modes of presentation are typically incorporated into belief (or other cognitive) contexts. Within this cognitive context, the causal history of the mode of presentation fixes the referent of the belief. The mode of presentation does not function *descriptively* to fix the reference (e.g., "the train that appears to me now as I look out the window"). Rather, it serves as a mental *indexical*, whose indexical function is completed via the causal aetiology of each (token) mode of presentation. Bach, arguing against a descriptivist view of reference fixation (in which the referent would be the unique object "satisfying" the description), appeals to a causal relation (relation "C") to fix the object of perceptual belief:

to believe something of an object one is perceiving does not require thinking of it under any description—the object is already singled out perceptually. By suggesting that there must be an individual concept, formed from the percept, that determines (satisfactionally) the object of belief, the descriptive view gets things backwards. For by having the percept, the perceiver is already in a position (assuming the percept is appropriately caused by the object) to form beliefs about the object, which is determined relationally. Percepts function in belief as mental indexicals, and the object of a percept token is whatever bears C to it. To be the object of a perception-based belief, an object need not be represented as being in that relation; it need merely be in that relation. (1987, 21)

Perception suffices to "single out" objects, about which we can then entertain beliefs. The percept serves as a mental indexical: it enables the belief to be about whatever object is causing the percept, just as "here" or "now" refer to the area around here and the present time. The mode of presentation under which the object is presented must segregate the object from its surroundings: otherwise, the idea that the object is causing "the percept" would not suffice to single out the object. If we don't assume perceptual segregation, then a single percept (i.e., the whole visual field) would usually be in a causal relation with many objects.

We see both factors at work here, conceptual and perceptual. The perceptual factor fixes the individual referent, and the conceptual factor (in Bach's example, the belief context) is what makes it appropriate to speak of reference (or cognitive contact) at all. In fact, Bach (1987) and Recanati (1993, ch. 6)—who approvingly invokes Bach's notion of a mental indexical—do not spell out in any detail the conceptual aspects that are involved when percepts serve as mental indexicals (their further discussions of indexicals focus on linguistic cases). We may assume that they did not hold these perceptual indexicals to be "pure indexicals" (e.g., "I") whose referents are determined by linguistic meaning (Recanati 1993, 81). Rather, the percept as indexical should function as a demonstrative, that is, as something whose target is partly established by what Kaplan calls *directing intentions* (Kaplan 1989b, 588; also Perry 2000, 317–18). The directing intention would be part of the conceptual and cognitive factor in reference.

Although neither Bach nor Recanati gives details concerning the cognitive factor in perceptual reference, Evans (1982, ch. 6) devotes an entire chapter to "Demonstrative Identification." Much of the chapter defends his view that in acts of linguistic direct reference we must suppose that the speaker knows which object he intends to refer to. In elaborating this principle, Evans invokes spatial location as playing a fundamental role in singling out objects. He also addresses the question of whether, in singling out an object by means of perception, the cognitive factor includes subsumption of the object under a sortal concept. Although his discussion is tentative, he concludes that no specific sort (*human being*, *cherry pitter*) is needed, but perhaps only a generic sortal such as *material object* is needed for standard cases.

I am sympathetic to the need for a cognitive factor in establishing object perception and object reference. Before examining that topic (in Secs. 8–10), I want to consider further the role that causation allegedly plays in the accounts that Evans and Bach (and Dretske, too) offer concerning the perceptual factor.

Causation seems to me to be insufficient for fixing reference in the basic perceptual cases. In the accounts of basic perceptual reference just reviewed, the percept plays a crucial role in presenting the object as segregated from the surrounding region. For Bach (1987, 21), the percept "singles out" the object by providing a segregated percept. For Evans (1982, 124–5), it seems that the "information system" is already working with segregated representations, in that he invokes photographs and percepts as being *of* individual objects, even if several are present.[15] Percepts enter into demonstrative acts, in which the

---

[15] Dretske (1995b, 34) retains, or tacitly relies on, his earlier notion that objects are visually differentiated in the preconceptual (sensory) act of seeing them. Unlike Bach (1987) and Recanati (1993), whose theories of *de re* representation Dretske invokes (1995b, 24), he only hints at an indexical component to *de re* perceptual reference (1995b, 33); the notion of directing intentions seems foreign to Dretske's insistence that a contextual (causal) relation can fix reference by itself if it merely acts on a representational system (1995b, ch. 1). Dretske's "reference" amounts to a bare intentional or "aboutness" relation.

object segregated by the percept is made the focus of reference by a directing intent—which, in this context, we may call a *referring intent*. At this juncture, it strikes me that the causal relation does no work for basic perceptual reference. Perceptual processes typically segregate and perceptually present things that are objects in locations; referring intent singles out that segregated entity (whatever it may be) as the intended object of reference. The object itself, considered as an object, enters into the content of the referring act through the structure of the referring intent: the perceiver intends to focus on that *object*, there. In such acts of referring intent, the concept of a material object is required (at a bare minimum). This concept does not enter into a standard descriptivist account of fixing reference; but it is required as part of the referring intent.

Up to this point, I have allowed myself to speak, with Dretske and Recanati, of "perceptual reference" when considering what Kaplan, Evans, and Bach describe as an "of-ness," "aboutness," or "representational" relation between image and object or between perception-based thought and object. Having rejected the causally based two-factor theories of *de re* object representation developed by Evans, Bach, and Recanati, I want now to develop my own two-factor theory. In so doing, I distinguish between object perception proper and the further act of cognitively attending to a specific object. Henceforth, when speaking in my own voice, I describe only the latter cognitive act as *perceptual reference*. I distinguish such acts of reference from the more basic case of *object perception proper*, which I describe as perception with object content, or as perceiving an object as an object. I believe that object perception proper rests on the psychological capacities to segregate objects and to conceptualize them as objects. So I look first to the psychology of perception for help in understanding how things that are objects become segregated in the subject's visual experience. Subsequently, I turn to the question of what is needed in order to perceive an object as an object, and to refer perceptually to the objects that we perceive.

7. Object Perception and Perceptual Segregation

When psychologists write about object perception, they describe various aspects of vision that present us with a segregated world, that is, with a world segregated into "objects" (Palmer 1999, chs. 6–7; Peterson 2001). Some of the phenomena they discuss are:

Figure/ground contrast
Grouping through motion

Amodal completion
Illusory contours
Size and shape constancy
Tracking behind occluders.

Figure/ground contrast was made famous by the Gestalt psychologists, and has many illustrations (see Fig. 7.1a). Grouping through motion indicates that whatever moves together is perceived as a unit. Amodal completion refers to the perceptual presence of the occluded portions of partially visible objects: in Figure 7.1b, we "complete" the black circles. Illusory contours, as illustrated by the white triangle in Figure 7.1b, exhibit the tendency of perception to present coherent surface structures. Size and shape constancy yield perceived objects with constant properties (perhaps "contractively" scaled—see Ch. 6). Tracking behind occluders means that the visual system keeps track of a moving target that disappears behind something and then reappears.

Through these factors, vision presents us with a world of segregated volumes. When these volumes move, they are visually presented to us as following continuous motion paths, even when they are momentarily hidden from view and subsequently reappear.

These factors are certainly the beginning of object perception, but are they enough? That, of course, depends on what it takes to perceive an object. And that in turn depends on what an object is. Metaphysically, P. F. Strawson

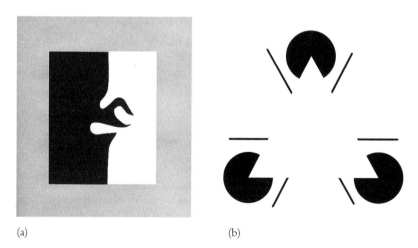

(a)   (b)

Figure 7.1. Examples of two perceptual phenomena that illustrate perceptual organization into bounded areas. (a) is figure/ground segregation (reproduced from Rubin 1921, Plate 2). (b) provides examples of amodal completion and illusory contours, after Kanizsa (1979).

(1959, 31–6) stressed the notion of objects as reidentifiable individuals, Enç (1975) investigated criteria of numerical identity, and Hirsch (1982) appealed to spatiotemporal segregation and continuity as criteria of objecthood. On these views, a paradigmatic material object is something that persists through time, retains its structure, and is continuously locatable in space, so as to be the same individual, and so as to be reidentifiable as that individual and not merely as having the same structure or being of the same kind. With relatively unchanging objects, such as rocks, this description works well. Living things are also reidentifiable objects, but they go through a process of growth and development in which their size and shape change in characteristic ways. Even here, we can admit such change into our notion of a persisting object, as long as we can retain spatiotemporal locatability and reidentification of the individual.

Psychologists too are interested in object classification and the recognition of individuals. But they are also interested in the most basic instance of object perception, which involves treating a present individual, even if otherwise unknown as to kind or identity, as an individual material object. Again, we may ask what it takes to perceive such an individual as an object. I join some psychologists in believing that, although perceptual segregation and attentional tracking of unified spatiotemporal regions put us into a perceptual relation with things that are in fact objects, they do not by themselves achieve object content, that is, the perceptual content that something is an individual object.

In a series of studies of adult perception, Ken Nakayama and his colleagues have argued that initial segmentation of the world into bounded volumes is a perceptual process that occurs prior to object perception itself. Nakayama et al. (1995) rely on both phenomenology and experimental studies in drawing attention to what they term an "intermediate" level of processing: more integrative than the mere reception of the local features of the retinal image, but not yet including object knowledge or other cognitive factors. They call this level "the level of visual surface representation" (1995, 9), which they describe as follows:

It is a general purpose, intermediate representation in that it codes enduring aspects of our physical world yet is not concerned with detailed specifics. This surface level determines whether surfaces are seen as connected or disconnected; folded, straight, or curved; whether they pass in front of or behind; whether they are transparent or opaque. Again, we see this level as distinct from object-level processing, which requires knowledge of specific object[s] or object classes. (1995, 9–10)

The specification that the surfaces are "seen as" connected or disconnected (and so on) does not denote conceptual seeing, but is a report of phenomenal spatial structure. It is "seeing as" of the sort that occurs in figure/ground organization, which does not require identification or conceptual classification (see Fig. 7.1a here, and Nakayama *et al.* 1995, 7–9).

Nakayama *et al.* (1995) emphasize that intermediate-level perceptual processes segment the world into three-dimensional spatial structures bounded by surfaces. They extend this analysis to motion, including the motion of items that appear to be partially covered by an occluder. In this case, the visual system apparently follows a rigidity constraint. In the apparent motion of intermittently flashed shapes, some of which extend perceptually (but amodally) behind an occluder, they consider cases in which potentially "spurious" and "nonrigid" completions of such motion might occur, and they find that the visual system instead presents rigid structures that undergo translation: "the visual system codes, and we see, motion of a surface, not the motion of isolated fragments" (1995, 40). These intermediate processes of perceptual organization track spatial structure that is bounded by surfaces, completing them when they move behind occluders.

Given that the perceptual processes postulated by Nakayama *et al.* are preconceptual and pre-attentive, in what sense can such processes "track" bounded volumes? They do so by responding to retinal features in such a way as to solve what is called the "correspondence problem" regarding motion (Nakayama *et al.* 1995, 34–8). As multiple elements move across the retinas and exhibit discontinuous motion at the edges of imaged occluders, there may be more than one way to represent them in three-dimensional space. Nonetheless, the visual system assigns the elements to distinct bounded volumes possessing some specific structure or other. More generally, Nakayama *et al.* contend that their surface representations can attract attention (1995, 40–5). Once the intermediate-level system has presented the visual system with segregated surface structures in a location, attentional processes may track individual bounded volumes. (Of course, there is no need to suppose that the perceiver wittingly focuses on "surface structures," so conceived.)

8. Perceptual Qualities as Abstract Particulars

Sensory perception presents segregated spatial structures, and tracks these structures across motions. Does this amount to representing the structures as individual objects? I think not. Spatial structure is particular, but need not be singular. It is sortal and permits occurrent counting, but it need not represent particular structures as individual things. My point here is conceptual. When we perceive a spatial structure, usually we see non-epistemically (see$_n$) things that are in fact individual objects. The question is whether the perceptual representation of a trackable spatial structure in itself yields the content that an object is present, or even yields an intentional relation to an individual. I think not, because I take it that the perceptual content in question may only be that of an abstract particular, even though it is determinate and countable.

The notion of an *abstract particular* was developed in twentieth-century philosophy by G. F. Stout (1923), D. C. Williams (1953), and Keith Campbell (1990), who advanced the notion as part of a general analysis of what there is. According to one ontological thesis, everything that exists is composed of abstract particulars, which are instances of properties. There are no universals, there is no substratum; there are only instances of properties. An individual apple is nothing over and above a collection of properties at a location (where location is also a property): shape, color, flavor, firmness, and so on. An appropriate collection of co-located ("compresent") properties yields a concrete particular, an individual.

Since I'm concerned with abstract particularity only as a form of representational content, I need not consider the legitimacy of this ontological thesis. What matters for my analysis is that perceptual representations can present abstract particulars as countable instances of property instantiation, and that such representations need not determine unique individuals (because they present only one or a few properties, which are insufficient for objecthood).

To see this, consider the spatial structure of a specific type of right triangle (with angles 30-60-90). Here is one, there is another (Fig. 7.2, (a) and (b)). Are these individuals? We accept that they are; they are here on the page, two to them, countable, for all to see. Now consider the perceptual representation

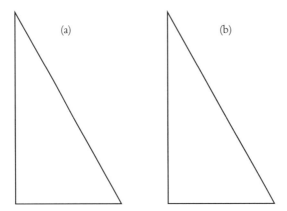

Figure 7.2. Structurally identical 30-60-90 right triangles, to exemplify abstract particulars.

of these triangles as spatial structures, leaving aside further cognitive responses that introduce the full content of thought. The perceptual image presents each triangle as a spatial structure with a size and at a distance, and exhibits it in relation to other spatial structures. But it does not by itself bear the content that these triangles are here at these very global positioning coordinates, or that their structure was created in Philadelphia in a computer program that provided the code used to print them in the umptieth copy of this book. Such facts about global position or book-specific causal ancestry *would* provide sufficient information to designate the individual triangles as unique individuals. But the perceptual image, unconnected with additional knowledge, does not contain this specificity. It presents a determinate spatial structure, but even determinate spatial structure is abstract. There can be many 30-60-90 triangles of this size and in this local spatial relation to the perceiver. There is no way to tell from local spatial structure itself which individuals are being presented on any given occasion. Thus, mere (local) particularity of spatial structure does not yield individualizing content.[16] Genuine individuation would require further content, most likely conceptual in nature. The fact that these very triangles are causing your current perceptual state would, of course, fix individual reference, but so far we have found no way to get this information into the perceptual system.

The matter is not helped if we track the triangles over brief motion paths, such as would occur if we fixated one of the triangles and slid the book away. Motion through space instantiates a particular structure, but again this structure is abstract. Each motion path in perception is an abstract particular. It is a particular in that it presents a specific geometric structure. It is abstract in that this same type of structure can be realized by any number of individuals. We are looking for what serves to specify a particular instance as a singular thing.

Adding sortal notions need not yield individuality (especially in a developmental context). Suppose we have twenty yellow teacups. Identifying them by their kind as teacups allows us to distinguish them from the bread plates. But by itself it need not specify them as individuals. Object-kinds, such as *teacup*, can serve as abstract particulars, too (albeit complex, conjunctive ones). To perceive an instance of a teacup requires identifying the complex of spatially compresent properties that make for a teacup; but it doesn't require representing this

---

[16] My emphasis on spatial structure at a location in describing bounded volumes that are perceived nonconceptually bears some similarities with Clark's (2000, 2004) view that sentient representations assign features to places. Clark's theory differs from mine in that he ascribes nonlinguistic referential apparatus to his purely sensory representations, sufficient for the identification of space–time regions (where I require mere abstract-particular, viewer-relative spatial structures); additionally, he denies the existence of a visual space (2000, ch. 3), which I affirm (Chs. 5–6).

complex as a concrete, unique individual that has the properties of an object, including unique spatiotemporal location over a long stretch of time. In representing the teacups at local (but still abstract particular) spatiotemporal locations, we can count the twenty cups. But occurrent countability doesn't entail individual objecthood. You (or I) can count all the self-connected patches of red currently visible from your (or my) viewing position. But the patches of red need not be coterminous with individual objects, and even if they were, the representational content you use in counting need not assign individual objecthood to the red patches. For both the teacups and the colored areas, counting them only requires that we can for a short while keep track of them as spatially distinct instances of kinds.

In seeing teacups, we as adult perceivers typically see them as individual objects. We could if we wanted give them names, creating singular terms for them. As adult thinkers, that would come easy (even if we had to mark them on the bottom in order to keep their identities straight). But the mere combination of spatial structure and sortal specification does not of itself yield individualization or objecthood. Representing objecthood, as happens in adult perception, requires added content. At a minimum, it requires perceiving the teacups as individual material objects (not as mere local collections of properties), including the background knowledge that garden-variety objects such as teacups occupy distinct spatiotemporal locations (or space-time worms, for the sophisticate) throughout their existence as teacups.

In any event, I affirm that adults regularly think of the solid objects that they see as individuals. Further, the adult concept of an object-kind most likely includes the conceptual content that instances of such kinds *are* individuals. It might be an empirical fact that many adult sortal concepts include the notion that instances of the sortal are persisting objects. But the representing of a particular space-time structure, even adding sortal designation, does not by itself attain that level of conceptual content or individual reference. Representationally, there can be particularity without individuality.

9. The Object Concept and the Competent Infant

For much of the twentieth century, researchers in cognitive development accepted something resembling William James' characterization of the world of the infant as a "blooming, buzzing confusion" (1890, 1:488), spatially amalgamated and awaiting conceptual differentiation. As the century wore on, various perceptual constancies were attributed to ever younger infants. Still, many thinkers accepted the view of Jean Piaget, that "during the first months of existence, the primary universe is an objectless one formed of perceptive scenes which appear and disappear by reabsorption" (1971, 16).

During the past twenty years, Elizabeth Spelke and her colleagues, including more recently Susan Carey and her collaborators, have strongly challenged the notion that infants develop their object concept late. Their work explores what they term the "physics" and "metaphysics" of infant perception.

In her early work, Spelke showed infants a straight rod, the middle segment of which was occluded by a screen so that only its upper and lower ends were visible. If the rod remains still, infants give no evidence of perceiving the two ends as connected. But if the visible ends move, then even four-month-old infants perceive the two ends as parts of a single connected entity (Kellman and Spelke 1983). In other studies of partially occluded, hidden, and reappearing objects, Spelke found ever more sophisticated object content in infant perception. This led her to formulate the thesis that infants begin with an initial "theory" of the physical world, a theory informed by an "object concept" (Spelke 1990). The target objects in her experiments were mid-sized dry goods, rigid material objects smaller than a baby but larger than a baby's hand. These were the prime instances of the alleged "object concept."

Spelke's empirical work led her to conclude that the object concept is applied after three-dimensional surface structure and motion have been recovered from stimulation and perceptually represented. She proposes that in infants the object concept is applied centrally to these already formed spatial representations. Four initial principles guide the application of the concept: cohesion, boundedness, rigidity, and no action at a distance (Spelke 1990). Cohesion implies that all the points of an object exist simultaneously (even if they can't all be seen), and that they move together. The boundedness principle implies that objects have boundaries, and that distinct objects cannot occupy the same space (cannot share points that are part of each object). According to Spelke, infants apply the rigidity principle wherever they can; that is, if a transforming spatial structure can be interpreted as a rigid moving object, the infant's perceptual system will do so. Finally, "no action at a distance" says that spatially separated objects are interpreted as moving independently from one another if they can be; but if they move together rigidly, they are perceived as separate objects only if a gap between them can be detected.

Although Spelke's principles accurately describe aspects of infant perception, that fact does not require us to grant that they describe *object perception*. Using the work of Nakayama *et al.* (1995), we can reinterpret her principles as preconceptual principles of perceptual organization, principles that yield the perception of coherent spatial structures without invoking an object concept.

As I summarized it in Section 7, the work of Nakayama *et al.* describes cases of perceptual organization with amodal completion for moving elements; these findings might account for cohesion, boundedness, and rigidity as principles of the perceptual organization of bounded spatial structures. Further, their principles for solving the correspondence problem are akin to Spelke's principle of no action at a distance. Perceptual processes that yield bounded, trackable volumes that engage the attentional mechanisms of infants might account for Spelke's empirical results, without needing to attribute object content to infants, as she does.

Using the notion of an abstract particular, we can further reinterpret Spelke's principles as applying to the organization of spatial structure, including moving structures that pass behind occluders. Spelke's principles can thus be treated as applying to abstract particulars, presented preconceptually as three-dimensional spatial volumes. So construed, these principles need not invoke the concept of an object as a reidentifiable, persisting concrete individual. The less sophisticated notion of a moving and trackable spatial volume with cohesion and boundedness will do. The impenetrability aspect of boundedness would simply be a rule for the perceptual interrelation of bounded volumes, as would rigidity and no action at a distance (which is similar to the Gestalt principle of "common fate").[17] In short, we can account for the phenomena that support Spelke's principles by attributing to the infant an ability to detect the property-kind *bounded trackable volume* (BTV). BTVs are abstract particulars.

To see how this can work, let us consider some *prima facie* strong data for infant object perception. Spelke and Kestenbaum (1986) presented four-month-old infants with two different scenarios (Fig. 7.3, top). In (a), a single rod moves continuously from left to right, passing behind two occluders (shown as solid black rectangles). In (b), the left-hand rod moves from left to right, stopping behind an occluder; after a pause, another rod appears from behind the right-hand occluder, moving from left to right. The infants then saw the test displays. Spelke (1990) interpreted their responses as indicating that they perceived a single moving entity in (a), and two entities in (b). Let us focus on (a). She concluded from the data that infants "are able to apprehend the persisting identity of objects that move fully out of view" (1990, 46). Suppose, as seems plausible, that the infant represents the spatial structure in (a) as following a path of continuous motion behind the occluders. Does he need to have the concept of an individual material object to do so (as "persisting

---

[17] Spelke (1990) argues that Gestalt principles cannot account for her findings; however, she restricts her argument to what she calls "static" Gestalt principles, and within these she does not include figure/ground organization. In contrast, the Gestalt and other factors I rely on for segregating bounded volumes (Sec. 7) include dynamic factors and figure/ground organization.

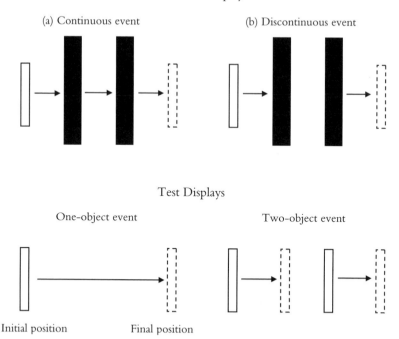

Figure 7.3. Habituation displays and test displays for Spelke and Kastenbaum (1986). The moving bars that served as stimuli are represented by the smaller, unfilled rectangles; solid lines indicate their initial positions and dotted lines their final positions. In the continuous event (a), the bar moves continuously behind two occluders (the solid black rectangles) and is visible as it moves between them. In the discontinuous event (b), one bar stops behind the first occluder, and a second bar appears moments later from behind the second occluder. Separate groups of four-month-old infants were habituated to (a) and to (b), and then each group saw both test displays. The infants who were habituated to the continuous event (a) generalized to the one-object event, and those habituated to (b) generalized to the two-object event. Spelke (1990, 48) concluded that the discontinuous motion led infants to perceive "two distinct objects." After Spelke (1990), fig. 9.

identity" implies)? Evidently not. A locally determinate, abstract-particular spatial structure will do; the infants may simply be tracking a continuously represented BTV of cylindrical shape (i.e., having the spatial structure of the rod's surface). They would need to represent it as a particular volume, but the data do not require that they possess the richer content of objecthood, of a persisting unique individual. The experiment may provide evidence of the role of amodal perception in filling in the motion path, and of the ability of the representational system to track BTVs. But full object content is not required.

More recently, Susan Carey and her collaborators have extended Spelke's research to investigate more closely the notion of objects as individuals. Xu and Carey (1996) showed infants either one or two objects, then hid them behind screens, and subsequently removed the screens. Sometimes, when they showed and then hid two objects, only one object reappeared. The infants were surprised by such inconsistent outcomes (as measured by looking times). Xu and Carey concluded that the infants subsumed the objects under the general sortal "object" and that they "identified" the objects as individuals.

Xu and Carey have again imported more of the apparatus of adult cognition than is needed. They see themselves as applying Spelke's notion of an object concept. But that notion (as reinterpreted above) doesn't require the full concept of an individually persisting concrete material object. An abstract particular spatial structure will suffice. Carey and her colleagues further conclude that when infants show evidence of counting, they are in effect invoking singular terms to "quantify" individuals (Huntley-Fenner *et al.* 2002; Van de Walle *et al.* 2000). But again, abstract particulars, or instances of property-kinds, are countable. We can include the property-kind BTV among potential countable property-instances in infant perception. Its instances are countable occurrently and over short periods of time (during which the BTV may be amodally represented).

Xu and Carey (1996) also showed that although ten-month-old infants can count such BTVs when the BTVs occupy distinct locations, they apparently cannot use color or shape to keep track of similar-sized BTVs that are placed behind a screen one at a time. When presented with an occluding screen from behind which the experimenters successively extract and replace (one at a time) a red toy truck and a blue rubber elephant, the infants may count only one item (Xu and Carey 1996)—either one object, or one BTV (depending on one's interpretation). A subsequent study by Tremoulet *et al.* (2001) found that ten-month-olds could keep track of objects placed behind screens by their shape (triangle or circle), but not by their color (red or green), whereas twelve-month-old infants could use either shape or color. The use of various properties to track objects (as the experimenters call them), or BTVs (as I call them), develops late in the first year of life.

Zenon Pylyshyn (2003, 259–68) interprets these and other data in a manner that is partly friendly to the position I have been developing. He argues that the early visual system is able to track individual things, which he calls "proto-objects," by visual indexes. A central case is tracking spatially distinct items along their motion paths. He regards this as a capacity that could occur in the absence of an object concept. He thus acknowledges that the infant-data on object tracking does not require us to ascribe an object concept to infants.

Pylyshyn regards the object concept as something that develops. Spelke *et al.* (1995) allow that sophisticated object concepts (as are found in philosophical discussions of object persistence) develop during childhood and even into adolescence or adulthood. Pylyshyn in effect is saying that even the most basic aspects of the object concept may develop throughout infancy.

However, Pylyshyn's view differs in an important respect from the position that I am proposing. He does not think that perception of spatial structure, or of any other property, mediates reference to objects. Rather, like the *de re* theorists, he regards the causal relation between an object and a conceptual representation (mediated by the object's effects on the retina) as in itself sufficient to establish a reference relation (2003, 269; 2007, 39, 58). How it could do so is difficult to understand. Figure 7.4 is redrawn from Pylyshyn (2003, fig. 5.4). It shows objects *x*, *y*, *z* in causal relations (indicated by the solid arrows) to retinal elements *r*, *s*, *t* and concepts X, Y, Z; and it presents (through the dashed arrows) the relation of reference that (allegedly) is thereby established between concepts X, Y, Z and objects *x*, *y*, *z*. In his account, this referential relation arises as if by magic. The visual system has no access to what is causing the retinal stimulation, except as a result of perceptual processes such as those described by Nakayama *et al.* (1995). These processes of early vision should not be construed as attempting to trace back the path of causation; rather, they take retinal structures as input and yield the representation of

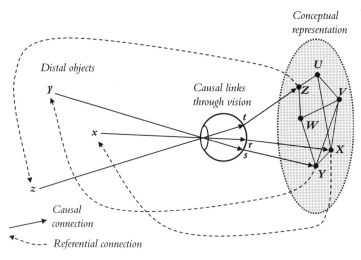

Figure 7.4. A sketch of the causal relations between distal objects and retinal elements, showing postulated causal relations between retinal elements and conceptual representations, and postulated referential relations between conceptual representations and distal objects. After Pylyshyn (2003), fig. 5.4.

three-dimensional visual structures as output. The products of these processes permit the attentional tracking of bounded volumes (and they could thereby serve as a basis for subsequent deictic acts of reference); but reference to an object is not required in order for attentional tracking to occur. This can be true even though the perceptual system usually tracks what are in fact objects, and does so nonaccidentally. The perceptual system may well have evolved to track things that are in fact objects by segregating them as BTVs. Further, although causal relations obtain and are necessary in order for perception to occur, the basic perceptual processes in vision do not represent such causal relations. These processes produce representations and experiences that segregate the world into volumes arrayed within the three-dimensional visual world of the perceiver.[18]

The importance of the experiments and theories of Spelke, Carey, or Pylyshyn is not at issue, but rather their *interpretations* of their experiments, and especially the kinds of object content that they attribute to infants. I don't claim to have shown that their attributions are incorrect—only that the data do not compel us to accept them. In this subject area, that's where the action is. As Spelke *et al.* (1995) observe, this work hopes to uncover in the infant the origin of the principles that inform adult cognition. I have been cautioning against finding adult cognitive capacities in the infant by projecting them there from underdetermined data.[19] Are infants just born with the concept of persisting concrete individual? Or does this concept develop out of more primitive abilities for representing spatial structure, recognizing sameness of spatial structure, and tracking the motion of spatial structures?

---

[18] Pylyshyn himself, when he provides a concrete description of how the tracking of his proto-objects occurs, invokes the continuous motion path of the objects: "if visual elements follow certain kinds of (perhaps smooth) space-time trajectories, they are more likely to be treated as the movement of a single individual object" (2003, 212). He also speaks of the need for parts of the visual field to become "segregated" if objects are to be perceived (2003, 210). These achievements—tracking a smooth motion path and segregating a bounded volume—are products of visual processing. These processes do not have access to the *de facto* causal relations between distal objects and retinal stimulation; it is only as a result of perception that perceivers (or vision scientists) can seek to investigate such *de facto* causal relations. Such investigations of course reveal that the successful operation of the visual system depends on certain causal regularities being in place, and the processes of the visual system may have become tuned to such regularities through evolution or learning. But that is different from the visual system itself representing or seeking to represent or trace causal pathways (see Ch. 5).

[19] I am in effect suggesting that Spelke and her colleagues (along with *de re* causal theorists) may be guilty of what William James (1890, 2:196) described as the "psychologist's fallacy": "The great snare of the psychologist is the *confusion of his own standpoint with that of the mental fact* about which he is making a report. ... The psychologist ... stands outside of the mental state he speaks of. Both itself and its object are objects for him. Now when it is a *cognitive* state ... he ordinarily has no other way of naming it than as the thought, percept, etc., *of that object*. He himself, meanwhile, knowing the self-same object in *his* way, gets easily led to suppose that the thought, which is *of* it, knows it in the same way in which he knows it, although this is often very far from being the case."

These questions are worthy of empirical investigation. Clearly distinguishing among the variety of hypotheses that are consistent with the data can only aid such investigations.

10. Toward a Biofunctional and Developmental Account of Object Perception

From our first year, our perceptual system represents the layout of the world spatially and chromatically, presenting us with bounded volumes having a size, shape, color, at a distance, and moving or still. These surfaces and volumes arrayed in space are typically caused by objects, but that fact alone is powerless to make the perceptions be *of* the objects. Granted, in order for us to see things that are objects, the objects must cause some (distinct or segregated) aspect of our visual experience. But our ability to perceive the objects as *objects* and to refer to them as *individuals* is a further achievement that relies on but goes beyond the mere perceptual having of these segregated and bounded visual structures.

The psychological capacities of the early visual system move us toward the abilities to perceive and to refer to individual objects. Basic visual perception segregates the world into BTVs. The underlying perceptual mechanisms, which we may consider to be preconceptual, track bounded volumes across space and behind occluders. They index these BTVs, and allow them to become objects of attentional focus. BTVs are segregated and trackable; someone who can keep track of them over a short period of time can count them. But these capacities do not yet manifest or require an object concept or the ability to refer to individuals.

To attain the level of objects, we must at a minimum add the capacity to represent an otherwise unknown individual material object (e.g., a cherry pitter). Merely indexing a BTV and tracking it does not yet specify that it is a unique, persisting object. For that, the background conceptual capacity to regard something as an individual object must be added. The subject needs to have within its horizon of possibilities some notion that there are unique individuals to be tracked, that they retain their identity over time, and that they may be bearers of other (as yet unperceived) properties. The infant's visual system may already be tracking things that are in fact individual objects. But for a perception with object content to occur, the infant's visual system must apply the concept *material object* (or the like). For a pure deictic act of referring to occur, the intending agent needs be able to want to refer to *that material object, whatever it may be.* The developmental evidence suggests that the notion of an individual material object with persisting properties, such as a stable color, arises after ten months. Conceptual investigations by philosophers (see Enç 1975) suggest that this notion involves believing that two solid things can't be in the same place at the same time.[20] So perhaps true perceiving and indexing of individual objects is a fairly late achievement: maybe you need to be two years old, or even older, to possess the requisite notions.[21]

With the background concept of *individual material object* in place, subjects are in a position to engage in direct reference. The background conceptual ability does not need to function in a definite description that is sufficient to pick out the object. That is, I am not proposing that descriptions of things mediate our reference to those things in the most basic cases, as Schiffer (1978) suggested. On Schiffer's account, except for the indexicals "I" and "now," even demonstrative thoughts always have a descriptivist core that serves to fix the object of reference, as in:

(16) the only red thing in my field of vision.

Although such descriptions may be used to single out an intended object of reference, as in,

(17) the cherry pitter that Norman gave to Holly,

the most basic referring acts will not be mediated by description. They will be demonstrative acts of referring:

(18) that, there,

which I take in typical cases to be short for

(19) that thing there,

and therefore to require the concept *thing*, and indeed *thing as individual*, where the first concept we have of *thing as individual* may well be the concept of a

---

[20] In the philosophical literature, some authors argue for a distinction between a sortal object, such as a statue, and its material constituents (see Thomasson 2007, chs. 4, 10, for a critical discussion). If such a distinction is available, it presumably comes later in conceptual development.

[21] Although, on present evidence, I favor a view that the object concept develops in the first several years of life, my criticisms of Spelke and Carey do not rely on this assumption. My position does imply that, if the object concept is innate, it must have more content than Spelke's principles describe, and that any evidence for this content's being innate must go beyond what Spelke, Carey, and their collaborators have demonstrated with their experiments. (Their experimental results require nothing more than the ability to track and count BTVs.)

material object as a persisting, cohesive, unitary, individual.[22] In any event, it can be true that such concepts are needed in order for referring to occur, without its being the case that these concepts thereby descriptively mediate reference. Rather, they serve as the needed background to allow demonstrative acts to be targeted at material objects *as* objects, and therefore for demonstrative acts to reach the level of referring to objects. In the visual case, we need (at a minimum) the object's location in order to refer to it directly, and in the typical case, we use at least some of its spatial and chromatic features to cognize it as an individual and hence as an object of reference.[23]

The concept of causality need not enter into these acts of reference. A pure attentional act of singling out a BTV can mediate the demonstrative relation. Someone can demonstratively refer to the cherry pitter in front of himself without knowing or conceiving the causal processes that mediate vision. Nonetheless, those who possess the causal concept might put it to use descriptively in an act of reference that also includes a demonstrative element, as in:

(20) whatever is the cause of this segregated appearance,

which might determine singular reference. The act of reference incorporates the demonstrative element "this," and the causal relation enters as a description that completes the referring link.

Beyond referring to otherwise unknown individuals, human subjects (at least) are able to perceive and refer to known individuals (recognition), otherwise unknown individuals of a certain kind (classification), and to known individuals of a kind (recognition with classification). There are competing theories of how this occurs, and the relevant psychological mechanisms may differ depending on the domain. Face perception may be done by holistic spatial structure (Yue *et al.* 2006); other objects may be recognized by pattern matching of constituent parts (Biederman 1987). Our mature abilities to recognize and to name individuals arise from the prior ability to refer to material objects.

---

[22] The literature extensively discusses whether the notion of *physical object*, or, as I prefer, *material object*, is a sortal suitable for counting instances of individuals. Xu (1997) argues that it is a sortal; Hirsch (1997) agrees, for "basic objects." Of course, even if *material object* is a sortal, knowing that a thing falls under this concept is not sufficient for identifying that thing or re-identifying it perceptually; for that to occur, the thing's spatial location or other specific attributes are needed. My use of the word "thing" in the discussion above is not intended to assert that *thing* is a sortal, but (minimally) that it is a generic concept for individuals that includes the sortal *material object* as a species. In contexts such as (19), "thing" most likely acts as an equivalent to "material object."

[23] I thus treat *perceptual reference* to a material object as a three-place relation among object, percept, and referring intention. (See n. 3.) I treat object perception proper as a two-place relation between a conceptualized percept and an object.

The basic (nonconceptual) content of the senses, the representation of size, shape, color, and so on, provides the materials for further, more sophisticated, referential, and conceptual capacities that mediate the work of object perception, reference, recognition, and classification. I am thus proposing a concept-mediated view of object perception at its most basic level. *De facto* causal relations do not get us object perception. Rather, in the visual case, we (or our visual systems) must subsume a visually segregated thing under an object concept. For reference to occur, we must be able to single out a visually segregated thing as an individual through a referring act (although we need not be able to recognize it as a known individual). The cognitive acts of recognizing and classifying individuals on the basis of their appearances go beyond such bare perception and bare reference. However, it is conceivable that the classification of abstract particulars by sortal concepts precedes the perceptual representation of unique individuals. That is, a child might be able to classify BTVs (e.g., as red balls), and even to count the number of instances of the sortal, before she understands that each ball is a unique individual.

On this view, it may turn out that some animals do not perceive individual objects as individual objects. They perceive a spatial and chromatic layout that allows them to navigate. They may even develop concepts or protoconcepts that allow them to recognize kinds of stuff in their world: food, predators, conspecifics. Do they represent their reproductive mates as their mates? Here perhaps chemical labeling may come into play, and may allow them to detect an individual by a unique chemical marker. But if they don't have the representational capacity to represent the individual as spatiotemporally locatable and re-identifiable, then they don't perceive their mates as objects. (They might, of course, still recognize them as instances of the complex abstract particular, *my mate*.) We, in a reporting mode, may speak of the objects that other animals (or human infants) perceive, but short of attributing to them the conceptual capacities just enumerated, we shouldn't describe them as object-perceivers themselves. Which doesn't mean that, in tracking BTVs, their perceptual systems don't track things that are in fact objects.

Seeing individual objects in a cognitively relevant manner, hence seeing them as potentially re-identifiable things, requires a certain level of conceptual development. In consequence, seeing objects is a cognitive achievement, for us as for other higher mammals. It isn't free—but it needn't be. It is work we can do. Simple, honest, conceptual, recognitional, and classificatory work. The kind of work that our highly articulated spatial and chromatic representations enable us to perform when joined with appropriate conceptual resources.

11. Conclusions

Naturalistic accounts of object-perception proper cannot rely solely on causal or other contextual relations in order to fix the object-referent of perceptual states. We need to invoke conceptual capacities in order to account for contentful perceptions of objects, that is, of things as persisting, re-identifiable, continuously spatiotemporally locatable entities. I suspect that the tendency in analytic philosophy—represented by Dretske, Burge, Bach, and others—to suppose that perceptual reference can be fixed causally arises from their concern with language and belief, including their analyses of the sentences used to describe perceivers, their perceptions, and the role of those perceptions in linguistic acts. They have thereby imported one or another set of background beliefs or practices into the analytic situation for describing perception, and they have relied on our tacit knowledge and abilities as fellow participants in these linguistic practices in making their arguments seem plausible. But the aspects of our linguistic practices that make *de re* referential assignments plausible in the cases of language, belief, and third-person perceptual reporting do not obtain for our initial sensory contact with the world. We are not justified in reading the sophistication of thought into the basic operation of the senses. Rather, individual subjects must possess (presumably, develop) some basic conceptual resources in order to engage in pure or direct acts of reference.

I also contend that object perception proper is something that needs an explanation built upon our fundamental perceptual capacities and invoking conceptual abilities. The perceptual system segregates volumes for us, and naturally tracks such segregated volumes over short periods of time. These are the beginnings of object perception, but they do not yet yield the content of a persisting, re-identifiable, continuously spatiotemporally locatable entity. For that, we need conceptual structures that take us beyond episodic perception to conceptual or at least protoconceptual cognition. Object perception is not free: beyond the sensory representation of surfaces and volumes, it requires cognitive structure and ability.[24] We must be able to take the locally available

---

[24] In Sec. 6, I describe the two-factor theories of object cognition of Evans (1982), Bach (1987), and Recanati (1993), and I interpret their appeals to mental indexicals or demonstratives as requiring conceptual abilities. Thus, it may seem as if their accounts of object reference also imply a conceptual factor. This is true of their accounts of object cognition, but these authors invoke an of-ness relation between percept (and perhaps other images such as photographs) and objects that does not depend on a conceptual relation, and this of-ness relation either constitutes a noncognitive form of object reference (for Recanati 1993 and Dretske 1995b) or is deemed an essential component of perception-based object reference (Kaplan 1969; Evans 1982; Bach 1987; Recanati 1993). By contrast, I require a cognitive

spatiotemporally segregated volumes and cognize them as unique entities that can persist and that we might re-identify as the same individual. In this way, presently perceived spatiotemporal features become the basis for perceiving a present thing as an object. Our exploitation of this basis may be effortless and automatic. For that very reason, we need to turn to theoretical analysis to discern the requirements of object perception. I've sketched those requirements here.[25]

I want now to list some things I am *not* saying. I am not saying that all seeing is seeing as. The perception of BTVs is apparently nonconceptual or preconceptual. Moreover, in the context of ordinary language, Dretske's seeing$_n$ (or "simple seeing") has its place when we report what someone saw on a given occasion, including which objects the person saw, without attributing to them knowledge of what he or she saw. What I have denied is that such simple seeing by itself establishes either object reference or perception of something as an object. I therefore do affirm that all perception of objects that makes cognitive and referential contact with them as objects is seeing as. At the same time, I do not require that, in order to perceive and to refer to objects, one must have a philosophically sophisticated notion of an object. What I claim is that, in the core cases, perceivers must conceptually subsume a thing under the concept of persisting individual material object; and also that this conceptual content is not required for the perception and tracking of BTVs. Together, these assertions mean that the perceptual tracking of BTVs alone is not evidence for the possession of an object concept.

Further, although I have emphasized the imagistic and nonconceptual nature of the perception of BTVs, I am not saying that language or concepts never influence the imagistic aspects of perception. Nor am I claiming that as adults we have introspective access to the pure case of perceiving a BTV (without seeing it as a concrete individual). I also doubt that we have introspective access to the automatic processes or background assumptions that guide our

component in object perception of any kind that is deemed to bring perceivers into an intentional relation with objects as objects. I distinguish such intentional relations from cases in which a third party, using his or her own knowledge, describes which object a perceiver is in fact perceiving (a description that does not reveal the perceiver's own intentionality).

[25] In this and the preceding paragraphs, I have hinted that mine is also a naturalistic account of object perception. However, given my appeal to referring intentions to fix reference, my account is naturalistic only if such cognitive capacities count as "natural." They do count under the "inclusive naturalism" of Chs. 1 and 10, which denies that intentionality must be reduced to non-intentional terms for it to be a natural phenomenon. Dretskean (1981, 1995b) naturalism hopes to reduce intentionality to the allegedly "physical" notion of information, and some *de re* theorists may be attracted to causal theories of reference in the hope of a reductive naturalism. I prefer not to require of naturalism the reduction of the intentional.

perceptions of objects, or that underlie our various linguistic practices for describing objects and perceivers. But I have no need to claim that we have such access in order to hold the position I have put forward.

Additionally, I am not saying that description usually fixes reference. Demonstrative reference has a nondescriptive component, in the act of indicating or focusing attention on a perceptually segregated target of reference ("*that* thing *there*"). I do say that indexical reference requires background concepts that place the target object under a description ("that *material object* there"). But applying the concept of material object is not sufficient in itself to establish direct perceptual reference; the object's spatial location or other perceived spatial and chromatic features must come into play. These need not be sufficient for us to classify the object as a known individual, but merely as an (otherwise unknown) individual of occurrent perceptual acquaintance. Further, I am not denying that we may engage in referring acts in which causation helps to fix the referent. Such referring acts may and do occur. When they involve referring to an object demonstratively via its causal relation to a percept, the role of the causal concept in the act of reference is mediated by description ("whatever is causing this percept"). Moreover, the facts of perceptual causation may enter into philosophical analyses that describe the perceptual situation of other perceivers; in that case, such facts may be deemed philosophically relevant to determining what object someone is seeing$_n$, or what object they have in fact brought under a referring intention. In each case, the causal facts become relevant in a manner that is mediated by theoretical understanding.

Finally, I am not saying that the development of the object concept stops with the sortal *material object*, or even with other basic sortals such as animal kinds and food stuffs. As our object concepts develop, we can bring finer distinctions into play. For the young child, stone and moss may be part of one otherwise unknown type of material object. For an adult, the stone may be one object, the moss an attachment. Similarly, the adult may distinguish between the table and the dried avocado sauce adhering to it (even if the table is green and the color matches). We may even come to intend that our singular acts of referring are filled out by the causal or other contextual relations that obtain between us and the intended objects of our reference. The *de re* intuitions that accompany sophisticated language use exhibit our conceptual development.

The relations among thought, language, and perception are rich and complex. We will not understand those relations by favoring any one factor to the detriment of the others. What we take for granted in our linguistic practices may in fact depend on highly structured nonlinguistic psychological capacities.

In both our linguistic practices and our more basic perceptual capacities, we may rely on certain background concepts and knowledge in ways that are not immediately apparent. It is the job of philosophical analysis to tease out such reliances. My analysis indicates that object perception isn't free, even if objects seem to us to be there for the perceptual taking at every moment.

PART II
Color Perception and Qualia

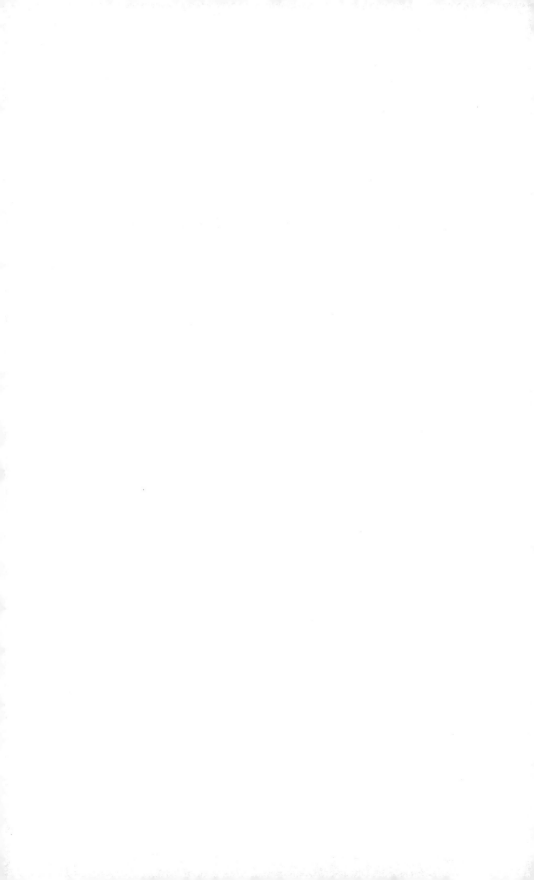

Introduction

The status of sensory qualities has been a topic in philosophy since the ancient Greeks. In the history of thought about color, scientific theories were formed in relation to a background of philosophy, and philosophical theories often arose in conjunction with or as a result of scientific work (as in the cases of Aristotle, Ibn al-Haytham, Galileo, Descartes, Boyle, Locke, and Newton). Through the end of the nineteenth century it was usual for color scientists, such as Helmholtz and Hering, to address the philosophical assumptions and implications of their work. They engaged such assumptions directly, and examined them with philosophical thoroughness.

During the middle of the twentieth century philosophical and scientific thought about color separated. Especially in the decades after 1950, philosophers offered "physicalist" theories of color without engaging seriously with the physics, physiology, and psychology of color vision (e.g., Smart 1961). Other philosophers examined in great detail linguistic statements about color, placing great emphasis on what they imagined the "ordinary" person would say about color perception (e.g., Austin 1962). But this imagined "ordinary" person usually advanced theses recognizable from previous, or old, philosophy and science (and was again not acquainted with up-to-date science, on which, see Russell 1953).

At about the same time, many color scientists came to believe that they could proceed without philosophy, or without themselves adopting philosophical assumptions. In this they were mistaken. In any area of active science that moves at the border of the unknown, there is no such thing as doing science without philosophy. To attempt to do so simply means that one's philosophical assumptions go unexamined. That may not cause much damage locally and in the short term, but it can limit scientific imagination if one is stuck in old philosophy. It can be damaging to color science if one's philosophical assumptions, imbibed in the final decades of behaviorism and expressed through an unthinking commitment to physicalist reductionism, lead one to be suspicious of phenomenal experience and biological function, and hence of the very substance of color vision.

During the 1970s and 1980s, philosophy of science—led by the subfields of philosophy of biology and philosophy of physics, but including philosophy of psychology as well—re-engaged the scientific literature. In philosophical theories about color, this meant coming to terms with the physics, physiology, and psychology (including the phenomenology) of color vision. That was a good thing. But it was not decisive, since scientific theories do not have the status of authoritative heralds in deciding how to think about the metaphysics and epistemology of the sensory qualities. Nonetheless, they do have weight. In this area, as in many other areas of philosophy, one can't make philosophical progress without knowing anything else, that is, without engaging with what others know about color. That's how it should be. Philosophy aims at generality, but must earn its broad perspective one step at a time, working from the bottom up, while keeping in sight the general vista it demands of itself. Workers in philosophy, as in other areas of the humanities, must earn their abstractions, rising up from the details.

These various currents—appeals to science (e.g., Hilbert 1992, 2005), appeals to previous philosophy (often to disparage "sense data" approaches), and appeals to "ordinary" intuitions or "common sense" (e.g., Stroud 2000)—remain at work in the philosophical literature. Appeals to common sense have led to a revival of naive realism about color, that is, of the view that objects just have the color properties they appear to have (e.g., J. Campbell 1993, 2005).

As is evident from the tenor of the essays in Part I, I am not sympathetic to appeals to "what we ordinarily say," or think, in attempts to develop a philosophical account of perception. It is not that I disparage nontechnical discourse or believe that sentences such as "the ball is red" are false when uttered by the uninitiated—on the unconvincing grounds that they don't have a sophisticated understanding of the object property *red*—or indeed when uttered by the philosophical sophisticate. As discussed in Chapter 11.5, I find that appeals to "ordinary" discourse often attribute more theoretical structure to such discourse than it plausibly contains or can bear. More generally, I would cite the fact that various aspects of human understanding of the natural world, and even of the most fundamental aspects of human life, have developed over the millennia of human theoretical discourse. Consider how much weight should be given to the claim that since the Earth seems stable to "ordinary" common sense, *it really doesn't rotate*; or to view that since ordinary folk don't believe that gases can be combined via a flame to make a liquid, then *hydrogen can't really burn to yield water droplets*. In the domain of fundamental human experience, the inner mechanisms of human reproductive processes were unknown until the twentieth century, and they were not revealed by a careful consideration of human reproductive phenomenology. Similarly, although most humans are well acquainted with seeing colored objects, there is no reason to believe that this experience should reveal what colors are, metaphysically. Which, again, does not mean that everyday utterances about the colors of things by the philosophically and scientifically unsophisticated are false. They just aren't the basis for metaphysics.

During the 1990s, several prominent philosophical accounts of color perception were influenced by a particular strand of color science: accounts of constancy that saw the function of color vision as that of extracting the physical reflectance properties of object surfaces from the light reaching the retinas. These objectivist accounts of color perception are discussed throughout Chapters 8–11. Prominent scientific accounts of the phenomenon of color constancy (e.g., Maloney and Wandell 1986) had the implication (discussed in Ch. 6.2) that full constancy would yield a chromatic homogeneity that is not characteristic of human visual experience; the mismatch with experience was chalked up to a failure to achieve the targeted full constancy. Some philosophical accounts adopted this interpretation of full constancy as the aim of color vision (Hilbert 1987, 1992; Dretske 1995b, ch. 3.4; Tye 1995, ch. 5.3).

Within the scientific community, the standard objectivist theories underwent criticism from several directions. A common theme in such criticisms was that the senses should not be viewed as instruments for recovering physical values (Jameson and Hurvich 1989; Gilchrist 1994; Mausfeld 1998, 2003). In particular, critics observed that it may be useful for the perceptual system to provide phenomenal access to the illumination of a scene, instead of discounting illumination as in the traditional objectivist accounts. Philosophical objectivists have not been silent in response. Hilbert (2005) argues that objectivism can simply be revised to view the task of color vision as detecting the precise physical characteristics of both the surface reflectances and the illuminant (see also Matthen 2005, 159).

That might be the case, but in Chapters 6.3 and 8–9 I provide an alternative account of the functions of color vision, which suggests that objectivists are using the wrong vocabulary and conceptual matrix for describing color vision. This alternative account views color vision as functioning to make objects discriminable and identifiable by color. For these purposes, full color constancy is not required. It is an implication of my view that producing color experiences (or at least color representations) in perceivers is an essential component of what it is for an object to be colored. I also take color qualia to be real items in nature, in virtue of being real features of experience.

My account shares something of the perspective of Mausfeld (2003), but it differs in two related respects. First, whereas Mausfeld (2003, 400) sees color science proper as describing only the internal processing mechanisms of organisms and views discussion of what perceptual states "represent" in distal objects as merely "metatheoretical" and heuristic, I view such talk as part of an essential description of the function of sensory systems as serving to represent external (in vision, distal) objects. Second, whereas Mausfeld (ibid.) believes that the functions of color vision should be specified by describing internal processing mechanisms without appealing to the broader context of evolutionary adaptation, I believe that comparative and evolutionary perspectives provide important insights into the functions of color vision. Mausfeld (ibid.) opines that in discussions of the digestive system, "no one would maintain that in order to understand its function one has to take into account its evolutionary history, or physical or chemical regularities of food composition in a certain environment." As explained in Chapter 1.3, appeals to ecological and evolutionary considerations do not require that a full selection history has been ascertained. Even so, appeals to evolution and ecological context can guide functional thinking. In fact, alimentary scientists do concern themselves with ecological pressures and the evolutionary history of digestive processes (e.g., Brena *et al.* 2003; Mackie 2002; Tokuda *et al.* 2004). Mausfeld and I agree in rejecting what I call the "physical instruments" approach (Ch. 8.2), an approach which holds that the language of physics provides the correct vocabulary for describing both visual stimuli and the representational primitives of color perception.

Color experience is, it seems to me, phenomenally determinate: hues and achromatic colors are phenomenally definite, even if the standard descriptive vocabulary we have for the various dimensions of color experience is incomplete (see Gilchrist 1994; Mausfeld 2003). Most objectivist and dispositionalist theorists make a second assumption: that a determinate color experience signals an equally determinate color property in objects, so that we should expect that sameness of phenomenal hue (in standard conditions) indicates sameness of color property. I worked under this assumption in Chapter 8.

In Chapters 9–11, I reject the assumption that a determinate color property must yield a single phenomenal hue under standard conditions. Instead, I present a conception of the color property which acknowledges that color experience interacts with conditions of illumination and other contextual factors. As all grant, such experience does not directly correspond to the product of illumination and surface property, or else color experience would be directly determined by the proximal stimulus (the light reaching the retina). But a full discounting of variations in illumination to achieve full constancy does not occur, either. Nonetheless, despite the fact that the same object yields different phenomenal hues under the range of variation within natural daylight, we are able to identify it as being "of the same color." Moreover, human color receptors, the retinal cones, are polymorphic, yielding different mappings between physical stimulus and phenomenal hue within the range of "normal" trichromats and for "anomalous" trichromats. These facts have been seized upon by some philosophers, who argue that colors aren't real but are instead subjectively produced illusory contents, albeit useful ones (Hardin 1988). I view colors as dispositionally defined properties of objects, but I also argue against the view that object colors should yield the same determinate hue experiences, even under "standard" conditions: variation is to be expected and is consistent with color being a dispositional property of object surfaces (see also Hatfield 1999, 266–7). The fascination with color determinacy in the dye industry and other technological contexts has led to a false conception that if they are object properties, colors should always look the same (at least in standard conditions).

My approach to color vision and color qualia is broadly naturalistic, but, as mentioned in Chapter 1, I include the intentional and the phenomenal within nature. That is, I take it that subjective human experience is a natural phenomenon (Ch. 10.5). I do not intend my *inclusive naturalism* to be all-encompassing. I am generally sympathetic to a nature–culture divide, which recognizes distinct methodologies in the natural and the human sciences (Hatfield 1990b, ch. 7.2).

The chapters were produced for various occasions, which accounts for some terminological variation: for example, spectral reflectance distributions (SRDs) are also labeled as surface spectral reflectances (SSRs). Chapter 8 originated as a talk entitled "Why I Am Not a Barlowist," which arose from discussions with Gershon Buchsbaum and was presented to Peter Sterling's Laboratory of Neural Microcircuitry at Penn in 1991. That talk formed the basis for presentations on "Representational Content and Environmental Context" at the Cornell Cognitive Science Symposium and as an Austin–Hempel Lecture for the Departments of Psychology and Philosophy at Dalhousie University, also in 1991. A subsequent version was presented as a contributed paper at the Philosophy of Science Association meeting in 1992. Despite the use that Dretske (1995b, 92) makes of it, I did not intend that paper to suggest that color vision aims to discriminate *as SRDs* the environmentally present SRDs of objects of differing behavioral significance (e.g., plant leaves and bark); instead, I proposed that color vision might function so as to represent such objects differently without specifically representing the underlying SRDs that differently affect the retinal cones. Chapter 8 mentions "red," "green," and "blue" cones in shudder quotes; on the advice of Ed Pugh and the late Leo Hurvich, in subsequent chapters I dropped even the shudder-quoted use of those labels and adopted the ever-more-standard labels of LWS, MWS, and SWS cones.

Early versions of Chapter 9 were presented in 1994 at the University of Notre Dame and at the conference on Color Science and Philosophy at the Institute for Research in Cognitive Science of the University of Pennsylvania; a subsequent version was presented in 1996 at the CUNY Graduate Center and in the colloquium series of the Center for Interdisciplinary Research in Bielefeld (to the group on Perception and Evolution). I gave an earlier version of Chapter 10 at the Humboldt University Symposium on Mental Representation and Reality in 2001 organized by Ralph Schumacher. I presented an earlier version of Chapter 11 at the conference on Perception and the Status of Secondary Qualities, University of Bielefeld, September 2003 (also organized by Schumacher), with Rolf Horstmann commenting.

I note two terminological points in connection with Chapter 11, both concerning variants of the term "representation." First, in the present version I describe my position as "critical realism" rather than "representative realism" (Ch. 11.7). In the previously published version, I undertook a quixotic quest to define a *direct* "representative realism." This quest unnecessarily sought to expand the standard usage of "representative realism," when all I needed was recognition that some direct realisms treat perception as representation-mediated. Hence, in the present version, I uphold a representation-mediated *critical direct realism* (see also Ch. 1), which does not posit sense data proper, and which I compare to the critical realism of R. W. Sellars (1916). I now believe that *representative realism* should be restricted to positions which hold that external objects are *inferred* from sense data or other mediating representations; the most usual form of representative realism in the twentieth century also held that such representations *literally possess* qualities such as color and shape (e.g., on the most common view of sense data). Second, in Chapter 11.1–4, I follow Dretske (1995b) and Tye (1995) in labeling as "representational theories" their views that the phenomenal content of perceptual experience is exhausted by perceptual information about physical-object properties. Tim Crane (1992a, 8–9, 12) happily calls such views "pure information theories," which correctly (in my view) puts the focus on informational content. I consider Dretske's (1995b) and Tye's (2000) preferred name, "representational" theory, to be unhappy, because it takes a general notion, representation, and uses it too specifically, threatening to preclude uses of "representation" that don't mean "informational representation" in their specific sense. But their usage has become standard as a label for their type of theory, and so I've noted and used their terminology, while feeling free to use the term "representation" elsewhere in a more generic sense.

8

Color Perception and Neural Encoding

DOES METAMERIC MATCHING ENTAIL A LOSS OF INFORMATION?

It seems intuitively obvious that metameric matching of color samples entails a loss of information. Metamers are distinct distributions of wavelength and intensity (or *spectral energy distributions*) that perceivers cannot discriminate. Consider two color samples that are presented under ordinary white light and that appear to all normal observers to be of the same color. It is well-established that such color samples can have quite different surface-reflective properties; e.g., two samples that appear to be the same shade of green may in fact reflect strikingly different patterns of wavelengths within the visible spectrum (see Fig. 8.1). In this case, sameness of appearance under similar conditions of illumination does not entail sameness of surface reflectance. Spectrophotometrically diverse materials appear the same. It would seem then that information has been lost, that the visual system has failed in its task of chromatic discrimination.

This intuition implicitly relies on a conception of the function of color vision and on a related conception of how color samples should be individuated. It assumes that the function of color vision is to distinguish among spectral energy distributions, and that color samples should be individuated by their physical properties. I shall challenge these assumptions by articulating a different conception of the function of color vision, according to which color vision serves to partition visible objects into discrimination classes. From this perspective, objects are chromatically individuated by their membership in a

First published in David Hull and Mickey Forbes (eds.), *PSA 1992*, 2 vols. (East Lansing, Mich.: Philosophy of Science Association, 1992), 1:492–504, copyright © 1992 by the Philosophy of Science Association. Reprinted with permission.

particular equivalence class. Spectrophotometric diversity may in some cases (though not in all) be consistent with sameness of class membership. Metameric matching need not entail a loss of (pertinent) information.

My argument requires the articulation and adjudication of competing conceptions of the function of color vision. For my stalking horse I will examine the conception of color vision advanced by Barlow (1982c) and his followers (Buchsbaum and Gottschalk 1983). I will contrast this conception with one derived from an approach to vision in the spirit of Marr's (1982), though it will turn out that it is not Marr's own analysis of color. My argument presents a function-based analysis of the content of color sensations (thereby extending Ch. 2, consistently with Matthen 1988); however, someone who accepted function-ascription in biology but was squeamish about content-ascription could reformulate the argument using only function-ascriptions.

1. Task Analysis and Perceptual Content

In recent years there has been increasing attention to the role of task analysis in the investigation of psychological systems. A task analysis specifies what it is that a particular system does, where this "doing" cannot be captured through mere behavioral description; it is a specification of the function of a given system, or of its task within the economy of the organism. To take a nonpsychological example, there are many things that the digestive system "does," including producing growling noises when inputs have been light. But its function, its contribution to the economy of the organism, is to break down nutrients for distribution in the body. In psychology, the task-analysis approach seeks to determine the functions of various psychological systems, or their contributions to the psychological or cognitive economy of the organism.

Teleology lingers in the background of task analyses (sometimes being brought into plain sight). Such teleology is underwritten by appeal to natural selection. In the popular Wrightian analysis of functions (and its descendants), a function is ascribed to a type of system through an etiological analysis: a system's function is whatever it does that explains (evolutionarily) its presence in organisms of a certain type (Wright 1973; Matthen 1988; Millikan 1984). To ascribe a function is to make a conjecture about the adaptive significance of a given structure, and hence about the characteristics of the structure that led to its fixation and subsequent maintenance in a (temporally persisting) species of organisms. Such conjectures are difficult to confirm or disconfirm, but they are not totally immune from empirical evidence (and science is in the business of venturing beyond the data). In any event, task analysis is central to physiology and psychology, and an appeal to adaptation and evolution currently offers the most promising means of legitimizing the latent teleology of such analyses.

When applied to representational systems such as the visual system, task analysis provides a means of ascribing representational content to states of the system. Matthen (1988) makes this point in treating perceptual systems as systems that have the function of detecting the presence of certain environmental conditions; the "on" state of the detector mechanism is then ascribed representational content in accordance with the environmental condition it serves to detect. Thus, the "on" state of an edge detector has the content *edge*. More generally, various states of the visual system are assigned content in virtue of the environmental characteristics it is their function to represent: determinate shapes, sizes, motions, positions, and colors, to name a few (Chs. 2, 3).

The notions of task analysis, etiological function-ascription, and function-based content-ascription have not received universal endorsement. But for present purposes I will take them as given. My aim is to show how competing task analyses have been given for the function of the visual system and in particular for the reception and postretinal transmission of information about color. These competing analyses lead to different conceptions of the content of color perception, or of the function of color detecting mechanisms in the visual system.

2. Contrasting Task Analyses of the Visual System

Marr (1982) should be credited for drawing attention to the important role of task analysis in the investigation of perceptual systems. But he did not invent task analysis. Visual theorists have proposed (or presupposed) conceptions of the function of vision from earliest times (Aristotle 1984*b*, 436^{b}18–437^{a}9; Ptolemy 1989, bk. 2), and more recently Gibson (1966) made investigation of the natural functions of the senses central to his *perceptual systems* approach. Marr's own analysis, which assigns to human "early vision" the function of producing a representation of the spatial and chromatic properties of the distal scene, shares much with Gibson's (1950, 1966) analysis of the visual system. According to this conception, the perceptual apparatus is "distally focused," that is, it is tuned toward representing structures at a distance, and is not particularly tuned toward the representation of its own proximal states (e.g., the state of the retina).

Marr contrasts his approach with that of Barlow, and he criticizes the latter for merely describing the activity of single cells without addressing the question of the function of that activity (Marr 1982, 12–15, 19). In their work on space and color coding Barlow and his followers have emphasized the problem of the encoding and neural transmission of the physical characteristics of the retinal image, as opposed to the problem of representing distal scenes. This is not, as Marr charges, because Barlow failed to appreciate the importance of task analysis itself. Rather, it is because he (and his followers) gave a different task analysis than that favored by Marr. Examination of these contrasting task analyses will bring into relief the issues about metamers in color vision that I wish to address.

Far from failing to appreciate the notion of task analysis, Barlow explicitly proposes to analyze the functions of the sense organs. Thus, in an early paper he asserts that birds' wings are for flying, and asks, in effect, what sensory relays are for (1961b, 217). Indeed, his early work on fly detectors (Barlow 1953) led him to formulate the "password" hypothesis, according to which certain physical characteristics of stimuli act as "releasers" to initiate adaptively appropriate behavior, such as tongue-shooting (1961b, 219–20). But by and large, Barlow and his followers have emphasized the function of the senses as recorders of the physical properties of the image on the retina. Barlow described the function of the retina as follows: "The retina is a thin sheet of photoreceptors and nerve cells lining the back of the eye where the image is formed. It is obvious that its functional role is to encode the image falling on the retina as a pattern of nerve impulses in order to transmit the picture up the optic nerve to the brain" (Barlow 1982b, 102). More recently, Sterling has written that "the retina's task is to convert th[e] optical image into a 'neural image' for transmission down the optic nerve to a multitude of centers for further analysis" (1990, 170).

Although these authors are analyzing the function of the retina, not of the visual system as a whole, their conception of retinal functioning is part of a larger conception of how the visual system works. According to this conception, the retina records the physical image for efficient transmission to central visual centers (Barlow 1961a; Woodhouse and Barlow 1982), where subsequent processes "interpret" the neurally encoded image (Barlow 1982a, 31–2). Barlow in fact conceives of the senses as *physical instruments* designed to accurately encode the physical properties of the proximal stimulus; remarking on the familiar practice of labeling the external senses as "exteroceptors," he observes that "these so-called exteroceptors are really specialised interoceptors; they sense the outer world only by means of its physical and chemical influence on the special sense cells of the nose, the ears, or the eyes" (Barlow 1982a, 1).

De facto, he has adopted what Gibson once labeled the conception of the senses as "channels of sensation" (1966, 3), by which he meant that one conceives the sense organs as recording their own state, rather than as components in a system that has the function of perceiving the distal environment. (Of course, all concerned agree that sensory transducers are affected by physical energy; the matter in question is the functional analysis of the detection and representational systems in which the transducers serve.)

Marr, by contrast, conceives vision—or at least early vision in primates—as having the function of generating a representation of the distal layout (1982, 41–2, 268–9). In connection with this conception of early vision, he considers the transduction process from the standpoint of the reception of stimulus characteristics that will allow recovery of distal properties. In considering the coding of spatial information on the retina, he focuses on the problem of detecting the aspects of the image that are informative of distal spatial structure. He thus looks for aspects of the image that "correspond to real physical changes on the viewed surface" (1982, 44). Hence, he emphasizes zero-crossings because of their correlation with physical edges in the world (49–50, 54). Similarly, in considering what encoding of the retinal image might best serve as input for stereopsis and detection of directional motion, he emphasizes that "by and large the primitives that the processes operate on should correspond to physical items that have identifiable physical properties and occupy a definite location on a surface in the world" (105); again, Marr proposes that zero-crossings might be appropriate (106). A Barlowist might object that detection of zero-crossings is not a good idea because it does not lead to an efficient encoding of the retinal image (Eckert *et al.*, unpublished). But Marr would be nonplussed: he did not view the visual system as having the function of encoding the retinal image for transmission to higher centers. Rather, he saw the retina as detecting distally relevant features of proximal stimulation. In Marr's analysis, the image is not conceived simply as a two-dimensional pattern that must be encoded with minimum loss of information about the image itself, as if the problem of retinal encoding were one in video engineering.

An important moral of this brief comparison is that, depending on one's conception of the function of vision, one will have differing conceptions of the properties that are encoded and hence represented in the process of neural transmission. Barlow, reflecting the inspiration of his approach in engineering and communication theory, emphasizes the reliable coding of generic physical properties present at a sender (such as spatial frequencies on the retina) so that the physical properties could be reconstructed at the receiver (in the visual cortex). Ultimately, he suggests, a completely reversible code, in which one could fully specify the causes of sensation, would depend upon a completed scientific (read: physical) description of sensory energy (1961*a*, 354–9). Detection of physical properties is primary; information about such properties subsequently enters into inferential reasoning about distal causes, and only through such "interpretation" does it yield representations of the distal (behaviorally relevant) world. Marr, by contrast, reflecting the inspiration of his approach in biology and psychology, looks to the biological significance of sensory systems and hence conceives of them as systems for representing organismically significant properties of the distal environment. These properties are described in a biological vocabulary: Marr (1982, 32) describes the functional organization of spider vision to detect mates by detecting a pattern of light characteristic of a conspecific of opposite sex; in early human vision, he emphasizes the representation of distal spatial structures of human scale. These biological properties of course have a physical realization; indeed, the physical properties of light, distal objects, and optical media place constraints on the mechanisms of visual representation and detection. Nonetheless, in Marr's conception, as in Gibson's, the senses are taken to be detectors of biologically relevant properties. And the regularities upon which sensory systems depend for their functioning—Marr's "physical assumptions" (1982, 44–51) and Gibson's ecological regularities (1966, ch. 1)—are not laws of physics, but local (earthly, or even niche-specific) regularities in the relations between organism and environment. The difference between the *physical instruments* and *perceptual systems* approaches can be articulated more fully by returning to the case of color.

3. Competing Task analyses of Color Vision[1]

What is the function of color vision? No single answer can be given for all organisms. Even if the question is narrowed to the function of color vision in vertebrates, it still admits a variety of answers, depending on how widely one construes "function." Here I intend to leave aside various functions that color vision has assumed in complex human societies and to focus on conceptions of the function of color vision explicit or implicit in the literature associated with the Barlow and Gibson/Marr approaches. These competing conceptions of the function of color vision lead to differing task analyses and hence to differing conceptions of the content of color perception, and in particular of the properties in the world that perceived colors represent.

---

[1] For the purposes of this section, as in the rest of the chapter, "color" is used to mean what color scientists call "hue," or "chromatic color" (Boynton 1990, Hurvich 1981).

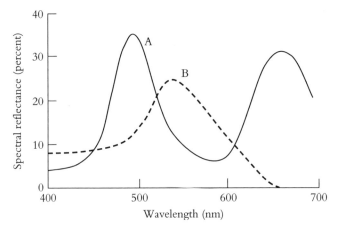

Figure 8.1. Two spectral reflectance distributions that produce matching greens in daylight for normal human observers. After Hurvich (1981), 207.

Barlow and his followers ascribe to the color receptors in the retina, and to color vision itself, the function of encoding accurately (and hence discriminating among) spectral energy distributions in the visible range of the spectrum. As Barlow puts it, "For colour vision, the task of the eye is to discriminate different distributions of energy over the spectrum" (1982c, 635). Buchsbaum and Gottschalk echo the same point: "The visual system is concerned with estimating the spectral functional shape of the incoming colour stimulus" (1983, 92). A spectral energy distribution is a well-defined physical magnitude mapping wavelength against intensity within a given sample of light, and thereby producing a particular "spectral functional shape." According to Barlow's conception, an optimal color system would encode each spectral energy distribution differently. Our trichromatic system is good, but not perfect, at encoding various distributions. It discriminates many distributions, but for some physically distinct combinations of wavelengths it gives the same response. This is the phenomenon of metamerism, illustrated in Figure 8.1.[2] According to Barlow (1982c) and Buchsbaum and Gottschalk (1983), metameric matching (same response to distinct energy distributions) is a failure of the visual system, a loss of information. It counts as a failure in the context of a specific conception of the function of the color system: to discriminate among spectral energy distributions. This approach to color vision is consonant with Barlow's conception of the visual system as a physical instrument. It treats

---

[2] Metamerism can be defined for samples of light received at the eye, or for surfaces illuminated by a given light source; my discussion takes surface metamers as its primary example.

the problem of color encoding much as a video engineer might treat the problem of building a good television camera: as the problem of accurately encoding the physical characteristics of a signal within given dimensions of variation. It may not be the happiest conception of the task of vertebrate color vision.

Marr's (1982, 250–64) brief treatment of color is an extension of his general program: he ascribes to the color system the function of determining the color of a distal surface, where "color" is defined as the spectral distribution of the surface reflectance. Although he differs from Barlow and his followers in emphasizing the distal focus of color vision, he nonetheless adopts the common attitude that color is to be understood as a physically defined property of the distal stimulus, in this case, its surface-reflective characteristics. As far as can be told from Marr's analysis, he considered it the function of color vision to represent each physically distinct surface reflectance differently. Hence, he too might consider surface metamerism to reveal a deficiency in color vision.

In this case Marr has not been true to the spirit of his approach, which enjoins the investigator to reflect upon empirically given regularities of the visual environment (as extant during the evolution of the visual system) in seeking to understand the functioning of the visual system. That is, he does not provide a set of "physical assumptions"—ecological regularities pertaining to the earthly environment—for color vision, corresponding to those he provided for the recovery of the spatial structure of distal surfaces (1982, 44–51). His analysis of color vision does not analyze the characteristics of the distal stimulus as fully as it might; rather, it simply accepts the usual spectrophotometric description.

What would correspond, in the case of color, to the "physical assumptions" of Marr's analysis of spatial perception? Consider the spatial case more fully. Marr's analysis sought to discover regularities of reflective surfaces in earthly environments that a visual system might be built to exploit in reducing the informational equivocation of the retinal image. Marr conjectured that the visual system might have evolved to make use of certain surface regularities, such as evenness of grain, which allow it implicitly to restrict the domain of permissible perceptual outcomes, thereby allowing the system, in environments for which the regularities hold, to recover successfully surfaces that it otherwise could not. In the case of color, a similar restriction would occur if it were supposed that the function of the color system is not to discriminate all possible spectral energy distributions, or surface reflectance characteristics, within the range of the visible spectrum, but rather is to permit useful discriminations among determinate, environmentally given classes of surface reflectances. Adjudication of the functional adequacy of color discrimination would require consideration of the actual distribution of surface reflectances and of the organismic significance of differences among objects with differing surface reflectances for a token species in its characteristic environment; it could not be carried out by an abstract analysis of spectral resolving power alone. (This is not to deny the usefulness of analyzing the system's abilities in this regard, on which see Section 4.)

Assume that one function of color vision is to enhance the discriminability of objects and surface features, and that a particular color system serves to promote the discrimination of healthy green plants from soil and rocks. Such a color system must be able to discriminate the surface reflectances of green plants from other reflectances. In evaluating the proficiency of the system, it would be of no consequence if there were physically possible but not actual (nonplant) metameric matches to green plants that the system could not discriminate. As long as such potentially equivocal stimuli were not extant in the environment, the fact that the color system could not discriminate them would not imply a functional deficiency. Similarly, for the purpose of enhancing the discriminability of foliage, it would be of no consequence if various types of soil and rocks possessed metameric surface reflectances. Indeed, it might well be an advantage if classes of surfaces that were biologically equivalent in relation to a given organism appeared to be of the same color to that organism, despite spectrophotometric variations in surface-reflective properties (an advantage consisting in fewer irrelevant differences among sensory representations). Under this analysis, an adaptively better color system would be one that allowed the organism to do a better job of discriminating environmentally significant objects or surface characteristics than could a conspecific with less sensitive or no color vision.

An approach to color vision of the sort just canvassed has in fact been taken by investigators who adopt a comparative and evolutionary approach. Jacobs (1981) is one such investigator. He approaches color vision with the working hypothesis that its primary function is to enhance object discrimination, and ultimately, object recognition, by providing an additional source of information, beyond achromatic differences in surface reflectances, for discriminating objects with characteristic surface compositions. He reports that achromatic luminance discrimination is very good in vertebrates, but that discrimination is enhanced by as much as one third when color is added (1981, 168–9). He repeats the familiar conjecture, described by Polyak (1957), that one function of color vision might be to aid in the discrimination of ripened fruit (taking on a red, orange, or yellow color) from the surrounding green foliage (Jacobs 1981, 160, 179). He concludes that "it is hard to believe that color visual systems did not evolve in concert with the particular spectral energy distributions that are critical that each species be able to discriminate," though he adds that firm evidence for this view has yet to be found (174). In any event, the implied conception of the function of color vision is clear: its function is to facilitate discrimination among biologically relevant, environmentally given classes of object surfaces.

Jacobs (1981, 160) distinguishes three uses of color perception in the cognition of objects: (1) object detection, by which he means the discrimination of separate objects (say, a red object from its green surroundings), (2) object recognition, or the recognition of an object as being of a certain kind (say, an apple), and (3) signal properties of color, or the use of color to discover further properties of a kind of object (that the apple is almost ripe). Each of these uses goes beyond the bare perceptual representation of color itself; each involves further representational or cognitive capacities, from the simple cognition of something as an object, to its cognition as an object of a certain kind, or as an object of that kind possessing one variable property rather than another. These are all cases in which the perception of color aids in a further cognitive achievement, involving additional representational content beyond that of mere color perception. I wish to ask about the representational content of perceived colors (or of color sensations) themselves.

The preceding analysis of the function of color vision suggests that color perceptions have as their content classes of object surfaces. Let us say that the content of our color perceptions is various object surface colors. "Surface colors" themselves are determined in relation to a particular kind of visual system: to have the same surface color is to appear the same to normal observers under prevailing conditions of natural illumination. As metamerism reveals, surface color cannot be equated with a physical property such as spectral reflectance, because, under the present definition, two objects can have the same surface color but different reflectances. Color, as a property of the surfaces of objects, is that group of (often physically disjunctive) surface reflectances that form an equivalence class in relation to a given visual system in its characteristic photic environment.[3] It is a relational property, which must be defined in relation to a specific type of visual system, and it does not constitute a well-formed physical kind. Indeed, from the point of view of physics various equivalence classes are heterogeneous; they are only grouped together as color

---

[3] This conception of color as a property of objects is similar to Beck's definition of color as "the property of light by which two objects of the same size, shape, and texture can be distinguished" (1972, 181; his definition extends to achromatic color). It is opposed to the philosophical analyses of Hilbert (1987, 99), who equates colors in objects with individual physical surface reflectances, and of Hardin (1988, 111–112), who contends that, failing a reduction of color to a physical property such as surface reflectance, it should be categorized as an illusion.

kinds because of their effects on a token kind of visual system. Color shares this relational aspect with other biologically constituted properties, such as *nutrient*.

On this conception, color sensations have their own representational content, prior to the subsequent cognitive categorization of objects into kinds. Color vision functions to enhance the discriminability of surfaces of objects of different kinds, but it falls to higher cognitive processes to recognize those objects for the kinds of objects they are, and hence to perceive their utility or lack thereof. For surface-perceiving visual systems such as those of primates, presumably this is so even if in a given environment the only reason to discriminate red from green is in order to be able to discern ripe fruit amidst foliage. Differences of surface color are represented in the processes of early vision, which are processes for representing the surface layout of the environment. The content of the representations produced by such processes is limited to surface properties. Color adds a new dimension of discriminability, or a new class of represented surface differences. But even if only ripe fruit is red, the bare perception of *red* doesn't mean *ripe fruit* unless the system it is part of is itself specialized for fruit detection. But presumably, if detection of ripe fruit was a selective pressure on the development of color vision, the animals in question could already discriminate fruit on the basis of other surface-reflective properties (shape, texture, achromatic luminance). Adding color gave them an added surface feature to use in discrimination. The content assigned to perceived colors in this case pertains to the surface feature, not to the more sophisticated cognitive achievement of recognizing an object as food of a certain sort.

As this sketch makes clear, content assignment to color sensations relies on a task analysis of the color system, and this analysis itself implicitly contains and is guided by evolutionary conjectures. The disparate tendencies of Barlow's physical-instruments approach and of the perceptual-systems approach as developed in this chapter are rendered explicit in their respective analyses of the evolution of trichromacy.

4. Evolution, Optimization, and Trichromacy

The physical-instruments and perceptual-systems approaches adopt quite different analyses of the shift from dichromacy to trichromacy during the course of mammalian evolution. Barlow and his followers address this topic by asking how well trichromatic systems discriminate among all possible spectral energy distributions within the visible spectrum. Trichromatic systems do well, though not perfectly, as metamerism shows. On the ecological conception adopted by the perceptual-systems approach, the relevant query is not how good trichromacy is at covering the spectrum; rather, one should ask what new (or improved) discriminations of environmentally significant object surfaces trichromacy allows. Both approaches appeal to evolution, for Barlow couches his analysis of trichromacy in terms of optimality, and he assumes that evolving systems are driven toward optimal performance (within resource constraints). Comparing Barlow's appeal to evolution with other evolutionary accounts of color vision will allow us to see both the usefulness and the limitations of his physical-instruments approach.

Barlow and his followers evaluate trichromatic systems for their efficiency in coding color information. They ask, in effect, what the optimal coding for discriminating among spectral energy distributions might be, and then they test various assortments of receptors—mainly, trichromatic and tetrachromatic—for their sensitivity, concluding that a trichromatic system does remarkably well (Barlow 1982c; Buchsbaum and Gottschalk 1983). The analysis is rigorous and ingenious. Thus, Barlow considers various ways in which distinct sinusoidal functions of wavelength and intensity ("comb-filtered" spectral energy distributions) can be resolved by color systems with various receptor properties. He concludes that, given the broad receptivity of human cones, little or no advantage in resolving such functions would be gained by having four types of cone rather than three. He offers this finding as an explanation for why trichromacy might have evolved in mammals (1982c, 641).

Barlow's argument appeals to the controversial notion that evolution optimizes. Recent work cautiously endorses the claim that optimizing selection has played a role in evolution (Travis 1989). Careful statements of the optimization approach, such as that of Maynard Smith (1978), avoid the assumption that organisms are in some general sense optimally designed. Maynard Smith characterizes optimization theories as attempts to formulate concrete hypotheses about the selective forces at work in shaping the diversity of living things. He contends that, when properly formulated, such hypotheses make specific assumptions of three kinds: (1) about the kinds of phenotypes that are possible given present species characteristics, (2) about what is optimized, and (3) about the mode of inheritance of the trait in question. As Maynard Smith (1978, 33–4) stresses, point (2) is a conjecture about the selection forces that have been at work in fixing a trait. He argues that candidate optimizing-explanations must include as part of the hypothesis under test a specification of the trait that is being optimized and of the selection forces that operate upon it.

Optimization arguments have been applied to the evolution of the visual system with apparent success. Thus, Woodhouse and Barlow (1982, 136) have found that the spacing of receptors in the fovea is very near the theoretical limit set by the physical optics of the eye; they offer evolutionary optimization as the explanation. Others have found that photoreceptors in deep-sea fish have absorption properties that maximize photic sensitivity in a light-starved environment (Lythgoe 1979, 82–3). It is important that optimization arguments be constrained by assumptions of type (1), pertaining to possible phenotypes. Barlow (1982c) explains the lack of optimal spacing among the three types of cones in mammalian trichromats by appealing to the tradeoff between optimizing color sensitivity and spatial resolution. For the purpose of sampling spectral energy distributions, even spacing among the peak sensitivities would be desirable. As it happens, the "red" and "green" cones cluster at 565 and 535 nm while the "blue" cone is at 440 nm. Barlow speculates that the close similarity between red and green cones allows them to be pooled for the purposes of spatial resolution, thereby effectively doubling the number of foveal receptors (1982c, 642). Goldsmith (1990), in an extensive review of the interplay between optimization and constraints on phenotypic possibilities, offers a quite different explanation. The distinction between red and green cones is relatively recent (65 million years), and presumably stems from a mutation in the gene for an ancestral green cone. In some dichromatic species of New World monkeys, a related gene for the green cone regularly produces variants with a spread of 30 to 35 nm. Goldsmith conjectures that molecular genetic constraints fix the possible red and green cone variation in the range of 535 to 570 nm, and that this variation set the phenotypic boundaries within which selection for trichromacy could act. He concludes that "the capricious course of mammalian evolutionary history, rather than adaptation by natural selection, is probably primarily responsible for the spectral positions of the long- and mid-wavelength cone pigments" (1990, 317). While further work may be needed to determine the relative roles of genetic constraint and selection pressures in this case, it is clear that optimization arguments should seek to specify the domain of phenotypic possibilities.

As Section 3 has shown, characterization of what is being optimized may be even more fundamental. The optimization arguments of Barlow and his followers suggest that in color vision the trait to be optimized is the power to resolve individual spectral energy distributions or physical surface reflectances. They present no argument that the adaptiveness of color vision depends on this ability; indeed, they provide no argument that this ability would be biologically adaptive. Instead, they simply assume that spectrophotometric resolution is the appropriate measure of performance. By contrast, I have emphasized the adaptive feature of color vision suggested by Jacobs (1981), namely, increased discriminability of object surfaces. The appropriate measure of the adaptiveness of trichromacy over dichromacy on this conception hinges on new or enhanced discriminability of surfaces in an animal's environment.

The extant studies of the relation between environment and evolution in color vision do not support the Barlow approach. The evolution of distinct cone pigments, a prerequisite for color vision, probably was not initially driven by a demand for spectral differentiation. Pigments with a range of sensitivity maxima would increase the range of optic sensitivity of the eye, thereby permitting increased discriminations among surface reflectances without necessarily permitting differential spectral sensitivity. (In order for multiple cone types to be exploited for color discrimination, the available neural machinery must be sensitive to differences in activity between or among cone types; a system that summed across cone types would enjoy enhanced optic range without color vision—see Goldsmith 1990, 301–4; Jacobs 1981, 178–9.) In an extensive study of the relation between environmental conditions and cone types, McFarland and Munz (1975) concluded that in certain tropical fishes, a system of two cone types evolved in order to enhance the contrast between objects and their background in spectrally restricted underwater photic environments. In such environments, dark objects can best be discriminated with a receptor whose sensitivity matches the peak spectral transmission of sea water (which, at a depth of 25 m, is nearly monochromatic). Light objects can best be discriminated with a pigment whose sensitivity is offset from the background light. On the basis of comparing several species with different feeding habits and inhabiting different photic environments, McFarland and Munz argued that "the evolutionary selection of multiple photopic systems, and of color vision itself, is probably related to the maximization of contrast against monochromatic backgrounds" (1975, 1045). Although little work has been done measuring the environment in which primate trichromacy evolved, Jacobs reports that investigation of the environment of one South American primate supports the view that the principal color discriminations are "among subtle shades of green or between contrasting colors and green" (Snodderly 1979, as quoted in Jacobs 1981, 175). Here, ecological considerations suggest that the finest discriminations are needed within the greens, and otherwise between the greens and the entire red–yellow end of the spectrum.

The physical-instruments approach of Barlow and his followers is not without its place. Optimization arguments can help to guide the formulation of functional and evolutionary hypotheses; maximization of sensitivity to various physical properties of stimulation is one form of optimization. Rigorous specification of the physical capacities of sensory systems can thus arm the investigator with candidate hypotheses about function. It would be a mistake, however, simply to assume that there has been evolutionary pressure to optimize sensitivity for the stimulus dimensions of greatest interest to physicists or to video engineers. Judgments of function must be tested by taking the animal–environment relation into account. Only by learning how sensory systems actually are used can we determine what they are for.

5. Conclusion

Assume that the function of early vision in primates is to provide representations of adaptively significant features of the distal environment. The task of the system should then be described by denominating the adaptive significance of the distal properties. On this conception, the visual system is not a physical instrument for recording the values of proximal stimulus as described in physical optics. Rather, it is a perceptual system with the function of representing surfaces as an aid to detecting food and other significant objects. Extended to the case of color vision, this approach suggests that metameric matching need not entail a loss of information. If color vision has the function of discriminating particular environmentally given classes of object surfaces, the mere possibility of metamerism may be irrelevant to an assessment of its performance. Further, environmentally extant metamers need not entail a discriminatory deficiency if their discrimination would not yield a biologically significant partition of environmental surfaces. The representational content of color perception might best be conceived in terms of partitions of object surfaces into discrimination classes that are conjoined with adaptively significant objects, and not in terms of a physical specification of spectral energy distributions.

9

Objectivity and Subjectivity Revisited

COLOR AS A PSYCHOBIOLOGICAL PROPERTY

1. Introduction

Philosophical theories of color divide into three. There are the so-called objectivists, who argue that color is a mind-independent property of objects. There are the subjectivists, who argue that color is not a property of objects, but an internal state of the perceiver or the subjective content of a perceiver's experience. And there are the relationalists, who argue that color, considered as a property of objects, is a relational property; it is a property that surfaces and light sources have of causing experiences with various phenomenal characters in perceivers.

These philosophical theories differ on the question of what color is. Objectivists think of color as a physical property, which is in principle independent of color experience and visual perception. Subjectivists make color experience primary in their conceptions of color; indeed, they think that the notion of color has primary reference only to visual experience. Relationalists also define color in relation to color experience; however, they are able to define color as a property of the surfaces of objects by considering the relation between objects and color experience.

Proponents of all three positions marshal the available scientific evidence in their support. To support objectivism, Hilbert (1987, 1992) appeals to

First published in Rainer Mausfeld and Dieter Heyer (eds.), *Colour Perception: Mind and the Physical World* (Oxford: Oxford University Press, 2003), 187–202, copyright © 2003 by Oxford University Press. Reprinted with permission.

Maloney and Wandell's (1986) analysis of color constancy as an inference to the spectral reflectance distribution of a given surface. The objective colors of things are equated with individual surface reflectance distributions. In arguing for a subjectivist position, Hardin (1988) points to facts of perceiver variability and variety in the physical causes of color phenomena. He argues that because color cannot be equated with a specific physical kind, color experience is a (useful) illusion. The relationalist uses similar sorts of data to argue that color as a property of objects is constituted by the fact that illuminated objects have a disposition to cause perceivers to experience color visually (J. Campbell 1993; Harman 1996; Johnston 1992). Some relationalists appeal to a functional notion of color perception, perhaps supplemented with data concerning interspecies differences, to argue that color is a psychobiological property, and that a primary function of color perception is discrimination among objects (Ch. 8; Thompson 1995).

The frequent appeal to the facts of color science in the philosophical color literature is a good thing. It is an instance of the more general trend in philosophy of science to expect that the philosopher's examples and arguments are responsive to actual scientific positions and to common features of scientific practice (see Hatfield 1995a). At the same time, attention to scientific practice reveals that interesting questions at the forefronts of science typically are not resolved by a bare appeal to facts, but to facts in relation to a background of scientific theory and philosophical assumption. The same feature is present in philosophical debates on color. The three major positions just named depend heavily on background understandings of theoretical terms from both science and philosophy; two of the most important are the terms "objective" and "subjective" themselves.

In this chapter I will focus on the notion of color as a property of the surfaces of objects. Examination of the arguments of the objectivists will help us understand how they seek to reduce color to a physical property of object surfaces. Subjectivists, by contrast, seek to argue that no such reduction is possible, and hence that color must be wholly subjective. I will argue that when functional considerations are taken into account, a relationalist position best accommodates the primary data concerning color perception, and permits a better understanding of the ways in which color is both objective and subjective. The chapter ends with a reconsideration of the notions of objectivity and subjectivity themselves, and a consideration of how modern technology can foster misleading expectations about the specificity of color properties.

2. Objectivism

Traditional objectivists hold that color is a mind-independent physical property of objects. The most likely candidate for such a property is the surface spectral reflectance (SSR) of an object. The SSR is the percentage of the light at each wavelength across the visible spectrum that is reflected by a surface. The amount reflected depends on the percentage of the light absorbed by the surface, the remainder being reflected. Figure 8.1 provides examples of two surface spectral reflectance distributions (or reflectance functions). The most important characteristic of such distributions for our purpose is that they tend in natural objects to be relatively smooth functions, which differ in shape. As we will see, the relation between such distributions and perceived color can be complex. But there are some regularities, such as that typical red objects will reflect more light toward the long-wavelength or red end of the visible spectrum, and typical blue objects will reflect more light toward the short-wavelength or blue end of the spectrum.

Sophisticated objectivists such as Hilbert (1987, 1992), Maloney (2003), and Wandell (1995, ch. 9) identify object colors with surface spectral reflectances. They see the visual system as seeking to develop a stable representation of the surface reflectance (or a more basic physical property related to that reflectance, such as Maloney's bidirectional reflectance density function). The ability to develop a stable representation of surface color under variations in ambient illumination is known as *color constancy*. The light received at the eyes from an object is a function of both the object's reflectance properties and the spectral composition of the illuminant (e.g., dawn sunlight, incandescent light, midday sunlight, all of which differ). Therefore, if constancy is to be achieved, the illuminant properties must somehow be accounted for. As traditionally conceived, this would require solving an equation with two unknowns (surface reflectance and illuminant) by contemplating only the value of their product (the light received at the eyes); so stated, the problem cannot be solved. Additional information of some sort is needed. Maloney and his colleagues have developed ingenious linear models of color constancy that attribute to the organism some engineering assumptions concerning candidate spectral reflectance distributions and the candidate illuminants, making the problem soluble within certain ranges of accuracy. Further, some objectivists, including Barlow (1982c), Hilbert (1992), and Shepard (1992), see color constancy as the driving force behind trichromacy (the three-pigment system in human and some other primate eyes). That is, they think that trichromacy evolved because it allows the eye to serve as a better instrument by which the visual system can recover information about SSRs.

Two aspects of the objectivist stance are of interest here. First, its overall conception of the task of color perception is what I have called a *physical instruments* conception (Ch. 8.3). Objectivists see the perceptual system as seeking a representation of a distal physical property, such as the SSR. Mausfeld (1998, 224) criticizes this view of perception for treating the visual system as a "measurement device." On such a conception, physics provides the appropriate concepts for describing the representational task in color vision, which is to achieve a representation of physical properties described as such. The relationalist functional view presented below offers an alternative to this conception of the visual system's function in color perception.

The second point of interest concerns the objectivist's response to the fact of metamerism. Metameric surface colors occur when different SSRs yield the same perceived color under specified conditions of illumination. This means that physically distinct stimuli, which exhibit different functions relating wavelength to the absorption and reflection of light, yield phenomenally indistinguishable color experiences. The phenomenon of metamerism is well established. The interesting question is how to interpret it.

Objectivists such as Hilbert (1987, ch. 5) and Barlow (1982c) conclude from metamerism that there are many more colors than we perceive. Having defined surface color in terms of SSR (or a related measure), they identify each SSR as a distinct color. If the human visual system, or any visual system, fails to discriminate among SSRs, then it fails to discriminate all the colors there are. Consonant with their physical-instrument conception of the function of color vision, the physical description of surface properties provides the standard for individuating colors, and not the facts of color experience.

3. Subjectivism

The position of subjectivism is most prominently associated with C. L. Hardin's 1988 book, *Color for Philosophers*. This book raised the standard of philosophical discussions of color by paying close attention to scientific work. Hardin examined the various objectivist and dispositionalist theories. (Dispositionalism is a type of relationalist theory.) He rejected objectivism and physicalism on the grounds that there is no single physical property corresponding to the colors we experience. In so doing, he adopted a phenomenalist stance: he took it that a theory of color should be driven by the facts of color perception. To this extent, he made color experience, or at least color response, fundamental in color theory considered as a part of the theory of vision.

Hardin argued that if physical properties cannot be put into sufficiently direct relation to color experience, the notion that colors are objective should be rejected (see also Boghossian and Velleman 1991). He disposed of an objectivism similar to Hilbert's (1987) by appealing to metamerism and certain other higher-order properties of color, such as the finding that red, green, yellow, blue, black, and white are the primary colors. Hardin contended that since objectivists cannot explain the special status of these primaries by appeal to physical properties alone, their attempted reduction fails. (Jackson and Pargetter 1987, though not responding specifically to Hardin, provide the basis for an objectivist reply that allows subjective variability but identifies color as the physical property that causes experience in individual perceivers in specific circumstances. This position, though interesting for its admission of the variability of relation between physical properties and color experience, fails to respond adequately to the objectivist desideratum of making color a mind-independent physical property, on which see Hilbert 1992.)

In addition, Hardin (1988) moved against dispositionalist theories of color vision, which he characterized as a variant of subjectivism. A common form of dispositionalism—descended from the natural philosophies of René Descartes and Robert Boyle, and made prominent in the philosophy of John Locke—holds that colors are secondary qualities (for a review, see Hilbert 1987, ch. 1). A secondary quality is a property of an object that is defined by the object's standard effect on something else. In the case of color, the standard effect is the "idea" or experience of color. In more recent language, the position holds that for an object to be a certain shade of blue is for it to produce a specific experience of blue in standard observers under standard conditions. The appeal to standard conditions takes account of differences in illumination; objects that look white in daylight may, in certain conditions, look red under red light. A dispositionalist theory might make daylight the standard condition, in which case the object would be classed as white. The notion of a standard observer rules out color blind observers, or observers in special states of adaptation or in drug-altered states.

Boyle and Locke expressed this position using the language of primary and secondary qualities. Primary qualities are physically basic. For Boyle and Locke, they include the size, shape, position, and motion of the microscopic corpuscles that they held to constitute matter. Candidates for the relevant primary qualities today might be the absorption and reflectance properties of surfaces, or the underlying atomic and molecular properties that determine those properties. Colors, sounds, tastes, odors, and tactual qualities such as hot and cold are secondary qualities. Physically, they are constituted from primary qualities (for Locke and Boyle, configurations of corpuscles). But they are defined as powers to produce sensations or ideas in the minds of observers. In this sense, they are relational properties. If there were no (actual, or perhaps possible) observers, there would be no secondary qualities—the existence of the secondary qualities depends upon there being observers in which the experience of color can be caused.

Hardin (1988) sought to show that the notions of standard conditions and standard observers cannot support a view that colors are stable dispositions of objects to produce experiences. The scientific literature shows that color constancy is not perfect. So if color in objects is the disposition to produce color experience of a specific hue (or shade of color) in standard observers under standard conditions, nature does not cooperate. Under any natural (i.e., not artificially restricted) interpretation of what might count as standard conditions or standard observers, the conditions and observers can be fixed and yet the color response vary (among standard observers and within the class of standard conditions). If the dispositionalist wants to assign to objects specific, stable, intersubjectively common hues using the relation between surface reflectance properties and the color experience of observers, the evidence Hardin presents poses a serious problem.

In the end, Hardin argues that close scrutiny of the notions of standard conditions and observers reveals that color is an interest-relative and subjective notion with no objective basis. He concludes that color experience is a useful illusion; it presents objects as having properties they do not have. The illusion results from properties that objects and perceivers do have, hence it has some foundation in reality; it is persistent, and so permits the use of color appearances in the classification of objects (Hardin 1988, ch. 2). But, Hardin thinks, these findings undermine any attempt to ascribe color as an objective property to objects (see also Boghossian and Velleman 1989).

In my view, Hardin's response to the scientific evidence is too extreme. By re-examining the notions of subjectivity and objectivity and reflecting further on the notion of property, I think we can find a place for a relationalist functional theory of color that permits color to be a *subject-relative*, but in important respects *objective* psychobiological property of objects. These reflections will not require that we examine or qualify the empirical results that Hardin describes. Rather, we will look at the theoretical context and philosophical assumptions that he and others use to interpret those results.

4. Relational Functionalism

I agree with Hardin that color experience should be an important component in any analysis of color as a property. My analysis therefore begins from the place of color in perception. From this position one might or might not come to reduce color as a property of objects to a mind-independent physical property. In fact, I also agree with the tenor of Hardin's response to physicalist objectivism (Ch. 8). However, I think that the sort of facts he presents can be made consistent with a certain kind of objectivist view of color, a relational functionalist view. My view is relationalist in that, like the dispositionalist, it accepts that color as a property in things consists in the disposition of things to cause experiences of a certain sort in perceivers. It is functionalist in that it looks to the biological function of color vision for guidance about what sort of property is constituted by the relations between objects and perceivers.

The analysis I will present disagrees with the physicalist objectivists on four important points. I will argue that:

- Color constancy need not be the driving force toward trichromacy.
- To possess color an object need not be assigned a precise shade of color.
- Properties can be species-relative.
- Objectivity is not always incompatible with subjectivity.

These points taken together are consonant with a view that trichromatic color vision evolved in primates as a means for discriminating objects by their surface properties, for which exact constancy is not needed. In opposition to Hardin's (1988) subjectivism, these points can serve as the basis for assigning color to objects as an objective, subject- and species-relative property.

One way of asking what property colored objects have is to ask what representational content is found in color experience. That is, what does experienced color represent about objects? The physicalist objectivist thinks that it does or should represent individual SSRs, and then concludes that to the extent that color experience does not uniquely reveal SSRs, it falls short of its representational task. My approach is that color experience represents surfaces as having properties that make them instances of a hue class. It may do so by representing the surface as having a specific hue, but this does not mean that the object can or should be assigned that particular shade as its color. Rather, the object is assigned a color type, in relation to its appearance to color observers of a specific type (e.g., normal human observers) under ecologically standard conditions (e.g., daylight viewing). If an object appears green, blue, red, yellow, etc., in daylight, then it is assigned that color, but need not be assigned (as a stable, objective property) the particular shade it appears as having to an individual observer under a given instance of daylight.

This position arises from a functionalist conception of assigning representational content in perception. A functional approach assigns content in relation to a task analysis, or an analysis of the function of the representational system in question (Chs. 2–3; Matthen 1988). Thus, one function of vision is surely to represent the spatial layout; various spatial structures would be assigned as contents of visual experiences under this analysis. In the case of color vision, to apply this sort of analysis one would seek to determine what the (or a) function of color vision is for a given species. (There need not be only one function in a given species, or across species.) Ascriptions of such functions are based in biology, and typically appeal to evolutionary theory. The basic idea is that a structure or system is assigned a function in accordance with the selection pressures that lead to its evolution and maintenance in a type of organism. Consequently, if color vision has come to have other, culturally defined functions that have not been active in natural selection, those functions are described as artifact-functions and are left out of the primary analysis of color as a naturally occurring property. (More on this below.)

The long history of the evolution of eyes shows that visual pigments are adapted to prevailing light conditions. The pure rod retinas of deep-sea fish are adapted to the small segment of the visible spectrum that penetrates to their depth (Lythgoe 1972; Lythgoe and Partridge 1991). In those with only one type of rod pigment, the wavelength of maximum light sensitivity of the rods closely matches the peak ambient light. That sort of match would be effective for fish who hunt from below, seeing their prey as dark areas against the downward light.

Many fishes are dichromats. Investigators have wondered how a two-cone system could evolve. They have considered evolutionary scenarios in which a stable two-cone retina might evolve prior to the development of dichromatic color vision itself. (The possession of two types of visual pigment is not sufficient for color vision; the visual system must compare the outputs of the two types for color discrimination to occur.) McFarland and Munz (1975) argue that the original selection pressure for two types of cones in ocean fish that hunt near the surface might have come from the demands of two sorts of discriminatory tasks. For hunting from below, such fish would be well served by cones with maximum sensitivity matching the peak wavelength in the available downwelling light, as for the deep-sea fish. That would make any object seen from below dark against a bright background. Along the horizontal line of sight, the peak available light is of shorter wavelength than the broad spectrum downwelling light (within several meters of the surface). Hence, for hunting objects along that line of sight, it is better to have a cone type with maximum sensitivity offset toward the long wavelengths. In that way, the ambient spacelight of the background would appear darker, and objects reflecting the broad-band downwelling light would stand out.

McFarland and Munz (1975) contend that two-pigment cone retinas might have evolved so that both sorts of discrimination could be served by a single eye. That would require separate visual pathways for each cone type, a precursor to color vision. They conjecture that "the evolution of high visual acuity with maximum contrast under varied photic conditions would favor the selection and maintenance of separate visual pathways for these different cases. In other words, we have described the elements necessary for color vision" (1975, 1073). Color vision would not be needed initially to explain the advantage of this system, and could evolve subsequently, once the two visual pathways were available to allow further selection on neural wiring.

Adopting a biofunctional and comparative attitude, we may ask what color vision is "for" in (at least some) mammals. After a thorough review of the literature, Jacobs (1993, 456−7) concluded that color vision serves the following functions:

(1) to provide contrast not based on achromatic brightness or lightness;
(2) to aid in the detection of small objects in a dappled environment, where lightness cues are largely masked (e.g., fruit in trees);
(3) to aid in segregation of objects divided by occlusion (e.g., fruit seen through leaves, see Mollon 1989);
(4) to identify objects by their stably perceived color (requires something approaching color constancy).

Only item (4) requires something approaching color constancy, and even it does not require perfect constancy; it would suffice if environmentally salient objects could be stably re-identified by color class. The fineness of the partition of the hue space needed to achieve this task would depend on the characteristics of the objects to be sorted (Ch. 8; Hatfield 1999). That of course is an empirical matter that would require analysis of the photic properties of biologically significant objects on a species by species basis.

Much of the literature on comparative color vision, and on the evolution of trichromacy in primates, stresses functions (1) to (3). Mammalian trichromacy is comparatively recent, having evolved in the Cenozoic era, after the adaptive radiation of mammals some 65 million years ago (Goldsmith 1990). Genetic analysis suggests that it evolved through selection on naturally occurring polymorphism in the middle-wavelength sensitive (MWS) cone. Thus, the short-wavelength cone is thought to have been stable, but the MWS cone to have exhibited polymorphic variance that provided instances of the MWS and LWS cone types, in relation to which selection for neural wiring to permit trichromatic color vision might occur. Trichromatic color vision of this sort would allow better discrimination of yellow, red, and orange objects found among green leaves. For such discrimination to occur, perfect or near-perfect color constancy would not be needed. Rather, it would need only be the case that yellow, red, and orange fruit was more easily discriminable to a trichromat (by comparison with a dichromat) across a significant range of natural lighting conditions. This "fruit detection" hypothesis has long been favored as the explanation of the development of color vision (e.g., Allen 1879, ch. 6; Walls 1942, ch. 12) and trichromacy (Polyak 1957, 972–4), and receives support from recent empirical studies such as those reported by Mollon (1989) and Jacobs (1996).

According to this analysis, when trichromacy evolved things gained new colors, as the visual system became able to group things using a more fine-grained partition of the chromatic appearance of surfaces. Thus, fruit and leaves came to appear more distinctly different, chromatically, than before. For tasks (1) to (3), there is no need for precise color constancy, nor any need that color properties be equated with specific shades (that is, highly determinate hues).

5. Color as a Psychobiological Property of Surfaces

Color is an attribute of objects that makes surfaces visually discriminable without a difference in brightness or lightness. Focusing for the moment on human color vision, it makes objects discriminable because they appear with differing hue or chromaticity. More generally, ascriptions of color vision to various animals can be made by finding that the members of a species (or a subpopulation of the species, e.g., normal trichromatic humans) can discriminate independently of brightness or lightness in E (an environment, which normally is specified by ecologically typical conditions).

Under this analysis, color is a relational attribute, analogous to being a solvent. The existence of color as an attribute of objects depends on the normal effects of objects on perceiving subjects. In humans, these effects include a phenomenal or experiential component. Accordingly, for an object to possess color is for it to have a surface reflectance that produces a phenomenal chromatic visual presence that permits discrimination among objects independent of brightness or lightness by members of a type of population in E.

The colors under which objects appear can serve as the basis for categorizing objects. However, qualitatively similar clusters of color experiences are not themselves categories (*pace* Thompson 1995, 184, 196). For the colors of objects to be useful for categorization, the same object should appear with the same hue-type under a variety of conditions, but it need not appear with the same specific hue. It is consistent with an object possessing color that it appear differently under differing conditions (of the perceiver, and/or the environment); such differences would be multiplied if there were no color constancy, but objects would still possess the attribute of color. Even with some degree of color constancy, the expression of the attribute of color can be affected by environmental conditions and the state of the perceiver.

Modern color science has developed colorimetry, or the alignment of color judgments with combinations of wavelengths, into an exact art (Kaiser and Boynton 1996, 25–6, and appendix). This art is made possible by severely restricting the conditions under which color observations are made by test observers. The high degree of accuracy achieved makes possible standardized dyes, and serves engineering functions such as the production of color television sets. The specificity found in laboratory colorimetry should not result in our treating the color attribute as if it were realized by a set of finely differentiated color properties (corresponding to the range of highly specific hues). For certain cultural, scientific, or industrial purposes, such specificity is desirable. However, when color vision is regarded as a biological capacity of sighted animals, the resulting functional approach to the color attribute suggests it is realized by surface characteristics that yield varying color responses across differences in ambient conditions and type and state of perceiving subject.

This variation also is recognized in color science. The attitude toward it varies. We have seen that many objectivists view "the color of an object" as a highly specific physical property that may be recovered with more or less success by natural visual systems under ecological photic conditions; under this conception, the same response to differing SSRs, or differing responses to the same SSR, indicate error. Subjectivists have concluded that the extant variation undermines the very notion that objects are really colored (have a color property). In my view, the subjectivist gives up on color properties too quickly, while the objectivist divorces the color property from color experience and misdescribes the function of color vision.

There is a prejudice in ordinary philosophical uses of language against relational attributes and properties, and against attributes that don't stably possess determinate values. Yet there are perfectly good relational property types that, in virtue of their relativity, may be differently assigned to one and the same object at the same time. An example is the biological property of being nutritious. To be nutritious is to be usable in metabolism. The property of being nutritious is species-relative. Wood is nutritious for termites, not for humans; that is, it possesses the property of being nutritious for termites, but does not have a nutritive property in relation to humans. Its being nutritious depends on its physicochemical properties. These physicochemical properties have effects on all sorts of things, and interact with other chemicals during metabolism. Being nutritious does not add anything to the chemical constitution of wood. Yet it is a property that wood might or might not have. If there could be no wood-eating animals, wood would not be an animal nutrient. It would not be altered physically by facts about its being or not being a nutrient. But it would have, or not have, a biological property.

Color as an attribute of objects is analogous to the property of being nutritious, except that the effect it has on organisms has a mental component. Hence, I denominate color a psychobiological attribute. It is a property objects have, in relation to perceivers, of being visually discriminable by phenomenal hue rather than lightness or brightness. (Notice that I take phenomenal hue, color, or chromaticity as primitives, and do not try to define them in terms of something else; that is a characteristic of theories that make color experience, or color discriminatory capacities, theoretically primary.)

Because color properties are individuated in relation to perceivers, objects might be described under more than one color name at the same time, in relation to various populations of seers. That is fine, because they have as many instances of the relational color property as there are distinct classes of perceivers to which objects are related. Objects that may be assigned more than one color name (e.g., they are yellow to certain dichromats but orange to trichromats) possess two (or more) distinct color properties at the same time, depending on how many type-distinct classes of color perceivers there are for whom they appear chromatically distinct. This does not of course imply that they simultaneously possess mutually exclusive properties (being yellow and being orange in the same respect at the same time); they have as many different color properties as there are types of perceiver in which they cause type-distinct color responses. Moreover, if there were not (and could not be?) any chromatically endowed perceivers, there would be no colors. There would of course still be photons and reflectances.

The metaphysics of relational and dispositional properties is intricate (see McLaughlin 2003). When I say that color is a relational property that involves the disposition of objects to cause experiences of certain sorts in a population of perceivers, I am telling you what kind of property it is. I am not trying to capture ordinary language talk about colors. (Philosophical color theories—see, e.g., Jackson and Pargetter 1987, Johnston 1992—are often driven by "ordinary" intuitions about property and causal talk, but such language has no special metaphysical authority in my view.) In particular, I am not trying to capture language about the causal relation between objects and color experience, or about the notion of "property" as distilled from ordinary talk of objects. My aim has been to locate the color property within a biofunctional conception of the senses.

Once the basic notion of color as a psychobiological property is in place, there is no reason to preclude use of a notion of *physical color* that is independent of color as a visual property. Visually, color is a relational property involving both objects and perceivers. But we could also speak of "physical color" as a property of reflecting light according to a specific SSR. Even while granting that the relational notion of color as a psychobiological property is primary, we might choose to develop a perceiver-independent notion of physical color as a means of describing the reflective properties of objects, or the spectral composition of light. To avoid confusion, it would be necessary to keep in mind that such physical colors would be defined without relation to color experience or color perception; they would be defined in a purely physical vocabulary of wavelength or frequency.

Whatever language we choose for describing the physical properties of light and of surface reflectances, it is in virtue of its physical SSR that an object is able to affect light and produce a color response in an observer. But the colors of objects cannot be reduced to or identified with SSRs. Rather, object colors are to be identified with properties objects have of causing color experiences in perceivers. A physical SSR may help us identify this class, but using it alone, independent of the color discrimination capacities of organisms, we could not define real colors. There would be no physical reason for marking off the "visible spectrum" or carving it into color regions independent of the visual capacities of organisms. Color is a perceiver-dependent property of objects.

6. Objectivity and Subjectivity Revisited

Hardin (1988) opposed his brand of subjectivism to the sort of objectivism espoused by Hilbert 1987 (Hardin in fact addressed earlier forms of the position, as in Armstrong 1961 and Smart 1961). The arguments of the various objectivists and subjectivists share a common conception of objectivity, according to which objectivity requires mind-independence. This conception of objectivity allows Hardin to argue that if there is no candidate color property individuated by purely physical criteria independent of effects on perceivers, color is not an objective property, but is wholly subjective or illusory. In my view this particular dichotomy of positions into objectivist and subjectivist relies on an overly coarse analysis of the notions of objectivity and subjectivity themselves.

The notion of objectivity is complex and many faceted. It can include at least the following aspects:

(1) pertains to a mind-independent reality;
(2) pertains to the object;
(3) sustains factual claims;
(4) pertains to publicly available states of affairs;
(5) is real.

Item (1) is often invoked in discussions of color, but the other factors are important, too. Moreover, most or all of the other aspects are independent of (1). Although some philosophers still question whether there can be factual claims about mind-dependent or mind-supported states of affairs, such as the sensations, thoughts, and feelings of individual subjects, experimental psychology has been offering measurements of psychological states for more than 150 years. Of course, those psychologists who consider themselves to be determining the experiential sensory states of their subjects may be wrong, in the general sense that all science is fallible and not absolute. However, in what follows I will explore the implications of thinking that they are right.

The notion of the subjective also is complex and many faceted. It can include the following:

(A) is dependent on the mind alone (with no dependence on objects);
(B) pertains to the subject;
(C) varies idiosyncratically (no intersubjective agreement);
(D) pertains to experiential, private states of affairs;
(E) is not real.

The root notion of "subjective" is that it pertains to the subject (B), which need not entail that it depends on the mind alone (A). A feeling of hunger pertains to the subject and involves a mental state, but it may depend on the state of the digestive system and blood chemistry. Students who accuse professors of "subjective grading" have aspect (C) in mind. Aspect (D) is sometimes thought to preclude intersubjective knowledge of a subjective state, but that depends on what grounds there might be for inferences across subjects. It is sometimes suggested that something wholly mind-dependent "is not real" or does not belong to the world (E). On the other hand, one might argue that minds (or brain-dependent experiential mental states) exist and so must belong to the world—that is, must be real. (Indeed, even dualists such as Descartes typically thought of the mind as existing in the natural world, and hence did not exclude dualistically conceived mental states from the "reality" of the natural world; see Hatfield 2000a.)

Color as a psychobiological property of objects is "objective" in senses (2) to (5). It lacks only (1), mind-independence. But even if (1) is denied, we can retain (2) to (4), which allow a robust notion of objectivity. Items (2) to (4) include pertaining to the object, sustaining factual claims, and pertaining to publicly available states of affairs. They permit a notion of objectivity including publicly available facts. I like item (5) as well; even though the relational notion of color depends on mental experiences for its paradigm statement (in the case of human beings), one might well assert that human phenomenal experience is nonetheless "real" (i.e., a part of the world).

Colors as relational properties of objects are objective in that they

(2) pertain to the object;
(3) sustain factual claims;
(4) pertain to publicly available states of affairs;
(5) are real.

But this is not inconsistent with their:

(A′) being dependent on the mind, because they are attributed to objects as a result of the objects' effects on experience;
(B) pertaining to (an experiential effect on) the subject.

(A′) is rewritten from (A) to make explicit that mind-dependence can involve relations between mental states (such as color experiences) and extra-mental or extra-brain states of affairs (such as the object surfaces that standardly cause color experiences).

Even when color is defined in relation to phenomenal experience, then, it has elements of both objectivity and subjectivity. It is subjective in senses (A′) and (B), but not (E). As regards (C), some intersubjective variation occurs, but it often (and increasingly with the growth of knowledge) can be explained in a systematic fashion by taking into account physiological differences among subjects. Sense (D) should be divided. Color defined in relation to experience is subjective in sense (D′): the experiences of individuals are ontologically private, that is, a given instance of a color experience can be "had" by only one person. But it need not be, and typically is not subjective in sense (D″): epistemically private. Third parties can make reasonable claims about someone else's color experience, arguing from analogy with their own experience (and, if needed, pointing to species-shared biological characteristics). Hence, the subjectivity of color experience in senses (A′), (B), and (D′) is not inconsistent with the public availability of color as a species-relative property.

7. Culture, Naming, and Property Specificity

Culturally, we have exploited the chromatic sensitivity of our visual systems to develop finely divided color categories, and we exploit visual sensitivity to use color in systems of identification and contrast, which we rely on for many practical purposes. Color coding is used in medical and engineering contexts where life-or-death outcomes depend on color discrimination. Artists and decorators rely on the availability of stable, reproducible paints and dyes exhibiting a highly specific hue under a range of conditions. Such scientific and cultural uses of our abilities for fine-grained color discrimination have led some to mistakenly concretize the color names as well-behaved color predicates for which we should expect to find a corresponding mind-independent physical property in the world. This has resulted in misplaced demands on candidate color "properties," as in expectations of transitivity of color matches, excessively stable possession of determinate color values, and so on.

These are unreasonable expectations about color, which may come from supposing that if color is to be a property it must be a mind-independent property and behave like a physically measurable state of an object, taken in isolation. Such unreasonable demands on analyses of color as a property can be avoided by recognizing that:

- Color as an experience is a way our visual system presents objects.
- Color as an attribute of objects is defined in relation to the ways objects produce in us representations of their surfaces, discriminable by hue class.
- Biologically, color attributes are broadly tuned dispositional relational attributes of objects.

Not every property is a physical property. The property of being nutritious is not. Neither is color. They are both biofunctional properties. Color, as a property defined in relation to phenomenal experience or psychological discriminatory capacities, is a psychobiological property. As such, its basis may be found in the relation of subjects to objects. It is in relevant respects both subjective and objective. As explained, there need be no paradox in that.

10

Sense Data and the Mind–Body Problem

In the latter part of the nineteenth century, philosophers, physicists, and the new psychologists agreed to this extent in their conceptions of the mind–body problem: they all had a healthy respect for the integrity of both the mental and the physical domains. Whatever their particular commitments, whether phenomenalist, dualist, or materialist, they all accepted the reality of both mental and physical phenomena—where mental phenomena are, in the first instance, phenomenally characterized and perhaps equated with the contents of consciousness, and physical phenomena abstract from the knowing subject and sustain laws governing changes in spatiotemporally characterized objects. This acceptance of the mental domain held for physicists such as Ludwig Boltzmann, Ernst Mach, and Hermann Helmholtz no less than philosopher-psychologists such as Wilhelm Wundt and William James (despite their other differences).

In the early and mid twentieth century the situation changed, at least for certain psychologists and philosophers. There arose a stringent skepticism toward—or even a fear of—the mental, initially in all its guises, then later with respect to the phenomenal. This attitude at first expressed itself in Watson's and Skinner's behaviorisms, which shared the aim of eliminating all mental notions from cognitively serious discourse, and Carnap's and Hempel's physicalism, which aimed to reduce all talk of mental states to a purely physical language (or, subsequently, an observational physical thing-language). These movements were driven by conceptions of objectivity that seemed to exclude the *phenomenal* from the domain of the *objective* on grounds of privacy and subjectivity. The subsequent "linguistic turn" favored language, as public and

First published in Ralph Schumacher (ed.), *Perception and Reality: From Descartes to the Present* (Berlin: mentis Verlag, 2004), 305–31, copyright © 2004 by mentis Verlag. Reprinted with permission.

social, over the contents of experience as the locus of cognitive content. If the language were restricted to a physical (or physical thing) discourse, then the mental and the phenomenal might be rejected outright, or what was legitimate in mentalistic discourse might be reduced to physical talk (or physical thing talk).

The outright rejection or reduction of the mental was tempered through further development of the linguistic turn, in which cognition and thought came to be conceived linguomentalistically. As information theory and the computer analogy arrived, language was conceived as providing a model for mental states and processes (inclusive of intentionally characterized thought). In the second half of the twentieth century, there arose the linguistic model of cognition and perception. In its extreme form, it reduced all cognitive states to linguistic states, or formulae in a language of thought (Fodor 1975, 1987). In a slightly more relaxed version, it assimilated all mental content to propositional content, reducing or denying the phenomenal character of perceptual experience (Dretske 1981, 1995b; Tye 1995, chs. 3–6).[1]

The ongoing flight from the phenomenal was driven partly by the epistemological factors already mentioned—the notion that, by contrast with (allegedly) private phenomenal experience, language is a public medium, and that statements about physical objects concern publicly available states of affairs (e.g., Dummett 1993, ch. 9). It was also driven by a metaphysical thesis concerning the domain of the natural: that the natural is the physical or the material, so that mentalistic notions, especially those connected with the qualitative character of experience, do not sit easily with, or are precluded by, a proper naturalism.

These contrasting attitudes toward the phenomenal were both driven by problems arising from the mind–body relation. The earlier scientists and philosophers, including Helmholtz, Mach, and James—and subsequently Russell—acknowledged the difficulty of explaining mind in terms of body or bodily states, physically described. Mach, James, and Russell opted for a phenomenal realism, according to which phenomenally characterized entities are more basic than either physical objects or the psychological "subject" or "self." This position reached its fullest expression in the neutral monism of

---

[1] Dretske of course does not think of information as, in the first instance, carried by "natural" languages (such as English or German), which he views as artificial or "conventional" representation systems (1995b, 8, 19). He considers the contents of natural representations (including perceptual representations) to arise from indicator information; but this information is itself propositionally characterized (1981, 65–8, 176), or (equivalently) is characterized as the representation of a fact (1995b, 9). Such propositional content is conceived to exist independent of natural language. Tye (1995, 101, 121–3, 134–43) also treats sensory representations propositionally and symbolically, while distinguishing them from beliefs and conceptual content.

James and Russell, which treats Mach's elements, James' primal stuff, and Russell's momentary particulars (his successors to sense data) as neutral but real elements, out of which the derivative domains of the mental and the physical are to be constructed. These elements are phenomenally characterized, for example, as color patches, and so are modeled on perceptual states. But they are intrinsically neither mental nor physical (see Hatfield 2002c). They can be regarded as falling in the domain of either the mental or the physical depending on the context in which they are viewed: as a part of a series of elements exhibiting a physical process, such as the flowing of a stream, or as part of a series of individual experiences, such as a walk in the park (including a pass by the stream).

This neutral monism, though admirable in its respect for the phenomenal, is in the end a crazy position. The physical world can't be constructed out of color patches, or colored points. One well-known problem here, which beset later attempts to construct knowledge of the physical out of talk of color points and the like, is the complexity of the logical constructions involved and the failure fully to reduce the meaning of physical object statements to statements about elementary experiences.[2] Although such problems might well lead one to abandon the phenomenal as an adequate basis for analyzing talk of the physical, in my view the really big problem for neutral monism is that physical objects just aren't made of perception-like entities, of color patches or colored points. They are not made of sensational or phenomenal elements, but of the chemical elements in the periodic table, which are themselves composed of subatomic particles, which are in turn composed of yet more basic particles or energy packets or what not.

[2] Carnap's attempt in the *Aufbau* to reconstruct cognition on an "autopsychological" basis is a late expression of the phenomenalist epistemological tendencies found in Mach, James, and Russell. Indeed, he (1928/1967, §162) explicitly aligned himself with Russell's (1921) position, as reportedly derived from James (also noting similarities with Mach's position), though under a strictly "constructionist" or "constitutional" interpretation (which differs from Russell's ontological concerns, and focuses on accounting for intersubjective knowledge—see Richardson 1998). In introducing his "autopsychological" basis of "elementary experiences," he referred (1928/1967, §65) to the work of Moritz Schlick, Wilhelm Schuppe, Hans Cornelius, Heinrich Gomperz, Hans Driesch, and the Gestalt psychologists Max Wertheimer and Wolfgang Köhler. While the use of logical construction was his original methodological contribution in the *Aufbau*, the appeal to a Gestalt conception of "whole experiences" was his leading substantive contribution to the constructive project. He considered the position he developed to be compatible with materialism (1928/1967, §59), conceived scientifically rather than metaphysically. Later philosophers (e.g., Quine 1953; Putnam 1981, 181) considered the failure of phenomenalist construction programs like that of the *Aufbau* to motivate adoption of a physicalist language, or (subsequently) an "observational thing-language," as the reduction basis for all science and any cognitively significant talk (discussed below). Carnap himself, as late as 1961, endorsed the possibility of epistemic reconstruction on the basis of sense data, but stated a preference for an observational physical thing-language as affording greater intersubjective agreement (1928/1967, vii–viii; also 1963, 19).

In the first two sections of the chapter, I characterize the nineteenth-century respect for the phenomenal by considering Helmholtz's position and James' and Russell's move to neutral monism. Then in the third section I want to show a moment's sympathy with those who recoiled from the latter view. But only a moment's. The recoil overshot what was a reasonable response, and denied the reality of the phenomenal, largely in the name of the physical or the material. In the final two sections of the chapter, I develop a third way, which retains a healthy respect for the mental and for the mind–body relation, does not attempt to equate objects with congeries of sensations, and does not attempt to deny the reality of the phenomenal. In fact, I claim that on some conceptions (and not merely idealist-phenomenalist conceptions), the phenomenal is a fact of nature, and hence a part of the natural world. Some aspects of this third way are familiar in the various representative and critical realisms of the twentieth century. But the realization—or, more neutrally, the conception—that the natural might include the phenomenal is less familiar. Yet this position has its predecessors, too, not only among the physicists and psychologists of the nineteenth century, but among major physicists (as opposed to physicalist philosophers) and psychologists of the twentieth.

1. Respect for the Phenomenal

For physicists, philosophers, and psychologists of the nineteenth century, the existence of a domain of mental phenomena, phenomenally conceived, was a fact. By "phenomenally conceived" I mean conceived in such a way that (at least some) sensations present qualities that are considered to be peculiar to experience, in the sense that they cannot be literally identified with the intrinsic properties of physical objects. For philosophers today, one way to put this point is to say that nineteenth-century physicists and philosophers accepted, as a matter of course, some version of the distinction between primary and secondary qualities. They held that phenomenal color is found only in perceptual experience, and that its causal basis in objects must be described in the wholly physical language of wavelengths and electromagnetic energy. This did not necessarily mean that they denied that bodies may truly be *said* to possess colors,[3] but it did mean that they analyzed

---

[3] The assimilation of scientific and philosophical theoretical positions concerning secondary qualities to a context of ordinary language, so as to have such positions say, in ordinary terms, that bodies "are not really colored," simply creates a red herring. Hacker (1987, 2, 39–40, 55–60) claims that scientists and philosophers asserted, in an ordinary-language context, that "what we see ... is not (objectively,

what it is for a body to be colored either in purely physical terms alone (appealing solely to wavelengths and so leaving color perception and color experience aside), or in relation to the character of experience that objects and light cause in perceivers. They did not attempt to reduce the latter factor, involving appeal to phenomenal experience, to statements about physical properties alone.

A characteristic statement of the acceptance of the mental or the psychological into the domain of natural science may be found in Helmholtz's *Physiological Optics*. In that work the nineteenth-century physicist and physiologist examined not only the physical properties of light and the anatomy and physiology of the eye, but also the "sensations of sight," including experiences of light and color, and the "perceptions of sight," including the experience of size, shape, and distance, single or double vision, and depth perception. At the end of the work, in discussing whether to accept physiological explanations of the latter phenomena (the perceptions of sight, and especially the facts of single and double vision), he wrote:

I acknowledge that we are still far from a natural-scientific understanding of psychic phenomena. We may agree with the spiritualists that such understanding is absolutely impossible, or we may take precisely the contrary view along with the materialists, according as we are inclined toward one speculation or the other. For the natural philosopher, who must stick to factual relations and seek their laws, this is a question for which he possesses no basis for choice. It must not be forgotten that materialism is just as much a metaphysical speculation or hypothesis as is spiritualism, and that it therefore does not provide one with the right to choose between factual relations in natural science without a factual basis. (1867/1910 3:432)

Three points are of interest here. First, Helmholtz allows that there are factual relations in the domain of the "psychic phenomena" (*psychischen Erscheinungen*). Second, he characterizes the "materialists" as those who hold that a (presumably "full") "natural-scientific" understanding of such phenomena is possible, which would result from explaining the phenomena by appeal to brain processes. But, third, he contrasts the natural philosopher (that is, the natural scientist) with the materialist, and characterizes materialism as a metaphysical speculation.

publicly) coloured" (56). Scientists and philosophers have made verbally similar claims, but the context was theoretical, not ordinary. They were making a claim about a certain theory of the physics of sensory qualities—a theory that denied that color is a "real quality" (by contrast with Aristotelian theories, which survived into the nineteenth century, according to which color is a real quality, that is, a primitive physical property that is "like" our experience of it). Distinguishing phenomenal qualities from their physical bases (which ground secondary qualities) does not preclude one, in an ordinary context, from speaking of matching the color of one's socks with the color of one's pants, any more than did the acceptance of the proposal that the earth rotates diurnally preclude one from speaking of the sunrise.

Now it may be thought that Helmholtz is proposing that we simply bide our time until a materialist understanding of sensation and perception becomes available. That is, it might seem as if he were saying that, short of a materialistic explanation of the mental, there is no natural-scientific work to be done with the psychical phenomena at all. But that is not the attitude he took, either in this work or in his subsequent publications (e.g., Helmholtz 1878, 1894). In the continuation of the above passage, he made clear that the actuality of the psychic is to be accepted, whether one shares the metaphysical aspirations of the materialist or not:

> But no matter what view is taken of the psychic activities, and no matter how hard it may be to explain them, they are in any case actually extant, and their laws are to a certain extent familiar to us from daily experience. (1867/1910 3:432)

These laws include what Helmholtz termed the "association of ideas" (*Ideenassoziation*). In his view, such laws operate over phenomenally characterized sensations, that is, sensations characterized by (experiential) quality and intensity. In perception, they yield phenomenally characterized experiences of objects at a distance, perceived with a certain color, and so on.

In the continuation of the passage, Helmholtz showed skepticism about employing the materialist hypothesis in a natural-scientific account of sense perception (1867/1910 3:437–46; see also Hatfield 1990b, ch. 5). Together with the quotations given, this yields two conclusions. First, he had a healthy respect for the domain of the phenomenal. Second, he had a healthy respect for the mind–body problem itself, and for the difficulty of attempting to explain the phenomenal by appeal to neural structures and processes. In both respects he was (or came to be) in good company. Of the physicists and philosophers mentioned above, Mach, James, and Russell (in the teens and twenties) agreed with both points; among the rest, only Boltzmann (1897) advocated a materialist perspective and asserted the identity of sensations and other mental processes with brain processes; but he did not deny the reality of the phenomenal, which he had no intention of reducing away.

2. Sense Data and Neutral Monism

In the last decades of the nineteenth and first decade of the twentieth century, this appreciation of the reality of the phenomenal spawned a position that Russell (1914a/1956, 129) termed "neutral monism." It is the position that there is only one stuff in the world and that it is to be characterized in phenomenal terms (in the case of vision, phenomenal color is used), in other words, in terms of the content of perceptual experience. This position is expressed in the following series of quotations, the first from Mach:

> As soon as we have perceived that the supposed unities "body" and "ego" are only makeshifts, designed for provisional survey and for certain practical ends (so that we may take hold of bodies, protect *ourselves* against pain, and so forth), we find ourselves obliged, in many profound scientific investigations, to abandon them as insufficient and inappropriate. The antithesis of ego and world, sensation (phenomenon) and thing, then vanishes, and we have simply to do with the *connexion* of the [previously mentioned] *elements*. (Mach 1886/1897, 11)

Mach analyzed the concept of body into a series of "elements" characterized in terms of the phenomenal properties of sensation. "Bodies" are convenient makeshifts cobbled together out of certain series of such elements. The ego is another makeshift, specified by focusing on a different series of elements.

James, who was familiar with Mach's work, later adopted a similar position, cast as a thesis about the basic "stuff" of the world:

> My thesis is that if we start with the supposition that there is only one primal stuff or material in the world, a stuff of which everything is composed, and if we call that stuff "pure experience," then knowing can easily be explained as a particular sort of relation towards one another into which portions of pure experience may enter. The relation itself is part of pure experience; one of its "terms" becomes the subject or bearer of the knowledge, the knower, the other becomes the object known. (James 1904/1996, 4)

In speaking of "subject" and "object," James is identifying relations that occur within the sequences of pure experiences. As he had put it in the *Principles*, in which his later position was adumbrated but not fully adopted, "If the passing thought be the directly verifiable existent which no school has hitherto doubted it to be, then that thought is itself the thinker"—by which he meant that no separate subject, distinct from the stream of thought itself, need be posited (James 1890, 1:401). His pure experiences, like Mach's elements, account for both physical object and knowing subject. The knowing subject is reduced to a set of pure experiences that may take other experiences as objects.

Finally, Russell adopted the position of James (which he also attributed to Mach):

> William James, in his *Essays in Radical Empiricism*, developed the view that the mental and the physical are not distinguished by the stuff of which they are made, but only by their causal laws. This view is very attractive, and I have made great endeavours to believe it. I think James is right in making the distinction between the causal laws the

essential thing. There do seem to be psychological and physical laws which are distinct from each other. We may define psychology as the study of the one sort of laws, and physics as the study of the other. (1919/1956, 299)

For Russell, the world is to be viewed as constituted from the momentary "particulars" of perception. These are modeled on perceptual experiences: they have the properties of being, say, roundish and reddish—which means that they literally are instances of the phenomenal quality red, this particular patch of which is round. They are presented, as we would ordinarily say, from a "point of view." They thus have the properties Russell had earlier ascribed to sense data—though he now withholds that term from them. He does so because he takes the term "sense datum" to imply a datum *for someone*, that is, for an experiencing subject. But he, with James, has given up the subject. Although momentary particulars are in the first instance found in perception, they are not "given" to a persisting subject; rather, a series of such particulars constitutes the subject. Further, Russell was willing to extrapolate from the series of experienced particulars to other series of unexperienced momentary particulars, which are nonetheless ascribed properties such as those met with in the phenomenally present instances. These would be unsensed sense data, but for the abandonment of that term.

The perception-based character of Mach's "elements," James' "primal stuff" of "pure experience," and Russell's "particulars" is apparent. Because of the temptation to see the elements and particulars as sensations or mental-like entities, all three authors were charged with idealism. (Sometimes in-house: Russell 1945, 813, later charged James with a tendency toward idealism.) They saw themselves as avoiding idealism, and also avoiding an independent, non-phenomenally-characterized "thing in itself."

We can sketch the considerations that led these authors to their shared position in four steps. They each held the empirically plausible view (E) that phenomenally characterized perceptual objects are salient in human cognition. They then confronted the worry (S) that if these are seen as subjectively dependent states which merely represent (or phenomenally *present*) a mind- or perception-independent world, skepticism about knowledge of that external world may arise—or, less dramatically, an external world would have been posited unnecessarily. But, having been convinced of the reality of the phenomenal on empirical grounds, they also acknowledged (D) the great theoretical difficulty in reducing the phenomenal to the physical. Hence, to avoid (S) while acknowledging (E) and (D), they adopted (P), the limitation of world as it *is* (or, less dogmatically, as it is *known*) to Russellian momentary particulars. These (presumably) cannot be relegated to the "merely subjective," since they are prime reality, and constitute the epistemic basis for all knowledge claims.

3. Physicalism and Exclusive Naturalism

Although phenomenally characterized states retained currency in philosophy into the second half of the twentieth century (in various sense-data theories and their successors), within the science of psychology there arose a sustained effort—marching under the flag of behaviorism—to dispense wholly with phenomenal experience as both an object of explanation and a source of empirical data. Though the behaviorist campaign was not absolutely successful (perceptual psychology and psychophysics continued to be pursued, relying on phenomenal reports), behaviorism set the dominant tone in American psychology well past mid-century.

The original champion of behaviorism was John Watson, who had been trained as a comparative psychologist. He endeavored to bring to the study of human beings the rigor of an animal psychology that relied exclusively on behavioral evidence. He intended to show that a behavioral psychology of human beings could dispense with introspective methods (broadly conceived, to include all phenomenal reports), and with mentalistic concepts of any kind. He offered two principal reasons for rejecting phenomenal reports and mentalistic concepts:

(1) lack of intersubjective agreement in phenomenal reports;
(2) embroilment in the mind—body problem.

To support (1), he pointed (1914, 6–8) to the controversy over imageless thought, the disagreements among introspectionists over the degrees of clarity associated with the focus of attention, and disagreements over the dimensions of variation in sensation (e.g., whether sensations include an internal element of spatial order, or how many basic color sensations there are).

Watson considered problem (2), the mind—body problem, in connection especially with the functionalist movement in psychology (which arose in the decades prior to behaviorism).[4] The functionalist focuses attention away from

---

[4] This early American functionalism is to be distinguished from the "functionalism" in philosophy of mind and philosophy of psychology that arose in the 1960s. The main branch of the more recent functionalism is an input–output or input–internal state–output functionalism, in which the notion of "function" loses its biological connection and is reduced to the mathematical or logical notion of a function as relating one state to another (on which, see Shapiro 1994). Only those recent functionalists who conceive "function" biologically can claim descent from the earlier functionalism.

the analysis of consciousness in introspection, toward the functioning of mental states in the adjustment of organisms to the environment. Prior to the rise of behaviorism, functionalist psychology had already treated behavior as an object of explanation and source of data in psychology. But the functionalists retained a mentalistic framework of explanation, freely exploiting (according to Watson, and in fact) terms such as sensation, perception, affection, emotion, and volition. This brought them face-to-face with the mind–body problem. Watson observed that if the functionalist wants to "make mental states really appear to function, play some active role in the world of adjustment, he almost inevitably lapses into terms which are connotative of interaction" (1914, 9). As he saw it, functionalists tended to fall back on the language of mind–body interaction in practice, while stating their "official" position in the allegedly less problematic language of parallelism; this official position causally insulates their posited mental states from the bodily and behavioral activity they were intended to explain. In his view, both interaction and parallelism were problematic.

Watson was in sympathy with the biological flavor of functionalism—that is, with its notion that the organism, through the formation of habits and the like, becomes adjusted to the environment. But he rejected the functionalist's mentalist remainder.

We advance the view that *behaviorism* is the only consistent and logical functionalism. In it one avoids both the Scylla of parallelism and the Charybdis of interaction. Those time-honored relics of philosophical speculation need trouble the student of behavior as little as they trouble the student of physics. The consideration of the mind–body problem affects neither the type of problem selected nor the formulation of the solution of that problem. (1914, 9)

The mind–body problem doesn't arise, because the behaviorist does not characterize the states of the organism in mental terms at all. No mentalistically conceived states are permitted in his scientific domain, and so there is no occasion to ask how such states might be related to neural or bodily states.

The final comparison in the quoted passage, between the behaviorist and the student of physics, reveals a third factor in Watson's brief against mentalism, though one that functioned more by rhetorical implication than explicit argument. Watson contrasted introspective psychology, which "failed to make good its claim as a natural science," with properly scientific behaviorism: "Psychology, as the behaviorist views it, is a purely objective, experimental branch of natural science which needs introspection as little as do the sciences of chemistry and physics" (1914, 26, 27). Part of his point here has been expressed in (1), the alleged lack of intersubjective agreement, hence lack of objectivity, with introspection. But that is not the whole point. Watson's behaviorist program sought to restrict descriptions of the organism to a language that was continuous with the other natural sciences, by contrast with the (allegedly problematic) mentalistic language of even the biologically inclined functionalists. Behaviorism, by eschewing mentalistic language and restricting itself to descriptions of observable stimuli and observable responses characterized in physical and chemical terms (or in descriptions of observable motions), removes any barriers between its descriptions and those of the other natural sciences. We thus have a third rationale for rejecting phenomenal reports and mentalistic notions:

(3) The exclusion of mentalistic conceptions from the world as described by natural science.

Behavioristic psychology becomes continuous with paradigmatic natural sciences such as physics and chemistry. Watson was in fact a materialist reductionist, who held that in the end all sciences must reduce to physics and chemistry.[5]

Although Watson's was not the only form of behaviorism in the teens and twenties (see Roback 1923, and Ch. 14, herein), it was the version that captured the attention of philosophers such as Russell, Carnap, and Hempel. Russell (1921, 5-6) sought to reconcile the physicalism of Watsonian behaviorism with his view that physics no longer required matter (a reconciliation to be mediated by James' neutral monism); he used phenomenally characterized particulars as the basis of both physics and psychology. Carnap, after the phenomenalism of the *Aufbau*, adopted a position of physicalism according to which all psychological statements can be translated into statements about the physical states of an organism. He expressed the position as follows: "Every psychological sentence refers to physical occurrences in the body of the person (or persons) in question" (1932/1959, 197). He allowed that we may (provisionally) need to describe organisms at

---

[5] Watson made the point as follows: "This suggested elimination of states of consciousness as proper objects of investigation in themselves will remove the barrier which exists between psychology and the other sciences. The findings of psychology become the functional correlates of structure and lend themselves to explanation in physico-chemical terms" (1914, 28). Watson's explicit pronouncements, like Skinner's later, focus on the "methodological" point that consciousness and the phenomenal are not susceptible to scientific study (1914, 27-8); but it is clear from his discussion of images that he intended to reduce all allegedly mental phenomena to implicit or explicit behavioral responses (1914, 16-21), and that he intended to eliminate "mind" from the domain of what can be known and therefore from what can be said to exist from a rational, scientific perspective (the only cognitively serious perspective, by his lights).

the level of molar behavior, because we are (for now) unable to determine or measure the relevant neural states. Such descriptions should be seen as coarsely portraying the organism as a physical system, short of the ultimate description through "systematic assignments of numbers to space-time points." Assuming that these ultimate descriptions are properly "physical," "we can rephrase our thesis—a particular thesis of physicalism—as follows: *psychology is a branch of physics*" (197).[6] Soon thereafter, Hempel expressed the physicalist thesis as follows: "All psychological statements which are meaningful, that is to say, which are in principle verifiable, are translatable into propositions which do not involve psychological concepts, but only the concepts of physics. The propositions of psychology are consequently physicalistic propositions. Psychology is an integral part of physics" (1935/1949, 378).

Among the motivations for Carnap's and Hempel's physicalism (and their subsequent thesis of the logical reducibility of psychological statements to an observational, physical thing-language) was the conception that the mind–body problem was a metaphysical pseudoproblem and that any mentalistic talk not translatable or reducible[7] to physical (or observational thing-) language must be rejected. We have seen Hempel claim that there are no meaningful statements in psychology that include terms not translatable into the concepts of physics—as, presumably, the notion of phenomenal content alluded to earlier in this chapter would not be. Carnap also, even after weakening his post-*Aufbau* physicalism, expressed grave reservations that purely mentalistic notions, not logically reducible to the physical thing-language, could be sustained. He characterized the distinction between bodily and mental processes as arising from "the old magical and later metaphysical mind–body dualism" (1938/1955, 47). While allowing that this distinction might be of practical use in the early stages of scientific development, he suggested that a developed psychology would go behavioral, dropping mentalistic talk (47–9). Indeed, he purported to show

---

[6] Carnap's physicalism of the early 1930s involved assigning determinate physical magnitudes to space-time points (e.g., 1932/1959, 197). Ironically, he adopted this form of physicalism just a few years after physicists had concluded that quantum theory precludes such assignments. Carnap (1963, 14–15) later recalled that he had not kept up with physics after the 1920s (thus, after his work on relativity theory), and had been informed of the developments in quantum theory by Reichenbach. He does not make clear whether his learning of quantum theory was a factor in the rejection of classical physicalism in favor of a middle-sized object "thing-language" and talk of observables (talk that echoed the language of the Copenhagen interpretation of quantum theory). However, he later affirmed that quantum theory precludes classical physicalism (1966, ch. 30).

[7] Reduction in this case did not entail (but permitted the search for) the reduction of psychological laws to biological or physical laws; rather, it implied the translatability, or the even weaker conditional definability, of all psychological statements into statements about observable thing-predicates (Carnap 1928/1967, §§2, 35; 1938/1955, 49–60).

that "there is a behavioristic method of determination for any term of the psychological language" (59).[8]

The suggestion that mentalistic notions, including references to peculiarly phenomenal contents, are at odds with the concepts and attitudes of natural science has become widespread. All of points (1) to (3) above—lack of objectivity, difficulty in solving the mind−body problem, and the incompatibility of mental concepts with the point of view of natural science—have continued to fuel skeptical or even eliminative attitudes toward the mental. Indeed, according to a widespread conception of naturalism, by definition the natural excludes the (unreduced) mental. On this conception, for a mentalistic notion, such as phenomenal content, to be naturalized is for it to be analyzed into the nonmental (or nonphenomenal) terms of a "naturalistic" vocabulary. Because it excludes the mental and the phenomenal from the core notion of naturalism, this attitude may be termed "exclusive naturalism."[9]

At first, consonant with Watsonian (and, later, Skinnerian) behaviorism, the result was a continued rejection of all mentalistic notions. But with the development of information theory, the construction of digital computers, and the resulting computer analogy for mental processes, many philosophers and some psychologists came to believe that although the phenomenal should be rejected, there was hope for integrating mental content, propositionally conceived, into a naturalistic outlook. The ultimate result was a view that the phenomenal must either be eliminated or reduced to propositional content. We will return to this conception, and challenge it, in Section 5. Meanwhile, let us consider more fully point (3), focusing on the (alleged) incompatibility of naturalism, or of the outlook of natural science, with a conception of the mental inclusive of the phenomenal.

4. The Physicists and the Phenomenal

The tendency toward physicalism and exclusive naturalism in the middle decades of the twentieth century (carried on by Quine 1974 and others after

---

[8] Carnap's notion of "behavioristic" explicitly included, besides observations of molar behavior, processes internal to the organism (e.g., nervous processes), dispositions to behave, and environmental effects of behavior (1938/1955, 48−9).

[9] For characteristic recent statements of "exclusive naturalism," according to which, for the intentional or the phenomenal to be natural it must "really" be something else (something material), see Dretske (1981, x; 1995b, 28, 65) and Fodor (1987, 97−9). Dretske and Fodor are of course not physicalists, for they allow the possibility that reduction will not be forthcoming; but they are materialists, and use materialism as their criterion of the natural. For criticism of this theme in recent philosophy of psychology, see Hatfield (1990b, ch. 7) and Shapiro (1996).

Carnap and Hempel moderated their early physicalism) was motivated by a sense of the epistemic solidity of the science of physics. Physicalist philosophers held that physics should provide our basic view of what there is, and that phenomena that cannot be described in physical terms should form no part of our conception of reality.

Interestingly, the central members of the group that created the most profound change in physics of the twentieth century—the developers of quantum theory—did *not* share this physicalist outlook. That is, philosophically reflective physicists such as Max Planck, Erwin Schrödinger, Niels Bohr, and Werner Heisenberg did not think that the phenomenal (if unreduced) should be excluded from a complete account of reality. The particular form in which they expressed this attitude varied, as did their own philosophical outlooks (whether representative realism, neutral monism, or inclusive naturalism). But they were agreed on rejecting the demand, or even expectation, of physical reduction (whether of laws or entities) in all areas of reality, or of making physics the ultimate arbiter of what there is.

Planck was the most classically oriented of the originators of quantum theory. (He, like Einstein, held out for the retention of a classical realism and strict causal determinism underlying quantum probabilities.) Epistemologically, he adopted a representative realism. He rejected what he termed the "positivist" conception that the aim of science is merely to concatenate and report the immediate data of the senses (1932, 68). Within a positivist perspective,[10] one stays close to the phenomenal:

The whole world around us is nothing but an analogue of experiences we have received. To speak of this world as existing independently of these experiences is to make a statement that has no meaning. (1932, 70)

Planck rejected this outlook, as inadequate to the notion that scientists make discoveries pertaining to independent structures and entities. We need not rehearse those arguments, as interesting as they may be. The point of importance is that Planck intended to retain, in his conception of reality, both the immediate data of sensory experience and the commitment to an independent world that physics seeks to describe in abstraction from the qualities found in sensory experience.

In describing the data of immediate experience and the independent world of physics, Planck employed the vocabulary of the late nineteenth-century philosopher-psychologists such as Franz Brentano (1874). He spoke of an

---

[10] Planck's unnamed positivist (1932, 67–90) holds a position like that of Machian phenomenalism.

"inner realm" of experience, and an independent "outer world," posited through a metaphysical hypothesis:

We have taken a jump into the metaphysical realm; because we have accepted the hypothesis that sensory perceptions do not of themselves create the physical world around us, but rather that they bring news of another world which lies outside of ours and is entirely independent of us. (1932, 82)

Below, in Section 5, I will qualify talk of perceptual experience as "inner." For now, we may simply note that Planck adopted a framework of representative realism: our experiences inform us of a world whose underlying physical properties must be inferred, and in constructing a picture of that world we depart ever further from the givens of experience (to a description of subatomic particles and forces, curved space-time, and so on).[11]

Schrödinger endorsed a similar picture of the relation between the world as described by physics and the world of immediate experience, but he drew a different conclusion (similar to Russell's neutral monism). He described previous scientific thought as tending toward or expressing a "principle of objectification." As science developed, it systematically excluded "the Subject of Cognizance from the domain of nature" (1958/1967, 127). Citing A. S. Eddington (1928) and Charles Sherrington (1940), he described the course of science as excluding phenomenal qualities from the world, and ultimately excluding mind itself, with the consequence that no mind—body relation can be found in a scientific picture of the world, because mind finds no place in nature.

Schrödinger rejected the exclusion of subject and mind from nature. While admitting the practical utility of a distinction between a subjective domain of experience and an "objective" picture of physical reality, he believed that "in philosophical thought" we should "abandon" that distinction (1958/1967, 137). He contended:

It is the same elements that go to compose my mind and the world. This situation is the same for every mind and its world.... The world is given to me only once, not one existing and one perceived. Subject and object are one. (1958/1967, 137)

His belief that subject and object are one did not lead him to deny the difference between a purely physical view of the world and a larger view that would

---

[11] Einstein, who was the least philosophically loquacious of the quantum masters, appears to have adopted (after a purportedly Machian youth) a representative realism, which may be exemplified by the following quotation: "The belief in an external world independent of the perceiving subject is the basis of all natural science. Since, however, sense perception only gives information of this external world or of 'physical reality' indirectly, we can only grasp the latter by speculative means" (1934, 60).

include the phenomenal qualities. He maintained that neither physics nor physiology could account for the phenomenal qualities. Taking the experience of yellow as an example, he noted that the physics of wavelengths does not account for phenomenal yellow. Nor does physiology:

> We could at best attain to an objective knowledge of what nerve fibres are excited and in what proportion, perhaps even to know exactly the processes they produce in certain brain cells—whenever our mind registers the sensation of yellow in a particular direction or domain of our field of vision. But even such intimate knowledge would not tell us anything about the sensation of colour, more particularly of yellow in this direction. (1958/1967, 168)

He did not therefore conclude that phenomenal yellow doesn't exist, or that perceptual experience of phenomenal qualities cannot serve as a basis for objective knowledge. Indeed, he maintained that all scientific knowledge ultimately must be based on observations, which "are always of some sensual quality" (1958/1967, 178).

Schrödinger recognized that the scientific outlooks of Eddington and Sherrington opened an impassable gulf between subject and object. But he refused to conclude that the experiencing subject and the world of phenomenal qualities should therefore be dispensed. Rather, he looked for a philosophical position capable of reconciling subject and object. In 1925 and again in 1960, he endorsed a position like that of Mach and Russell. But he added the proviso that if forced to choose between either the material or the psychic as the basis for what is real, we would have to opt for the psychic, "since that exists anyway" (1961/1964, 63; also 15–17).

Bohr and Heisenberg offered the most original view of the relation between mental experience and the rest of science, and of the relations among the sciences themselves. They both characterized the now-rejected perspective of nineteenth-century physics as having (mistakenly) excluded mind or subject from nature. In a lecture given at Leipzig in 1941, Heisenberg described this exclusion as the product of seeking a methodologically unified science, inspired by a mechanistic or Newtonian outlook: "Nature consisted of matter subjected, in conformity with natural laws, to change in time and space by action and reaction" (1948/1952, 81). This problematic outlook was unable to accommodate all the phenomena of nature, inclusive of biological and mental phenomena. Biology presents concepts not readily expressed in the Newtonian framework, such as "growth, metabolism, heredity, etc."[12]

---

[12] In placing concepts such as growth, metabolism, and heredity beyond the domain of classical mechanics, Heisenberg (1948/1952, 82) and Bohr (1934, 117–19) were not endorsing vitalism. Rather, they suggested that the description of living things, including the functional language of biology,

Further, "no suitable place could be found in this view of nature for that great realm of reality comprising mental processes." Such a state of affairs was not acceptable in Heisenberg's view: "we can understand that this view of nature could never be fully convincing" (1948/1952, 82). Bohr, too, lamented the inability of the classical picture to incorporate consciousness and the data of psychology into its view of nature, and for that reason he described the classical picture as inadequate.[13]

The position articulated by Bohr and Heisenberg may be dubbed "inclusive naturalism." It includes the mental (and, as we shall see, the phenomenal) within the domain of reality, and suggests that any view of nature which excludes such phenomena is unacceptable. Heisenberg observed that classical physics was doomed as a general scientific outlook because it could not include the mental in its conception of nature:

Of course such a methodological unity cannot justly be called a unity of the scientific conception of nature. Such a conception must, at least in principle, be able to accommodate *all* parts of nature and it must be able to allot a definite place to each sector of reality. It was precisely this demand which so clearly demonstrated the shortcomings of the views based on classical physics. In that picture of nature the mental world figures, so to speak, only as the opposite pole of a material reality incapable of accommodating it within its bounds. (1948/1952, 92)

Heisenberg agreed with Schrödinger that the picture of the world offered by classical physics excluded mind. For that reason (among others), he, like Schrödinger and Bohr, found that picture unacceptable.

cannot be wholly translated into the language of particles and forces. While this matter has not been settled, today even reductionistically inclined philosophers of biology acknowledge that reduction seems unlikely (see Rosenberg 1985).

[13] Bohr wrote: "Even though it was, to some extent, possible within the frame of classical physics to compare organisms with machines, it was clear that such comparisons did not take sufficient account of many of the characteristics of life. The inadequacy of the mechanical concept of nature for the description of man's situation is particularly evident in the difficulties entailed in the primitive distinction between soul and body. The problems with which we are confronted here are obviously connected with the fact that the description of many aspects of human existence demands a terminology which is not immediately founded on simple physical pictures. However, recognition of the limited applicability of such pictures in the account of atomic phenomena gives a hint as to how biological and psychological phenomena may be comprehended within the frame of objective description" (1958, 91; also 1934, 117−19). Bohr obviously was not endorsing the notion of the soul, but he equally was not suggesting that the difficulty of integrating mental phenomena into the classical picture of nature was a problem for mental phenomena. The "hint" from quantum atomic theory was the notion of complementary description. The inability of physical modes of description to deal with consciousness and the mental does not entail that either description is false, just that neither provides, by itself, a complete description of nature (on which, see 1958, 92−3). (This question of completeness with respect to all phenomena in nature is of course distinct from the question of the completeness of quantum theory as a description of a specifically "physical" reality—i.e., the reality described by quantum physics itself—on which see Bohr 1935/1998.)

Heisenberg was willing to allow that further scientific developments *might* eventually yield a unified description of nature that included consciousness and mental processes. But in the meantime, he had no doubts about the reality of consciousness and mentality, or about the need to include them in any conception of nature. In thus advocating an inclusive naturalism he came into agreement with an earlier conception of nature, which held sway from the time of Aristotle into the mid eighteenth century, according to which mind is part of nature. Having contemplated the failed attempt to make classical mechanics into a theory that was adequate for all nature, he opted instead for a pluralistic attitude toward the domains of nature:

> We are now more conscious that there is no definite initial point of view from which to radiate routes into all fields of the perceptible, but that all perception must, so to speak, be suspended over an unfathomable depth. When we talk about reality, we never start at the beginning and we use concepts which become more accurately defined only by their application. (1948/1952, 93)

In other words, we no longer can take the particles and forces of classical physics as the ultimate starting point for all explanation. We must include all domains of reality in our starting point and attempt to make progress in understanding each domain by beginning with its proper concepts and seeking to make them more precise.

The club of physicists whose work brought about the most far-reaching changes in physical theory since Newton were not physicalists. Their conceptions of reality included the contents of phenomenal experience. Bohr and Heisenberg went the furthest in articulating a novel position. They characterized the exclusive naturalism of physicalism as the quaint heritage of the old atoms-in-the-void picture of the world, and they insisted that the contents of consciousness (phenomenally conceived) be brought into the domain of the natural.

There is of course no *refutation* of physicalism here, and no inconsistency on the part of those philosopher-physicalists who might grant epistemic authority to physics but disagree with the leading physicists on the philosophical upshot of their discipline. The philosophers might simply hold that the physicists should stick to physics and stop talking about the mental and its place in nature. They might think that the physicists had gotten out of their depth, and that they, as philosophers, were better suited to drawing out the philosophical implications of physics.

At the same time, we might ask what attitude allowed the physicists to be quite comfortable and self-assured in making the pronouncement (*a*) that physics as classically conceived cannot explain the phenomenal, and (*b*) that the phenomenal will not and should not go away. We can expect that Planck, Schrödinger, Bohr, and Heisenberg (among others) were well versed in the power and limitations of physical theory (old and new). We may expect that they, better than many philosophers, would be able to extrapolate the explanatory power of physical concepts. While not according their pronouncements an absolute authority, we might nonetheless expend some effort taking into account their considered judgment about the inability of physics to explain the phenomenal. Further, given their experience with pursuing and extending an empirical attitude toward nature and with holding theory accountable to fact, we might also take seriously their conception that the phenomenal constitutes its own empirical domain, which, at least by Bohr's and Heisenberg's lights, must be incorporated into any acceptable conception of nature.[14]

The pronouncements of the physicists, though not having absolute authority, should easily counterbalance the unsubstantiated hopes and predictions of the ordinary physicalist that the mental and the phenomenal will be reduced or eliminated through the march of science. A more properly empirical attitude might embrace the various domains of phenomena (including the atomic, the biological, and the mental, by Heisenberg's count), and leave open, pending further inquiry, the question of how they are ultimately to be related. Accordingly, a properly empirical attitude would start from an inclusive naturalism, that is, a naturalism inclusive of phenomenally characterized mental states.

5. The Phenomenal and Inclusive Naturalism

Leaving aside the antiphenomenalism of earlier behaviorism and physicalism, we can ask what reasons are now given for being wary of or rejecting the phenomenal. Such reasons may be metaphysical or epistemological. On the metaphysical side, a concern about fitting the phenomenal into nature has led some philosophers to seek to replace phenomenal conceptions with ones allegedly more compatible with physicalism or materialism. Such efforts include the attempts by U. T. Place (1956), J. J. C. Smart (1962), David Armstrong (1968), and others to reduce the concept of "sensation" to the

---

[14] Bohr and Heisenberg referred to the extant sciences of biology and psychology in justifying their claims about the empirically suitable concepts of those natural sciences. Among their contemporaries, the Gestalt psychologists (e.g., Koffka 1935, chs. 1–3) made a case for regarding phenomenal experience and perceived meanings as natural phenomena, subject to natural scientific investigation (see Epstein and Hatfield 1994).

having of a certain sort of brain state;[15] P. M. Churchland's (1979, ch. 2) and P. S. Churchland's (1986) eliminative materialism; and Dretske's (1995b) and Tye's (1995) reduction of sensory qualities to informationally characterized material states. Dennett's (1978, 1988) reduction of the phenomenal to the content of certain sorts of "myths" or stories we tell ourselves conforms to the more widely held view that intentionally characterized content (propositionally conceived) is easier to square with standard naturalism than would be "qualia" or other phenomenally characterized contents.[16]

On the epistemological side, Shoemaker (1996), Dennett (1988), and others have charged that phenomenal experience has characteristics of internality, privacy, and subjectivity that make it difficult or impossible to justify knowledge claims about the phenomenal, and that make phenomenal experience unsuitable as a basis for knowledge of a publicly available, intersubjectively discussable world of objects and events. Further, Shoemaker (1996, 25–7, 224–5) has argued that claims to know the contents of phenomenal experience presuppose a "Cartesian" conception of the mind, according to which the contents of consciousness are known infallibly and with complete transparency. "Refutation" of this extreme position may then be taken as grounds for rejecting a "perceptual model" of knowledge of phenomenal states. On the further (questionable) assumption that the perceptual model is the only model of knowing (unreduced) phenomenal experience, such knowledge is precluded.

A full characterization of and response to these metaphysical and epistemological objections would be a topic unto itself. Here I can merely indicate the direction such a response might take. Regarding the epistemological worries, the charge that perceptual states are "internal" and divorced from a world of intersubjectively available objects draws upon terminology used by some late nineteenth-century adherents of phenomenality: that phenomenal experience is "inner," as opposed to the "outer" experience of objects themselves (an "external world"). Allegedly, these theorists posited an "inner world," to be

---

[15] It might at first seem questionable to classify Place, Smart, and Armstrong among the antiphenomenalists, for they viewed themselves as *reducing* mental concepts, including that of sensation, to states of the nervous system, and (technically speaking) reduction does not eliminate the reduced entities (see Rey 1997, 22–3). But in fact the physicalism of Place, Smart, and Armstrong forsook phenomenal aspects of sensation, and reduced sensations wholly to brain states caused by paradigmatic external stimuli, so that an "orange sensation" becomes the sort of brain process we have when we "really see an orange" (Smart 1962, 167). Such a reduction was in effect an elimination; for discussion, see Cornman (1971, pt. 1).

[16] The view that informationally characterized representations are easier to accommodate into a materialistic naturalism is widely held; it funds the approaches of Dretske (1995b, xiii–xiv) and Tye (1995, ch. 5); see also Rey (1997, 6–10).

accessed by a special "inner sense." But this characterization is incorrect. Talk of "inner perception" was not used to characterize the spatial location of the perceptions themselves, but to focus on the relation of such perceptions to the subject experiencing them. As Wundt put the point, "the expressions outer and inner experience do not indicate different objects, but different points of view from which we take up the consideration and scientific treatment of a unitary experience" (1901/1902, 2–3). The expression "point of view" might seem to bring us back to a spatial comparison, but Wundt clearly used it in the sense of mental attitude, not literal standpoint. Thus, in describing objects on the table, we may either focus on the objects themselves—a cup, a book, a pen—or on the fact that in seeing them we also have experience of a certain character, as of a cup, a book, and a pen. The experience is phenomenally "of the world" from the outset, and so does not seem to be located "internally." We do not need to take up a special attitude to externalize our sensations, or to make them seem to be of a world. Nor do we need a special "inner sense" to experience them. Simply by having the experiences we are put in a position to describe their phenomenal character (the cup appears bright red, it visually overlaps and so obscures one corner of the book, the pen is seen parallel to one edge of the book, the table top appears smooth and grey, etc.).[17]

But even if, as various perceptual psychologists have contended, the world of immediate experience is as of a world of objects, there remains the objection that each individual's experience is private, and therefore epistemically impotent. In their strongest versions, such objections rely on the problems of solipsism and skepticism about other minds. Such extreme forms of skepticism are, however, of little use in a context in which one wishes to contrast perceptual knowledge with intersubjective knowledge of a world of objects. The latter sort of knowledge can also be undermined by extreme skepticism—such as the skeptical position that all factual knowledge about objects and events more than five minutes old is negated by the skeptical "possibility" that the world came into existence five minutes ago, with all our (apparent) memories and physical records intact. Solipsism and skepticism about other minds are

---

[17] In suggesting that phenomenal aspects of experiences can be thus described, I do not suggest that such phenomenal contents are special non-intentional "internal objects." Some authors (e.g., Robinson 1994, chs. 5, 8) have characterized sensations as "non-intentional" and therefore "internal"; they instantiate properties such as redness and roundness that serve as inner objects of perception. In my view, one can avoid this classical sense-data position while treating phenomenal qualities as representational, without having to reduce them away by equating them with informational states (in the manner of Dretske and Tye); the phenomenal qualities found in experience may be thought of as *presenting* the surfaces of objects under a certain phenomenal aspect, which is what constitutes our *seeing* that object-surface.

no more pressing than this sort of skeptical worry. And more generally, we typically are in a good position to use others' experiences to know what sort of experience we might expect in given perceptual circumstances, and hence also to know what their perceptual experience is like. As members of the same species, with like perceptual experience (subject to known and detectable differences, such as the various color deficiencies), we naturally and rightly suppose that if, when out on a walk, we indicate the color of the leaves, or point to the shape and color of the rising moon, our companion can share our experience (i.e., will experience very similar colors and shapes). Even if our experience is private in the sense of being individual, a public world is available to us because we share similar perceptual mechanisms, which yield coordinate perceptual experiences.

There remains the problem of subjectivity. It is a commonplace that when several persons view a complex event, such as an automobile accident, from different or even quite similar spatial standpoints, they may report conflicting and inconsistent descriptions of the events. In dealing with such situations, we would of course need to disentangle memory effects, emotional salience effects, and response biases (e.g., one person lives with the driver of one of the cars involved, the other was a neutral passerby). Free perception of uncontrolled events by multiple observers is not the paradigm for intersubjective agreement. Nor do the physical sciences hold up such conditions of observation as likely to produce intersubjective agreement on even the properties of middle-sized objects; observation in the physical, chemical, and biological sciences is highly structured and controlled. Lack of agreement in uncontrolled observation must be accepted by both friends and foes of phenomenal experience. The fact is that when the circumstances are controlled, as in color-matching experiments (testing qualitative matches of isolated color samples), the intersubjective agreement is quite high for phenomenal properties. In these circumstances, the charge of subjectivity collapses back on extreme skepticism, such as the inverted spectrum scenario, or other variants of solipsism and the problem of other minds.

Turning to the metaphysical side of things, let us consider first the weakness of purely propositional accounts, such as those of Dretske and Tye. Here, perception of phenomenal red is reduced to the occurrence of an informational state in the visual system that represents an objective surface property of a certain type in a location. Qualia allegedly drop out. But such accounts run afoul of the known facts about color vision, that there is no single physical property that we detect when we perceive several instances of phenomenally indistinguishable greens or reds. In color science, it has been determined that physically heterogeneous spectral properties can appear phenomenally identical (or be judged identical, to adopt nonphenomenal language). If information tracks physical states, then the spectrally heterogeneous samples should be perceived (judged) differently. But they are not in the case of "metamerism" just described.[18] For the friend of the phenomenal, this scenario simply presents a case in which identical or extremely similar phenomenal characters are produced by distinct physical stimuli. From a phenomenal perspective, the quality of the experience depends upon the peculiar apparatus of the human perceptual system. Because the appearances (and judgments) are the same for normal perceivers in similar circumstances, this response creates no special problem of subjectivity. The physicalist may hope to explain away the facts of metamerism, perhaps by adopting a revised version of what it is to be a physical property (e.g., so as to allow a disjunctive property that comprises the physically heterogeneous metamers). But *prima facie* plausibility is on the side of unreduced phenomenal experience.

I suspect that the most persistent reason for philosophical resistance to qualitatively characterized phenomenal experience is the belief that it cannot be integrated into a naturalistic picture of the world. This is the problem of fitting, say, phenomenal red into one's ontology. It is sometimes called the "hard problem" (e.g., Chalmers 1996, xii–xiii; also Levine 2001) because of the apparent conceptual or explanatory gap between phenomenal red and a physical description of the stimulus or a physicochemical description of brain activity (say, neurons firing in the visual cortex).

There are some conceptions of the status of phenomenal red that are implausible on the face of things. For instance, if it is supposed that phenomenal red is a property of a sense datum, or of a Russellian "momentary particular," a property of "being red" must be ascribed to an experienced item distinct from the physical stimulus. This item cannot literally be identified with neurons, for they do not themselves take on the various colors of seen objects, but remain whitish or grey. As indicated at the outset, I affirm that a position attributing the property of being red to a phenomenally present item—in the same way in which the property would be ascribed to physical objects if naive realism were true—is at best implausible. Still, it may seem that in speaking of "phenomenal red" as something that exists, I am obliged to provide up front an ontology of

---

[18] The informationalist might argue that there is in such cases a single physical property that the perception of red is supposed to pick out (or has the function of indicating, in Dretske's terms), and that all other metameric matches are cases of misperception. This response relies on a "physical instrument" conception of the function of vision, according to which vision tries to track physical properties. It can be countered by a conception of color vision (derived from comparative study of color vision in other mammals) according to which heightened discriminability of object-surfaces, not property-detection *per se*, is its primary function (see Ch. 8).

qualitative content. I have said it is unsatisfying to say that qualitative character must really be "something else," in the spirit of Dretske and Tye. So, what is it, on my view?

I am not prepared to answer this question here, but would suggest that lack of an immediate answer should not lead one to repudiate phenomenal red. Instead, I suggest we take a hint from the original quantum physicists, and adopt an empirically based liberal attitude toward what may be found in nature, the attitude of inclusive naturalism. We should, on this view, simply include phenomenal red among the phenomena of nature, and thus accept that the phenomenal is itself real. From there, we might ask how its existence and characteristics are to be explained. If we don't accept substance dualism (a position that doesn't really help in explaining phenomenal qualities[19]), we should assume that phenomenal red depends on brain activity. In my view, we should accept the dependence of phenomenal red on brain activity as a working hypothesis, but not set it down as a condition on the acceptability of including phenomenal red in the domain of natural phenomena. As I see things, at present no one has any idea of how to explain phenomenal red in terms of brain activity. There is some knowledge of the brain correlates of sensations, but no direct explanatory relation or intelligible connection between brain activity and phenomenal content (of the sort that statistical mechanics provides between the kinetic energy of the atoms or molecules of a gas and the temperature of the gas). At the same time, our theory of matter offers no assurance that we have discovered the most basic properties of matter itself—that we have found the ultimate particles and forces, or characterized the ultimate field structure, or even determined that particles and fields provide the ultimate conceptualization of matter. Further, we have no settled framework for delimiting the emergent properties, if any, of complex material systems such as the brain.

I suggest that it is preferable to adopt an investigative attitude toward the relation between the phenomenal and the brain, rather than attempting to exclude phenomenal qualities from the domain of nature because they don't match our intuitions about what is consistent with present physics and our imagined extrapolation of that physics. The empirical liberalism of inclusive

---

[19] Although dualism may seem to help the cause of phenomenal qualities by providing a nonmaterial home for them, it doesn't solve the problem. Dualists do not (like sense-datum theorists) think that the mind is (or is confronted with an item that is) literally red (see Hatfield 2003*b*, 324–5). Hence, dualists are left with a seemingly unsolvable problem of accounting for the phenomenal content of sense experience, as are materialists. To allow for phenomenal qualities, each must simply accept that states of the mind or brain are such that phenomenal red occurs within our sensory experience, and continue to look for an explanation or account of that fact.

naturalism is consonant with a pluralistic attitude toward the domains of properties to be found in the natural world, and their interrelations.

The idea that the natural excludes the mental, or some aspects of the mental, is itself recent (see Ch. 14). It was not the dominant conception in the seventeenth or eighteenth centuries (despite potted histories to the contrary), when the mind was regarded as part of nature. Here, the historical sense of physicists such as Planck, Schrödinger, Bohr, and Heisenberg was on target. The conception of exclusive naturalism arose among those for whom classical physics provided a clear and adequate picture of a physical world bereft of sensory qualities, thereby making mind the (suspect) repository of what was left over. Behaviorism and physicalism (later joined by materialistic functionalism) then attempted to outlaw the mental (or merely the phenomenal) remainder.

With the demise of the classical physicalist picture of nature and the rise of a biological perspective on the senses, we are well positioned to reconsider the place of phenomenal experience in nature. We might simply accept as a fact of nature that organisms with sensory systems like ours are constituted so that at least part of our perceptual take on the world is presented via consciously available, phenomenally characterizable perceptual experiences. Psychologists would have as part of their task describing such experience, detailing its causal conditions, and ascertaining the role it plays in cognitive and affective lives of organisms. Philosophers might try acknowledging the phenomenal as a natural fact, integrating the descriptions of psychologists or observationally astute philosophers into their descriptions of the mental, and situating that domain in a larger naturalistic and philosophical landscape, in accordance with the liberally empiricist outlook recommended by our physicists in Sections 1 and 4. We would thereby avoid the unsavory situation of allowing largely unexamined metaphysical assumptions about "the natural" to back us into the position of denying the obvious presence of phenomenal experience. We could then seek to construct a picture of human mentality and cognitive achievement that started from the fact that we are biological creatures endowed with a physiology that supports various cognitive states and capacities, including those of having something appear to us in some way. To paraphrase Schrödinger, we might as well acknowledge the existence of the phenomenal. It's there anyway.

11

The Reality of Qualia

1. Introduction: Qualia Realism and Color Ontology

I am a qualia realist. I believe that specifically phenomenal qualia are present in perception. Thus, when we see a yellow lemon in good light, we typically see that it is yellow by experiencing a yellow quale. We can experience (an instance of) the same yellow quale in the absence of the lemon, or of any yellow object. In my view, not only is the experience of the lemon's quality real—something many will grant—but the experienced quale is real, in the sense that it exists as perceiver-dependent phenomenal content.

I am a qualia realist because I think this position permits the best account of visual perception, for both spatial and color perception—although in this chapter I focus on color, and, more specifically, on surface color. We experience surface color in experiencing colored objects, and we experience such objects as if color were simply a property of the surface, on a par with its shape. I think that qualia realism gives the best account of what it is to see surfaces that are colored. Thus, *qualia* realism is, in my view, part of an account of *quality* realism about the colored surfaces of objects. We see the colors of objects in virtue of having visual experience that contains phenomenal color as a subject-dependent phenomenal content.[1]

First published in *Erkenntnis* 66 (2007), 133–68, copyright © 2007 by Springer. Reprinted with permission and edited for length and terminological consistency (see the Introduction to Pt. II).

[1] There is great terminological variety in discussions of qualia and phenomenal experience. I use the term "qualia" to denote subject-dependent phenomenal contents, which are subject-dependent not merely for their existence (as phenomenal experience must be on *any* theory except James–Russell neutral monism and its kin) but also for their phenomenal character. When I wish to describe contents of consciousness without implying that these contents are qualia, I use the term "phenomenological experience" (by contrast with "phenomenal experience," which I take, for vision, to be spatially and chromatically determinate). In this paragraph and at some other places in the chapter (which will be clear from context), I use the term "quality" to refer to properties of objects (whether relational or

Philosophers have long been concerned with the status of color. The Greeks asked whether material objects are really colored or color arises only with human or animal perception. Aristotle thought that color is a real quality, and that, during perception, the "form" of that color is transmitted from the object to the sensitive soul. Democritus held that the atoms that compose things aren't really colored, but that color arises as a merely subjective effect of atoms on perceivers. Philosophical reflections on color properties and color experience intensified during the early modern period, when Descartes and Locke (among others) developed a distinction between primary and secondary qualities. Discussion has again intensified in recent years, raising issues in metaphysics, epistemology, and philosophy of mind.

Visual scientists, who sometimes were philosophers as well, have also investigated color and color perception from the early days of visual theory. They have discovered many things about color, and continue to do so. The scientific book on color and color perception is not closed. To my mind, that means the philosophical book should remain open as well.

I have claimed qualia realism gives the best account of what it is to see colored objects, which implies that it is part of the best philosophical account of what color is. The main accounts of color ontology currently fall into three general types: objectivism, subjectivism, and dispositionalism (Ch. 9). *Objectivists* argue that color is a mind-independent property of objects. They say that, when we perceive a colored object veridically, we perceive a physical property that the object possesses independently of all perception or experience of it (ours or any other). They identify this physical property with the object's color. Currently, the most popular form of objectivism is called "representationalism," according to which the phenomenal content of color experience is nothing but the representation of a physical property (Dretske 1995*b*; Tye 1995, 2000, 2003); such representations *constitute* phenomenal experience, which contains no subjectively supplied content. *Subjectivists* argue that color is not a property of objects, but an internal state of the perceiver:

not). However, I use "qualitative" to suggest phenomenal content. I also use "red-experience" to refer to a red quale, by contrast with the potentially neutral term "experience of red," which sometimes is used technically to denote the experience of a physical property that is alleged to be a thing's redness. The terminological diversity in this field creates some potential traps: "representative realist" theories of perception tend to adopt views on color ontology that are *opposite* to those of recent "representational" or "intentional" or "pure information" theories. "Intentional" is sometimes used as a synonym for "representational transparency" (under this usage, my theory of color qualia would *not* be intentional), but at other times it is used in Brentano's original sense (Section 6). Finally, although the dispositional account I develop here focuses on surface colors (since surfaces are the primary objects of mammalian vision), it could easily be extended to include radiant light from an energy source.

color reduces to the subjective content of a perceiver's experience. By contrast with objectivists, they think that the notion of color has legitimate reference only to *visual experience*, and they deny that objects are really colored. In their view, color experience is a kind of standing illusion, although a useful one (Hardin 1988). *Dispositionalists* also define color in relation to color experience, but that definition allows a notion of "object color" that ascribes a color property to the surfaces of objects in virtue of the relation between objects and the color experiences they produce. They argue that color, considered as a property of objects, consists in a relational disposition, or its causal basis;[2] it is a property that surfaces (and light sources) have of causing perceivers to have experiences that exhibit various phenomenal characters (Johnston 1992; Peacocke 1984). For dispositionalists, color as a phenomenal feature of experience is conceptually primary; they then use experienced color to define the related notion of color as a property attributed to objects (Chs. 8–9).

My arguments focus primarily on the objectivists and the dispositionalists, and favor dispositionalism. If a convincing version of either of these positions were established, that would remove the motivation for retreating to a purely subjectivist account. In focusing on color properties and color experience, I leave aside (for the most part) questions of color categories or color concepts. In the primary instance, we presumably categorize colors of objects in accordance with how the objects look. Along with the authors I discuss, I assume that objects can look a certain way as regards color independently of whether we have the concept of that color, or have any concept of color at all.[3] At the same time, I don't believe that my specific arguments for dispositionalism depend on this assumption; that is, I believe that someone who held a different view about the relation between color concepts and the phenomenal experience of color could adapt and use my arguments.

---

[2] Some philosophers distinguish between a *disposition* and the *causal basis* of the disposition in the actual physical (or other) properties of a thing (e.g., McLaughlin 2003, 479), whereas other philosophers contend that a disposition *is* a causal power of the actual properties of things (e.g., Armstrong 1999, 62–4). I avoid needlessly taking sides on this issue, and I sometimes remind the reader of that by speaking of "a disposition or its basis."

[3] In distinguishing phenomenal color from color categorization or color concepts, I do not assert that conceptualization of phenomenal experience has no phenomenal effects. Such effects are, I suppose, many and varied. Expectations or conceptual identifications may influence color appearances; conceptual identification itself may change the overall phenomenological feel; and, in certain cases, adopting an introspective attitude (which brings its own conceptualizations) may affect our phenomenal experience by directing our attention to hitherto unnoticed features or aspects of that experience (see Ch. 16). What I deny is that color experience is *constituted* by its conceptual (classificational) content.

2. Physics and Biology of Color

In my view, any account of color as a property of objects should relate that property to color perception and color experience in some way. This relation need not *necessarily* be dispositionalist; it may simply be explanatory, so long as the account of color as a property of objects gives, or is working toward, an explanation of color perception. This desideratum is widely shared by philosophers and color scientists. If some philosophers and scientists do not endorse it, I think of them as having changed the topic (to a purely physical discussion of light and wavelengths, perhaps), and I am not addressing them here.

My aim is to articulate a conception of colors in objects as dispositions of objects to cause color experiences in perceivers. Consequently, to understand what color *is* as a property of an object (or of an object's surface) requires that we understand object surfaces, illuminants, eyes, brains, and color experiences. One doesn't need to reflect on or understand any of these things in order to *have* color perceptions or to classify things by their colors. But in order to understand what color is in objects, and how it is involved in color perception, we must consider these factors.

From the perspective of the physics and biology of color properties, it is interesting to consider color perception as a capacity that has evolved in sighted animals. Not all animals are sensitive to color, that is, not all of them can distinguish between the total amount of light energy (in the visible spectrum) that they receive at a given location in their eyes, and the distribution of that energy across the visible spectrum (Jacobs 1981, ch. 2). Only animals possessing eyes that are differentially sensitive to wavelengths can discriminate color (or colored surfaces).[4] Among color-sensitive animals, some are called "dichromats" because their retinas possess only two types of light-sensitive receptors, which means that they can discriminate fewer color qualities (say, blue and yellow, plus gradations) than can other animals, the "trichromats," whose retinas contain three types of light-sensitive receptors that allow them to discriminate more color qualities in objects (say, blue, yellow, green, and red, plus gradations).

[4] The fact that an animal is not sensitive to variations in the wavelengths of light does not prove that it has no color phenomenality. An animal that could discriminate only light intensities might (conceivably) experience those intensities chromatically, say, by experiencing brighter shades as yellow and darker shades as blue (thanks to Don MacLeod, personal communication). In this chapter I am concerned with color experiences that arise from spectrally based sensitivities, that is, with cases in which an organism can discriminate surfaces by spectral differences (as opposed to mere intensity differences) in the light reflected to the eyes.

Among mammals, humans and some other primates are trichromats. The three types of receptors in their retinas, called *cones*, are maximally sensitive to light in the short-, middle-, and long-wavelength regions of the visible spectrum, and these three types are therefore called S, M, and L cones. Primate trichromacy evolved from short- and long-wavelength dichromacy some tens of millions of years ago, when the longer-wavelength cones separated into middle- and long-wavelength types, thus yielding three types in all (Goldsmith 1990). This development permitted greater discrimination among surfaces that reflect light predominantly from the middle- and long-wavelength portions of the spectrum (such as green leaves and yellow or red fruit).

Color and color perception have their basis in the physical properties of the world and in the biological and psychological capacities of organisms that are sensitive to color, not all of which are sensitive in the same way. The fact of biological diversity by itself suggests relativity between organisms and colors, but I won't rest my case for dispositionalism there.

The case for dispositionalism arises from a scientific analysis of the causal basis of color perception, starting with the "new science" of the seventeenth century. The genesis of dispositionalism as a theory can best be understood against the background of the theory that it supplanted. The standard view had been that color is a real property or quality in the Aristotelian sense. This meant that in the surfaces of things there is a property, color, that is transmitted to the mind "without its matter" during perception (Simmons 1994). On this view, the mind receives a copy or instance of the color property that inheres in the surfaces of things. Once transmitted into the brain (according to medieval Aristotelian accounts), this instance expresses itself as a color experience (Hatfield 1998).

Aristotle's physics of color was a plausible account of the facts as known, but it was wrong. Early modern philosophers and scientists picked away at the Aristotelian view that things contain different "forms" that account for their effects, ultimately replacing it with a view that there are a few basic physical properties that account for all the physical effects of material things (on each other, and on perceivers). According to the mechanical philosophy of the seventeenth century, these properties were (primarily) size, shape, and motion. Color as a "real quality" was banished from a world of particles in motion; color as a property in objects was reconceived as a physical disposition to affect light in such a way as to cause sensations of color (phenomenal experiences) in perceivers. In this way, physical colors came to be denominated in relation to color sensations or color experiences.

Dispositionalism was enshrined in the distinction between primary and secondary qualities, according to which color in objects is a secondary quality.

Contrary to some common (and recently repeated) misconceptions, secondary qualities as Locke construed them are not "in the mind"; rather, they are physical properties of objects (properties consisting in configurations of the primary qualities such as size, shape, and motion) that have the "power" to cause specific types of color sensations in perceivers (Locke 1690, II.viii.10–13). For an object to possess color as a secondary quality is for it to possess a power to cause the sensation or experience of color in perceivers (Ayers 1991, vol. 1, ch. 23).

Newton subsequently reconceived the basic physical properties of things in terms of mass, force, and their distribution. Light was reconceived as consisting of rays (analyzed as either particles or waves, and more recently as exhibiting aspects of both) with differing refractive properties that correlate with the color of the light. Newton's discovery of the refractive properties of lights of different colors did not by itself yield an adequate theory of color vision. Modern theories of color vision arose in the nineteenth century, with the discovery of the three types of color receptors mentioned above. Color vision occurs because the nervous system compares the responses from the three cone types, thereby allowing the visual system to respond differentially to stimuli that reflect differing wavelengths of light into the eyes.

From a biological and psychological perspective, sensory systems allow organisms to navigate their environment and to discriminate and detect what's in it. In this functional context, we can distinguish the environment and its properties from the ways that perceiving organisms represent them (without yet deciding whether some sensory properties are defined relationally and dispositionally). We may then ask both *what* gets represented in perception and *how* it gets represented. The features of objects that are represented by human vision include spatial properties and colors.

Let us consider various answers to the question of what color experience represents in the environment. Subjectivists maintain that color experience has no representational content, or else has only an illusory one. Objectivists say that the phenomenal content of color perception is nothing but the representation of a physical property: the bare (visual) representation of the physical surface property by itself constitutes phenomenally experienced red or yellow. (If one experiences an illusory color, then one's color experience mistakenly presents it as being the case that a certain physical property is present when it isn't; the mistaken representation of the physical property creates the phenomenal experience of the illusory color.) By contrast, dispositionalists ascribe phenomenal red or yellow to perceptual experience as an intrinsic feature of experience itself, and they hold that perceivers are so constituted that light stimuli of various kinds cause various kinds of color experiences.

Although dispositionalists may speak of phenomenal color as representing the surface properties of an object, they (unlike representationalist objectivists) do not think that the phenomenal content of color experience is reducible to the bare representation of a physical property.

In thinking about what color experience represents, it is useful to ask what color perception is good for. We've seen that color perception allows perceivers to respond to more than the lightness and darkness of objects. Further, because objects look different, colorwise, organisms are better able to tell them apart visually. The physical basis for the objects' looking different as regards color (when seen under the same viewing conditions) is that they reflect light differently.

The comparative amount of light of various wavelengths that a surface reflects is called its *spectral reflectance distribution* (SRD). An SRD describes the percentage of light reflected by the surface of an object for each wavelength in the visible spectrum. Perfect reflectance would be 100 percent; complete absorption by the surface would yield zero percent. Natural surfaces typically reflect varied percentages of light in the visible spectrum from any given point on the surface. The peaks and valleys, the shape of the SRD, determine what color a surface region is perceived to have under a given illumination and with other conditions held constant. Generally speaking, a surface that predominantly reflects light of short wavelengths will appear blue, while one that mainly reflects long wavelengths will appear red. However, the relation between SRDs and color perception is complex, as I will discuss in greater detail.

The color properties of surfaces depend on their SRDs. Objectivists and dispositionalists disagree over whether color amounts only to the SRD (or to a grouping of SRDs, perhaps along with relations to SRDs of neighboring surfaces), or whether color must be analyzed relationally and dispositionally. Representationalist objectivists hold that colors in objects *just are* their SRDs, and that color experience is constituted simply by representing an SRD (Hilbert 1987) or a grouping of SRDs (Dretske 1995b, 88–93; Tye 1995, 146–7). They may claim that color experience is "transparent" (Tye 2000, 45–51), by which they mean that there is no mediating subjective element of experience that constitutes phenomenal color. Rather, the physical property, present to the mind representationally, constitutes the phenomenal color (Dretske 1995b, 88–93).

The dispositionalist posits phenomenal reds and yellows as subjective features of experience that the SRDs of object surfaces cause in accordance with the laws of color perception. Dispositionalists may even think that these phenomenal colors *represent*, in some way or other, a surface property of objects (in a more generic sense of "represent"). Some dispositionalists hold that phenomenal color represents its physical basis in things (Peacocke 1984). I prefer a version of dispositionalism according to which phenomenal color stands as a *sign* for an unanalyzed surface property (as discussed below). In either case, dispositionalists are committed to there being a relation between two distinct things: a phenomenal color and a surface property. They think that the phenomenal color is causally correlated with physical surface properties, and that it represents or signifies the surface properties of things, without making those properties "transparently" present in consciousness so as to constitute phenomenal color.[5]

Objectivists and dispositionalists agree that color experience permits us to discriminate physical objects with different SRDs. Without yet trying to settle whether to take a *transparency* or a *sign* view of this representational relation, we can ask what kinds of discriminations color vision makes possible. By studying how color vision helps various species, scientific work in animal color vision has suggested that the capacity for discriminating the surface colors of objects serves the following functions (Jacobs 1993, 456–7):

(1) to provide contrast not based on achromatic brightness or lightness;
(2) to aid in the detection of small objects in a dappled environment, where lightness cues are largely masked (e.g., fruit in trees);
(3) to aid in segregating objects that are partly occluded (e.g., fruit seen through leaves);
(4) to identify objects by perceiving their color stably across varying conditions of illumination (requiring something approaching color constancy).

I have already discussed (1). In (2), the chromatic contrast mentioned in (1) enhances the salience of small objects (red or yellow fruit) in a field

---

[5] Arguments concerning "transparency" often confuse two issues: one phenomenological, the other, metaphysical. Phenomenologically, the friends of representational or information theories claim that a qualia realist or other friend of subjective content should hold that color qualia seem to be "internal" or "in the mind" as opposed to seeming to be present in the surfaces of objects (Dretske 1995b, 162; Tye 1995, 30–1; 2000, 51–2). They then rightly observe that colors seem to be in the world, not in the head, and claim an argumentative victory for representationalist transparency. In fact, this argument is based on a caricature of the notion of introspective awareness of subjective mental contents (Ch. 16). Indeed, dispositionalists can agree that phenomenal colors seem to be properties of surfaces (see Secs. 3–4). The second issue concerns the metaphysics of phenomenal experience. Objectivist representationalists contend that phenomenal color is constituted by having a visual representation with a certain physical property as its content; there is nothing more to the color: the physical property is "transparently" present in experience as a phenomenal color. Dispositionalists contend that phenomenal color is a subjectively based mediating content by which we see the colors of objects. Phenomenology will not settle this metaphysical dispute (see also Crane 2000), and this second issue is independent of the phenomenological point. Henceforth, I use "transparency view" only in relation to the second issue.

of differing color surrounding them (green leaves). In (3), chromatic unity (having a single hue: red, yellow) permits a surface to be seen as continuous even though, from a specific locus, only parts of it are seen (intervening objects occlude some parts of the surface). Finally, in (4), the hues that are stably perceived in specific objects or kinds of object permit those objects to be identified or reidentified by color.

The literature on comparative color vision, and on the evolution of trichromacy in primates, stresses functions (1) to (3). Genetic analysis suggests that mammalian color vision evolved through selection on naturally occurring variation in what are now the middle-wavelength-sensitive (M) cones. The short-wavelength cone is thought to have been stable, but the M cone is believed to have exhibited variations that in time became the M and L types of cone (Goldsmith 1990). Trichromatic color vision of this sort would allow better discrimination of yellow, red, and orange objects found among green leaves. This "fruit detection" hypothesis has long been favored in explaining the development of trichromacy (Jacobs 1993, 457). For a visual system that compares the outputs of the M and L cone variants, some objects become easier to discriminate on the basis of color.

Accordingly, objects "gained" new colors when trichromacy evolved and the visual system came to partition the chromatic appearances of surfaces more finely. Fruit and leaves now appeared chromatically more distinct and hence were easier to discriminate than before. On this view, the function of color experience is to represent surfaces in distinctive ways so as to enhance their discriminability and perhaps to aid in the identification of object kinds. Any such account assumes that perceived colors correlate with the reflective properties of objects, even if evolution acts opportunistically to change some of those correlations (by adding new ones). However, it remains to be seen whether such accounts must regard color experiences as specifically *representing* physical reflective properties such as SRDs.

3. Color as a Psychobiological Property of Objects

With this primer in place, my reasons for preferring dispositionalism can be stated briefly, in terms of comparative advantages. Objectivists seek a single physical property to be identified with the color of an object. This property then constitutes the content of color-perceptual representations of surfaces. As objectivists, they must seek a mind-independent property. I don't believe that they have or will find any good candidates for a categorical (or intrinsic) physical property that is the color of a thing; the only properties that are good candidates for object color must be defined relationally with reference to visual experience.

The best contemporary reason for this conclusion is the phenomenon of metamerism. For natural vision systems, such as the human perceptual system, each SRD does not yield a unique color perception (under a given illuminant). Rather, many SRDs, even those whose graphs exhibit widely divergent shapes, may yield the same perceived color: they are "metamers" of one another (see Ch. 8). Although "metamerism" means etymologically "sameness of parts," here it means "sameness of color response" to physically distinct SRDs. The SRDs that group metamerically do not constitute a *physical kind* independent of color vision; there is no strictly physical property or principle that relates them. From the fact that we (normal perceivers) perceive objects having physically distinct SRDs as instances of the same surface color, I conclude that the quest for a single mind-independent color property fails.

Objectivists of course know about metamerism, but they don't agree with my conclusion. The objectivist representationalist Michael Tye (2000) seeks to address this problem by adopting a physicalist dispositionalism, one that defines object colors by their tendencies to affect other physical objects. Tye (2000, 160–1) groups metamerically matching SRDs together so as to form a *disjunctive* physical property to serve as the mind-independent property that the visual system detects in color perception. Accordingly, he defines object colors through their effects on the S, M, and L cones. A red object is one that, *ceteris paribus*, causes a certain pattern of relative activation across the three types of cone; metamerically matching red objects would all cause the same relative activation. This renders surface colors as dispositions, but the reference to cone types ostensibly is a way of defining these dispositions as existing independently of minds. Hence, Tye holds out hope for a reductive physicalist dispositionalism (2000, 149–50).

While it is true that we can define surface colors relative to the physical effects of incoming light on the three cone types, we cannot do so without appealing to color experience. We can isolate the pattern of cone firing that signals (to the theorist) the presence of a red object only by noting that this pattern of cone firing causes a red-experience. That is, we can isolate the pattern only by appealing to phenomenal or psychological facts. The "disjunctive properties" that the objectivist tries to use as a physical basis for reduction have no interest or significance from a purely physical point of view. Such properties can be defined only in relation to the responses of color perceivers: they are not mind-independent.[6] Hence, Tye's position fails as a version of objectivism.

Another objectivist response is to say that each SRD is actually a distinct color, and that the human visual system is simply incapable of resolving all the colors there are. So, if two SRDs produce exactly the same perception of green, this just shows that the normal human visual system is blind to some colors (Hilbert 1987). For a committed physicalist, such talk of illusion or misrepresentation makes some sense. However, from a biological and psychological perspective, it is problematic, if we accept that a function of color vision is to enable us to tell things apart. In fact, from such a viewpoint it presumably is better *not* to discriminate each SRD, since that would create too vastly a variegated color world. That objects are grouped into a small number of hue ranges, rather than each SRD producing a distinct hue, presumably makes our color world more useful and manageable. Further, since SRDs are grouped relative to the color experience that they produce, it is not objectionable for dispositionalists to define the physical color property as an arbitrary disjunction (from a physicist's point of view). The groupings of SRDs are conceived as driven evolutionarily by enhanced discriminability for objects (and not by the search for a chromatic partition of object surfaces that coincides with a physically precise description of the surfaces' reflective properties).

Since physicalism does not otherwise have much going for it (as I have argued in Ch. 10), I take it that the comparative advantage goes to the biological and psychological perspective. Color perception is, after all, an evolved psychological capacity of biological systems.

There is, however, a variant of the "one SRD per color" position that seeks biological plausibility. If we assume that in ecologically pristine environments there is only one naturally occurring SRD per hue or shade, then we could define that as the "real" physical color (Dretske 1995*b*, 89–93). Suppose that tomato red has only one SRD, strawberry red another, geranium red another,

---

[6] Tye (2000) seems to acknowledge this fact in his analysis of color as a disposition to cause cone firings, in analyzing a surface's being pure red: "we may now propose that a surface is (pure) red, for example, so long as it has a reflectance that, *ceteris paribus*, under normal viewing conditions, enables it to reflect light that produces opponent processing distinctive of the experience of (pure) red" (160). Although he subsequently attempts to drop the reference to the experience of red in favor of the pattern of cone firings, the cone firings can be color-typed only by their experiential effects. That being accepted, Tye's analysis is the same as that of the subjective dispositionalist: for a surface to be red is for it to cause a red-sensation or experience in normal perceivers under standard conditions. He might of course argue that the pure red in question is transparently the representation of the physical property of the surface that causes it. But notice that he is now defining the physical property in relation to the red-experience, as the property having the disposition of causing a red-experience. He has not reduced the experience to the representation of the property, but instead has in effect defined the property in relation to the independently specified subjective experience.

and so on. By hypothesis, there would be no natural metamers; metamerically matching SRDs, if artificially produced, would yield color experiences deemed to misrepresent, for they would yield a color experience that, according to nature, should signal the presence of a specific biological kind.

This conjecture is interesting (see Ch. 8.3−4), but problematic. It has not been established that, in the ecological circumstances in which trichromacy evolved, there were unique SRDs for each distinguishable shade of red and green. In this regard, there needs to be more sampling of extant SRDs in natural environments. Moreover, even if a one-to-one correspondence provided the original selective pressure (in the fruit-detection scenario), that does not entail that primate populations have maintained color vision *because* distinct hues signal distinct biological kinds. The general enhancement of discriminability across various chromatic circumstances might well be responsible for the maintenance of trichromacy. More significantly, there are important challenges to the one-SRD/one-shade hypothesis. All pieces of ripe fruit of a given kind do not have the same SRD: they vary in appearance. So there is no single SRD to signal each type of fruit. Moreover, because color constancy is not perfect and natural lighting conditions vary, a given SRD does not always produce a unique phenomenal shade, and may under some conditions appear the same shade as does another SRD under slightly different illumination. Color vision does not achieve the presumed goal of recovering unique SRDs, nor is it apparent that that is or should be its goal.

If there is no well-conceived physical property that can on its own serve to partition colors as properties of objects, what is the basis for color properties? I maintain that color properties should be classed relative to color perception or color experience. This means that theories of color as an object property must begin (conceptually) with color experience. Given that there is no way to reduce the phenomenal content of color experience to a representational content that transparently presents a distal property,[7] both the existence and character of the object quality must depend on the experience itself. By saying that the object quality depends on experience, I mean that the phenomenal characters of color qualia are features of how colored objects appear to us, that is, they are features of the experience by which we see colored objects. I also mean that we should construe the qualitative character of color experience as developing out of the subject's capacities for phenomenally presenting objects.

---

[7] I use the term *presents* to emphasize the sense in which phenomenal experience makes its objects present to consciousness. Presentations that make external objects present to consciousness (or that purport to do so) are also *representations* (of the distal object).

We might think of it this way. Mammalian visual perception presents the spatial properties of things. It is initially specialized for presenting surfaces phenomenally to perceivers. It presents surfaces as spatial structures, and also as colored. If there were no chromatic color perception, all surfaces would appear with shades of grey, from black to white.[8] But, with the development of color vision, surfaces came to be presented with one or another phenomenal color. Because of the spatial structure of experience, these colors are presented as being properties of the surfaces. There is no need to "refer" or "project" the color experience outwardly. Evolutionarily, color experiences are a kind of phenomenal infusion into pre-existing perceptual presentations of surfaces in locations. The phenomenal character of this infusion is not generated by its representational content (as in objectivist representationalism). Rather, we may imagine that mutation generates it, and that its etiology lies in the capacities of neural structures to generate phenomenal characters.

From a phenomenological point of view, and from the standpoint of ordinary experience, objects are presented as if color were a simple categorical property of the surface. That is the manifest representational content of color experiences: they present objects as having a (categorical) color property. The phenomenal content of the color experience makes no further comment on the color property in the object. Color experience simply presents the object surface as having a distinctive character. Beyond the implication that, with conditions held constant, surfaces that look different chromatically are different in some way, color qualia of themselves don't contain further content about the properties of surfaces.

As theorists, we can now seek a further characterization of the relation between phenomenal color and the physical object-surface. The phenomenal color presents the object surface under a minimal characterization, compared to the physicist's description of the surface.[9] The capacities of the brain for

---

[8] This speculative description of monochromatic color vision (either with one cone type, or with multiple cone types but no comparison of outputs) is used for illustrative purposes; there might be phenomenal colors that represent light and dark (see n. 4).

[9] If we use the convenient metaphor of characterizing representational content through propositions, then we can say that according to an objectivist representationalist such as Dretske, color perception carries the content "that such-and-such physical property is present" (using the notion of natural "information," Dretske 1995b, 2–4, effectively builds this sort of content into nature's nomic relations among properties and then uses it to construct representational content). By contrast, I ascribe unsophisticated content to phenomenal color, on the order of "an (unanalyzed) color property is present of type x," where x ranges over shades of color (this is the content of phenomenal color, independent of any categorization of the color shade). This content presents the object surface "under a description," albeit an unsophisticated one. Such representations have intentional opacity, as normally understood; thus, if there were a single physical property of the object surface that were nomically related to a type of color experience, a description of that property could *not* be substituted into the

presenting phenomenal character do not arise from conceptually sophisticated physical descriptions such as are embodied in color experience according to the representationalist. From the present theoretical point of view, color experiences are blank signs for the color properties of objects. They contain the content that a thing has a color property of a specific kind (yellow, red, etc.), but they do not provide any further details. We, as theorists, can correlate the signs with their causal conditions under a physical description and we can determine that the color property in objects is a disposition to produce color experience. However, evolution established those correlations in the visual system through the trial and error of natural selection. It did not build into color experiences the content that they result from dispositional properties.

Phenomenal colors are aspects of our experience under which we experience surfaces, and they are arbitrary signs by which we distinguish surfaces. Such signs represent things that in fact have causally relevant physical properties (SRDs or disjunctions of SRDs), but they are not *representations of physical properties* as such: they do not carry in their representational content a specification of the SRDs that cause them. They serve to group surfaces according to their effects on perceivers, and so as to enhance the discriminability of objects. They present the surfaces of objects *in accordance with* the distinctive dispositional bases objects have for producing color experiences, but we need not construe them as *representing* the specific physical properties that constitute a particular dispositional basis. Color qualia, as signs, simply present the object as having a color property of a kind that differs from other color properties.[10]

characterization of the representational content of a phenomenal color. (Note: the present-day concept of intentionality I have just invoked differs from the original Brentano intentionality that I describe in Section 6; also, I truly hold that propositional characterization of nonconceptual content is merely metaphorical.) By contrast with Dretske's approach, I avoid commitment to natural information and am forced to build representational content out of the representational capacities of the organism. In this chapter, I have merely gestured toward the evolved representational capacities of the brain, which I see as biological functions for representing (see Chs. 1–3).

[10] The terminology of color sensations as "signs" for "external qualities" comes from Hermann Helmholtz (1868/1995, 166–8). (However, Helmholtz, as many dispositionalists, shares the determinacy assumption discussed at the end of the present section, on which I differ from him.) Helmholtz contrasted "sign" with "image"; a perception that was an image would represent its object through the same type of property that is in the object (say, physical spatial relations through phenomenal spatial relations). By contrast, a sign does not intrinsically reveal through its own character the character of the external qualities it denotes, which is one sense in which such a sign is arbitrary: its phenomenal content bears no intrinsic connection with what it signifies in objects. Colors may be arbitrary signs in a further sense: it may be contingent that red-experience was selected for long-wavelength colors, and blue for short-wavelength; indeed, for all we know, the kinds of phenomenal colors we experience may be one group out of a range of possible phenomenal palettes. Here, our ignorance is great, for we have no grip on the capacities of brain structures for generating phenomenal characters. Finally, it can be imagined that the initial sign-relations were not arbitrary in one limited sense: that phenomenal color originally signaled specific object properties such as nutritional or sexual readiness (in the case of red). I would

Accordingly, phenomenal colors are arbitrary signs for the properties of surfaces. Neither we nor our visual systems—nor the visual systems of our trichromatic primate ancestors—need to know this or to be able to reflect on this in order for it to be the case. Indeed, as previously noted, objects are presented phenomenally as if color were a simple property of a surface. Evolution need not have built into color experiences the content that they are produced by dispositional (relationally defined) properties of objects for it to be the case that they are so produced. It is as theorists, not as bare perceivers, that we discern that the dispositional account provides the best color ontology.

On this view, things are red, blue, green, and yellow because they produce red-, blue-, green-, and yellow-experiences in normal perceivers under standard conditions.[11] I thus disagree with the third major position, subjectivism, by maintaining that we can use the dispositional basis for things to produce such color experiences in defining color as a property of objects.

Subjectivists reject dispositionalism largely because they don't think that the notions of *normal perceivers* and *standard conditions* can be made good. They base their argument on the variability among perceivers who are classed as "normal" trichromats, and on the variability of even the same perceiver to the same SRD under conditions that would all be classed as "standard." They reason that such variability is inconsistent with construing relationally grouped SRDs, or metamers, as instances of a dispositional color property in objects (Hardin 1988).

The subjectivists are right about the variability, but I don't accept their conclusion. Their argument tacitly relies on an assumption about what kind of property a color property would be if it were actually a property of objects: that the relevant property would be the disposition unvaryingly to produce a determinate shade or hue. Thus, on their interpretation of dispositionalism, for a given SRD to be an instance of yellow a perceiver would always have to see it (under standard conditions) not merely as in the yellow range, and not merely as some determinate shade of yellow (because phenomenal color shades

argue that, even if this were so, the function of phenomenal red became generalized to present bare color properties as well (or instead), thereby rendering the representational content of a red-experience independent of the nutritional or reproductive properties of red objects.

[11] I use the language of "yellow-experience" here, rather than "looks yellow," because some philosophers, including some dispositionalists, hold that talk of "looks" typically or always implies a suspected contrast between how a thing *looks* and how it *is* (between *mere appearance* and *reality*). Peacocke (1984) offers yet other reasons for contrasting "looks yellow" with his preferred notation for yellow-experience: "yellow′." Nonetheless, there are other senses of "looks" that do not imply an appearance/reality suspicion, including a *phenomenal reporting* sense. Elsewhere in this chapter, I use "looks" in the reporting sense, which aims to describe the character of our experience rather than to express our judgments concerning the actual properties of the things we look at (Ch. 16.2, esp. n. 5).

are determinate), but as the same determinate shade each time. Subjectivists attribute to the dispositionalist the view that colors in objects are dispositions uniformly to produce experiences of particular determinate shades of color (rather than, say, a range of shades).

Many dispositionalists make this assumption, but they needn't and shouldn't. The functions of color vision are served merely if color vision enables us to better discriminate some objects from other objects, and enables us to reidentify them as those objects when we encounter them again. Thus, a lemon would not always need to appear with the same determinate shade of yellow in order to be better discriminable from green leaves. And for us to re-identify it by color as a lemon as opposed to an orange or a ripe tomato, it need not appear with exactly the same determinate yellow, so long as it falls in the range of yellow. If we take the biopsychological account seriously, it leads us to view object colors as mapping one–many onto the experience of hues, within a range of shades (see Hatfield 1999, and Ch. 9, for further discussion). This would be a kind of reverse metamerism. Of course, there would need to be boundaries: if a yellow object is seen under aberrant lighting conditions (say, under monochromatic blue light), then it appears dark bluish grey and not yellow, and so it doesn't appear to have the object color that it in fact has. Or if a red object is seen by a nonstandard observer (say, someone with a form of red–green colorblindness), then it may not generate a red-experience. These are violations of standard conditions and normal observers.

If we reject the assumption about hue determinacy, the subjectivists' arguments lose their force. Dispositionalism thereby gains the comparative advantage over subjectivism because it avoids treating a functionally successful mode of perception as inherently illusory.

4. Epistemological Worries

Dispositionalism, as I have developed it, is an account of how we see surface colors. It affirms that objects have colors and that we see them. For us to see a surface color is for an object's surface to cause us to have a visual experience of a phenomenal color through which we represent the surface of the object (for normal observers under standard conditions).

Be that as it may, dispositionalist positions have been charged with the same offense that characterizes subjectivism: that they render color experience illusory. The charge arises from the fact that objects appear as if phenomenal color is an inhering categorical property in things. Dispositionalism renders color experience illusory because it tells us that things aren't colored in the way that they appear to be. After all, things don't appear to us as possessing dispositional bases for causing phenomenal experiences of color in us; they just look colored.

This objection rests on two assumptions that I will challenge. The first assumption concerns what it means for things to look colored; the second concerns what ordinary observers should be able to tell about their own experience. I call the first assumption the *simple property* view. I call the second the *metaphysical transparency* view.

The simple property view holds that for a thing to look colored is for it to look like it has a property, color, in or on its surface. Objectivist representationalism embraces this assumption, and proudly proclaims that its own analysis of color phenomenology asserts that the color experience just *is* the representation of a surface property. However, dispositionalism can also say that object surfaces are colored and that they are presented in visual experience as being colored. Its analysis of what this means, however, differs from that of objectivism. The dispositionalist says that the property of color in an object is a dispositional basis of its surface for causing experiences of phenomenal color of a certain kind. (If illumination or surrounding colors are allowed to vary, then the *kind* of phenomenal experience might comprise a *range of shades* rather than a single shade.) This phenomenal color is an experience of the object's color; in my version of dispositionalism, phenomenal color represents the surface as having an unanalyzed color property. So far, both positions permit one to speak of "the surface colors" of objects, and of the ways those colors appear to observers.

The metaphysical transparency view comes into play at this point. Tye claims (1995, 146; 2000, 146) that the dispositionalist view makes our perceptual experience of color illusory. He argues that, if color in objects is a disposition to cause color experiences of certain kinds, then we should be able to discover this by simple inspection. That is, if dispositionalism were true, then objects should manifestly appear to have the disposition to cause color experiences in us, instead of simply looking colored. Since they don't so appear, dispositionalism allegedly renders color experience illusory.

Tye is assuming a lot. First, regarding illusion. Tye seems to adopt a notion of illusion such that if things don't look *as they are* in some respect, the appearance is an illusion. But "looking as they are" is a notoriously slippery notion. From the window of a jetliner in midflight, the roads and houses below look smaller than they usually do. Is that an illusion? As we look down a highway, the sides of the road appear to converge in the distance (even though we know they don't, and even though we know that highways of constant width look just like this). Is that an illusion? Clearly, the notion of illusion needs further specification. Normally, we take it that an appearance is illusory if objects appear otherwise than we expect them to appear in those circumstances (Hatfield 1986a). Thus, close at hand we expect lines that are straight to appear straight, and lines of equal length (presented in plain sight) to appear of equal length. The various line illusions provide instances in which these expectations are not met: we call the resulting appearances "illusory."

But how should we expect a dispositional property to appear to us? Should we expect it to be obvious to all normal perceivers that color in objects is a disposition to produce color experiences? Given the functions of color vision sketched above, there is no reason for us to expect so, any more than we should expect water to appear really to be H_2O, or lilies to appear to be of the same botanical family as onions and garlic. We do accept that some substances smell like they would be good to eat, and that such odors are a generally reliable guide to nutritional properties; but we don't expect to be able to find the biochemistry of nutrition directly revealed by phenomenal odors.

At stake here are differing conceptions of what we should expect our sensory experience to reveal to us about itself. Philosophers who complain that colors in objects don't appear to be dispositional properties seem to expect our sensory experience to be *metaphysically transparent*: if we attentively inspect our sensory experience, it will reveal its real nature to us.[12] However, there is no reason to suppose that the senses have evolved in order to reveal the principles of their own operation, or to suppose that the true physical descriptions of the object properties that cause (and are signified by) our sensory representations should be transparently available in consciousness. Assuming that the function of the senses is to allow us to navigate the environment and that the function of mammalian color vision in particular is to enhance the discriminability of surfaces, then, if the senses present us with colored surfaces that appear the way they should given their object colors, there is no illusion.

On the dispositional account offered here, a colored surface *should* appear as if the phenomenal color were in or on the surface, because the function

---

[12] The notion that colors should "reveal" their intrinsic character as properties to reflective perceivers has been widely endorsed. Boghossian and Velleman (1989) reject dispositionalism because it does not account for color phenomenology (colors don't *seem* to be dispositional properties) and adopt projectivism (a form of subjectivism). Johnston (1992) echoes G. Strawson's (1989) desire for "Revelation" of the color property in experience in arguing *for* a secondary qualities account of color (a form of dispositionalism). As will become clear, I do not think that the notion of "revelation" provides any constraint on the correct theory of color ontology: object colors could be dispositions even if no one knew it. I agree with Johnston (1992) that any correct analysis of color ontology should acknowledge that normally sighted subjects can tell on the face of it that phenomenal blue differs from phenomenal red, but I do not treat this as "revelation" of the color property *per se*, even if it is "revelation" of an aspect of colors (viz., phenomenal colors as regards their intrinsic quality).

of color experience is to present the surface in a manner that enhances its discriminability. This account distinguishes between a surface looking *as if* it possesses a disposition to cause color experiences in us, and looking *as it should look* if it has such a disposition. Color experience will serve its function, and will fit the dispositional account, if a surface looks however it should given its dispositional color properties. In this regard, it is not illusory if objects are presented phenomenally as if color were a categorical property of the object surface.

The account takes for granted that there are regular relations between color experience and physical properties that underlie object colors.[13] It also takes for granted that color experiences fall into phenomenally distinguishable groupings. Thus, observers can readily distinguish phenomenal yellows from phenomenal reds. To this extent, color properties are partially revealed in experience. From our color experience (in standard conditions) we can tell that two objects have different colors (yellow vs. red). We know *how* yellow and red look. We can't tell, just by looking, *what* yellow and red are as properties of an object surface. But that's alright. It is too much to expect of color experience that a surface transparently look as if it possesses a disposition to cause color experience in us—even if, given the proper theoretical knowledge, a perceiver may come to see that a surface has such a disposition.

5. Analytic Objections from "Our Ordinary View"

Some philosophers who write about color think that conclusions about what color is must be responsive to our "ordinary" ways of thinking about things. According to such philosophers, if a particular metaphysical thesis about "what color is" does not "capture the content of our everyday beliefs about the colors of things" (Stroud 2000, 189), that constitutes grounds for rejecting that metaphysical thesis. This approach holds that it would be unacceptable

[13] Many discussions of qualia employ examples that permit the relations between object surfaces and color experiences to vary, as in "inverted spectrum" cases: I see a red object as you do, but Jones experiences green when looking at the same object under the same conditions (Kriegel 2002; Shoemaker 1996, Pt. IV). I find such cases to be of limited use. When philosophers faced verificationist objections to the very notion of phenomenal experience, the inverted spectrum offered a useful thought experiment for conceiving how two observers might be *behaviorally identical* and yet *psychologically different* (assuming Jones has learned to say "red" when she has a green-experience). But on the assumption that psychophysical laws (which relate stimuli to phenomenal experience) are indeed *laws*, such inversion is *physically* (naturally) *impossible*. Indeed, in the usual form of the thought experiment, in which molecule-for-molecule identical individuals are attributed inverted spectra, the principle that color experience supervenes on brain states renders spectral inversion *metaphysically impossible*.

to find that many of our ordinary ways of thinking are in error. Accordingly, metaphysics must accommodate "who we are" into "what there is."

I have no trouble with the claim that metaphysics must accommodate human beings, including their thoughts, feelings, and experiences, into what there is. I take it as obvious that human beings exist, and that they think, feel, and experience many things. Any view that tried to deny this would put itself into a pretty big hole, as regards credibility. It would need a powerful argument to lift itself out, and I at least have never seen such an argument on behalf of this sort of eliminativist metaphysics.

But to acknowledge this much is not to give our "ordinary" conceptions the kind of metaphysical authority that these philosophers give them. The notion that human beings should be accommodated into a philosophical view of the world does not of itself entail that "ordinary" beliefs should decide metaphysical questions. Ordinary beliefs should constrain metaphysics in some areas. For example, I'd grant that ordinary beliefs about what a family portrait should look like, or how a lawn should be kept, can and should have some impact on the metaphysics of family portraits and of lawns. But when we are trying to understand color as a property, I see no reason to give "the ordinary" much weight. Indeed, in this context I'm not sure what "the ordinary" is. At the University of Pennsylvania, where nearly all undergraduates take courses in introductory psychology, the "ordinary" understanding of color theory among people on the street might be fairly sophisticated, at least to the point of understanding basic scientific findings. On other streets, "ordinary" people might never have thought about what kind of property color is, and might simply think that being colored is just a matter of being colored.

In philosophical circles, "ordinary conceptions" about color tend to be conceptions about what kind of property color is—most usually, that it is a categorical property rather than a relational one. To my mind, framing such a distinction is not really "ordinary" at all: it is the product of previous philosophy, embedded in unexamined (philosophical) "common sense" (see also Russell 1953).

It seems to me that philosophers should be prepared to find that science tells us things about color that we didn't know or even believe before. Philosophers should be willing to have it turn out as a matter of scientific discovery that, say, color is a useful illusion, so that, technically speaking, things aren't really colored, or perhaps that color is a perceiver-relative property. They should be prepared to accept these findings as proposals about what color is, from the perspective of current scientific theory. In ontology, we should give considerable weight to evidence supplied by the best current science (subject, of course, to philosophical interpretation).

This does not mean that the findings of science or of metaphysics should automatically be taken as proposals about how to talk. Someone could propose the theory that things aren't really colored, but do so only for the purposes of metaphysics and science and not expect that people more generally would stop talking about the colors of things. (I don't, of course, interpret the results of science as actually implying that things aren't really colored.)

To see that scientific advances need not change entrenched forms of speech, consider a famous development in the history of astronomy. When the Copernican theory of the solar system was accepted, it became the proper scientific account of what happens at dawn and at dusk: the earth's rotation brings the sun into view, and subsequently the rotation causes part of the earth to occlude the sun. Yet, nearly five centuries later, we continue to talk about "sunrise" and "sunset." That is, when scientists discovered and ordinary folk came to believe that the sun doesn't really rise, that was not taken as a mandate to stop saying "the sun rises." Nor was continuing use of "sunrise" taken as a threat to Copernican theory.

Here I find myself at odds with some recent philosophical arguments concerning the relevance of ordinary beliefs to color metaphysics. Barry Stroud (2000) urges that we should give due consideration to the predicative implications of our "ordinary" perceptual talk. He offers the following eight sentences that express a perceptual or cognitive relation to color and colored things (2000, 103–4):

(1) Jones sees yellow.
(2) Jones sees something yellow.
(3) Jones sees something to be yellow.
(4) Jones sees a yellow lemon.
(5) Jones sees a lemon to be yellow.
(6) Jones sees that a lemon is on the table.
(7) Jones sees that there is a yellow lemon on the table.
(8) Jones believes that there is a yellow lemon on the table.

Although Stroud uses these eight sentences for a variety of purposes, the main drift of his discussion is to consider how sentence (1) can be related to the others. His aim is to test the credibility of various interpretations of what (1) describes as "seen," and what (2) to (8) attribute to the lemon on the table. In particular, he is concerned with interpretations of (1) that attribute to Jones the experiencing of a sensation, that is, of a phenomenal yellow that is intrinsic to that experience and yet is distinct from the physical properties of the surface of the lemon and of the light reflected from it. He believes that such interpretations of (1) are in tension with what sentences

(2) to (8) imply, because these latter sentences attribute "yellow" to the lemon as a property. In Stroud's view, if sentences such as (8) are true, then we must take seriously the view that yellow is a (categorical) property of the lemon on the table (2000, 114–16). Taking ordinary talk seriously yields a presumption in favor of naive realism about the color property.

I am not inclined to think that ordinary talk can bear even this much metaphysical weight as regards the color property. Consider what conclusion we might draw by applying a similar analysis to the Copernican case and taking seriously the ordinary talk of "sunrises":

(A) Smith believes that the sun rose at 6 a.m.
(B) What Smith believes is true.
(C) We must grant that the things mentioned in Smith's true beliefs have the properties that Smith predicates of them.
(D) Therefore, the earth doesn't turn; rather, the sun rises.

The conclusion (D) is ludicrous. But why so? Because we are well educated about the solar system and the diurnal rotation of the earth, and yet we are willing to talk of "sunrises" without supposing that, in so doing, we contradict scientific theory.[14] We are able to let ordinary talk play its ordinary role, without supposing that our use of an antique expression from an earlier conception of the solar system commits us to those earlier views.

In order to investigate further the use of "ordinary" talk in metaphysics, I want to focus on a problem that allegedly arises from taking sentences (2) to (8) seriously while also holding that sentence (1) reports Jones' experience of a merely phenomenal quality. According to Stroud, if we take Jones to believe that "yellow" is a phenomenal quality and that "yellow" is possessed by objects, we must ascribe to Jones the "unintelligible" thought that a "sensation" has been "transferred" to the object. This ascription is unacceptable, says Stroud, on the principle that "someone could perceive something to have a certain

---

[14] What one finds plausible to assert about colors can be heavily influenced by one's understanding of color theory. Thus, at the conference on secondary qualities in Bielefeld at which this essay was first presented, another presenter found it plausible to assert that "Yellow lemons look green in blue light." If "blue light" is taken to mean monochromatic blue light (or perhaps blue light composed only of lights having wavelengths such that, if any individual wavelength is viewed on its own, it appears as a shade of blue), then yellow lemons in blue light appear black or dark bluish grey because yellow lemons absorb nearly all blue light (thanks to David Brainard and Feng Gai for use of their monochromators). If one adds some greenish light of wavelength 480 nm and higher to otherwise blue light (e.g., by producing a light composed of all wavelengths from 450 to 490 nm), then the light still appears bluish and the lemon takes on a greenish cast in "blue" light (because only the green light is reflected in a significant amount). Of course, if one mixes yellow and blue pigments, one gets green: but that is a *subtractive* color mixture, rather than an interaction between colored light and a pigmented surface (such as the lemon's).

property only if the thought of its having that property made sense to him" (Stroud 2000, 111). Stroud asserts that it is "unintelligible" to suppose that subjective properties of sensation "belong to" external objects (113). That is, if (2) to (8) ascribe a categorical property of yellowness to the lemon, and if (1) refers to a sensation, then these sentences, taken together, allegedly ascribe the quality in the sensation to the lemon in an "unintelligible" way.

My problem here is: "unintelligible" to whom? Consider a set of corresponding sentences pertaining to the feeling of heaviness.

   (1′) Smith feels heaviness.
   (2′) Smith feels something heavy.
   (3′) Smith feels something to be heavy.
   (4′) Smith feels a heavy book.
   (5′) Smith feels a book to be heavy.
   (6′) Smith feels that a heavy book is in his hand.
   (7′) Smith feels that there is a heavy book in his hand.
   (8′) Smith believes that there is a heavy book in his hand.

Sentences (2′) to (8′) seem to ascribe heaviness as a property to the book. (1′) can be read as the report of a feeling or sensation. If these sentences are all true, must we say that Smith can "make sense" of the property of being heavy?

I want to consider two cases. In the first case, some of us believe that Smith has "spread" a felt quality on the world, even though Smith himself doesn't believe that. In the second, we ask whether it is necessary that Smith be able to "make sense" of what heaviness *is* in order for us to think that he believes true sentences ascribing heaviness to things.

In the first case, let us suppose that Smith is Aristotle, who believed that objects have an absolute, tangible quality of heaviness. Aristotle considered that this quality is "expressed" in our sense experience of heaviness, as a case of "like knows like": it is as if the quality of heaviness in the object has migrated into the sense experience (and subsequent intellectual representation). Later philosophers who disagreed with Aristotle described this relation between the qualitative "form" in the object and the subsequent sensory representation as one of "resemblance," but Aristotle's own followers used the term "similitude" (see Hatfield 1998; Simmons 1994). Aristotle further held that things having the absolute quality of heaviness seek the center of the universe, which, for that reason, is the center of the Earth. Things would seek that center even if the Earth were not already in place.

Aristotle and his followers held beliefs that Stroud finds that "we" cannot even think: that qualities as experienced in sensation are in things, that an object would be drawn toward a region even though no matter like it (and no matter at all) was already there, and so on. We might believe that Aristotle and his followers believed these things because they reasoned by analogy directly from their experience of heaviness to the properties of heavy things. Holding up a heavy thing requires an exertion of effort; we feel our effort in lifting and holding the thing. Perhaps Aristotle or his followers (wrongly) ascribed something like that effort to heavy things, in their strivings to reach the center of the world.

What we take to be "intelligible" depends on what we already believe. And what "we" believe changes. Today, we think that books are heavy because of their comparative mass in proximity to a much larger mass. This is thought about in two ways: a gravitational field of attraction exists between the book and a larger mass, say, the Earth; or the book has a tendency to move along a certain line in curved space-time that leads it toward the large mass.

Does Smith need to be able to "make sense" of the force of gravity and of action at a distance, or of curved space-time, in order to have the belief asserted in (8′) and for that belief to be true? I think not. We can allow Smith to have true beliefs about states of affairs even if he does not really understand the property that the object has or that he ascribes to it. If we attribute a specific false belief to Smith, such as that heaviness is an internal striving downward (or centerward) of an object, we still can allow him to believe truly that books are heavy, even though he doesn't understand what heaviness is. Presumably, we allow that Aristotle could believe truly that logs (or stones) are heavy. Despite his grossly false understanding of heaviness, Aristotle surely knew something about heavy things, such as that marble is heavier than timber. We should be prepared to allow that his talk can function for everyday purposes, and that (8′) can be true, even if his way of talking and thinking implicitly contains a bad theory about how things are. But we ought not to search for acceptable metaphysical theses by analyzing such a person's presuppositions when he talks about heavy things.

In my own dispositionalist account, Jones can believe (8), that the lemon is yellow, without knowing *what yellow is* as a property of objects. Suppose that yellow in objects is a disposition to cause an experience of phenomenal yellow in a perceiver. Then Jones believes truly of a lemon that it is yellow just in case the lemon in fact possesses this disposition (whether or not she has any beliefs about dispositions or even possesses the concept of a disposition). In order to have a true belief about a colored thing, Jones no more need understand the metaphysics of the color property than she need understand the physics (and metaphysics) of gravity in order to have a true belief about a heavy thing. Further, we need not conclude that she is using the term "yellow" equivocally in (1) and in (8), because we need not consider Jones to be thinking like Aristotle. She might, in (1), simply be talking about the yellow color of an object. In contrast, we, as theorists, may suppose that Jones sees yellow objects in virtue of having an experience of phenomenal yellow, and so we might use a sentence like (1) to describe Jones as experiencing a phenomenal quale. But we, as (dispositionalist) theorists, distinguish "phenomenal yellow" from "yellow as a property of objects," and we use the former to analyze the latter. We are not guilty of equivocation, because we understand the two different senses of "yellow."

In this regard, dispositionalists violate another aspect of (allegedly) "ordinary" talk. Stroud (2000) and others (e.g., Austin 1962) believe that "is yellow" is conceptually prior to "looks yellow" or "is a yellow-experience." They support their contention by appealing to phenomenology and to the context of learning. Yellow *seems to be* a simple, categorical property. Children learn the word "yellow" by perceiving things that *are* yellow (lemons, color samples). Yet dispositionalists claim that "yellow-experience" is *conceptually prior* to "object-yellow," because they analyze object-yellow as a disposition to cause yellow-experiences. Nonetheless, dispositionalists can grant that "is yellow" *does have priority* phenomenologically and in the order of learning, while still holding that "yellow-experience" is conceptually prior for the purposes of color ontology. We learn to apply "yellow" to yellow objects (which usually look yellow). In so doing, we need not learn what (metaphysically) yellow *is*. Later, as dispositionalist theorists, we come to understand that yellow-experience is conceptually prior to being yellow, even if we have already learned a wide variety of correct applications of "is yellow" without knowing what yellow (as an object property) really is.

"Ordinary" talk should certainly be preserved in many domains. Ordinary talk can even set strong constraints on metaphysics in some human domains, such as in talk of human institutions and artifacts. But it does not provide the grist for metaphysics in general, including the metaphysics of the biologically based perceptual capacities of perceivers.

6. Phenomenal Color and Intentional Existence

Many philosophers find it difficult to grant the existence of qualitatively characterized phenomenal states, or "qualia." If we suppose that phenomenal red is real, they want to know what phenomenal red is a property of, and where it is located.

Early twentieth-century realists about perceptual qualities had ready answers to such questions. Sense-data theorists such as Russell (1914c, 1915) believed that, if we experience a red round thing, a red round sense datum exists that possesses the property of redness in the same way that that datum possesses a round shape. Both are properties of the thing we see. Russell called the thing a "momentary particular," and he considered it to be real; at the same time, he regarded physical objects as described by physicists to be logical fictions, constructions out of sense data (see Hatfield 2002c). According to him (and to some but not all sense-data theorists), our sense data are literally red and round. They possess the quality red in just the way that we experience them to possess it.

I am not a quality realist in Russell's sense. I do not hold that phenomenal red is a property of our experience as Russell did. Nor do I believe that our experiences are red in the same way that I believe objects have the property of being round. Like many philosophers today, I don't subscribe to the sense-data project. But I do think that qualitatively characterized phenomenal experiences are real, and that their qualitative characters, such as red, are aspects or features of perceivers' experiences.

Many philosophers who object to qualia set up "natural science" as the prime arbiter of what is real. They then resist granting existence to qualitatively characterized phenomenal experience because they think that it cannot be integrated into a "naturalistic" picture of the world. This is the problem of fitting phenomenal red (say) into one's ontology. In its general form, as a problem of integrating visual consciousness with brain activity, it has been called the "first and greatest problem" (Sherrington 1951, 109, 113) and, as a general problem about conscious experience, the "hard problem" (Chalmers 1996, xii–xiii). The problem arises because of the apparent conceptual and explanatory gap between phenomenal red and a physical description of the stimulus or a physicochemical description of the relevant brain activity (neurons firing in the visual cortex).

One of the chief sources of this problem comes from thinking that, if phenomenal red is real, then we must ascribe the property of being red to some thing, according to a normal substance/property ontology. So, if phenomenal color is real, something must really be colored, or have the color property, in just the way that the surfaces of things have the property of being red according to a kind of naive realism or updated Aristotelianism. If a sense datum does not bear the property, then a brain state or some other entity must have it, or so the reasoning goes.

I find a home for qualia in experience: I construe them as intentional contents, in Brentano's original sense. Brentano originally posited the relation of intentionality to obtain between an act of perceiving and an entity that is present to consciousness (1874/1995, 88). According to Brentano, this entity exists "in" the perception, whether it exists externally to the mind or not. Thus, the fact that we can be aware of phenomenal red as a qualitative content of our experience entails that phenomenal red exists intentionally: it is "presented" to us in consciousness. Brentano held that our being aware of the phenomenal red in this way is neutral with respect to the further question of the relation between mental contents and "external" physical objects (1874/1995, 92–100). For the purposes of his "empirical psychology," he was interested only in mental phenomena as present to consciousness.

I adopt Brentano intentional entities as a phenomenological description of existent "qualia," that is, of phenomenally characterized features of experience. I, too, intend this description to be neutral about how these features are ultimately realized (say, by brain states) and I will return to the ontological status of qualia in a moment. At present, I want to recall the point from Section 4, about the lack of metaphysical transparency. As applied here, that point entails that a quale such as phenomenal red can be presented in experience without our being aware that it is a quale, or a peculiarly mental item. In being aware of phenomenal red, the theoretically uninitiated (or the holder of an alternative—and, in my view, incorrect—theory) may experience the phenomenal red simply as a property of the surface of an external object. Something that is in fact a phenomenal entity need not be experienced as being "in the mind" or as being "merely subjective"—even if it is a subject-dependent mental entity. Furthermore, such phenomenally present qualia may serve to present, or represent, the surface properties of external objects in ordinary acts of seeing such objects, and they may do so without subjects' being aware that they see external objects by means of a subjective phenomenal content. To repeat, the phenomenal content may seem to the perceiver simply to present a categorical property of an object, rather than to be a phenomenal feature in a perceptual process through which a dispositional property of an object causes us to see the object in virtue of our having phenomenal experience of a certain kind.[15]

In the view on offer here, the mind and brain are such that our experiences present us with objects in the world under some phenomenal aspect or other

---

[15] The term "intentionality" in Brentano's original sense is more specific than recent uses of that term to denote a generic representational relation. Hence, my treatment of qualia as intentional entities is opposed to so-called "intentional" or "representational" theories of phenomenal qualities as proposed by objectivist representationalists (e.g., Dretske 1995b; Tye 1995, 2000). These latter theorists use the term "intentional" simply to describe a representational relation between a state of mind and an object or object property, and they equate phenomenal content with representational content in order to do away with the dispositionalists' phenomenal qualia and with the Brentano intentionality of such qualia. I of course also use "intentional" in this more generic sense, to mean an "aboutness" or "representational" relation. (The different uses are clear from context.)

(and usually more than one at a time). Among these aspects are both shape and color. As I would develop the theory further, both shape and color present external properties under a subjective aspect: both show subjective characteristics. In the case of shape, we can observe the subjective aspect in the compression of Euclidean space with distance from the standpoint of the perceiver, as when viewing a road with parallel sides whose sides nonetheless converge phenomenally within the visual field (Chs. 5–6). These "phenomenal aspects" are characteristics of our experience, but neither our brains nor external objects possess the properties exactly as presented. That is the wonder of Brentano intentionality. In accordance with the inclusive naturalism of Chapter 10.5, I assign these phenomenal contents, or "qualia," to the domain of the natural, even in the absence of reduction.

7. On What We See

At least one line of objection remains to the view that we see the surfaces of objects by having a subject-dependent phenomenal experience that mediates our perception of the object. This view may remind some philosophers of "representative realism." In standard versions of representative realism, we are said to "see our sense data" or to "see our representations," and to infer the external world from them. But, a common objection runs, the objects that we perceive in our everyday encounters with the world are surely external objects, not subjective entities in our heads. Surely we see people, trees, and cars, not sense data or representations from which we merely infer these other objects.

The way of talking that this objection criticizes, according to which what we "really see" are sense data (or the equivalent), was Russell's mature position on perception. He (along with William James and others) came to believe that we should restrict our ontology to "momentary particulars" (Hatfield 2002). On this view, we see only momentary particulars, because what we think of as "external objects"—human bodies, trees, cars, and glasses of mango juice—are in fact constituted out of such particulars. Although the mature Russell was not a representative realist, in an early discussion of sense data he endorsed a representative realism in which we "see" our sense data or representations (Russell 1912, 11–12 and ch. 2), and this form of representative realism came to be widely discussed (e.g., Ayer 1958, chs. 2–3).

My position does not endorse neutral monism or sense data, nor does it imply that we "see our representations." I endorse a realism in which representations mediate our perception of objects, but it is a *critical realism*,[16] rather than a representative realism. According to this view, we see the properties of objects by having phenomenal representations of certain sorts. These representations, these phenomenal experiences, are not *that which* we see, but *that by which* we see. This turn of phrase is an old response to the facile criticism that perceptual mediation entails that we see our own experience and not the objects that such experience phenomenally presents to us (Hatfield 1990*b*, 54). The response avoids the implication that in perception we are not aware of objects themselves; we are aware of them via mediating phenomenal experiences. This position also allows that, in seeing objects by having phenomenal experiences, we are aware of the phenomenal experiences themselves—though, as explained earlier, pretheoretically we need not be aware of the phenomenal experiences *as* phenomenal experiences. In an attitude of theoretical reflection, we can attend to the phenomenal experiences themselves, but that does not involve turning our attention to a special inner object. It is a matter of attending to the same experience by means of which we see objects (Ch. 16).

I remain committed to the view that phenomenal qualities exist (intentionally) as mediating experiences by which we see the colors of things. There is more to say by way of explaining intentional existence. In the meantime, I hope that this chapter has removed obstacles that have hindered acceptance of what I believe to be the best position on what color in objects is: it is a disposition (or its basis) for producing subject-dependent experiences of certain kinds in perceivers, which experiences may properly be called "qualia."

---

[16] "Critical realism" (so named) was developed as an alternative to standard sense-data theories by several philosophers in the early twentieth century, including Roy Wood Sellars (1916) and the authors in Drake (1920). My own position shares much with this earlier one.

PART III

History and Philosophy of Perceptual and Cognitive Psychology

Introduction

The papers in this third part consider aspects of the history of psychology in relation to the philosophy of psychology. These chapters examine theoretical concepts in cognitive and perceptual psychology, underscore the autonomy of psychological theorizing from physiological reduction, and make a case for the methodological priority of psychology over physiology and physicalistic description.

The first two chapters establish connections across historical periods within theories of spatial vision and of attention. Chapter 12 seeks the origin, in the theories of Ibn al-Haytham (Alhazen), Descartes, and Berkeley, of two-stage theories of spatial perception, which hold that visual perception involves both an immediate representation of the proximal stimulus in a two-dimensional "sensory core" and also a subsequent perception of the three-dimensional world. The works of Ibn al-Haytham, Descartes, and Berkeley already frame the major theoretical options that guided visual theory into the twentieth century. The field of visual perception was the first area of what we now call psychology to apply mathematics, through geometrical models as used by Euclid, Ptolemy, Ibn al-Haytham, and Descartes (among others). The chapter shows that Kepler's discovery of the retinal image, which revolutionized visual anatomy and entailed fundamental changes in visual physiology, did not alter the basic structure of theories of spatial vision. (On the sensory ontologies of Ibn al-Haytham and his followers, especially their use of Aristotelian "forms," see also Hatfield 1998.) Chapter 13 examines aspects of the history of theories of attention from antiquity to the present. It introduces the notion that natural scientific psychology originated prior to the usual nineteenth-century starting dates. This chapter charts the introduction of various phenomenological descriptions and theoretical concepts into discussions of attention and compares the structure of recent theories of attention with earlier theories, again demonstrating significant theoretical and observational continuity in this area of psychological inquiry. Since this essay was originally written, new work has appeared on medieval theories of attention (e.g., Pasnau 1997, ch. 4; Leijenhorst 2007). These studies do not alter the overview provided here.

The remaining three chapters use historical analysis to draw implications for contemporary philosophy and psychology. Chapter 14 examines the origins of psychology as a natural science and its various relations to philosophy, cognitive science, and neuroscience. More particularly, it critically examines the views that psychology first came into existence as a discipline around 1879, that philosophy and psychology were estranged in the ensuing decades, that psychology finally became scientific through the influence of logical empiricism, and that psychology should now disappear as a distinct discipline, in favor of cognitive science and neuroscience. It argues that psychology had a natural philosophical phase (from antiquity) that waxed in the seventeenth and eighteenth centuries. While the later nineteenth century saw new methods of experimentation and a surging number of experiments, systematic observation and experimental reports were extant from the eighteenth century (and quantitative models of vision, from antiquity). Natural philosophical psychology transformed into modern experimental psychology c.1900. From about that time, especially in North America, psychology separated institutionally from philosophy. But, contrary to many accounts, philosophers and psychologists collaboratively discussed the subject matter and methods of psychology throughout the first four decades of the twentieth century. Often, the main interaction with philosophy during this period is reckoned as an influence of the logical empiricism of the Vienna Circle on neobehaviorism. In fact, the leading neobehaviorists, Tolman, Hull, and Skinner, rejected logical empiricism as too restrictive methodologically. This chapter also considers the commonplace notion that all perceptual and cognitive psychology of a phenomenal or mentalistic bent was excised during this period, only to be revived through the combined influence of a reformed linguistics and the new field of artificial intelligence, with its attendant computer analogy for psychological processes. In fact, phenomenally oriented perceptual studies, and theories that posited internal cognitive states, continued in psychology through the middle decades of the twentieth century, despite the prominence of behaviorism in both psychology and philosophy. Subsequently, although some psychologists adopted the language-of-thought approach of traditional cognitive science, many did not. The chapter concludes that psychology should not and will not be subsumed by cognitive science and neuroscience.

Chapter 15 considers more closely the relations between psychology and neuroscience. There is a strong philosophical intuition that direct study of the brain can and will constrain the development of psychological theory.

When this intuition is tested against case studies from the psychology of perception and memory, it turns out that psychology has led the way toward knowledge of neurophysiology. The chapter presents an abstract argument to show that psychology can and must lead the way in neuroscientific study of mental function. The opposing intuition is based on mainly weak arguments about the fundamentality or objectivity of physics or physiology in relation to psychology. The chapter argues that psychological phenomena are methodologically prior to neurophysiological concepts and descriptions, that psychology provides the functional descriptions that guide the behavioral brain sciences, that psychological concepts are not reducible, but that neurophysiological data and concepts are nonetheless evidentially and explanatorily relevant for psychology.

Finally, Chapter 16 surveys the role of introspective evidence as conceived in previous philosophy and psychology, including the views of Descartes, Hume, Kant, Wundt, James, and the Gestalt psychologists. It distinguishes successful from unsuccessful applications of introspection and contends that introspective evidence is legitimately used in perceptual psychology today. The chapter considers various metaphysical and epistemological arguments against the legitimacy of introspectively available phenomenal content, including the "transparency" arguments of Harman (1990) and Dretske (1995b). It argues that descriptions of phenomenal experience, such as are the basis for ascribing imagistic content to perception, are scientifically legitimate.

Collectively, these chapters exhibit the role that history can play in critically considering contemporary positions in the philosophy of psychology. Oftentimes, contemporary theorists partially define their positions in relation to historical landmarks. Frequently, such theorists seek a comparative advantage over "standard" positions from the past. In Chapter 16, the foes of introspection misdescribe its use in previous psychology, often taking the most discredited form of introspection, the "analytical introspection" practiced by some early experimental psychologists, as a kind of straw effigy that is easily pummeled. Chapter 15 finds that a prominent claim that neuroscience injected radically new ideas into the psychology of memory rests on mistaken history. In Chapter 14, those who argue for an imperialistic annexing of psychology by neuroscience use potted history to support their notion that psychology was rescued from behaviorism by the nascent stirrings of orthodox (language-of-thought) cognitive science.

The influence of historical considerations in shaping contemporary theorizing can be seen in Mohan Matthen's recent book (2005). The book admirably engages historical and contemporary work on perception in arguing for its own propositionalist, non-imagistic conception of perception. In arguing against imagistic perceptual content, it equates imagistic visual experience with a two-dimensional sensory core (Matthen 2005, 2–3, ch. 2). As Chapter 12 relates, the notion of a sensory core was prominent in visual theory from the seventeenth into the nineteenth century, as an initial phenomenal representation that subsequently yields three-dimensional experience. But from the latter nineteenth century, it was displaced by phenomenally based descriptions of visual experience as immediately presenting a three-dimensional visual world. Hering, James, and the Gestalt psychologists Köhler and Koffka criticized the earlier view in seeking to replace it. Some recent theorists, including the neo-Helmholtzian Rock (1975, 1983), retain a commitment to a two-dimensional sensory core. In fact, Helmholtz himself had rejected the notion (Hatfield 1990b, 177), as did prominent theorists of the twentieth century, including Gibson (1950) and Marr (1982, with his 2½-D sketch). If the preponderance of major theorists—including Helmholtz, Hering, the Gestaltists, Gibson, and Marr—sets the theoretical standard in vision science, then those parts of Matthen's book that seek to refute the notion of imagistic or pictorial visual content by undermining the notion of a two-dimensional sensory core are more than a century behind the times.

Matthen's equation of two-dimensional sensations with the imagistic content of perception invites further reflection on the history of the distinction between sensation and perception. As discussed in Chapter 4.2.1, earlier theorists treated *sensations* either as two-dimensional images, or as aspatial elements varying only in quality and intensity (color sensations that have a determinate degree of brightness), which were distinguished from *perceptions* of a three-dimensional visual world. This distinction assumed that sensations are the immediate product of neural activity, whereas perceptions arise through psychological activity. Because of the work of Hering, James, the Gestalt psychologists, and Gibson, the notion that vision starts from aspatial or two-dimensional sensations (perhaps internally localized) had been rejected by the latter twentieth century. Consequently, few theorists (save Rock) distinguished two-dimensional, subjective sensations from three-dimensional, world-presenting perceptions. Rather, recent theories tend to posit a threefold division: (1) registered information (whether retinal or regarding muscle activity), which is nonconscious; (2) world-presenting sense perceptual experience, which in vision is imagistic experience of a world in depth possessed of relatively stable characteristics such as size, shape, and color, which experience is usually regarded (by all save Gibson) as the product of psychological operations (cognitive or noncognitive, depending on the theory); and (3) cognitive perceptual achievements, such as the recognition, classification, and identification of objects, achievements that are phenomenologically available within our visual experience. The old sensation–perception distinction has been replaced by this finer division. The question of the extent to which item (2) is to be regarded as containing subject-dependent (i.e., subjective) elements depends on the theorist's particular bent (as discussed in Chs. 5–6, 8–11). No theorists regard sense perception as phenomenally located within the subject's head; the objects of sense perception are located distally, in the world.

The chapters arose on various occasions. Chapter 12, a collaborative effort with William Epstein, stemmed from our mutual interest in finding the historical source for the notion of a two-dimensional sensory core. Originally, we had expected to trace the notion back to the nineteenth or perhaps into the eighteenth century. We were surprised to find that, in order to discover its origins, we had to consider the transition from medieval to early modern visual theories. I have appended a postscript with a new diagram of Ibn al-Haytham's optical physiology. Chapter 13 was an invited presentation at the Vancouver Cognition Conference on attention in 1995; it circulated in manuscript form and as a videotape of the presentation. Chapter 13 was the fifth in a series of Millennial pieces that were commissioned by *Mind & Language*; authors were invited to offer personal views on issues that they deemed to be "important in the present context of cognitive studies." Chapter 14 grew out of a previous paper (Hatfield 1999) that was presented at the biennial meeting of the International Society for the History, Philosophy, and Social Study of Biology in 1997 in Seattle. The ideas were subsequently discussed, usually under a variant of the title "What Can the Mind Tell Us about the Brain?," at Philosophy colloquia at Penn, Western Ontario, and Rutgers in 1998–9, at the 1998 meetings of the Cognitive Science Society in Madison, Wisconsin, and of the Philosophy of Science Association in Kansas City (a version was published in the PSA proceedings), and at the Center for Moral and Mental Philosophy, Federal University of Rio de Janeiro in 1999. A more recent version, which in part provided the basis for the revised essay published herein, was given at the Minnesota Center for Philosophy of Science in 2005. Finally, Chapter 16 was invited for submission to a volume on evidence deriving from a conference at Johns Hopkins University, held in 2003.

12

The Sensory Core
and the Medieval Foundations
of Early Modern Perceptual
Theory

In the eighteenth and nineteenth centuries the majority of theories of visual perception were built upon the view that during the process of vision there occur two conscious states with quite different phenomenal properties. The first state is a mental representation of the two-dimensional retinal image. The second is our experience of the "visual world" of objects distributed in depth. According to the then commonly accepted theory, the mental correlate of the retinal image is the truly immediate component of perception, and it provides the raw material from which the mind generates the three-dimensional visual world. Yet this retinal correlate—the "sensory core"[1] of the perceptual process—typically goes unnoticed, and the percipient takes his experience of the three-dimensional visual world to be direct and unmediated.[2] Although it

Co-authored with William Epstein. First published in *Isis* 70 (1979), 363–84, copyright © 1979 by the History of Science Society. Reprinted with permission.

[1] We have chosen to use the term "sensory core" to refer to a conscious state with the phenomenal properties of the retinal image, without arousing unwanted connotations about its psychological status (as, say, a form of experience produced by a special attitude) and without implying anything further about its epistemological status (as, say, an incorrigible "given"). Our "sensory core" shares the phenomenal properties of James Gibson's "visual field" (1950, ch. 3). Our usage of the term "sensory core" is parallel to E. G. Boring's "core" of perception (1965, 69–70), a term which he derived from E. B. Titchener. Our usage does not correspond to Roderick Firth's (1965, 216–19), but our "sensory core" shares the phenomenal properties of the "sense-data" he attributes to Locke and Berkeley (215–16).

[2] The 18th-c. philosopher Thomas Reid summed up this position well in his discussion of "visible appearances" (his name for the sensory core). After remarking that these appearances "are never made

may seem odd that an unnoticed state of consciousness should be viewed as the psychologically fundamental component of the visual process, that which we have labeled the "sensory core" has played a prominent role in visual theory since Berkeley drew his celebrated distinction between the immediate and mediate objects of vision. This paper will explore the theoretical context within which the notion of a sensory core developed.

Historically, the motivation for assigning the sensory core a content distinct from the visual world has come from geometrical optics. Unless it were believed that the spatial properties of objects as represented in the sense organ (say, by the retinal image) are different from the spatial properties of objects themselves, there would be no reason to question that perception of the visual world is simply a matter of directly apprehending the optical stimulation available at the retina. Consider the perception of a circle oblique to the line of sight. The circle projects an ellipse on the retina, yet a slanted circle is manifest in the visual world; the sensory core, in representing the retinal projection, thereby differs from the phenomenally direct apprehension of the circle. The postulation, on optical grounds, of a difference between the spatial attributes of objects themselves and the representation of those attributes in the stimulus pattern is logically anterior to the concept of sensory core, for without the supposition of such a difference, mere reception of the stimulus (which would now be assumed to share the spatial attributes of the seen object) could be viewed as adequate for perception of the spatially elaborated visual world. However, adherence to this optical distinction (between an object and its retinal projection) is not *sufficient* motivation for the postulation of two phenomenally distinct conscious states (the sensory core and the visual world). For one thing, it might be maintained that the phenomenal character of everyday experience in fact corresponds to the spatial features of the retinal projection; this would amount to denial, on phenomenal grounds, that there is a visual world distinct from the sensory core. Or some other kind of two-stage theory might be maintained, for instance, that the stimulus representation (the retinal projection) never enters consciousness, but, say, is processed into the visual world through physiological

the object of reflection, though almost every moment presented to the mind," he explained that "the mind has acquired a confirmed and inveterate habit of inattention to them; for they no sooner appear, than quick as lightning the thing signified [a solid object] succeeds, and engrosses all our regard. They have no name in language; and, although we are conscious of them when they pass through the mind, yet their passage is so quick and so familiar, that it is absolutely unheeded; nor do they leave any footsteps of themselves, either in the memory or imagination" (1785, ch. 6, sec. 3; in Reid 1863, 1:135). Reid's views were not anomalous; Pastore (1971), esp. chs. 1–10, has shown that the concept of a mental representation of the retinal image was a central theme in 18th- and 19th-c. perceptual theory.

mechanisms.[3] Indeed, a survey of the history of the psychology of vision would reveal that theories of vision in which a sensory core is postulated are but one species of two-stage theories of vision, and that an initial stage in which spatial properties of objects are represented as they are projected upon the retina may be postulated without it being supposed that this initial stage is consciously accessible. In any event, it can be seen that a second precondition of the distinction between the sensory core and visual world is the conjunction of the following two beliefs: (1) that a projective representation enters consciousness, and (2) that nevertheless we typically do apprehend (in a phenomenally direct manner) the objective spatial properties of objects.[4]

Our paper will focus upon medieval and seventeenth-century theories of vision, culminating in the work of Berkeley. Thus, even though the concept of sensory core derives its historical significance from its widespread employment during the eighteenth and nineteenth centuries, the historical situation has dictated that we focus upon an earlier period, since the concept whose development we wish to understand has its foundations in an optical tradition stretching back to Greek antiquity and including both Arabic and medieval Latin components. Our investigations have led us to believe that the development of this concept resulted from alteration within, rather than the radical overthrow of, the psychology of vision as it had come to be conceived in this optical tradition. If our interpretation is correct, it was not a change in the theory of the psychology of vision that engendered the idea of a sensory core, but rather the introduction of the theory into a new metaphysical context.

1. Ancient and Medieval Optics and Theory of Spatial Vision

The discovery that the three-dimensional attributes of objects are not represented in the sense organ in a direct or simple manner was not trivial. In several types of ancient visual theory, no difference was postulated between the spatial properties of objects and those of the optical stimulus, because it was believed that the stimulus to vision shares the attributes of the seen

---

[3] These "physiological mechanisms" are to be understood as noncognitive; another possibility, one that we shall invoke below, is that the projective pattern is represented and processed cognitively, but that these cognitive operations are not even in principle available to consciousness.

[4] The importance of these two notions in 18th- and 19th-c. visual theory is evident from Pastore (1971), 11–13 and 178–81.

object. According to the extramissionist position, vision proceeds from the eye to the object, and the properties of the object are known by direct contact. Galen and some of the Stoics shared the view that something is extramitted from the eye into the air, transforming the air into an instrument of sensation (standing in relation to the eye as a nerve to the brain) and thereby allowing for direct apprehension of the object's spatial properties. For intromissionist theories, something proceeds from object to eye and represents the object to the sensitive soul. The *eidolon* of the ancient atomists, a film of atoms emitted from the surface of the object, was conceived to convey a three-dimensional representation of that surface directly to the sense organ and through the optic nerve to the soul.[5] According to the theories considered so far, whether the eye reaches out to the object itself, or something comes to the eye and stands for the object, the spatial attributes of the thing that is sensed are identical to those of the object.[6]

The ancient writers just considered were concerned either with explaining the physical process of perception (perhaps in the service of epistemology) or with providing a description of the optical process for medical purposes. There was a third tradition in antiquity, in which geometry was employed in the analysis of vision (Lindberg 1976, 1). This tradition, whose most prominent members were Euclid and Ptolemy, provided a geometrical analysis of the field of vision in terms of a visual pyramid formed by rays extramitted from the eye to points on seen objects. According to this analysis, information about the viewer-relative situation of objects with respect to the horizontal and vertical dimensions is provided by the ordering of the rays within the visual pyramid to the right or left of one another and above or below one another. Information about distance is provided by the length of each ray from the eye to the object. In other words, to each of the three dimensions of Euclidean space corresponds a dimension of the visual pyramid.[7] It follows that if a percipient is to receive determinate information concerning the spatial features of a seen object, all three of the dimensions of the visual pyramid must be

---

[5] For a summary of the theories mentioned in this paragraph, as well as other ancient theories, see Lindberg (1976), 2–11, and the references mentioned there.

[6] The idea that the eye receives three-dimensional copies of objects has its attractions, and as late as 1823, Lehot put forth the theory that "the points of the luminous cones which penetrate the eye form, in the vitreous humor, at a certain distance from the retina, images in three dimensions, and vision is effected by the perception of these images," the vitreous humor being the sensitive portion of the eye (1823, 42–3). Conversely, the idea that a mere image might be sufficient for the apprehension of the three-dimensional world has obvious difficulties, and in antiquity the equivocality of images for size and distance was used as an argument against the view that the proper object of vision is an image: Theophrastus (1917), 97–9 (the image in question was the pupillary image).

[7] Ptolemy (1956), 25 (bk. 2, sec. 26); Euclid (1959), 1–2. Euclid does not consider the lengths of the visual rays, but only their ordering within the visual pyramid. See Lejeune (1948), 89–95.

apprehended. Thus the objective size of an object is inadequately represented by visual angle; distance, the third dimension in the visual pyramid, must also be taken into account (Ptolemy 1956, 45–6; Lejeune 1948, 95–101). A similar point may be made about shape. The relative order within the visual pyramid of those rays that meet the edges of the object does not bear determinate information about the object's shape; information about the lengths of these rays is also required (Ptolemy 1956, 46–50; Lejeune 1948, 103–7). Here then is the sort of optical distinction between elements in the optical pattern (visual angle, projective shape) and properties of objects themselves (size, shape) that is logically prerequisite to the idea of the sensory core.

The observation that information about the lengths of the rays is required for the discrimination of size and shape is not present in Euclid's *Optics*. It is, however, present in Ptolemy, who went beyond the geometry of the relationship between eye and object to concern himself with the actual processes—physical, physiological, and psychological—that occur during vision.[8] Following Aristotle and others, Ptolemy held that light and color are the proper objects of vision and that the mediate objects of vision—size, shape, location, motion, and rest—are discriminated through the differentiation of light and color.[9] Yet, as we have seen, mere differentiation within the ordering of the rays forming the visual pyramid would not be sufficient for the apprehension of size and shape (and the same holds for location and motion). Ptolemy was not only aware of this geometrical fact, but he also realized that despite the inadequacy of, say, visual angle for size, observers typically do apprehend objective size (1956, 38–46). Hence he recognized not only an *optical* distinction between objective size and visual angle, but also a *psychological* distinction between the discrimination of visual angle and the visual apprehension of size. Moreover, he gave a psychological explanation (albeit a very sketchy one) of the process by which distance and visual angle are conjoined in size perception. Lejeune has characterized Ptolemy's view as follows: "The information furnished by visual angle is not accepted in its 'raw' form. Long practice has accustomed us to make an appropriate estimate of the effects of the distance and obliquity of an object upon its apparent size, and we manage to restore the true size of the object" (Lejeune 1948, 96–7).

---

[8] As far as can be determined, Euclid intended his work to present geometrical optics in a way that would be of use to scenographers. Lejeune says that the *Optics* of Euclid is "no more than a treatise on perspective. It systematically ignores every physical or psychological aspect of the problem of vision" (1948, 172, see also 93–5); e.g., as far as vision was concerned, Euclid identified size with visual angle (1959, 2–7, props. 2–8). Lejeune (1948, 172–7) stresses Ptolemy's concern for the physiological and the psychological as a way in which optics had progressed since Euclid.

[9] Aristotle (1984a), 418ª9–30; Ptolemy (1956), 13–16 (2.6–11).

One might wonder what led Ptolemy to characterize the psychological processes involved here as an estimation (*existimare*), and whether the observer is conscious, or at least potentially conscious, of the elements (distance and visual angle) upon which the corrective estimations operate. Lejeune has concluded that Ptolemy "did not consider this operation as a judgment fully conscious and distinct from sensation itself" (1948, 99), a turn of phrase that brings to mind the unnoticed judgmental processes described by latter-day theorists. It would, however, be hasty to identify Ptolemy's theory with more recent theory in all its essentials.

Between the time of Ptolemy and the seventeenth century, the most significant contribution to visual theory was that of the Islamic natural philosopher Alhazen (*c*.965–1039). He made the intromissionist theory viable by applying ray geometry to the problem of how the eye receives a spatially coherent impression despite the fact that each part of the eye is bombarded by entities transmitted from every part of the visual field. In addition, Alhazen integrated his theory of geometrical and physiological optics into a detailed account of the physiology and psychology of vision, including a thorough treatment of spatial vision.[10] Each of these achievements is germane to our inquiry.

Alhazen's establishment of a geometrical basis for the intromission theory depended on his argument that the arrangement of points in the field of vision is reproduced in the physiological process generated at the crystalline humor (which he, in the tradition of Galen and Ptolemy, considered to be the seat of vision) by incoming radiation. Essentially he adapted the visual pyramid of Euclid and Ptolemy to the intromissionist position. For Alhazen, the pyramid consists of those rays that fall at right angles to the surface of the crystalline humor.[11] As in the theory of Euclid and Ptolemy, the pyramid has its base on the objects in the field of view and its vertex in the eye; in contrast to the previous theory, the direction of the rays is from object to eye. A cross-section of the pyramid is physiologically received by the crystalline humor through an act characterized as a "sensing." Of the luminous rays received at the surface of the crystalline, only the luminosity and color of each ray—and not the arrangement of the rays or the spatial information conveyed by that arrangement—is sensed by the

---

[10] For an evaluation of Alhazen's role in the development of optical theory, see Lindberg (1976), ch. 4. On the physiological and psychological aspects of Alhazen's theory, see Sabra (1978). In constructing our summary of Alhazen's views we have used these authors as a guide to Alhazen (1572), 8–12, 24–57.

[11] The perpendicular is selected from the sheath of rays converging on a single point of the crystalline by a *weakening* of all but the unrefracted (perpendicular) rays, or by a *special receptivity* of the crystalline to perpendicular rays (Lindberg 1976, 75–8; Sabra 1978, 165–6). [See Postscript, Fig. 12.3.]

eye itself.[12] This act of sensing occurs through an alteration produced by each luminous ray in the "visual spirit" present in the crystalline humor, whereby the visual spirit takes on the *form* of light and color.[13] The alteration suffered by each punctiform area is transmitted, by a "quasi-optical" process involving refraction and rectilinear transmission, from the crystalline humor through the vitreous humor and down the optical medium residing in each of the optic nerves (which were believed to be hollow and filled with visual spirit).[14] This process is described as the transmission of a coherent "form"—bearing point-for-point correspondence to the objects in the field of vision—from the surface of the crystalline through the eye and optic nerve. In the optic chiasma the separate transmissions from each eye join to form a single impression, and this unified punctiform representation of the field of vision is received by the *ultimum sentiens*, the faculty of sense that completes the act of vision.[15]

The *ultimum sentiens* avails itself of the spatial information present in the cross-section of the visual pyramid in order to apprehend the objects of vision other than light and color (Alhazen listed twenty such objects in all, including spatial properties such as size, shape, solidity, and motion).[16] However, as the geometry dictates, the arrangement of points within the cross-section provides direct information about only two dimensions: the third dimension, depth or distance, is lacking.[17] In fact, Alhazen embraced the intromissionist counterpart

[12] Alhazen (1572), 26–7 (bk. 2, sec. 6). See Bauer (1911), 29–32, and Sabra (1978), 173–4. Alhazen thus adopted the traditional view that light and color are the proper objects of vision (1572, 35, bk. 2, secs. 17–18).

[13] Alhazen adopts an Aristotelian view of the reception process; Aristotle had maintained that the sense organ accepts the *form* (in this case color) of the sensible thing without the matter, thereby taking on the properties of the sensible thing (see Lindberg 1976, 8–9 and 78–9). Incidentally, the term "visual spirit" refers to a substance that serves as the soul's agent in the eye; it is not a "spiritual" (ghostlike) substance (Alhazen attributes density to it), but neither is it the inert matter of Descartes' "animal spirits," since it is endowed with sentience.

[14] The transmission within each eye proceeds rectilinearly, with one refraction at the posterior edge of the crystalline; this refraction, which is toward the normal (and hence away from the optic axis), serves both to keep the rays from crossing (which would produce an inverted ordering) and to direct the rays toward the opening of the optic nerve (which was thought to be centered at the rear of the eye, along the axis of vision). Because of the special efficacy of the visual spirit, within the optic nerve the transmitted entity follows the path of the nerve without its ordering being affected. Lindberg (1976), 69–85, provides a thorough treatment of the physiology of this process; see also Sabra (1978), 166–8. Fig. 12.1 (below) illustrates the path of transmission according to a follower of Alhazen. [See also Postscript, Fig. 12.3.]

[15] Alhazen (1572), 24–7 (2.1–6). The reception of the forms of light and color by the opaque body of the *ultimum sentiens* in the optic chiasma occurs by an "illumination" and "coloring" of this body (1572, 27, 2.6).

[16] Alhazen (1572), 34 (2.15). Additional objects of vision, or *intentiones visibiles*, include number, similarity, and beauty.

[17] Ibid., 39 (2.24): "Remotio rei visae non comprehenditur per se." Especially telling is Alhazen's treatment of the perception of solidity (or corporeity), in which he says that vision immediately

of Ptolemy's geometrical observation that elements of the visual pyramid such as projective shape are indeterminate for objective properties such as shape. He was aware that a circle oblique to the line of sight would produce an elliptical pattern at the surface of the crystalline, and that visual angle does not specify the objective size of an object (distance, too, must be taken into account). Furthermore, and of greater interest for our story, Alhazen saw that an account was needed of the phenomenal fact that we typically apprehend circles as circles, even though they are oblique to the line of sight, and that we typically are able to discriminate the sizes of objects, even though this discrimination requires taking distance into account.[18] His viewpoint thus included the two notions which historically have been associated with the concept of sensory core, that spatial properties as received at the eye (e.g., an ellipse) differ from objective properties (e.g., a rotated circle), and that we nonetheless apprehend the latter. In essence, we may say that Alhazen realized that a mere understanding of the geometry of visual stimulation is not sufficient to explain the perceptual achievements of the human percipient: psychological processes must also be invoked. While this realization was also implicit in Ptolemy, Alhazen went further in developing an account of these psychological processes.

Since, on Alhazen's account, only a two-dimensional arrangement of luminous points is represented in the cross-section of the pyramid transmitted to the *ultimum sentiens*, the apprehension of objects in three dimensions must involve more than the mere passive reception of the stimulation carried by the optic nerves. The activity by which the *ultimum sentiens* goes beyond the stimulation it receives consists of "reasoning" and "distinguishing" (*rationem* and *distinctionem*); these judgmental activities are performed by the *virtus distinctiva*.[19] Alhazen offered an extended treatment of the psychology of visual judgments, but it will suffice here to observe that in cases where the judgments are performed over and over again, the faculty of judgment need not go through the entire process of judging (by "iteration of arguments") each time it is confronted with a particular set of sensory data; rather it comes to perform these judgments through recognition (*cognitionem*) of significant features, or signs (*signa*), that lead it to assign a particular set of properties to the objects

---

apprehends the longitude and latitude of bodies opposite the eye, but not the third dimension: "visus ... comprehendet statim extensionem illius corporis secundum longitudinem & latitudinem, & non remanet nisi dimensio tertia" (ibid., 47, 2.31). See also Bauer (1911), 55–6.

[18] Alhazen clearly states that any pair of diameters on a circle are seen as equal even when the circle is oblique to the line of sight (1572, 51, 2.36). With respect to size, he says "virtus distinctiva distinguet quantitatem rei visae, non considerabit angulum tantum, sed considerabit angulum & remotionem simul" (ibid., 51, 2.38; on the *virtus distinctiva*, see below).

[19] Ibid., 30–1 (2.10).

seen. Judgment by recognition takes place so quickly that we do not perceive that we judge.[20] It is in this way that distance, size, and shape are perceived. Distance is apprehended through a judgment of the number of regular-sized intervals composing the continuous ground space between the observer and the distal object, or, since the process occurs frequently, through a judgment by recognition.[21] From the distance to an object together with visual angle, the size of the object can be apprehended, again through judgment by recognition.[22] Similarly, apprehension of the distance to various points in the field of vision can be used to apprehend the solidity and shape of seen objects.[23] Thus, in general, according to Alhazen the visual apprehension of the spatial properties of the visual world is made possible by an unnoticed process of judgment.

The essentials of Alhazen's theory of vision are, in fundamental ways, parallel to those of the standard theory of the eighteenth and nineteenth centuries. First, pertaining to the effective stimulus for vision: while the two-dimensional array of light and color transmitted to the *ultimum sentiens* is not an optical image (such as the real image formed by a lens or the virtual image of mirror vision), the geometrical qualities it shares with the retinal image are striking (e.g., point-for-point correspondence with luminous points in the field of vision and ambivalence with respect to actual size). One might choose to characterize the physiology of vision according to Alhazen as the transmission of an "image" or "picture" of the objects in the field of vision through the optic nerve to the brain. Such a characterization would serve to emphasize that the immediate object of vision according to Alhazen shares the essential properties of what was taken to be the immediate object of vision by Kepler: an arrangement of points of light and color reproducing the two-dimensional arrangement of points in the field of vision.[24]

But it is with respect to his thoughts about the psychological processes that occur during spatial vision that Alhazen's theory exhibits the most striking

---

[20] Sabra (1978), 171–9, gives a thorough account of Alhazen's statements on perceptual judgment in general (Alhazen 1572, 30–2, 2.10–12), but does not deal with particular cases such as distance, size, or shape. Our discussion of these cases is of course not exhaustive, and a thorough treatment of Alhazen's psychology of vision is much needed.

[21] Alhazen's discussion of the apprehension of distance is long and complex (involving a distinction between the apprehension of mere outness as opposed to location, ibid., 38–9, 2.23–4); we have focused upon the apprehension of the amount of distance for moderate distances, in which case distance is apprehended "per cognitionem" (ibid., 39–42, 53–6; 2.25, 39–40).

[22] Ibid., 51–3 (2.38).   [23] Ibid., 47–8, 50–1 (2.31, 36).

[24] Lindberg (1976, 86) has especially emphasized the degree to which Kepler's optical work remained within an intellectual framework provided by Alhazen. Incidentally, a second feature of standard post-Keplerian theory is found in Alhazen: the independent transmission of points of stimulation from the receptive surface of the eye into the brain, which is a key feature of the so-called "constancy hypothesis" (on the importance of this hypothesis in the history of perceptual theory, see Pastore 1971, 11–12 and *passim*).

resemblance to later theory: distance is not immediately perceived (i.e., is not perceived by sense alone) but is apprehended by means of a judgmental act; size is apprehended by means of a judgment that takes distance into account; a circle oblique to the line of sight is perceived to be a circle through a judgment concerning the distance to various parts of the circle. And so it is not surprising that Bauer, in his 1911 study of Alhazen's psychology, remarked that in the field of spatial perception Alhazen "touched upon a series of the most important psychological problems, and his explanations anticipate in a surprising manner thoughts that were again taken up only in the most recent development of psychology" (1911, 54). Bauer drew particular attention to what he characterized as Alhazen's theory of "unconscious inference" (1911, 56–7), a term that immediately calls to mind Helmholtz's nineteenth-century version of the psychology of unnoticed judgments. Is it true then that all of the central elements of later psychology of vision were present in Alhazen (or perhaps even Ptolemy)?

The one element not clearly present is the sensory core, where the referent of this term is taken to be a consciously accessible representation of the field of vision in two dimensions. The difficulty in deciding whether Alhazen (or Ptolemy)[25] employed the concept of sensory core lies deeper than a simple failure of these authors to state clearly an opinion on the matter. To ask whether sensory stimulation is, at a particular point in the process of vision that begins with the reception of light at the eye and ends with an experience of the visual world, experienceable or not, is to ask a question that makes sense only within certain intellectual frameworks. Among many authors in the seventeenth and eighteenth centuries, to ask this question would have been to ask whether something was an *idea*, since ideas were the only legitimate objects of awareness. It is not clear what the medieval equivalent to this question would have been. This lack of clarity probably results from the fact that in the psychology of the Middle Ages (at least as manifested in the optical tradition) there was no clear distinction between the physiological and the mental. As Bauer (1911, 11) has remarked, for Alhazen and other Arabic as well as Latin authors (who were following Aristotle in this regard), the mental was not limited to the conscious. Thus, if we ask whether the "sensing" of light and color by the eye and the "judging" of the pattern of stimulation by the *virtus distinctiva* are physiological or mental events (where these terms are restricted to something close to their modern significations), the answer comes out as a confused "both," or perhaps "neither." They are like mental events insofar as they are described in the mentalistic language of sensing and

---

[25] See Lejeune (1948, 99) for the ambiguities in Ptolemy on this point.

judging.[26] Yet they are like physiological events in that they take place at early or middle stages in the chain of physiopsychological processes that proceed from the eye toward the central cavities of the brain. The intuition that events characterized as mental (described in mentalistic language) should be accessible to consciousness is not fulfilled. One is led to believe that the attempt to apply the modern categories "physiological" and "mental" to medieval visual theory is misguided.

In sum, the explanation of spatial vision provided by Alhazen (and, to a lesser extent, Ptolemy) contained the central features of the standard eighteenth- and nineteenth-century explanation. Included in Alhazen's theory was an optical distinction between objective spatial properties and spatial properties as received at the sense organ, as well as a physiopsychological distinction between spatial properties as represented in the sensory processes transmitted from the eye to the brain and spatial properties as apprehended in experience. If, despite the parallels between his explanation of vision and that of later thinkers, Alhazen did not employ the concept of sensory core, the reason is to be found in his conception of mind, rather than in factors internal to his theory of vision.

2. Visual Theory after Alhazen

Alhazen's major work on vision was available in translation to the Latin West by the early thirteenth century; his theory and its derivatives dominated optical science until the time of Kepler. A rapid survey of the relevant texts has suggested that with respect to the psychology of vision, Alhazen's chief followers in the West—Bacon, Pecham, and Witelo—were in fundamental agreement with the master: "no visible intention except light and color is perceived by sense alone";[27] distance from the observer to the visual object "is not perceived by sight, but is determined by reasoning";[28] indeed, all of the objects of vision except light and color "are apprehended not by sense alone but by the cooperation of argumentation and the discriminative faculty,

[26] Alhazen remarks that the rational processes by which the act of vision is completed are of the same type as other rational processes, but that we are able to ascertain this only through a second reasoning process, which is a reasoning about the reasoning that occurs during vision (1572, 32–3, 2.13). But Alhazen's view that the rational processes in vision are properly cognitive processes is, of course, not evidence that he believed the premises of those operations (the transmitted "form") were ever phenomenally accessible.

[27] Pecham (1970), 139 (pt. 1, prop. 61).

[28] Ibid., 141 (1.63); also Bacon (1962), 523 (pt. 5.2, dist. 3, ch. 3), and Witelo (1572), 121 (bk. 4, sec.9).

intermingled almost imperceptibly."[29] As is illustrated by Figure 12.1, taken from Witelo but representative of Pecham and Bacon (and Alhazen as well), there was similar agreement on matters of ray geometry and the physiological process of transmission: vision takes place by a pyramid of rays reaching the eye (those rays received perpendicularly at the surface of the crystalline, which are represented in the diagram by the lines proceeding from *gbc*, the visual object, to each eye); a cross-section of this pyramid, the points of which stand

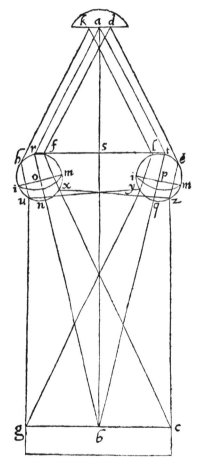

Figure 12.1. The visual system according to Witelo. The visual object is represented by *gbc*; the optic nerves are represented schematically by *hrf–kad* and *lte–kad*, and *kad* is the *ultimum sentiens*. From Witelo (1572), 103.

[29] Pecham (1970), 137 (1.56); also Bacon (1962), 497–500 (pt. 5.1, dist. 10, ch. 3), and Witelo (1572), 111–13 (3.60, 63).

in a one-to-one correspondence to points in the field of vision, is directed into the optic nerve by refraction of the rays traveling through the eye; and the impressions received by the two eyes are reduced to unity by being brought together in the nervous system (at *kad*).[30]

Remarkable as it may seem, there was nearly complete agreement on the principles underlying Alhazen's theory of vision among post-Keplerian visual theorists, including Kepler himself. Of special interest to us is the continuation of Alhazen's treatment of the psychology of vision, which we will examine presently. But the principles of Alhazen's optical analysis were also continued. This is not to say that Kepler and his followers believed the crystalline humor to be the seat of vision—all of the writers we will discuss accepted Kepler's view that vision takes place by means of the retinal image. It is rather that in terms of the analysis of the effective stimulus for vision, it makes little difference if the seat of one-to-one correspondence is moved from the crystalline humor to the retina. Assuredly, the retinal image is inverted and is a true optical image, but these facts do not change the principle of one-to-one correspondence. Viewed in terms of the overall process of vision, the Keplerian lens system simply functions to establish a one-to-one correspondence in a fashion different from Alhazen's selective reception of rays perpendicular to the crystalline.[31] Moreover, the essential features of Euclid's and Ptolemy's geometrical analysis of the field of vision were applicable in post-Keplerian dioptrics. Particularly, the relationship between objective size and shape and optically received size and shape remained the same: the static retinal projection is indeterminate for the objective properties.

The discovery of the retinal image did necessitate a change in the conception of the physiological transmission of stimulation from the eye to the brain. The notion that the stimulus to vision is an image formed across the posterior hemisphere of the eyeball is incompatible with the "quasi-optical" transmission of a cross-section of the visual pyramid directly into and through the optic nerve. Yet, as we shall see, the arrangements proposed by Kepler and his

---

[30] Bacon (1962), 449–53, 456–8 (pt. 5.1, dist. 5, and dist. 6, ch. 2); Pecham (1970), 117–23 (1.32–8); Witelo (1572), 92–4, 102–3 (3.17–20, 37). The diagram is from Witelo, ibid., 103, where it is introduced in a discussion of binocular single vision. It is clear from the text on p. 102 that lines *gu* and *cx* should be directed toward the center of the eye *o*, and *gy* and *cz* should be directed toward the center of the eye *p*, in which case the lines would be received perpendicular to the surfaces *unx* and *yqz*. This inaccuracy also occurs in a 14th-c. manuscript version of the drawing, reproduced in Crombie (1967), fig. 10.

[31] Kepler and later writers explicitly treated the lens system as a means of establishing a one-to-one correspondence between points in the field of vision and points on the surface of the retina: Kepler (1939), 153–6; trans. in Kepler (1964), 1:150–7; Descartes, *Dioptrique*, in Descartes (1969–75) (this edition of Descartes' works is hereafter cited as AT), 6:109; trans. in Descartes (1965), 91–5.

successors to effect this transmission did not deviate from the spirit of Alhazen's theory. Despite major alterations in the conception of the transmission process itself, the same characterization of post-ocular transmission as we have applied to Alhazen—the transmission of a "picture" or "image" through the optic nerve—remained applicable for at least two centuries after Kepler.[32]

Two views of post-retinal transmission are discernible in the seventeenth century. The first stems from Kepler himself. Kepler provided an interpretation of the transmission process that was consistent with his new understanding of the eye's structure and function but that remained within the ontological framework of the traditional physiology of nervous transmission. In both Kepler's account and the accounts of Alhazen and others, the key role in the reception of light and color and the transmission of the received impressions to the seat of visual judgment is played by "visual spirit."[33] Whereas for Alhazen the transmission could be seen as a direct extension of the received rays of light into and through the optic nerve, to Kepler it was clear that anything resembling an optical transmission had to end at the opaque surface of the retina. Kepler denied that visual spirit was an "optical body," but retained the view that the image or picture received at the eye is transmitted by means of the visual spirit to the seat of visual judgment, or, as he termed it (in Aristotelian fashion), the "common sense."[34] He described the transmitted entity as an "immaterial image" (*species immateriata*).[35] Both the affection (*passio*) of the visual spirit by light and color and the transmission of the immaterial image were considered by Kepler to be "occult" or "obscure" processes, belonging to "the realm of the wonderful."[36] The image itself was thought to be produced by and to correspond to the retinal image, and so to bear a point-for-point correspondence with the objects before the eye. Vision was pretty much equated with the immaterial image. Insofar as this was the case,

---

[32] R. Smith (1738, 27) provides a brief but representative statement of the 18th-c. view of post-retinal physiology: speaking of the "pictures" painted upon the retina, he says that "these pictures propagated by motion along the fibres of the optick nerves into the brain are the cause of vision."

[33] Kepler (1939), 152; (1964), 1:148–50; (1611), 23–5 (prop. 61), trans. in Kepler (1904), 28–30. Kepler shared the earlier view (n. 13 above) that visual spirit is the agent of the soul.

[34] In 1604, Kepler (1939, 152; 1964, 148–9) denied that visual spirit is an optical body, but he did not take a firm stand on post-retinal transmission (see also Lindberg 1976, 203–4); subsequently, he clearly stated that an image is transmitted to the common sense, but he equivocated on the role of the optic nerve in this transmission (1611, 23–4, prop. 61; 1904, 29–30).

[35] Kepler (1611), 24; (1904), 29.

[36] Ibid. Also, Kepler (1939), 152–3; (1964), 148, 150. While Kepler maintained that the process of transmission is beyond the scope of the *laws* of optics, he countered that since "optics" derives its name from "vision," it is "wrong to exclude it [the transmission process] from the science of Optics simply because, in the present limited state of our science, it cannot be accommodated in Optics" (1939, 152; 1964, 148).

there was no room in Kepler's views for the concept of a sensory core distinct from the visual world, since there was no basis for the distinction itself. The visual world was equated with a mental correlate of the retinal image.[37]

The second view of post-retinal physiology discernible in the seventeenth century stems from Descartes. It differs from the first view and from the position of Alhazen and his Latin followers, not in its conception of the psychologically effective features of the transmitted stimulus, but in the ontology of the physiological process. Descartes' physiological ideas often involve "adaptive modifications" of earlier ideas, and his views on the physiology of vision are no exception.[38] Indeed, his treatment of post-retinal physiology is essentially a recasting of the view shared by Alhazen and others into his new ontology, with its strict division between mechanistically conceived physiological processes in the nervous system and sensations in the soul. For the quasi-optical transmission of the forms of light and color through the efficacy of the visual spirit, or the transmission of an immaterial image through the special power of a mysterious spiritual agent, Descartes substituted the mechanical transmission of a "material image" to the seat of visual judgment. As illustrated in Figure 12.2, the transmission from the two eyes results in the formation, on the surface of the pineal gland (H), of a single "image" or "picture" composed of a pattern of motions (abc) that bear a one-to-one correspondence to the motions comprising the retinal image (1-3-5), and hence to points on the visible object (ABC).[39] Comparison of Figure 12.2 with Figure 12.1 reveals that although there are differences—primarily with respect to the anatomical destination of the transmitted entity (in the pineal gland as opposed to the optic chiasm) and the operations of the eye upon incoming rays of light (formation of a retinal image through the refractive power of the lens, versus the singling out of perpendicular rays)—the principle underlying the two views of postocular transmission is the same: the nervous system transmits the ordered array of stimulation received at the two eyes to the brain and combines the two transmitted impressions into one. Yet for Descartes the transmitted entity, just as the light proceeding from objects to the eye, is in the material realm; it has nothing of the character of sensation. The mind senses, rather than the

[37] Kepler (1939), 153; (1964), 150. See also Boring (1942), 223.
[38] On Descartes' "adaptive modifications" see Hall's commentary to Descartes (1972), xxxi–xxxiii and nn. 85 and 40.
[39] Descartes (1664; 1972, 83–6) describes the transmission process; also, AT 6:137 (1965, 100). The drawing is from Descartes (1664, 71); it was not done under the supervision of Descartes but was produced by Gerard van Gutschoven at the time of the posthumous edition, under contract from the editor, Clerselier (see Hall's commentary in Descartes 1972, xxxv). There is no mention in the text of the "reinversion" of the pineal image as suggested by the drawing; see Pastore and Klibbe (1969).

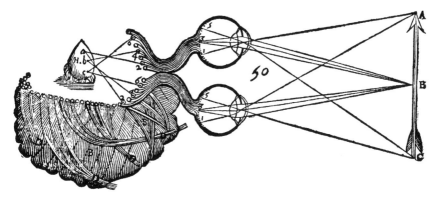

Figure 12.2. The visual system according to Descartes. From Descartes (1664), 71.

eye.[40] At the pineal gland body and mind are "united," so that motions in the material nervous system produce sensations in the mind.

These sensations serve for the apprehension of the qualities known by vision. In his *Dioptrique* (1637) Descartes listed six principal qualities: light and color, which alone are proper to vision, and four spatial qualities, location, distance, size, and shape.[41] Descartes made clear that these qualities are not apprehended by direct inspection of the pineal image, as if we had other eyes in our brain with which to gaze at this physiological "picture." The pineal image causes sensations only insofar as it acts upon the mind; the movements that constitute this picture, "acting immediately on our mind inasmuch as it is united to our body, are so established by Nature to make it have certain sensations."[42] He explained the sensing of light and color according to the principle of psychophysical correspondence: the nature of our mind is such that the "force" and "character" of the movements that affect the soul in the brain cause us to have sensations of light and color.[43] Similarly, through

---

[40] Descartes, AT 6:117–21; 1965, 87.   [41] AT 6:138; 1965, 101.

[42] Ibid. In applying the term "causes" to the relationship between the pineal image and the mind we do not mean to preclude the possibility of an occasionalistic interpretation of this relationship; indeed, there is strong evidence that Descartes was implicitly committed to an occasionalist metaphysics for both mind–body and exclusively material interactions, on which see Hatfield (1979), esp. n. 87, and the literature mentioned there.

[43] Descartes, AT 6:138; 1965, 101. Descartes points out that in order for us to have sensations, there need be no resemblance between the physiological event (motions in the brain) and the mental event (the sensation of light and color). He thus rejected the traditional physiology, derived from Aristotle, in which the form of the light and color is received by the visual spirit through a process which is an illumination and a coloring (see n. 15 above). In place of this view in which the sensitive soul takes on (comes to "resemble") the properties of the object, Descartes substituted his "no resemblance" theory of sensory physiology and psychophysical correspondence, on which see Hoorn (1972), 164–7, and Pastore (1971), 21.

an "institution of Nature," sensations of location and distance are produced directly in the soul by the arrangement and character of motions in the brain.[44]

In the case of the perception of size and shape, Descartes did not rely entirely on the principle of psychophysical correspondence, but rather invoked psychological processes of the sort described by Alhazen and his followers. He was aware that size and shape are not directly determined by visual angle and retinally projected shape. Rather, we must estimate or judge them: the size of objects "is estimated according to the knowledge, or the opinion, that we have of their distance, compared with the size of the image they imprint in the fund of the eye," and "shape is judged by the knowledge, or opinion, that we have of the position of various parts of the objects, and not by the resemblance of the pictures in the eye; for these pictures usually contain only ovals and diamond shapes, yet they cause us to see circles and squares."[45] In the *Dioptrique* Descartes did not provide a thorough analysis of these estimations and judgments. In particular, he did not reveal how the mind is able to base its judgments of the size of objects upon "the size of the image they imprint in the fund of the eye," even though the mind has no direct access to the retinal image. An answer that suggests itself on principle is that when Descartes spoke of the mind's judgments being based upon retinally projected size, he meant retinally projected size as it is represented in a mental correlate of the pineal image, since events at the eye affect the mind only by virtue of the intervening nervous transmission to the pineal gland, and then only insofar as the pineal events themselves cause the mind to have sensations.

Descartes' view that only a mental correlate of the pineal image is truly sensed found clear expression in a passage from the *Objections and Replies* (1641). In this passage Descartes distinguished among three grades of sense activity: (1) "the immediate affection of the bodily organ by external objects," which in the case of vision includes retinal stimulation and transmission to the surface of the pineal; (2) "the immediate mental result, due to the mind's union with the corporeal organ affected" (i.e., the pineal); and (3) "all those judgments

---

[44] Descartes, AT, 6:134–7; 1965, 104–5; also 1972, 94–100. Position is apprehended because the motions in the brain are uniquely determined with respect to both the position of the eyes within the head and the position of a luminous point upon the retina (by means of the latter we know that the object is situated at some point along the line of sight drawn from that retinal location). Furthermore, distance can be known through the effect upon the mind of brain states that mediate the accommodation and convergence of the eyes (in the case of accommodation, Descartes built upon the one important difference between pre- and post-Keplerian dioptrics, the necessity to provide an accommodative mechanism for changing the focal length of the eye; the potential use of convergence as a gauge of distance could, in principle, have been a part of pre-Keplerian psychology of vision). [On Descartes' psychophysical account of distance perception, see Ch. 4, n. 9.]

[45] Descartes, AT 6:140–41; 1965, 107.

which, on the occasion of motions occurring in the corporeal organ, we have from our earliest years been accustomed to pass about things external to us.''[46] Using the example of the perception of a staff, he clarified the relationship among the three grades:

But from this [the first grade of sensation] the second grade of sensation results; and that merely extends to the perception of the colour or light reflected from the stick, and is due to the fact that the mind is so intimately conjoined with the brain as to be affected by the motions arising in it. Nothing more than this should be assigned to sense, if we wish to distinguish it accurately from the intellect. For though my judgment that there is a staff situated without me, which judgment results from the sensation of colour by which I am affected, and likewise my reasoning from the extension of that colour, its boundaries, and its position relatively to the parts of my brain, to the size, the shape, and the distance of the said staff, are vulgarly assigned to sense, and are consequently here referred to the third grade of sensation, they clearly depend upon the understanding alone.[47]

The first grade of "sensation" comprises only the motions in the nervous system and so is not a true mental sensing. The second grade—the immediate mental result of nervous motion—is what properly belongs to sense. The mind cannot base its judgment of size directly upon the relative size of the retinal image (since this image is part of the first grade of sense), but rather judges from the extension and boundaries of the color patch present in sensation.

The distinction between the first and second grades of sense spans the boundary between body and mind. The distinction between the second and third grades is, interestingly, a distinction between types of mental events that occur during vision. The first term of the distinction—the second grade—is, however, unfamiliar to the ordinary observer, who takes the judgments of the third grade to be primary. Even though these judgments "depend upon the understanding alone" and therefore fall outside the category of sense, they are "vulgarly" considered to be sensations. This confusion results from the fact that, phenomenally speaking, we experience objects as being of a particular size and at a certain distance and are not aware that our ostensibly direct apprehension of objective size and distance is actually mediated by the second grade of sense and the judgments performed upon it. Descartes says that the reason we confusedly assign these judgments to sense "is just that in these matters custom makes us judge so quickly, or rather we recall the judgments previously made about similar things; and thus we fail to distinguish the difference between

---

[46] Descartes, AT 7:436–7; trans. in Descartes (1955) (hereafter cited as HR), 2:251.
[47] AT 7: 437–8, HR 2:252.

these operations and a simple sense perception."[48] Our experience of objects in space is determined by the outcome of judgmental processes. In spite of, or because of, our experiencing the outcome, we fail to notice the judgmental process itself, presumably including that upon which the judgment is based (spatial properties as represented in the second grade of sense). Thus, in the tradition of Alhazen and his followers, Descartes held that the judgments (or recollections of previous judgments) underlying spatial vision occur so quickly that we fail to notice that we in fact do judge.

There is a crucial difference between Descartes' treatment of these unnoticed perceptual judgments and that of previous writers. We have seen that for Alhazen it was difficult to decide—and most likely not appropriate to ask—whether the sensory impressions upon which judgments are made are in principle available to consciousness. With Descartes there is no doubt. The second grade of sensation is an event in the soul, an idea, and by virtue of this fact alone must be available to consciousness. Descartes identified the mental with the conscious; he contended that we can have no ideas of which we are not aware.[49] If percipients typically are not aware of the second grade of sensation, this fact is to be explained away by recourse to the habitual and rapid nature of the judgments, which entails a fleeting presence for the second grade of sense. But the second grade remains in principle experienceable.

It should now be apparent that Descartes' distinction between the second and third grades of sense corresponds to the distinction between the sensory core and the visual world. The second grade of sensation is a mental representation of the retinal image; the third grade is the ostensibly direct experience of solid objects at a distance, which actually results from unnoticed judgmental processes performed upon the unnoticed sensory core.

One might wonder what prompted Descartes to assert the existence of a mental representation of the retinal image and thereby to commit himself to a species of visual ideas that are distinct from ordinary visual experience and yet unfamiliar to the typical observer. Descartes' inclusion of the second grade of sensation in his analysis of vision does not seem to have resulted from an experiment in phenomenology. Nowhere does he claim to have experienced the second grade of sensation; we have seen that he was forced to explain why we typically do not experience it. Thus it seems unlikely that

---

[48] Ibid. The statement that we "recall the judgments previously made about similar things" is reminiscent of Alhazen's process of judgment through recognition.

[49] AT 7:246, HR 2:115: "there can exist in us no thought of which, at the very moment that it is present in us, we are not conscious." See also *Meditations*, AT 7:49, HR 1:169. Descartes used the word "thought" to signify "everything that exists in us in such a way that we are immediately conscious of it. Thus all the operations of will, intellect, imagination, and of the senses are thoughts" (HR 2:52).

Descartes' postulation of a sensory core was the product of new introspective techniques;[50] more likely, it was a hypothetical construction based upon Descartes' knowledge of the properties of the retinal image and his belief that the topological properties of that image are retained while being transmitted physiologically to the pineal gland where they become represented in sensation.

The belief that a mental correlate of the retinal image is available to consciousness was never central to Descartes' treatment of vision, and its introduction may be seen as a by-product of his separation of the physiological from the mental. This separation restricted the domain of the mental to events occurring in a substance that is divorced from processes in the eye or neural pathways (except at the pineal); taken together with the view that every state of this mental substance is a conscious state, this separation of mind from brain led to the implication that every truly sensory state is conscious. So the second grade of sensation, as a true sensory state, must (in principle) be available to consciousness. However, the postulation of a sensory core distinct from the visual world was in no way a *necessary* by-product of these factors. In principle, Descartes could have extended the principle of psychophysical correspondence to include all of our spatial ideas; that is, he could have imagined a mechanism by which the brain states bearing information about, say, distance and visual angle, interact with one another and with the mind to produce a sensation directly representing objective size. One could proffer a number of speculations about why Descartes did not do so, though it is enough here to remark that the distinction between the second and third grades of sensation was not merely, or perhaps even primarily, intended to capture a purely psychological distinction between two stages in the process of spatial vision; it also served epistemology in that it distinguished between passively produced sensations that are not susceptible to error and actively produced judgments, which are. Thus the distinction allowed Descartes to assign the error in spatial illusions to the fallibility of the judging intellect, a move that would have been more difficult on a purely psychophysical account of spatial vision.[51]

---

[50] We are not implying that phenomenal considerations never entered Descartes' thought on perception; indeed, his observation that objects appear of constant size at different distances (see above) is explicitly phenomenal. However, it is an observation regarding the *third* grade of sensation. We have found no instances of his speaking of direct phenomenal access to the *second* grade; when he wished to illustrate its properties, he used perspective drawings as an example (1972, 68; also AT 6:113, 147), an example that clearly depends upon the geometrical relationship (as specified by theory) between the retinal image and a perspective projection, rather than upon phenomenal considerations.

[51] The passages quoted above regarding the three grades of sensation arose in the context of considering the question of perceptual error, which Descartes assigned to the implicit judgments of the third grade of sensation (HR 2:252–3). On a purely psychophysical account, spatial perception would result from the lawful interaction of matter with matter and of matter with mind (the first and second grades of sensation, in which no falsity can reside, p. 252).

In any event, although the distinction between the second and third grades of sensation was not necessitated by Descartes' new ontology, the properties of the second grade of sensation may nonetheless be understood in terms of Descartes' assimilation of the traditional account of spatial vision to that new ontology.[52] The traditional view (of Alhazen and others) had it that during vision, unnoticed judgments are performed upon a sensory impression that represents the spatial properties of objects according to the projective geometry of optical stimulation. Descartes accepted both the traditional view of the geometry of the visual stimulus and the view that judgments serve to combine elements (such as visual angle and distance) that are represented separately in the optical array. His new ontology demanded that once the point-for-point transmission of the visual stimulus has its effect upon the mind (as it must if it is to serve as a basis for judgment), the resulting state is undeniably mental and therefore necessarily available to consciousness. And this state must in principle be available to consciousness even if Descartes did not draw attention to this fact. Such are the unexpected consequences that occur when explanatory schema cross the boundary from one ontology to another.

3. Berkeley's New Theory

While there were adherents of the concept of sensory core[53] between the time of Descartes and the publication of Berkeley's *Essay Toward a New Theory of Vision* (1709), Berkeley's work provided the first significant elaboration of the psychology of vision after Descartes' *Dioptrique* and was the primary vehicle by means of which the sensory core became a standard feature of visual theory for the next two centuries. Unlike the theories of the previous writers with whom we have been concerned, Berkeley's treatment of vision, where it

---

[52] It is not known whether Descartes was directly familiar with Alhazen's optical work. He was, however, familiar with Witelo (and hence with Witelo's version of Alhazen's theory), whom he mentioned several times (under the name "Vitellion": AT 1:239; 2:142; 3:483), and from whom he apparently copied a table of refractions (AT 10:8). It is likely that he was familiar with one of the Nuremberg editions of Witelo, and not Risner (AT 1:241). Descartes also knew of Roger Bacon's optical work (AT 2:447).

[53] Rohault (1735, orig. pub. 1671) espoused the Cartesian point-for-point transmission of the retinal image into the brain, where there arises "an *immaterial* Image, or that Sensation in which Sight properly consists" (1735, 1:248, pt. I, ch. 32, secs. 1–2); he contrasted this sensation with the judgments that lead us to think we directly apprehend objects at a distance (1:250–1, sec. 11) and with the judgments involving situation and distance, by which "we easily conceive what the *Bigness* of the Object is at a given Distance" (1:254, sec. 23). Malebranche also accepted the sensory core–visual world dichotomy (Pastore 1971, 46–9), as did Locke (1690), bk. 2, ch. 9, secs. 8–10.

was not epistemological or metaphysical, was psychological: it was primarily concerned with the associative connections among the *ideas* that comprise the immediate and mediate objects of vision.[54] The keystone of Berkeley's analysis of the psychological or ideational processes of vision was his theory of visual language, according to which the ideas of vision bear the same sort of relationship to the ideas of other senses, such as touch, as words bear to their referents.[55] Just as through a process of association words come to suggest their referents, the ideas proper to vision come to suggest ideas of the tactual properties, such as the idea of distance. These tactual ideas constitute our experience of a three-dimensional world and are commonly mistaken for ideas proper to the sense of vision. Berkeley (1709, §50) termed them the secondary objects of vision, thereby distinguishing them from properly visual ideas while recognizing that phenomenally these tactual ideas seem to belong to vision. And so according to Berkeley, our everyday experience of the visual world results from associative connections formed between properly visual ideas and tactual ideas, these tactual ideas being responsible for our perception of depth or distance.[56]

The proper or immediate objects of vision constitute the sensory core in Berkeley's theory and are therefore of primary interest in the present context. In the *Theory of Vision Vindicated and Explained* (1733), Berkeley explained that the proper objects of vision are pictures.[57] He did not mean that the mind directly contemplates the retinal image, for he denied that the images on the retina "are, or can be, the proper objects of sight"; these images are in the

[54] Berkeley (1733), §§37, 43. Berkeley contended that the psychological side of visual theory had been neglected by previous writers in favor of physical considerations (ocular anatomy, the nature of light) and the study of vision in connection with lenses and mirrors.

[55] Berkeley (1709), §§147–8; (1733), §§38–40. For a thorough discussion of Berkeley's linguistic theory of vision, see Turbayne's commentary in Berkeley (1963), vii–xlv.

[56] According to Berkeley the link between the proper and secondary (tactual) objects of vision is not mediated through active judgments of the intellect (as Alhazen and Descartes believed), but through a passive, associational process. Berkeley (1733, §§42, 16) clearly distinguishes the associational process of *suggestion* from the judgmental process of *inference*. He does speak of "sudden judgments" (1709, §20), but when he comes to explain the connection between the immediate and mediate objects of vision, he speaks of one idea "suggesting" another and not of inferences from one idea to another (1709, §§45, 47, 50, 51, etc.).

[57] Some passages in the earlier *New Theory* may suggest that Berkeley did not include form (retinally projected shape) among the proper objects of vision, from which it would follow that the immediate object of sight could not be a picture-like correlate of the retinal projection (e.g., 1709, §29; cf. Pastore 1971, 72–3). Berkeley (1709, §§127–43) denied that sight and touch perceive a common set of shaped and extended objects. Instead, he maintained that the *visual* shape and magnitude are ideas different in kind from *tactual* shape and magnitude, and thus that visual space (as represented in the immediate object of vision) and tactual space constitute separate, independent realms (§§136–43). Thus even though he denied that vision immediately apprehends the spatial world of touch, he did include peculiarly visual spatial ideas within the proper objects of vision.

tangible realm, being "tangible figures projected by tangible rays on a tangible retina" (1733, §50). While the images on the retina are sometimes referred to as pictures, Berkeley preferred to emphasize the distinction between the visual and the tactual by reserving that term for the visual ideas immediately present to the mind:

Pictures, therefore, may be understood in a twofold sense, or as two kinds quite dissimilar and heterogeneous, the one consisting of [ideas of] light, shade, and colors; the other not properly pictures, but images projected on the retina. Accordingly, for distinction, I shall call those "pictures" and these "images." The former are visible and the peculiar objects of sight. (1733, §51)[58]

But, as Berkeley tells us, while we do not perceive our retinal images, they nonetheless bear some correspondence to the pictures that constitute the proper objects of sight:

It is to be noted of those inverted images on the retina that, although they are in kind altogether different from the proper object of sight or pictures, they may nevertheless be proportional to them; as indeed the most different and heterogeneous things in nature may, for all that, have analogy, and be proportional each to other. (1733, §53)

Berkeley explained the nature of this proportionality by the extended use of an example involving a "diaphanous plane" divided into equal squares, similar to the painter's device. He compared the "image" that may be constructed upon this plane to the retinal image and explained that the visual "picture" itself (the proper object of vision) answers to the image on the diaphanous plane, in such a way that "what has been said of the images must in strictness be understood of the corresponding pictures" (1733, §57). Thus, according to Berkeley, the proper objects of vision are visual ideas of light and color, phenomenally present as a picture; this picture is correlated with the retinal image, but it is not our retinal images that we see.[59]

The fact that the ideas proper to vision are correlates of the retinal image while our everyday visual experience is of the visual world was not something

---

[58] Berkeley's statement that the proper object of vision is a picture should not be taken in a boringly literal sense to imply that the proper object of vision is planar and hence localized in three-dimensional space. It was perhaps to avoid the long arguments surrounding the problem of geometry in the *New Theory* (1709, §§149–58)—arguments easily misread as a denial that form is proper to vision—that Berkeley chose simply to characterize the proper objects as "pictures" in the more popular *Theory of Vision Vindicated*.

[59] Thus while we agree with Thrane's (1977, 255) assertion that Berkeley's proper object of vision is a "free-floating" bidimensional array, we cannot agree that Berkeley took the proper object of vision to be the retinal image itself (243, 255). On Berkeley's immaterialistic account, the flow of causality is not from the "photosensitive surface" of the retina to the mind, but from God to the mind; the surface of the retina is in the "tangible realm" and can be known only through tactual ideas.

that Berkeley could pass over without comment. As Berkeley admitted, "we cannot without great pains cleverly separate and disentangle in our thoughts the proper objects of sight from those of touch which are connected with them" (1709, §159). The result is that we do not experience the sensory core in its primitive form, but only its elaboration into the visual world. Yet a key premise in Berkeley's own polemic against the "received view" (that vision results from judgments of lines and angles) was that "no idea which is not itself perceived can be the means of perceiving any other idea" (1709, §10). An obvious tension arises. Berkeley surmounted this apparent embarrassment by drawing attention to a similar occurrence in the perception of speech: even though we must hear the words of the speaker in order to understand the thought that they convey, we hardly notice the words themselves, but pay attention to the meaning, and "even act in all respects as if we heard the very thoughts themselves" (1709, §51). The difficulty that we experience in separating the proper objects of vision from the ideas of touch

will not seem strange to us, if we consider how hard it is for anyone to hear the words of his native language pronounced in his ears without understanding them. Though he endeavors to disunite the meaning from the sound, it will nevertheless intrude into his thoughts, and he shall find it extremely difficult, if not impossible, to put himself exactly in the posture of a foreigner that never learned the language, so as to be affected barely with the sounds themselves and not perceive the signification annexed to them. (1709, §159)

While Berkeley is essentially repeating the argument from habit found in Descartes and Alhazen, the metaphor of speech perception provides concreteness to the claim that we perceive the proper objects of vision and yet are not aware of them as such. We give primary attention to the ideas of touch because, just as with the meanings of words, they are found to be functionally significant. It is the tactual world of mediate vision with which our tactual body must interact and from which it can receive injury (1709, §§59, 147).

The reasons that could be put forth for Berkeley's allegiance to the distinction between ideas of vision and touch, and thus to a typically unnoticed form of visual experience distinct from the visual world, would take us far into his immaterialism.[60] The particular form that Berkeley attributed to

[60] As an immaterialist, Berkeley could not allow that sight and touch perceive the same objects; he must show that the visual world that we seem to apprehend directly, and which agrees with our tactual ideas, is really mediately perceived by means of those same tactual ideas (or, rather, by means of associative connections established with previous tactual ideas), from which our properly visual ideas are really quite distinct. On his immaterialist account, each of the senses constitutes a separate realm, so that any regular connection between the ideas of separate sensory modalities is owing not to the fact that a single object is being sensed but to the benevolence of God in providing us with a coherent set

the proper objects of vision may, however, be understood in terms of the received tenets of visual theory. Berkeley found it to be "agreed by all that distance, of itself and immediately, cannot be seen" (1709, §2) and thus he could use tradition to support his view that the proper object of vision contains no direct representation of the third dimension and is a correlate of the retinal projection. In essence, he simply accepted from the optical tradition the theoretical postulation of a mental correlate to the retinal image. When he described the properties of the proper objects of vision in his *New Theory*, he described them in a manner that would be consistent with a mental correlate of the retinal image, but provided no argument for doing so (1709, §50). He apparently assumed the point would be obvious enough, as it would have been to anyone familiar with previous visual theory. He certainly did not provide an argument based upon an empirical confrontation with the pure proper objects of vision themselves, and in fact spent more effort than had Descartes in explaining away the lack of such confrontation. And when in *Theory of Vision Vindicated* he sought to provide a detailed explication of the proper objects of vision, he turned to the painter's device for constructing a projective drawing, not to any special phenomenal considerations.

In sum, even though Berkeley disputed many features of the received theory of vision, he did not dispute the view that our immediate visual experience is a picture-like correlate of the retinal image. In this sense Berkeley's proper object of vision may be identified with Descartes' second grade of sensation. There is, however, a shift in emphasis. With Berkeley the fact that the proper object of vision is potentially experienceable no longer remains in the background. This shift of emphasis was in part brought about simply by the fact that Berkeley devoted more effort than had Descartes to developing his psychology of vision, in which the key distinction was that between the immediate and mediate objects of vision (sensory core and visual world). But underlying Berkeley's special concern to treat vision solely in terms of ideational processes was his immaterialist metaphysics, in which *to be* is to be perceived is to be an idea in the mind of a perceiver (Berkeley 1710, pt. 1, §3). Insofar as Berkeley's metaphysics served to emphasize the distinction between the immediate and mediate objects of vision as two ideational states, it left its mark on subsequent visual theory. For after Berkeley the distinction between the sensory core and visual world became a widely accepted feature of visual theory, and remained so throughout the nineteenth century. While the view that the sensory core

of sensory ideas that exhibit cross-modal regularities (1709, §147; 1733, §§38–40, 29). On Berkeley's immaterialism and theory of vision, see Pitcher (1977).

is fundamental in the process of vision has been strongly challenged, it retains adherents even today.[61]

4. Conclusion

When the concept of sensory core emerged in the seventeenth century, it was a product of theory rather than of new phenomenological techniques. The crucial development was the inclusion in Descartes' visual theory of a distinction between two mental states, one corresponding to the retinal image, the other to experience of the visual world. Descartes' theory, however, was not uniquely responsible for the character of the sensory core—its two-dimensional, imagelike form—but only for the fact that it was conceived as available to consciousness (and hence conceived as the mental state we have named "sensory core"). Since the time of Alhazen (or, if we make allowances for differences owing to extramissionism, since Ptolemy), the effective stimulus for vision had been conceived as an entity that provided information about only two dimensions of the field of vision and which therefore required further enrichment by means of psychological operations in order to be elaborated into a world in depth. Descartes accepted this view of visual stimulation and the operations applied to it, and translated the view into his mechanistic physiology and particular form of mind–body dualism. A product of the translation was that the initial sensing of the two-dimensional stimulus pattern came to be viewed as a mental event in the Cartesian sense, and therefore as an event available to consciousness. Berkeley, who shared Descartes' view that all mental states are conscious, incorporated the accepted view of visual stimulation into an associative learning theory of spatial perception. His immaterialism led him to have a particularly heightened awareness of the distinction between the sensory core and visual world. Though later thinkers tended not to accept Berkeley's metaphysical views, his theory of vision had a lasting impact.

According to our analysis, Descartes' introduction of the concept of sensory core into the psychology of vision resulted in part from factors "external" to his visual theory. The argument is neither that Descartes' particular view of the

[61] The challenges to the concept of sensory core provide gauges of its prior acceptance: see James (1890), 2:203–82, and Köhler (1947), ch. 3. In the early development of the concept of "sense data" among philosophers, the sense data were attributed the phenomenal properties of the sensory core, and this seems to have been a borrowing from the psychologists (Russell 1914b, 68). A recent adherent to a notion that is reminiscent of the sensory core is Rock (1975, 562): "It is plausible to suppose that the first step in a very rapid process is a perception correlated with features of the proximal stimulus."

mind and body *demanded* the concept of sensory core—we mentioned above that conceivably he could have developed a physiological mechanism sufficient for the generation of the visual world—nor that the concept is inconceivable on any other view of mind and body. Rather we are arguing that in fact it was the Cartesian view of mind as applied to the traditional conception of the visual stimulus and the psychological process of spatial vision that resulted in the introduction of the concept of sensory core. While the current state of the historiography of medieval and Renaissance psychology does not allow us to delve further into the matter, it appears that the significant difference between Descartes' view of mind and that of his medieval predecessors was Descartes' unification of the mind into a single, rational, conscious entity. Medieval writers, including those in the optical tradition, generally followed Aristotle in dividing the mind into distinct powers, such as sensitive and rational, and further into several faculties or "internal senses."[62] Within this context it was appropriate to refer to events all along the chain of processes leading from the eye to the seat of visual judgment in mentalistic language, without conceiving of them all as belonging to consciousness. Descartes rejected the Aristotelian division of the soul. His unified conception of consciousness, which was dominant (though not unchallenged) well into the nineteenth century, provided a framework for continued adherence to the concept of sensory core.

   The reader may wonder why we have, in the course of this paper, focused our attention so steadfastly on the emergence of the concept of sensory core, and whether we have not produced a distorted picture by examining a question that does not obviously present itself upon an examination of either Alhazen's or Descartes' optical writings. We sympathize. One could write a history that emphasized the continuity and shared features of the psychology of vision from Alhazen to Descartes. Such a history would be a study of the development of one of the major viewpoints in the history of perceptual psychology: the view that the stimulus to vision is inherently impoverished with respect to the spatial properties of objects, so that the inadequate information contained in received stimulation must be enriched by judgmental or associative processes, or, to put it differently, so that the mind must construct the visual world by applying past experience to the inherently ambiguous sensory core. Our paper constitutes a portion of that history. If we have chosen to emphasize the concept of sensory core, it is because the notion that the psychologically fundamental component of the visual process is a conscious state representing the retinal projection

---

[62] Bacon (1962), 500, 543 (pt. 5.1, dist. 10, ch. 3, and pt. 5.2, dist. 3, ch. 8). On the partitioning of the mind into various internal senses, see Steneck (1974).

played such a dominant role in eighteenth- and nineteenth-century visual theory. Indeed, it was just that aspect of the sensory core which distinguishes it from Alhazen's transmitted "form"—its status as a conscious event—that became the target of criticism during the late nineteenth and early twentieth centuries.

Postscript (2008) on Ibn al–Haytham's (Alhacen's) Theory of Vision

Ibn al-Haytham—who was widely known in the Latin West as Alhazen, now often rendered as Alhacen—was the most important visual theorist between Ptolemy (second century) and Kepler and Descartes (seventeenth century). His work set the framework for visual geometry and the psychology of vision for more than six centuries after his death (*c.*1040–1).

The present chapter uses a diagram from Witelo to illustrate Ibn al-Haytham's visual geometry (Fig. 12.1). As explained in note 28, the diagram does not precisely render the geometry. The same holds true of the manuscript diagrams from the earlier Arabic editions, the oldest of which dates to 1083 (Sabra 1989, lxxxi), more than forty years after al-Haytham's death. I have thus thought it helpful to provide a more accurate rendering (Fig. 12.3), showing the reception of perpendicular rays at the surface of the crystalline humor (also known as the "glacial" or ice-like humor), the refraction of the rays at the rear of the crystalline (where it meets the "vitreous" or glass-like humor), and the quasi-optical transmission into and along the optic nerve. Al-Haytham's descriptions of the anatomy of the eye and of the geometry and physiology of vision are now readily available in the translation of the first three books of his Arabic treatise

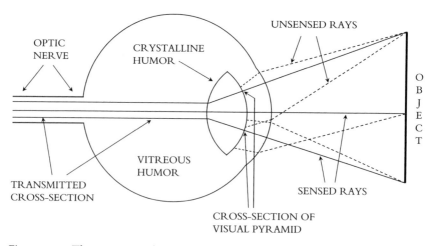

Figure 12.3. The geometry of sight according to Ibn al–Haytham. Only perpendicular rays are sensed at the surface of the crystalline humor; these proceed through the crystalline humor, are refracted at the boundary with the vitreous humor, and then proceed into and along the optic nerve.

(al-Haytham 1989, 55–100, 114–26). There is no need to revise the description of the eye and visual process as given in Section 1 (esp. nn. 11, 14), but Figure 12.3 supplements it. For additional discussion, see Lindberg (1976, 67–80) and Sabra (1989, 45–54, 73–8).

Since this chapter was originally published, these additional translations of optical works by authors it discusses have appeared: Bacon (1996), Ibn al-Haytham (2001), Kepler (2000), Ptolemy (1996), and Witelo (1991). Further, there have been new discussions of whether, and in what ways, various ancient and medieval authors, including scholastic Aristotelians, regarded the reception and judgment of sensory impressions to be accompanied by consciousness (e.g., Kaukua and Kukkonen 2007; Pasnau 2002, ch. 6.4; Yrjönsuuri 2008). These recent discussions do not challenge our conclusions in Chapter 12.

13

Attention in Early Scientific Psychology

Attention is a salient feature of human mentality, at least in its conscious manifestations. Yet attention became a central topic in psychology only recently by comparison with such areas as sensory perception, imagination, or memory. Descriptions of the chief characteristics of attention were built up from classical antiquity to the seventeenth century. But attention first became a chapter heading in standard psychology textbooks during the 1730s.

This chronology has an air of paradox about it because it dates the entrance of attention into psychology prior to the commonly accepted dates for the origin of psychology itself. The origin of natural scientific psychology is now typically dated to 1879 or to sometime in the two preceding decades. This dating reflects a certain perspective on "natural scientific psychology" that equates it with the experimental psychology of Wundt and Titchener. If one takes a broader perspective, permitting the definitions of the terms "natural science" and "psychology" to vary across the historical past (according to their interpretations by past thinkers), then *natural-scientific psychology* has a longer history than Ebbinghaus suggests in his celebrated contrast of its "short history" with the "long past" of psychological thinking in general (1908, 1).

It is from the perspective of this longer history that attention achieves chapter status in psychology textbooks only "recently." Section 1 sets this entrance, by sketching the historical contexts in which psychology has been considered to be a natural science. Section 2 traces the construction of phenomenological descriptions of attention, and then compares selected theoretical and empirical developments in the study of attention over three time slices: mid eighteenth

First published in Richard D. Wright (ed.), *Visual Attention* (New York: Oxford University Press, 1998), 3–25, copyright © 1998 by Oxford University Press. Reprinted with permission. Unless otherwise indicated, translations are the author's.

century, turn of the twentieth century, and late twentieth century. We shall find significant descriptive, theoretical, and empirical continuity when these developments are considered in the large. This continuity is open to several interpretations, including the view that attention research shows long-term convergence because it is conditioned by the basic structure of attention as a natural phenomenon. The less optimistic view would hold that theory-making in at least this area of psychology has been remarkably conservative when considered under large-grain resolution, consisting in the reshuffling of a few core ideas.

1. Attention and the Origin of Psychology as a Natural Science

The historical development of psychology as a natural science has not been treated adequately in contemporary histories of psychology. From the time of Boring (1929, 1950), such histories primarily have served the function of providing a strong identity for the discipline of experimental psychology. Boring and his followers (e.g., Schultz and Schultz 1987) have thus celebrated "foundings" and "founders," rather than explicitly posing and thoroughly investigating the question of whether scientific psychology should be seen as deriving primarily from the experimental psychology of Wundt and Titchener.

1.1. From psyche to mind

If "psychology" is considered in its root meaning, as the "science of the soul" (*logon peri tes psyches*), then it has been an autonomous discipline from the time of Aristotle's treatise *De anima*. In Aristotelian terms, the literal meaning of the word "psychology" is the science of the soul (*psyche*); the soul was considered to be a vital or animating principle, and hence to possess the so-called vegetative powers such as nutrition and growth. When psychology is so understood, the study of the soul's cognitive powers, including sense, imagination, memory, and intellect, is a subdiscipline. Within this Aristotelian subdiscipline, the emphasis was on providing a taxonomy of the cognitive powers, and on characterizing the "physical" or qualitative relation between object properties and sensory states that represent those properties. Study of the soul itself fell under the umbrella discipline of physics, considered as the science of nature in general, but this fact carried no materialistic or reductionistic implications. Paradoxically, from our point of view, quantitative investigations of vision, including discussions of the perception of size and distance, were carried out in the distinct discipline of optics, which did not fall under physics and whose subject matter was understood to be the complete "theory of vision" (Hatfield 1995b).

In the course of the seventeenth century, the dominant Aristotelian conception of the soul was replaced, primarily by Cartesian dualism. Descartes effectively equated soul with mind. He consequently redrew the line between body and soul, so that the functions of the vegetative soul were assigned to purely material processes, the sensory functions were attributed to the body or to the mind–body complex, and purely cognitive (and volitional) functions were assigned to the mind alone (Hatfield 1992b). Although this turn toward dualism is well known, less well known is that Descartes and his dualistic followers considered the immaterial mind to be a part of nature (Hatfield 1994). In particular, the influential Cartesians Le Grand (1694) and Regis (1691) explicitly placed the study of mental operations, including sense, imagination, and memory, under the rubric of "physics" (again conceived as the science of nature in general). The notorious Cartesian interest in clear and distinct perception, which elicited several analyses of the phenomenology of cognition, featured the role of attention in the act of judgment, especially in cases of allegedly self-evident cognition (Berlyne 1974).

1.2. Attention in the independent discipline of psychology

During the eighteenth century "psychology," understood as the science of the mind, was founded as an independent discipline. Professorships in psychology were established, textbooks were published, journals were started. As it happens, none of the chief practitioners of this new science of mind were materialists or reductionists: they were either dualists or were agnostic on ontology, adopting a position sometimes described as "empirical dualism" (Schmid 1796). They sought "laws of the mind" by analogy with Newton's laws of motion. Among the proposed laws, the most widely accepted were the famous laws of association (such as the associative law of simultaneity, or that of resemblance). Other explicitly stated laws pertained to memory: Christian Wolff, who apparently coined the word "psychometrics" (1738, 403, §522), proposed that "goodness of memory" can be estimated by such quantitative factors as: the temporary latency of response to a memory demand, the number of tries it takes to retrieve an item from memory, and the number of acts it takes to fix an item in memory (1738, 131, §191); however, none of these tests were operationalized in his textbook. Wolff (1740) also formulated several generalizations concerning attention. One described an inverse relation between the intensity of attention and the extent of the cognitive material that can be brought under it: the greater the attention, the smaller the part of the visual field to which it extends (§360). Another contended that, with equally distributed attention, that part of a whole which otherwise is cognized most clearly will come to the fore (§367). A third suggested that conscious attention serves the process of combining spatial representations and temporal processes into spatially and temporally ordered wholes (§§380–5). Several of his generalizations concerning memory and attention are formulated as proportions, but they are not accompanied by explicit quantitative data to support such relations.

Wolff's discussions of attention mark its introduction into psychology as a major topic. Comparison of the standard chapter headings from textbooks treating psychological topics supports this claim. In Table 1, a summary of main topics from the seventeenth-century works in the Aristotelian and Cartesian traditions is compared with a summary derived from surveying standard textbooks from around the end of the nineteenth century (Ebbinghaus 1911; James 1890; Ladd 1895; Wundt 1874). Many of the topic areas are identical or closely equivalent: the external senses, the physiology of nervous processes, the control of bodily motion, higher cognition, and appetite and will. But within one area there was considerable change. Authors in the Aristotelian tradition, and immediate subsequent authors as well, recognized "internal senses" in addition to the traditional five "external senses." The internal senses included memory and imagination, as well as other cognitive powers or capacities. Nineteenth-century works continue to have chapters on memory and on imagination, but they contain two new chapters in comparison with the seventeenth century: chapters on association and on attention. The latter topics

Table 1. Standard psychological topics in textbooks

On Soul or Mind (seventeenth century)	*Psychology* (1874–1911)
External Senses	External Senses
Neural Structures and Processes	Neural Structures and Processes
Internal Senses:	
Memory and Imagination	Memory and Imagination
	Attention
	Laws of Association
Higher Cognition:	Higher Cognition:
Judgment and Reasoning	Judgment and Reasoning
Bodily Motion	Bodily Motion
Appetite and Will	Appetite and Will

Note: Comparison of standard topics in textbooks treating psychological topics for the seventeenth century and the period 1874–1911. Attention and Laws of Association appear in the latter but not the former. Category labels signify topical areas that may be named otherwise in the original textbook. Only the main common areas are shown.

received only scattered treatment in the seventeenth century, in connection with other headings, including the senses, reasoning, and judgment. Wolff (1738) has a chapter on "attention and reflection," and his (1740) has one on "attention and intellect." Other works soon appeared with separate sections on attention, including Bonnet (1755, ch. 38) and Abel (1786, 81–106).

Any adequate explanation of the increased attention to attention in the eighteenth century would have to trace the discussion forward from seventeenth-century treatises on logic and mind. It is already known that the Cartesian doctrine that knowledge consists in clear and distinct ideas gave impetus to the investigation of attention itself and the empirical conditions in which it is exercised (Berlyne 1974). Clarity and distinctness, as understood in this tradition, are phenomenal characteristics. One recognizes clarity and distinctness, and even increases it, by paying attention to one's ideas. Descartes (1642) brought clarity and distinctness to the forefront of his own analyses of knowledge and cognition. The authors of the Port Royal *Logic* drew upon this analysis (Arnauld and Nicole 1683, 343, 363, 422; 2.19, 6.6), and Malebranche (1980, 79–81, 411–39; 1.18, 6.1.2–2.1) extended it greatly.

Careful study of the origin of attention as a topic in psychology would require a fuller examination of the development of psychology itself. At present, we have little knowledge of the development of either the theoretical or experimental side of psychology prior to the latter part of the nineteenth century. This means that we are lacking a good assessment of the relative roles of theory and experiment in the early development of psychology as an empirically based science. Although it is no doubt true that new experimental techniques were introduced to psychology in the latter half of the nineteenth century, it is also true that the theoretical formulations extant at that time show significant continuity with the early nineteenth and even the eighteenth centuries. Section 2 considers both empirical and theoretical continuity in the history of the psychology of attention.

2. History of Research and Thinking on Attention

Titchener (1908) credits the new "experimental psychology" with "the discovery of attention":

What I mean by the "discovery" of attention is the explicit formulation of the problem; the recognition of its separate status and fundamental importance; the realisation that the doctrine of attention is the nerve of the whole psychological system, and that as men judge of it, so shall they be judged before the tribunal of psychology. (1908, 173)

Titchener's claim about the "discovery" of attention becomes less interesting if we focus on the rhetorical excesses of the third point, that "discovery" implies bringing attention to the center of the "whole psychological system." If we just consider the first two points, Titchener's claim is clearly false: attention was noticed and discussed in the ancient and medieval worlds, and, as we have seen, had been introduced into the discipline of psychology by the 1730s. These developments can conveniently be traced under the rubrics of *phenomenological* descriptions of attention, *theoretical* analyses, and *empirical* investigations.

2.1. Phenomenological descriptions of attention

Neumann (1971) surveys the introduction of various descriptive or phenomenal characteristics of attention across the span of Greek, Roman, and European thought. His remarkable results, summarized in Table 2, indicate that the primary attributes of attention had been recorded by the seventeenth century. We need not endorse his taxonomy of attention fully; although it provides a reasonably comprehensive description of the conscious manifestations of attention, it fails to note phenomenal reports of involuntary shifts of attention as a descriptive category (an added item in Table 2). Nor should we suppose that in every case he is correct in identifying the "first" mention of each of these aspects (often he is not). His findings provide a list of early descriptions of the main conscious or phenomenal manifestations of attention, showing that the main features had been recorded by the seventeenth century, at the latest. We shall consider these attributes one by one.

Narrowing (Engeaspekt)   This first aspect of attention assigns it a narrow scope, such that stimuli are in competition to be perceived. Neumann attributes

Table 2. Phenomenological descriptions of attention

Descriptive Aspect	Neumann	Hatfield
Narrowing	Aristotle	Aristotle
Active Directing	Lucretius	Lucretius
Involuntary Shifts	— ——	Augustine
Clarity	Buridan	Aristotle/Lucretius
Fixation over Time	Descartes	Descartes
Effectoric Aspect	Descartes	Lucretius
Motivational Aspect	Leibniz	Augustine

Note: Early occurrences of phenomenological descriptions of various aspects of attention as reported by Neumann (1971) and found by Hatfield in the present study. Neumann does not include Involuntary Shifts as a category of phenomenological description. Neumann's original German terms are provided in the discussion.

this observation to Aristotle, who did not speak explicitly of attention, but who raised the following question about sense perception: "assuming, as is natural, that of two movements the stronger always tends to extrude the weaker, is it possible or not that one should be able to perceive two objects simultaneously in the same individual time?" (1984*b*, ch. 7, 447ᵃ11−14). That Aristotle had in mind the phenomena of attention is made clear as he continues: "The above assumption explains why persons do not perceive what is brought before their eyes, if they are at the time deep in thought, or in a fright, or listening to some loud noise." Aristotle accepts the assumption that the stronger sensory stimulus does indeed tend to extrude the weaker, but he does not conclude that therefore two objects cannot be perceived simultaneously. For, he observes, we can perceive white and sweet at the same time (449ᵃ11−19). He seems to have held, however, that only one object is perceived at one time by the same sense (e.g., vision). But in this case, the presence of weaker stimuli affects the distinctness with which the stronger one is perceived: "If, then, the greater movement tends to expel the less, it necessarily follows that, when they occur, this greater should itself too be less distinctly perceptible than if it were alone" (447ᵃ22−4). In any event, Aristotle fixed the question of whether there can be a single perceptual response to simultaneous stimuli, and hence of the scope of sensory awareness, in the literature of psychology for subsequent millennia.

Active Directing (Tätigkeitsaspekt)   Neumann attributes to Lucretius, in the first century BC, the observation that human cognizers actively direct attention. Lucretius offered two related phenomenological descriptions of the mind's activity in sense perception. First, he observed that things are not seen sharply, "save those for which the mind has prepared itself" (1965/1967, 6.803−4). Thus, "do you not see that our eyes, when they begin to look at something that is tenuous, make themselves intent (*contendere*) and ready, and that, unless they do this, it is not possible for us to see clearly (*cernere acute*)?" (4.808−10). Intentness and readiness, activities of mind and not simply external orientings of the sense organs, result in some things being seen rather than, or more clearly than, others. But, second, the mind can alter its perception of things already at hand by directing its perception: "Even in things that are plainly visible you can note that if you do not direct the mind (*advertas animum*), the things are, so to speak, far removed and remote for the whole time" (4.811−13). Consequently, Lucretius calls for "attentive (*attenta*) ears and mind" when he gives a long explanation (6.920). In both of the cases described, the mind (*animus*) actively directs (*advertere*) its perceiving toward objects of perception, whether these objects are merely anticipated (first case), or are present at the time. This "active directing" clearly implies the *voluntary* preparation or direction of the mind in attending to objects of perception, and in the anticipatory case, is an early description of a *priming effect* (Johnston and Dark 1987), though Lucretius did not use either of the italicized terms.

Though Aristotle did not use cognates for "attention" and Lucretius did so rarely, several cognate terms were entrenched in Latin vocabulary by the middle of the first century BC. These included *attentio* and related words, *intentio*, straining or directing the mind toward something or concentrating the mind on something, and *animadversio*, turning the mind toward, noticing something (Glare 1968, 132–3, 200, 938). In the middle of the first century BC, Cicero used these words regularly in his writings, including his work on oration, in which he, for example, opined that "with verse equal attention (*attendere*) is given to the beginning and middle and end of a line" (1968, 3.192). The Greek word for attention, *prosektikon*, apparently became common as the name of a faculty only with the writings of John Philoponus in the sixth century (see Hamilton 1895, 945).

Involuntary Shifts   Neumann credits Augustine of Hippo (354–430) with fixing terms cognate with "attention" (*attentio*, *intentio*) into the technical vocabulary used to analyze cognition. In a work on music, Augustine discusses the role of attention or alertness in perception generally (1969, 6.5.9) and in the perception of musical phrases (6.8.20-1). He describes the functioning of attention in religious experience (1991/1992), including cases in which attention is to be voluntarily directed (1991/1992, 3.11.19, 10.40.65), and he recognizes that attention can be involuntarily drawn. Augustine describes not only cases in which one is drawn toward objects of sensory pleasure, but also those in which objects of cognitive interest "tug at" one's attention (1991/1992, 10.35.56). Augustine thus described involuntary shifts in attention (without using the term "involuntary"), implicitly contrasting them with cases of voluntary control.

Clarity (Klarheitsaspekt)   Neumann credits Jean Buridan (14th c.) with the observation that simultaneous apprehension of more than one object decreases the clarity with which any of them is represented. Passages quoted above show that a relation between attention and clarity had been suggested earlier by Aristotle and Lucretius. Buridan (1518) presented a more varied description of this relation, using the terms "perfection" and "distinctness" to describe the dimension of perceptual cognition affected by stimulus plurality. Where Aristotle observed that the simultaneous presence of several objects reduces the clarity with which the "strongest" alone is perceived, and where Lucretius noted that attention or mental preparedness can increase clarity of perception, Buridan remarked that the relation between distinctness and plurality varies.

For a single object that is very large and wide, a lesser part of it is clearly visible though the whole is not, because it extends beyond the field of view. But for a middle-sized object near at hand, the whole may well be more clearly perceived than its many parts. And in some cases, though we perceive the presence of many objects, we perceive them less clearly than if only one of them were present (Buridan 1518, qu. 21, fol. 39v).

Fixation (Fixierungsaspekt)   In the seventeenth century, Descartes (1596–1650) described more fully the *Tätigkeitsaspekt* of attention by clearly distinguishing between the voluntary fixation of attention and involuntary shifts. As had Augustine, Descartes noted that attention may be involuntarily drawn to things. He described cases in which attention is drawn to what is novel, a phenomenon he attributed to the emotion of wonder: "Wonder is a sudden surprise of the soul which brings it to consider with attention the objects that seem to it unusual and extraordinary" (1985, §70). In such cases, attention is not under voluntary control, but is simply drawn to the novel thing. The mind can, all the same, choose to stay fixed on one object: "when we want to fix our attention for some time on some particular object," this volition causes physiological changes that maintain the relevant physiological state of the brain (§43) and that "serve to keep the sense organs fixed in the same orientation so that they will continue to maintain the impression in the way in which they formed it" (§70). We can also voluntarily fix our attention on mental contents in order better to remember something (§75). Finally, the mind or soul can avoid noticing some new things by fixing attention on others: "The soul can prevent itself from hearing a slight noise or feeling a slight pain by attending very closely to some other thing, but it cannot in the same way prevent itself from hearing thunder or feeling fire that burns the hand" (§46). Descartes here posits a balance between the power of fixation and the strength of involuntary changes in attention. He indicates that within limits we can retain our fixation, but that these limits can be surpassed by loud stimuli, and presumably by strikingly novel stimuli. Malebranche added that it is functionally appropriate that sensory materials should attract our attention because "the senses represent objects as present" and "it is fitting that of several good or evils proposed to the soul, those present should affect and occupy it more than absent ones, because the soul must decide quickly what it should do about them" (Malebranche 1980, 79–80, 1.18). The positions of Descartes and Malebranche presuppose a limited span of consciousness (*Engeaspekt*), the contents of which are subject to alteration by voluntary or involuntary shifts in attention (see also Locke 1975, 2.19.3).

Later authors, including Wolff (1738, §237) and Stewart (1793, 113), describe cases in which a cognizer can track one phenomenon, such as a conversation, while ignoring other sensory objects. Stewart argues that the ability to switch at will between two present conversations implies that the untracked conversation must be represented:

When two persons are speaking to us at once, we can attend to either of them at pleasure, without being much disturbed by the other. If we attempt to listen to both, we can understand neither. The fact seems to be, that when we attend constantly to one of the speakers, the words spoken by the other make no impression on the memory, in consequence of our not attending to them; and affect us as little as if they had not been uttered. This power, however, of the mind to attend to either speaker at pleasure, supposes that it is, at one and the same time, conscious of the sensations which both produce. (Stewart 1793, 113)

Stewart's suggestion that the unattended conversation is still present in consciousness, though remaining unnoticed, is related to the more recent distinction between automatic and controlled processing in relation to select-ive attention (Johnston and Dark 1987). Stewart (1793, ch. 2) discusses a version of the latter distinction at great length in connection with both the role of attention in memory fixation and the conscious, voluntary control of cognitive or motor tasks that later become habitual or automatic (though he counsels against use of the latter term).

  The ability to track either of two conversations implies the ability to shift attention without an accompanying change in the orientation or direction of the body or sense organs. Such a possibility was implied by earlier descriptions, from Aristotle on, of cases in which a person does not notice what is in front of him or her: in those cases, a person might attend to first one sequence of thoughts and then another, or switch from internal reverie to attend to a sound, while the gaze remains fixed (and blank). Wolff (1738, §256) provides the first explicit notice I have found of the ability to shift visual attention among the parts of a fixed perceptual representation without changing the total representation. He describes perceiving a whole tree (presumably in one glance, standing at some distance), and then shifting attention from leaves to branches to trunk; or perceiving a single leaf, and shifting attention from its shape to its color. It is not clear from these descriptions that Wolff envisioned a genuine decoupling of attention from the axis of vision, and he elsewhere maintained that the two are strongly coupled (1740, §§358−64).

Effectoric Aspect (Effektorischer Aspekt)   The effectoric aspect attributes to attention the power of making it "easier" for the sense organs to receive an impression through efferent effects (influence running from brain to nerve to end-organ). There are two related factors here that should be kept distinct. Some thinkers observed that one can prepare to perceive an expected object by pointing mobile sense organs, such as the eyes, in the proper direction. Although Neumann credits this observation to Descartes, it is implicit in Lucretius' earlier remark about the readiness of the eyes. A second type of effect arises with the hypothesis that attention can affect the sensitivity of the sensory receptors or nerves themselves. Strictly speaking, this is not merely a phenomenal-descriptive aspect of attention, because it posits hypothetical physiological changes in sensory receptors or nerves to explain how attention affects sensory acuteness (otherwise, the *Effektorischer Aspekt* would not differ from the *Klarheitsaspekt*). This hypothesis about receptor sensitivity is not found in the passage Neumann cites from Descartes (1985, §70) nor elsewhere in Descartes' works; Descartes simply claims that fixation of attention can keep the sense organs steadily pointed at a target object. But heightened sensitivity of the eyes is implied in Lucretius' remarks (1965/1967, 4.808–10).

Specific mention of heightened sensitivity in the sensory nerves is found in the eighteenth-century work of Charles Bonnet (1720–93), a Swiss naturalist. Bonnet (1769) described a situation in which he was paying attention to one object among several, each assumed to be simultaneously affecting the sense organs with equal force:

> Induced by some motive to give my attention to one of these objects, I fix my eyes on it. The perception of that object immediately becomes more lively: the perceptions of the neighboring objects become weaker. Soon I discover particularities in that object that previously escaped me. To the extent my attention increases, the impressions of the object become stronger and augment. Finally, all this increases to such a point that I am scarcely affected except by that object. (1769, §138)

Bonnet goes on to explain that the liveliness of a sense perception is expected to vary in direct proportion with the "movement" or activation of sensory nerves, and since in this case each of several objects is assumed to affect the nerves with the same force, the increased liveliness of the perception of the target object must be due to an increase in the activation of the relevant nerves owing to the influence of the mind upon them in accordance with the fixation of attention (§§139–41). He also produced a physiological explanation, involving the redirection of limited neurophysiological resources, for the reciprocal relation he described between the strengthened perception of the target object and the weakened perception of neighboring objects (§142).

Motivational Aspect (Motivationaler Aspekt)   Neumann credits Leibniz (1646–1716) with having introduced motivational factors to the description of attention, citing a passage in which Leibniz observes that "we exercise attention on objects which we pick out in preference to others" (Leibniz 1981,

2.19.1). Indication that one object can be picked out in preference to others through attention is found earlier in Augustine's mention of the voluntary direction of attention, and in Descartes' discussion of fixation, and perhaps implicitly in Lucretius' discussion of mental preparedness.

Overview   Some sense of how comprehensively these descriptions cover the domain may be gained by comparing them with a survey of the chief "processes" of attention (Parasuraman and Davies 1984) or "manifestations" of attention (LaBerge 1995) described in recent reviews. Parasuraman and Davies found that attention researchers had described three chief processes in attention: *selective, intensive*, and *alerting and sustaining* (1984, xii–xiii). To a first approximation, their selective process corresponds to the Active Directing category, intensive to the combined Narrowing and Clarity categories, and alerting and sustaining to a combination of Involuntary Shifts, the Effectoric Aspect, and Fixation. LaBerge (1995, 12–13) lists *selective, preparatory*, and *maintenance* manifestations of attention, which correspond respectively to the Narrowing and Active Directing, Effectoric, and Fixation categories.

2.2. Theoretical analyses of attention

The phenomenological descriptions of attention in the previous section are comparatively theory-free: they impose a descriptive vocabulary on the phenomena of attention, by classifying attentional acts as voluntary or involuntary, by relating attention to limitations on the momentary scope of sensory awareness, and by relating attention to phenomenal clarity and distinctness. Terms such as "voluntary" or "phenomenal clarity" are not, of course, theory-neutral. Still, the descriptive vocabulary used in the previous section, save for the invocation of receptor sensitivity and related hypothetical physiological mechanisms, does not engage in the theoretical activity of positing explanatory mechanisms or structures to account for the observed attentional phenomena. Moreover, the instances in which these descriptive categories were used arose in a variety of intellectual contexts, which only sometimes, as with Wolff and Bonnet, involved a systematic examination of the attentional capacities of the human mind.

On occasion, the ancients and early moderns did discuss theoretical frameworks for understanding attention. John Philoponus (6th c.) provides an early discussion of the concept of attention itself, considered as a lynchpin for all cognition. In his commentary on Aristotle's *De anima*, 3.2, he favorably reviews the following position, attributed to "recent interpreters" of Aristotle:

The attention, they say, assists in all that goes on in man. It is that which pronounces *I understand, I think, I opine, I resent, I desire*. The attentive function of the rational soul, in fact, pervades in all the powers without exception—the rational, the irrational, the vegetative. If then, they proceed, the attentive faculty be thus thorough-going, why not let it accompany the sensations and pronounce of them, *I see, I hear*, etc.? for to do this is the peculiar office of what is recognisant of the several energies. If, therefore, it be the attention which pronounces this, attention will be the power which takes note of the energies of sense. For it behooves that what takes note of all should itself be indivisible and *one*; seeing also at the same time that the subject of all these operations, *Man*, is one. For, if this faculty took cognisance of these objects, that faculty of those others, it would be, as he himself [Aristotle] elsewhere says, as if you perceived that, I this. That, therefore, must be one to which the attentive function pertains; for this function is conversant with the faculties—both the cognitive and the vital. In so far as it is conversant with the cognitive energies it is called Attention. (as translated in Hamilton 1895, 942)

Attention is assigned the function of unifying human consciousness, by "taking cognisance" of the materials provided by the various senses. Attention is not here portrayed as selecting, but rather as uniting and hence delimiting the momentary cognitive contents of any individual cognizer.

Although Philoponus assigned theoretical centrality to attention in the analysis of cognition, extended theoretical analysis of attention apparently did not soon become common. From antiquity through the seventeenth century, I have found that attention received the kind of hit-and-miss notice chronicled in the sequence of phenomenal-descriptive observations. Such theoretical analysis as did occur arose primarily in the contexts of applying terms and concepts developed elsewhere to the description of attention, of drawing variously phenomenally based distinctions, such as that between involuntary and voluntary attention, or of discussing the function of attention.

With the development of psychology as an independent science in the eighteenth century, attention came under more systematic theoretical and empirical scrutiny. In his *Psychologia empirica* (1738), Wolff defined attention as the "faculty of bringing it about that in a perception compounded from parts, one part has greater clarity than the others" (§237). What theoretical order Wolff brought to attention came in his chosen dimensions of empirical analysis. Having chosen cognitive clarity as the primary effect of attention, he set about to analyze the conditions under which clarity occurs. He found that attending to merely imagined representations is impeded by simultaneous sensory stimulation (§238), that attention to such representations is more easily conserved when fewer things act on the external senses (§240), that it is easier to attend to one image than to several (§241). He distinguished several dimensions in which attention admits of degree, including: *intensity* (not his term): attention is greater if it is harder to distract (§243); *longevity*: attention may last for longer or shorter periods (§244); *extension*: one may be able to pay attention to one or to several objects at once (§245); *voluntary control*: attention may be more or less subject to voluntary control (§246), and so on. In his *Psychologia rationalis* (1740), Wolff continued the same sort of analysis, now focusing largely on the relation between the direction of the visual axis and the focus of attention, describing the movement of the eyes in relation to voluntary attention and involuntary shifts of attention (§§358–65). He speculated on the physiological conditions accompanying and affecting attention (§§374–8), and he formulated the generalizations about attention mentioned in Section 1.2.

After Wolff, the literature on attention in the eighteenth century virtually exploded. This large literature has been the subject of a monographic study by Braunschweiger (1899), which remains useful. Braunschweiger divided the theoretical dimensions of this literature into several categories. He distinguished *sensory* and *intellectual* dimensions of attention in the literature: attention can select among external objects available for perception, but it can also direct "inner" cognitive states such as imagination and memory, or "inner" cognitive processes such as self-reflection or self-observation (1899, 25–31). In connection with this discussion, thinkers took various stances on the essence of attention itself (31–6), treating it either as a causal-explanatory factor in its own right, or as a phenomenon needing to be explained. Some treated attention as a *faculty* (i.e., as a mechanism that exists even when it is not in use), others as *mental effort* (i.e., as an activity of mind that exists only in its exercise), others as a *state of mind* (i.e., as a quality of sensations or perceptions, such as clarity). In the first two cases, attention exhibits causal agency; in the latter, it is an attribute of experience.

Braunschweiger (1899) analyzed eighteenth-century discussions along several other dimensions, which are: degrees of attention, which extended Wolff's treatment; the stimulus to involuntary attention and the control exercised in voluntary attention; the physiological correlate of attention; the effects of attention, from sensory acuity to memory and higher cognition; the means of improving attention; and limitations on or hindrances to attention. Throughout Braunschweiger's analysis, the primary theoretical results are manifested in taxonomies of the dimensions of variation in and conditions on the exercise of attention.

The main dimensions of theoretical variation attributed by Parasuraman and Davies (1984) and Johnston and Dark (1987) to late twentieth-century theories can be located within eighteenth-century discussions. Parasuraman and Davies found three main theoretical tendencies at work: the view of attention as a *selective* mechanism; the analysis of attention in terms of processing *resource allocation*; and the distinction between *automatic* and *attentional* processing. Wolff (1738) defined attention as a selectional process operating over degrees of clarity, though subject to both voluntary and involuntary control. As we have seen, Bonnet (1769, §142) explained the reciprocal relation between strengthened representation of a target object and weakened representation of neighboring objects by postulating that limited neurophysiological resources must be allocated, with consequences for subsequent perceptual representation. Finally, the distinction between processes that are under the control of voluntary attention and those that occur without even being noticed was commonplace in eighteenth-century psychology, partly as a result of the postulation of unnoticed and hence automatic inferential processes to explain size and distance perception (forerunners of unconscious inference, on which see Hatfield 1990b, chs. 2, 4, 5). Stewart reviews this distinction in the eighteenth-century literature (1793, ch. 2). Johnston and Dark (1987, 66–70, citing James 1890) divide twentieth-century theories into those that see attention as a *cause*, as opposed to those that see it merely as an *effect*. In Braunschweiger's (1899) terms, the *faculty* and *mental effort* positions correspond to the former classification, the *state of mind* position to the latter.

2.3. *Empirical investigations of attention*

It would be arbitrary to seek a firm dividing line between phenomenological descriptions of aspects of attention and empirical investigations proper. To suppose that the latter must involve experiment would only push the problem back one step, as the concept of experimentation has itself undergone considerable development since the rise of modern science. If we adopted too stringent an attitude toward experiment—say, restricting it to the standards of mid-twentieth-century journals of experimental psychology—we would be faced with the paradoxical result that much of Helmholtz's and Wundt's work on visual perception, as indeed much of Newton's work in optics, does not count as experiment. Consequently, here I will focus the discussion of empirical investigations on those empirical claims from the eighteenth century that are presented as part of a systematic scientific treatment of attention. My main primary sources will be Wolff's (1738, 1740), Bonnet's (1755), and Abel's (1786) eighteenth-century textbook treatments of attention and its empirical laws. As a standard of comparison with traditional experimental psychology, I return to Titchener's (1908) review of the results of the "new psychology" of the late nineteenth century, which will, to fix referents, be coordinated with the recent reviews of Johnston and Dark (1987), Kinchla (1992), and LaBerge (1995).

Titchener organized his review of the experimental psychology of attention around seven empirical "laws," or general (though not strictly universal) "statements of the behaviour of conscious contents given in the state of attention" (1908, 211). The first law states that "*clearness is an attribute of sensation*, which, within certain limits, may be varied independently of other concurrent attributes" (ibid.). Titchener takes this independence to be well confirmed for most attributes, though he cites considerable controversy with respect to intensity, finally concluding that clearness can vary independently of intensity (loud and soft sounds can be equally clear), but that clearness can affect intensity (an attended, and hence "clear" sensation may seem to differ less than stimulus intensity would suggest from an unattended, hence unclear, sensation produced by a tone of greater intensity). Earlier, Wolff held that we can voluntarily shift attention and hence affect the clarity of perceptions that otherwise would not be clear (1738, §§236–7). Bonnet, as quoted above, states a relationship between attention and the "liveliness" of perceptions, with their other qualities presumed to remain the same, and Abel (1786, §195) maintains that attention can be varied at will to affect the clarity of sensory representations. Clarity is only rarely mentioned in recent discussions of attention (e.g., LaBerge 1995, 27). The related notion of accuracy in perceptual judgment, usually not stated in phenomenal-descriptive terms, remains central (LaBerge 1995, 9).

Titchener's second law is the *law of two levels*, which accepts that "increased clearness of any one part-contents of consciousness implies the decreased clearness of all the rest," and asserts that only two "levels or degrees of clearness may coexist in the same consciousness" (1908, 220). Titchener reviews several opinions, including those that posit three or four levels of clearness, and sides with those that posit only two: focal attention, and what is outside it. (He confounds figure/ground reversal with clarity of representation in arguing for his position: 1908, 228–9.) Eighteenth-century opinion was divided on this question. Wolff did not address it directly, but *de facto* he spoke only of the focus of attention (which in vision may be larger or smaller, inversely with the degree of attention) and what is outside it (1740, §360), though in other contexts he allowed that attention may be divided among several objects, without stating whether each target has equal clarity (1738, §245). Bonnet (1755, 130–1) asserted an "infinity" of degrees of attention. In an example from vision, he described these degrees as falling off continuously from the center of the visual field to the boundary of peripheral vision. Abel observed that attention can be directed on one object, or divided among several, presumably in different degrees as the ideas themselves are livelier or more pleasant (1786, §§213, 237–41; see also Schmid 1796, 324–5). Recent spotlight metaphors suggest a two-level division (Johnston and Dark 1986, 50–6), though LaBerge interprets the zoom-lens metaphor as permitting a gradation (1995, 27). The conception of attention as a processing resource that can be allocated to one or more spatial positions in differing amounts is consistent with multiple levels of attention (Kinchla 1992, 712–13).

Titchener gives two laws in the third instance, both pertaining to the temporal relations of attention (1908, 242–7). The *law of accommodation* concerns the relation between cuing and reaction time: it takes a certain period (1–1.5 sec) to focus attention once cued; reaction time improves with cuing. The *law of inertia* states that it is more pleasing, or easier, to hold attention on one object than to shift it. Eighteenth-century literature does not contain reaction-time results, and so has no correlate to the first of these laws. As for the ease or difficulty of shifting attention, Wolff (1738, §§246–7) observed that in some instances attention tends to wander, and the problem is keeping it in place, and Abel (1786, §214) listed a number of conditions that affect the duration of attention.

Titchener's fourth is the *law of prior entry*, according to which "the stimulus for which we are predisposed requires less time than a like stimulus, for which we are unprepared, to produce its full conscious effect" (1908, 251). Although observation of the connection between attention and mental preparedness goes back at least to Lucretius, the eighteenth century made no advances here that I have found. In recent literature, the correlate to Titchener's *accommodation* and *prior entry* is the *priming effect*, which has been studied extensively (Johnston and Dark 1986, 46–7; Kinchla 1992, 724–33), along with the notion of attention as *preparatory* to perception (LaBerge 1995, 12–13).

Titchener's fifth is the *law of limited range*, which says that for brief (tachistoscopic) exposures of objects within the scope of clear vision, "a practiced observer is able to cognise from four to six of them 'by a single act of attention'" (1908, 260–1). In the eighteenth century, this question was not posed in connection with tachistoscopic presentation. The earlier question concerned the number of objects that can be held in clear consciousness, apperceived, or attended to, at one time. Opinions were divided. Krüger held that through attention the understanding is able to make just one of its representations clear at a time (1756, 228–9). Bonnet tested the question by seeing how many objects he could imagine at one time. He reported:

> I find considerable variety in this connection, but in general the number is only five or six. I attempt, for example, to represent to myself a figure with five or six sides, or simply to represent five or six points; I see that I imagine five distinctly: I have difficulty going to six. It is perhaps true that regularity in the position of these lines or points greatly relieves the imagination, and helps it to go higher. (1755, 132)

The task of determining how many items can be cognized clearly at one time was pursued with relative continuity over a period of 200 years. In the

1830s, the Scottish philosopher and psychologist William Hamilton proposed the following experiment to answer the question:

> If you throw a handful of marbles on the floor, you will find it difficult to view at once more than six, or seven at most, without confusion; but if you group them into twos, or threes, or fives, you can comprehend as many groups as you can units. ... You may perform the experiment also by an act of imagination. (1859, 177)

Hamilton controlled for time by fixing the onset of the task and operating under instructions that the number of marbles must be taken in "at once," that is, immediately and in one cognitive act. Later in the century, Jevons (1871) performed a similar experiment by throwing various quantities of black beans into a shallow round paper box and estimating their number as soon as they came to rest. His results, originally reported in *Nature*, are shown in Table 3. He concludes that since a 5 per cent error rate was obtained when the number of beans reached five, the proper figure for the limit of correct numerical estimation by a "single act of mental attention" is four. In the middle of the twentieth century, Kaufman *et al.* (1949) studied the discrimination of visual number using dots projected on a large screen, varying the instructions for speed and accuracy. They found no errors for two, three, or four dots. For both accuracy and speed instructions, error began at five dots; the errors were fewer

Table 3. Numerical estimation during a single act of attention

	Actual Numbers												
	3	4	5	6	7	8	9	10	11	12	13	14	15
3	23	—	—	—	—	—	—	—	—	—	—	—	—
4	—	65	—	—	—	—	—	—	—	—	—	—	—
5	—	—	102	7	—	—	—	—	—	—	—	—	—
6	—	—	4	120	18	—	—	—	—	—	—	—	—
7	—	—	1	20	113	30	2	—	—	—	—	—	—
8	—	—	—	—	25	76	24	6	1	—	—	—	—
9	—	—	—	—	—	28	76	37	11	1	—	—	—
10	—	—	—	—	—	1	18	46	19	4	—	—	—
11	—	—	—	—	—	—	2	16	26	17	7	2	—
12	—	—	—	—	—	—	—	2	12	19	11	3	2
13	—	—	—	—	—	—	—	—	—	3	6	3	1
14	—	—	—	—	—	—	—	—	—	1	1	4	6
15	—	—	—	—	—	—	—	—	—	—	1	2	2
Totals	23	65	107	147	156	135	122	107	69	45	26	14	11

Column header at left, rows labelled "Estimated Numbers".

Note: Data showing W. Stanley Jevons' estimates of the number of black beans thrown into a white paper box at the moment at which the beans came to rest, in comparison with the actual number of beans thrown.
Source: Adapted from Jevons (1871).

for accuracy instructions and reaction time longer. Kaufman *et al.* also reported reaction times from a similar experiment by Saltzman and Garner (1948), which showed that the times increase monotonically as the number of stimuli is increased from 2 to 10. Following Saltzman and Garner, they concluded that there is no such thing as a single "span of apprehension" or capacity of momentary cognition. They did not present their findings as bearing on attention, but they focused instead on the judgment of numerousness itself, and coined the term "subitizing" for cases in which number is determined "suddenly" (1949, 520). This "subitizing" literature is not commonly included in current discussions of attention. However, a correlate of Titchener's fifth law, and of the question posed by Bonnet, Hamilton, and Jevons, occurs in recent literature through comparisons of attention to a bottleneck (LaBerge 1995, 34).

Titchener's sixth law is the *law of temporal instability*, which says that attention is unstable in itself. Titchener cites Wundt (1902–3, 3:366) to the effect that attention is constantly broken, from moment to moment (1908, 263). However, Titchener himself considered the estimate of two to three minutes for the self-limiting duration of focused attention to be conservative (1908, 268). Wolff (1738, §244) noted that the ability to hold attention fixed varies from individual to individual, without giving a temporal estimate. Recent empirical work discusses this topic under the rubric of *sustained attention*, or the *duration of attention* (LaBerge 1995, 35–8), and suggests a duration on the order of hundreds of milliseconds.

Seventh and finally, Titchener expresses the wish that there were a law for measuring the *degree of clearness* or the degree of attention. Finding no single measure extant, he discusses several candidates, including the effect of distractors on some measure of performance (such as errors in a well-practiced sensory discrimination task). Other proposed measures of "attentional degree" or "attentional capacity" include measures of simultaneous range of attention (cf. law five), the effect of attention on sensory discrimination (cf. law four), the effect of attention on the formation of associations, and finally its effect on reaction time (1908, 279–80). In the eighteenth century, Wolff discussed several measures of degree of attention, including ease of distraction, capacity, and duration (1738, §§243–5). Contemporary work assesses various dimensions of attention through sophisticated measures of performance characteristics such as reaction time and performance error (Kinchla 1992).

These comparisons suggest that there is both continuity and divergence across the past 250 years of attention research: continuity at the global levels of theoretical conceptions and main dimensions of analysis, discontinuity in the development of sophisticated instrumentation for testing reaction time (late nineteenth century), and sophisticated approaches to measuring the fine-grained spatial and temporal characteristics of attention-based and un-attended processing (twentieth century). As elsewhere in psychology, current work on attention tends to be fragmented: there are traditions of work on attention as a selective mechanism (which might be early or late, voluntary or involuntary), as allocation of processing resources, and as something to be contrasted with automatic processing. Within these theoretical traditions, elaborate flow-chart models are being developed and tested. New empirical questions have arisen concerning the extent to which semantic as opposed to simple physical dimensions of stimuli are processed outside the focus of attention. New neural imaging techniques now make it possible to track the neurophysiology of attention more closely than before. At the same time, the question that was at the center of discussions in the eighteenth century and earlier, the cognitive function of attention, is less frequently posed, and the functioning of attention in higher cognition is less frequently discussed. As many authors have observed, "attention" now defines a complex field of research that may or may not be unified by a single underlying process or set of phenomena. It is less common now for a single author to attempt a systematic taxonomy of all the phenomena of attention. There is richness of results and of microtheory, but theoretical unification remains elusive.

3. Concluding Remarks

Examination of the early history of attention reveals that the chief phenomenal-descriptive aspects of attention had been recorded by the seventeenth century. The main overarching theoretical positions were formulated by the end of the eighteenth century, and the primary areas of experimental investigation by the end of the nineteenth. Experimental technique has been much refined, and new instruments make possible fine-grained analyses of the psychophys-ics of attention. These permit formulation of sophisticated questions about the temporal course, spatial distribution, and content-related characteristics of attentional processing.

Titchener's claim that research on attention was born with the "new" experimental psychology of the late nineteenth century is false. His claim in fact differs markedly from the attitude of William James, who is now cited more prominently than Titchener on attention. James (1890, ch. 11) referred freely to eighteenth-century works, including those of Wolff and Stewart. The extent to which the theoretical context set by eighteenth-century psychology conditioned and controlled the psychology of Wundt, Titchener, and indeed James, and thereby set the context for twentieth-century psychology, is at present unknown. This state of ignorance has largely resulted from the misbelief that scientific psychology is itself only slightly more than 100 years old. For the case of attention, I hope to have shown that that contention is at least 150 years off the mark.

14

Psychology, Philosophy, and Cognitive Science

REFLECTIONS ON THE HISTORY
AND PHILOSOPHY OF EXPERIMENTAL
PSYCHOLOGY

1. A Science of Psychology?

Psychology has been self-consciously trying to be a science for two hundred years, give or take fifty. In the meantime, it has developed a variety of laboratory techniques, collected much experimental data, shown some theoretical development, and undergone changes of opinion about whether its primary object of study is mind or behavior. Has it made its way to sciencehood? Some have thought psychology became scientific by freeing itself from philosophy near the end of the nineteenth century, while others make it wait for behaviorism and positivism. A few recent thinkers believe that psychology can remain scientific only by becoming something else: neuroscience, cognitive science, or those and more.

These various positions on psychology's sciencehood offer specific claims about the subject matter, methods, and explanatory adequacy of an autonomous discipline of psychology. The psychologists themselves have frequently affirmed that they became scientists when Wundt and others broke free from philosophy by establishing psychological laboratories and conducting genuine experiments on mental phenomena, using techniques and apparatus imported from physics and physiology. In a phrase once popular, psychology became a science by rising from the "armchair" of speculation and uncontrolled introspection, and

First published in *Mind and Language* 17 (2002), 207–32, copyright © 2002 by Blackwell Publishers. Reprinted with permission.

entering the laboratory to undertake controlled observation and measurement.[1] During the second quarter of the twentieth century, some psychologists and philosophers argued that these initial efforts had not resulted in a truly scientific psychology, because of a persistent mentalistic infection. Talk about mind or mental experience was, on this view, inherently subjective and unscientific. Accordingly, psychology was able to become a science only with the rise of behaviorism, as promulgated first by J. B. Watson under the influence of Jacques Loeb and other physiologists, and rendered genuinely scientific when Clark Hull and B. F. Skinner adopted the scientific methodology of logical positivism or logical empiricism.

The recent authors who believe that psychology should become something else grant that the discipline was propaedeutic to the scientific study of cognition, but deny that such a discipline should or will remain autonomous. Instead, neuroscience, cognitive science, linguistics, and others will partition its domain. Michael Gazzaniga, reflecting on the layout of the psychology building at Dartmouth College in Hanover, New Hampshire, concludes that there is no overarching discipline of psychology to hold together the various floors, devoted to social psychology, cognitive science, and cognitive neuroscience. In his view, "psychology itself is dead" (1998, xi). The cognitive and perceptual part of psychology has gone over to the "evolutionary biologists, cognitive scientists, neuroscientists, psychophysicists, linguists, [and] computer you name it" (xi). Howard Gardner sees the cognitive areas of psychology merging with artificial intelligence, to form "the central region of a new unified cognitive science" (1985, 136). The remaining discipline of psychology will be limited to various applied activities (in the clinic, the schools, and industry), and a few subject areas such as personality and motivation.

Who is right about whether, when, and how psychology became a science? That is a question for the history and philosophy of psychology, a blended mixture of historical scholarship and philosophical analysis. As a way of reflecting on mind and language in the past century or so of psychology, I want to consider some key themes and episodes in the history and philosophy

---

[1] It is typical to characterize early experimental psychology as simply introspective. But in fact early experimentalists such as Wundt (1902, sec. 3) and Titchener (1912b) were critics of uncontrolled introspection. They relied on subjects' (or self-) reports of perceptual experience, but they collected such reports in controlled circumstances in which the stimulus was known and the subject was focused on matching one stimulus to another, discriminating between stimuli, or estimating a value. The notion of skilled introspective analysis of sensations as developed by Titchener did come in for heavy criticism, but it was not the only or the primary notion of introspection in American psychology (on introspection in Wundt and Titchener, see Danziger 1980). And once the Gestaltists immigrated (Köhler 1929; Koffka 1935), phenomenally based reports of experience, distinct from the analytical introspection of Titchener, were well represented on the American scene.

of the experimental psychology of perception and cognition. These are the purported founding of scientific psychology *c.*1879, the relation of psychology to philosophy then and in the subsequent fifty years, and the rise of cognitive science in the 1960s and 1970s. These themes and episodes highlight aspects of the relations between scientific psychology and philosophy, as well as, in recent times, between psychology and cognitive science. In the end, I'll have my own prediction on whether psychology is going away.

2. The Founding of Psychology as a Scientific Discipline

Around the world psychologists celebrated the centenary of their discipline in 1979, a date chosen to mark 100 years since Wundt set up a laboratory at the University of Leipzig (having previously used his instruments at home). The celebratory literature was replete with knowing concessions that the precise date was somewhat arbitrary—one could look earlier to Fechner's experiments, or discuss whether Wundt's was really the first laboratory—but it nonetheless accepted the date as approximately correct.

In my view, the claim that psychology was created anew as a scientific discipline in 1879 or thereabouts is profoundly misleading. It obscures the disciplinary and theoretical continuity of the new experimental psychology with a previous, natural philosophical psychology. And it goes together with a story of rapid antagonism between philosophy and psychology at century's turn, which itself seriously misrepresents the state of play between philosophers and psychologists at the time.

Other natural sciences,[2] such as physics, biology, and chemistry, do not have a founding date. They mark milestones in their histories, but the study of the general properties of the natural world, of living things, and of chemical phenomena stretch back to the medieval period and, at least for physics and biology, back to Aristotle (though the term "biology" is an eighteenth-century

---

[2] With this phrase I render the question of when psychology became a science as the question of when it became a natural science. Most of the practitioners of the "new psychology" of the late nineteenth century considered their discipline to be, or to be trying to be, a natural science—though not all did. Wundt had at first thought of psychology as a natural science (in the 1860s), but later treated it as belonging to the "sciences of spirit" (*Geisteswissenschaften*), though with some methodological commonalities with natural science. In the first half of the twentieth century, the University of Pennsylvania (1938, 44) listed as one area of required instruction the "Natural Sciences": botany, chemistry, mathematics, physics, psychology, and zoology. The classification of psychology under natural science continues at Penn today. This classification was shared with Aristotle, Kant, and William James (see Hatfield 1997).

412   HISTORY AND PHILOSOPHY OF PSYCHOLOGY

coinage). The milestones they mark often involve radical transformations of the disciplines. These transformations may have brought into existence the modern form of the science, and so the modern discipline may see itself as having really sprung from these more recent achievements. But historians of the sciences, and practitioners themselves when they are thinking historically, allow that the study of their subject matter, considered generally, existed in antiquity.

Consider physics. As the study of the general properties of natural things —including living things and rational or minded beings—physics was a standard discipline in Aristotle's scheme of knowledge, a scheme that set the educational and theoretical framework for European universities from the thirteenth to eighteenth centuries. Physics was distinct from mathematical astronomy, a discipline that extended back to the ancient world and was represented by Ptolemy's *Almagest*. After some preliminary work by Nicholas Copernicus, Johannes Kepler, René Descartes, and others, in the late seventeenth century Newton propounded a new scheme of mechanics which could serve as the basis for astronomy, through the inverse-square law of gravitation and Newton's laws of motion. Newton's discoveries led to the development of modern physics, which leaves living things to biology and minded things to psychology. So Newton's achievement marks a kind of beginning that physicists can recognize. It was a big success that got them going on a track that led to where they are now (even though Newton's science was eclipsed by further radical transformations).

But it would be silly to say that Newton's work marked the beginning of physics as a discipline, for the discipline existed under that name from Aristotle's time on. In its Aristotelian form it was not, like astronomy, a mathematical discipline; physics dealt with the "natures of things," while separate mathematical sciences such as optics and astronomy described things using geometry. Some of the preliminaries to Newton involved bringing mathematics to bear on a wider range of natural phenomena, as in Galileo's "new" science of motion (which actually had medieval roots). But not all the conditions that made Newton's achievement possible involved mathematical applications or discoveries. There was also a conceptual background, ultimately derived (in function if not in content) from the "natural philosophical" approach of Aristotle. Natural philosophy was, even in Newton's time, another name for physics. It meant what it says: philosophy about nature. It was "philosophical" in that there was discussion of the basic classification of natural things into kinds, characterization of the properties of those kinds, and an explanatory framework invoking those kinds and their relations. This sort of natural philosophical work was performed by Descartes, who sought to replace the Aristotelian natural philosophy through the bold vision of a unified physics of heaven and earth governed by a few laws of motion (see Hatfield 1996). Historically, Newton's mathematical physics was a mathematized correction of Descartes' physics.

The point of this historical excursus is to introduce the notion of a natural philosophical background to a recognizably modern, mathematics-using, experiment-generating scientific discipline. The discipline of psychology also has a natural philosophical background. Its ultimate source is again Aristotle, through his *De anima* or "On the Soul." The Latin word *anima* translates the Greek *psyche*, which is the root for the modern term "psychology." For reasons that remain obscure, but may have to do with the awkwardness of the noun form "animistics" as opposed to "psychology," the discipline slowly changed its name from *de anima* studies to psychology across the seventeenth and early eighteenth centuries. But the study of the functions of the mind or soul was continuous. In the early period, Aristotelian psychology included the study of vital as well as sensory and cognitive functions ("soul" for Aristotle simply meant vivifying principle—though in fact Aristotle and his followers spent most of their time on the sensory and cognitive functions in the works entitled "On the Soul"). By contrast, Cartesian psychology (in its soul-related, as opposed to physiological, branch) included only the sensory, cognitive, and affective dimensions of mind: those that are available to human consciousness. This narrowing of the subject matter to the contents of consciousness took hold, and became a standard way of delimiting psychology in the eighteenth century.

Psychology, like physics, had a long history as a natural philosophical discipline. This history exhibits a second parallel with the history of physics. Just as Newton unified the mathematical treatment of nature with physics as the study of nature in general to form the modern discipline of physics, Descartes and his followers (with some anticipation by Ibn al-Haytham) brought a previously mathematical discipline into psychology: the discipline of optics, considered as the theory of vision (see Ch. 4). The field of optics, which had been cultivated by Ptolemy (2nd c.) and advanced by Ibn al-Haytham (11th c.) included geometrical theories of size and distance perception, to account for size constancy and distance perception. Descartes developed this theory in his work on *Dioptrics*, but also in the psychological portions of his *Treatise on Man*. His followers incorporated these perceptual theories into the parts of their textbooks on natural philosophy that treated the mind or soul (see Hatfield 1995*b*).

For reasons that have not been fully explored, calls for a more empirical, physics-emulating psychology came thick and fast around 1750. The

Swiss naturalist Charles Bonnet published his *Essai de psychologie* in 1755. Guillaume-Lambert Godart published his *Physique de l'ame*, or "Physics (i.e., natural philosophy) of the Soul" in 1755, and Johann Gottlob Krüger published his *Experimental-Seelenlehre*, or "Experimental Psychology," in 1756. Each of them called for application of the empirical attitudes found in other branches of science, whether physiology, botany, entomology, or Newtonian science, to the domain of the mental. None of them, least of all Godart, proposed to treat the psychological from a materialist standpoint. Their proposals were not about the ontology of the mind, and none of them saw any contradiction in allowing that the mind might be immaterial even while proposing to study its states and processes through observation and experiment. Krüger, especially, advocated what later was called "empirical dualism" (Schmid 1796, 189–90), the position that the phenomena of mind and body form distinct subject matters, whatever the underlying ontology might be. In any event, by the second half of the eighteenth century there was a thriving market for textbooks in psychology, so that even at that time one can find the standard prefatory remark offering justification for "yet another" textbook of psychology (Bonnet 1755; Krüger 1756). Further, these textbooks referred to some early quantitative experiments on sensory phenomena, including Patrick d'Arcy's (1765) determination of the rate of the decay of retinal stimulation, through a method of positive afterimages.

Psychology's long natural philosophical phase saw a slow growth in mathematically framed theories (as of the constancies) and in quantitative empirical work. Throughout the nineteenth century, there were more and more calls to make psychology into a true natural science. These were attempts to change it from a branch of the old natural philosophy (or from a "moral" discipline, as in Scotland and early nineteenth-century France) into a self-standing empirical science using up-to-date laboratory methods derived from physics and physiology. These results culminated in an explosion of new psychological laboratories during the 1890s and early 1900s (especially in North America, see Hilgard 1987, ch. 1). This stunning rapidity fed the idea that a totally new science had been "founded."

In fact the new science that took hold and developed in the late nineteenth and early twentieth centuries was a transformation of the old science (or old "natural philosophy"). This can be seen in the theoretical continuity between the old and new, especially in the core area of sense perception. The theories of spatial perception (including size and distance perception) of Wundt and Helmholtz take their theoretical bearings (directly or indirectly) from the earlier work of Johann Steinbuch, Caspar Tourtual, and Hermann Lotze, which relied on the theories of George Berkeley and William Porterfield, which in turn were framed by the work of Ibn al-Haytham and Descartes (see Hatfield 1990*b*; and Ch. 4, herein). Although the theoretical framework was refined and more fully articulated by the later generations, the basic description of size constancy (that for near distances we perceive things as having close to their true size, whether they are 5, 10, or 15 feet away), and the notion that constructive judgmental or associative processes underlie size constancy, were there from the start. The phenomena of distance perception had been studied experimentally in the eighteenth century. Subsequently, E. H. Weber, Fechner, Helmholtz, and Wundt successfully subjected yet further aspects of sensory perception to measurement, and developed precise methods for studying depth perception (see Turner 1994). But the theoretical notions they employed were directly continuous with previous work. Often, as in the case of James' *Principles of Psychology*, which set the framework for American psychology in the 1890s and beyond, the continuity was openly acknowledged. James showed appreciation for the descriptive and theoretical contributions of earlier writers, including not only mid nineteenth-century writers such as Alexander Bain and the Mills, but also the eighteenth-century German psychologist Christian Wolff (James 1890, 1:356–9, 409, 484–7, 651).

If all or most of this is true, then why the conventional story of psychology's novel founding *c.*1879? Several things explain this story, including ulterior motives and the conflation of coincidents. First the coincidents. The late nineteenth century saw a reorganization of American universities as they began graduate programs. Over the course of the century, the sciences, which had been included in the "philosophy faculty" in accordance with the Aristotelian classification of physics as natural philosophy, separated out into science faculties (though as they started offering the doctorate it was still called the PhD, or doctorate in *philosophy*). Psychology separated from philosophy proper a little later, due to the late arrival of the notion of "scientific psychology" (current in Europe from the eighteenth century) to the North American continent. Hence, the normal process of disciplinary consolidation could be mistaken in psychology's case for a totally new founding (more on this below).

But the primary reasons are ulterior. The discipline of psychology in the United States, Germany, and Britain retained a close connection with philosophy into the early part of the twentieth century. Although this connection was often amicable, some experimentalists saw it as a holdover of "metaphysical" and "armchair" psychology from the prescientific days. Moreover, the experimentalists then (as now) keenly feared that applied and clinical psychology would turn the discipline into a merely applied science. They therefore took action to consolidate the image of psychology as at core an experimental science, which meant distancing themselves from both philosophy and application. In the U.S., a first act of distancing occurred during the 1890s, as many departments of psychology were founded independently of philosophy. This allowed for comparatively amiable relations between philosophy and psychology in the first quarter of the twentieth century. But when E. G. Boring composed his *History of Experimental Psychology* (1929), he was intent on defining the new science through its experimental method (O'Donnell 1979); hence, connections with philosophy were relegated to a pre-historical phase from which psychology proper had emerged by freeing itself from philosophy, making it seem as though psychology were newly existent *c.*1879, instead of merely being transformed.

3. Behaviorism and Philosophy

For Wundt, James, and others, psychology was the science of mental life, or of conscious mental states. Behavior might provide a form of evidence, but there was no thought that psychology was aimed at predicting behavior. Wundt and James were in general agreement that conscious mental life might be explained via laws of mental life itself, and they both considered physiological conditions to be relevant—though Wundt would not allow physiological *causal* explanations in psychology, as opposed to mental causal explanations, which he did allow (Wundt 1902, 28). They further differed in that James, reflecting the Darwinian functionalism of American psychology, emphasized the explanatory power of viewing the mind teleologically, as functioning to adjust the organism to the environment (James 1890, 1:8, 79).

In the decades after the turn of the century, the focus on conscious states as the primary object of study in psychology was challenged. Several authors proposed that psychology should concern itself with explaining and predicting human "conduct," or the "behavior" of organisms more generally. Some early proponents of this attitude, such as William McDougall (1905, 1912), then at Oxford prior to moving to Harvard and then Duke, and Walter Pillsbury (1911) at Michigan, suggested that behavior should be explained using the mentalistic vocabulary of traditional psychology, and that introspection was among the methods to be used in discovering mentalistic explanatory facts. This was a behavioral psychology, but without a denial of mentalism. It was one of several forms of behavioral psychology, some of which denied the validity of introspection but retained mentalistic terms in the description of behavior itself, and the most radical of which sought to expunge every mentalistic concept, whether limited to behavioral description or not, from the language of psychology.

The most famous of the early radical behaviorisms was that of John B. Watson, erstwhile Professor of Psychology at Johns Hopkins University in Baltimore. Watson was a materialist who believed that the ultimate explanation of behavior would be physical and chemical (1913, 1914). Although in his view physiology would be the ultimate behavioral science, in the meantime a behavioral psychology might serve to explain behavior by charting stimulus—response relations, using Pavlov's conditioning theory and Thorndike's law of effect. Such a psychology could finally join the ranks of legitimate natural science, because it would reject all inherently unscientific (in Watson's view) mentalistic notions, whether introspective or descriptive of behavior itself. Stimulus, response, and measurable bodily states would be discussed using only the (presumably objective) vocabulary of physical description.

Watson saw himself as finally placing psychology on the road to scientific respectability. According to typical historical accounts (Boring 1950, 657; Koch 1964, 10; Leahey 1980, 303–6), the job was completed when the neobehaviorists Tolman (1932), Hull (1943), and Skinner (1938) married the focus on behavior and the rejection of introspective mentalism with the methodological sophistication of Viennese logical empiricism. Although Watson's form of behaviorism had remained metaphysical in its forthright materialism, Tolman and company allegedly rendered psychology into pure science by adopting the antimetaphysical methodological physicalism of Carnap (1932/1959) and Hempel (1935/1949). Carnap and Hempel proposed that all descriptions of behavior and its causes must be translatable into the language of physics.[3] Since the only affirmation here concerned the proper vocabulary of description and explanation, without endorsing "material mode" claims about ontology, logical empiricism allegedly allowed psychology to free itself of metaphysics and to gain methodological objectivity. Accordingly, American psychology came into its own by gaining a new rapprochement with philosophy—not with metaphysics, but with the logic of methodology, or the philosophy of science (L. Smith 1981).

There are two aspects of this standard story that I want to challenge. First, it accepts, either tacitly or explicitly, the common view that after

---

[3] Carnap put the point as follows: "Every psychological sentence refers to physical occurrences in the body of the person (or persons) in question" (1932/1959, 197). Molar behavioral descriptions might be used in our present state of ignorance, but they are to be regarded as coarse ways of referring "to systematic assignments of numbers to space-time points"; "Understanding 'physics' in this way, we can rephrase our thesis—a particular thesis of physicalism—as follows: *psychology is a branch of physics*" (197). Hempel summed up his point as follows: "All psychological statements which are meaningful, that is to say, which are in principle verifiable, are translatable into propositions which do not involve psychological concepts, but only the concepts of physics. The propositions of psychology are consequently physicalistic propositions. Psychology is an integral part of physics" (1935/1949, 378).

psychology separated itself from philosophy in the 1890s (or into the following decade), a state of hostility existed between the disciplines until the positivistic rapprochement. Second, it misdescribes the positions of the neobehaviorists themselves, imputing connections which did not exist between their work in the 1930s and that of the logical empiricists. Indeed, the neobehaviorists all rejected central tenets of the physicalist or logical behaviorism of Carnap (1932) and Hempel (1935).

The revisionist picture of the relation between behaviorism and logical empiricism has been forged through the work of Ron Amundson (1983, 1986) and, subsequently, Laurence Smith (1986). Through historical research, these authors have shown that the neobehaviorisms of Tolman and Hull were formed during the 1920s, each having felt the influence of American Neo-Realism, and Hull having developed a penchant for deductive explanation in science from his conversations with C. I. Lewis, A. N. Whitehead, and his study of Newton's *Principia* (L. Smith 1986, 165). Hence neither was influenced in their formative years by Vienna. Subsequently, in the 1930s, each had some contact with logical empiricism and the Unity of Science movement, and in the 1940s and 1950s each was interpreted as having adopted the logical analysis or the physicalism of Carnap and others. But in fact they each took little or nothing from Vienna. Tolman did not think that behavior could or should be interpreted in a purely physicalist language. He maintained that mentalistic notions such as goal and expectation could be used to describe and explain behavior when appropriately tied to responses, or response tendencies. Indeed, Tolman was willing to postulate intervening psychological processes involving "cognitive postulations" and "representations" (possessing the marks of intentionality) to explain the maze-running behavior of rats (1926, 1927; in 1951, 60, 65). These processes were realistically conceived but were not framed in the language of physiology (or physics). Tolman allowed psychology to posit explanatory intervening states described in a purely psychological language (even if it was assumed that the states had a neural realization).

Hull was also a realist, but of a different stripe. He was a materialist realist who wanted to exclude all mentalistic notions from the description and explanation of behavior. Like Watson, he felt that the ultimate explanations in psychology should come in neurophysiological terms. But he shared with Tolman a belief that at present it was premature to restrict the explanatory vocabulary of psychology in that way. Although rejecting Tolman's intentional or mentalistic notions, he identified himself with Tolman as a "molar" behaviorist, arguing that behavior theory could progress despite the lack of knowledge in neurophysiology, and granting behavioral science its own observational and theoretical vocabulary. He was willing to introduce undefined theoretical terms such as "habit strength," which he believed referred to unobservable internal states of the organism. He hoped eventually to define such terms directly, by using empirical data to determine the laws of habit strength. This approach was not in step with the ongoing Viennese accounts of theoretical terms as gaining meaning through their implicit role in a formal system so that theoretical terms are related to experience only remotely (see L. Smith 1986, ch. 7). Hull came away disappointed by his contacts with the Unity of Science movement. As he reached the limitations of his previously preferred Newtonian geometrical-style of formalized theory, he looked to Woodger's (1938) axiomatization of biology for help. But Woodger's adherence to the logical empiricist notions of implicit definition for undefined theoretical terms, and his unwillingness or inability to come to terms with Hull's realistically conceived intervening variables, led to a breakdown in their collaboration. Hull remained a materialist realist devoted to providing a realist interpretation of his unobservables. Nonetheless, Hull's students and colleagues, including Gustav Bergmann and Kenneth Spence (1941) and Sigmund Koch (1941, 1964), interpreted him as a devotee of logical empiricism. Koch (1964) used the presumed connection between Hullian behaviorism and logical empiricism as part of an argument to the effect that since logical empiricism had been discredited, Hull's behaviorism was discredited, too. This guilt by association failed to come to terms with Hull's own brand of materialist, realist, hypothetico-deductive science (on which, see Amundson and Smith 1984).

Skinner differed from Tolman and Hull in rejecting their realism, a position he cast as a rejection of *theory* in behavioral science. Skinner had been exposed to Machian positivism prior to 1930, and he adopted Mach's antimetaphysical inductivism, his focus on biological adjustment, and his suspicion of posited theoretical entities. In the early 1930s, Skinner had a favorable response to Carnap's (1932) early mention of behaviorism, and to Bridgman's (1927) operationism. After meeting Carnap in 1936, he expressed reservations about relying heavily on logic in the analysis of science, and he subsequently put aside both Bridgman's operationism and logical empiricism as overly formal and physicalistic (Skinner 1938, 1945). Although Skinner rejected mentalistic terms that could not be fully translated into neutral behavioral descriptions, he did not think that behaviorist psychology should be reduced to physiology nor that its descriptions could be restated in physical language. He did allow that one goal of science might be to discover connections among differing "levels of description" (such as the neuronal and behavioral levels), but he was unenthusiastic about the unity of science as a program. Emphatically, he considered discovery of such connections to be no part of the science of behavior as he understood it (1938, 418, 429), thereby rejecting the physicalist vision of psychology. He was also leery of materialism's tendency to overlook the behavioral level of analysis in favor of concrete physical states of the organism (1938, 440–1).

The standard story of a close alliance between logical empiricism and neobehaviorism turns out to be largely a retrospective fabrication. That does not, however, mean that there was no direct philosophical influence on the formation of behaviorism. Indeed, philosophers were involved in the formulation and discussion of behaviorism from the very beginning. And these philosophical discussions played a formative role in the development of Hull's and especially Tolman's neobehaviorism.

Nearly a century hence, when we look back at the formation of behaviorism, Watson's original manifesto (1913) and his subsequent books (1914, 1919) loom large. Some note might be taken of the inspiration Watson took from Loeb's (1900) tropistic approach to animal behavior, but the movement in psychology is laid largely at his door.

Things seemed different, and indeed were different, at the time. When A. A. Roback, then an instructor in psychology at Harvard, published in 1923 a book examining the recent history and present state of the behaviorist controversy, he identified no fewer than eight separate strands of behaviorism proper, as well as two versions of "psycho-behaviorism" (mixing some of the categories of introspective mentalism with behaviorism) and six varieties of "nominal behaviorism" (fully mentalist in orientation). In reviewing the rich literature of behaviorism, Roback looked not only to the *American Journal of Psychology* and the *Psychological Review*, but also to the *Journal of Philosophy, Psychology, and Scientific Method* and the *Philosophical Review*. Further, the books and articles he reviewed were written not only by individuals who are uncontroversially considered to be psychologists, such as Watson, J. R. Kantor, M. Meyer, A. P. Weiss, R. M. Yerkes, Tolman, Pillsbury, and McDougall, but also by philosophers, including E. A. Singer, R. B. Perry, E. B. Holt, and G. A. De Laguna. And the philosophers were not presented as simply reacting to the behaviorist writings of the psychologists. J. Dewey, G. Santayana, and F. J. E. Woodbridge were listed as "pre-behaviorists," presumably for their biological, functionalist attitude toward the organism as reacting to the environment. Singer (1911) was credited with having contributed "one of the earliest *explicit* behavioristic credos" (Roback 1923, 44).

Roback treated the philosophers as intellectual peers who contributed on equal footing to a discussion about the possibility, characteristics, and prospects for a behavioristic psychology. He considered psychology, once it entered the "experimental state," to have "emancipated" itself from philosophy

(1923, 97–8). But he also believed that every science, psychology included, was at all times subject to "philosophical audit," and that any science contemplating a shift in methodology and subject matter would of necessity engage in philosophical work, self-consciously so or not.

Roback's inclusion of the philosophers in his work was reasonable, for they had in fact informed and shaped the intellectual debate. Simply on the numbers, philosophical interest in behaviorism must be judged significant. Between 1911 and 1925, in the *Journal of Philosophy* alone there were fourteen articles with "behavior" or "behaviorism" in the title, beginning with a discussion note on Singer (1911). The contributors included the psychologists Watson and Tolman, and the philosophers Woodbridge and Stephen Pepper. Further, we have seen above that two out of three of the major neobehaviorists, Tolman and Hull, owed a major debt to the American Neo-Realists, who included Perry and Holt. Tolman retained strong ties to Perry, and frequently cited his work throughout the 1920s and into the 1930s (along with the work of Pepper and Singer). Further, Singer converted a fourth neobehaviorist, E. B. Guthrie, to behaviorism through his philosophy classes at the University of Pennsylvania. Hull was converted to behaviorism by teaching two seminars on it at the University of Wisconsin. He used Watson (1925) and Roback (1923) as texts, and reportedly stressed "the philosophical background of behaviorism" (L. Smith 1986, 152). While he found Watson's version of behaviorism wanting, he believed that the shift toward a nonmentalistic, behavioral psychology could succeed if it were better executed, both empirically and conceptually or philosophically.

This picture may seem historically anomalous, for two reasons. First, there is a working assumption that philosophy of science, or philosophical examination of the sciences, arose in America when the logical empiricists immigrated during the 1930s. Second, there is an even more widely held view that the disciplines of philosophy and psychology were estranged in the early decades of the century.

Neither of these assumptions bears scrutiny. In the period from 1890 onward, there was in fact considerable discussion of the relation between philosophy and science. The main streams of American philosophy, including Realism, Neo-Realism, and Critical Realism, all advocated that philosophy should take the results of the sciences seriously. Of the sciences, biology and psychology were given the most attention, though discussions of physical science were not rare. C. S. Peirce, Dewey, James, and J. Royce each had considerable scientific education and wrote about scientific topics, as did Singer, A. O. Lovejoy, M. R. Cohen, and of course A. N. Whitehead. Singer regularly taught a course in Philosophy of Science at Pennsylvania beginning in 1896–7, and in

Development of Scientific Thought from 1898–9; at Harvard, Royce taught courses pertaining to the criticism and examination of the special sciences (such as Cosmology or Philosophy of Nature) from 1885–6. Columbia was something of a center for the history and philosophy of science, study of which was encouraged by Woodbridge and Cohen, and later (from 1930) by E. Nagel. This program had already produced, as a doctoral dissertation in 1925, E. A. Burtt's *Metaphysical Foundations of Modern Physical Science: A Historical and Critical Essay*, which was an important stimulus to the further study of the history and philosophy of science in France by A. Koyré (on which, see Hatfield 1990a). The active interchange between philosophers and psychologists over the advent of behaviorism was an expectable expression of the prevailing naturalism and scientific interests of American philosophy in the first decades of the century.

The idea that philosophers and psychologists felt estranged in American universities after the turn of the century is if anything more fully an artifact of projective reconstruction. In the literature of the history of psychology there has been considerable examination of the situation in German universities during the late nineteenth and early twentieth centuries, where the philosophers and psychologists were battling over the appointment of experimental psychologists to chairs in philosophy. Such appointments were an outgrowth of the fact that from the late sixteenth century the discipline called "psychology" had been taught by philosophers (who also taught logic, natural philosophy, moral philosophy, and metaphysics). As psychologists began to do laboratory work, they naturally wanted to occupy chairs with appropriate resources for setting up a psychological institute. But the ministers of education created few new chairs, instead filling philosophy chairs with experimentalists. Tension between the two groups was manifested in the various charges of "psychologism" bandied about during the first two decades of the century (and catalogued in Kusch 1995).

A story of similar tensions on the American scene has been portrayed by the historian Daniel J. Wilson (1990). He speaks of the philosophers in America feeling "inferior" in their interchanges with psychologists, making up for this by founding their own society (the American Philosophical Association, or APA) in 1901 so that they wouldn't have to meet with the psychologists anymore (who had founded *their* APA, the American Psychological Association, in 1892), and then going into a crisis in the first decades of the twentieth century over their relation to science. But Wilson presents precious little evidence for this crisis. He also seems to have little understanding of the basic tenor of philosophy in every age, for he suggests (1990, 125) that philosophy's failure at discipline-formation was manifest in the lack of broad substantive agreement on matters philosophical among all practicing philosophers! More seriously, Wilson's claim that philosophers felt threatened by psychologists is belied by data in an article he cites. Ruckmich (1912), comparing the standing of psychology to philosophy and other fields in 1911 at thirty-nine institutions, found that in nearly every category of comparison, whether total budgeted faculty salaries, number of students taught, or number of students matriculated, philosophy ranked above psychology in most universities. For the nineteen schools that released budgetary information, the average total budget for salaries was $6,545 for philosophy and $5,285 for psychology (compared with $15,545 for physics and $11,090 for zoology). On these measures, philosophy and psychology both ranked below some sciences, and also below some departments of education, revealing the American penchant for practicality and application.

The actual relations between philosophy and psychology in American universities were reasonably amiable. The two disciplines typically were not set in competition for resources, and both experienced tremendous growth during the 1890s and into the first decades of the twentieth century. The situation was totally different from that in Germany. There had been no graduate schools in Arts and Sciences in America until late in the century. During the course of the century, and especially after the Civil War, instruction in science had increased at major schools, including Harvard College with its Lawrence Scientific School and the University of Pennsylvania with its Towne School. By contrast, both philosophy and psychology were typically taught by a man with religious credentials (often a reverend), who served as Provost or Vice Provost of the college or university. When doctoral programs in Arts and Sciences came to America in the 1880s and 1890s, many fields underwent an expansion of faculty (see Geiger 1986; Veysey 1965). Philosophy and psychology started with comparatively few faculty members (often the same person). But in the general expansion, both were allowed to grow. Equipment was cheap in both fields (cheaper in philosophy). Already in the 1890s separate positions were established in experimental psychology, and as universities organized into more fine-grained departmental structures, philosophy and psychology tended to go their separate ways. Of the thirty-nine psychology programs surveyed by Ruckmich (1912), twenty-one had completely distinct departments, and in the remaining cases, the affiliation with philosophy (or sometimes with education) was frequently characterized as "partial" or "theoretical" (i.e., notional), and in about half the cases the psychologists reported that they did not believe the affiliation posed a problem (Ruckmich did not collect data on how the philosophers felt). Overall, there was no need for war, for both fields were experiencing a rapid expansion of resources.

A genuine spirit of intellectual interchange pervades the discussions of behaviorism by philosophers and psychologists in the teens and twenties. Further interchange is evident from the Minnesota Studies in the Philosophy of Science volumes in the 1950s, and from books such as Hamlyn (1957). Philosophy and psychology remain in dialogue. And with the more recent rise of cognitive science, an especially close relationship obtains between philosophy and other disciplines that study cognition; indeed, a philosopher (Fodor 1975) offered the core statement of the assumptions that initially provided theoretical unity to cognitive science itself. Questions remain, however, about the relation between *psychology* and cognitive science.

4. Psychology and Cognitive Science

There is a general impression that during the period from 1920 to the mid-1950s, behaviorism succeeded in driving cognitive topics and cognitive theoretical notions out of experimental psychology in America. This impression feeds a story that as a result of symposia on neuroscience, artificial intelligence, and information theory in the period 1948 to 1956, cognitive science was born, which in turn allowed cognitive psychology to develop (Gardner 1985). Allegedly, in the meantime Chomsky (1959) finished off behaviorism with his review of Skinner's *Verbal Behavior*. Cognitive science, as a mixture of computational and linguistic models (with some hope for a connection with neuroscience), was here to stay.

In fact, each of these assertions should be questioned—and, in my view, rejected. Although behaviorism became strong or even dominant in the period 1920–60, it by no means was able to stamp out the study of cognition and perception in American psychology. For one thing, the Gestalt psychologists Wolfgang Köhler and Kurt Koffka—open opponents of behaviorism who studied thought and perception using phenomenological methods—immigrated during the 1930s and established the Gestalt viewpoint as one to be reckoned with. Further, investigators originally trained in the Gestalt tradition, such as Irvin Rock (1954) and William Epstein (1973), converted to a view of perceptual processing as a combining, through cognitive or noncognitive processes, of information registered (perhaps preconsciously) by the perceptual system.

But even beyond the ongoing work in perception, there remained a tradition of studying attention, memory, problem solving, and thought. Woodworth (1938), a popular handbook in experimental psychology, contained chapters discussing such behaviorist favorites as conditioning and maze learning. But it had many more chapters on perceptual and cognitive topics, including the use of reaction time to measure the "time of mental processes" (ch. 14), and separate chapters on attention, reading, problem solving, and thinking. The latter chapter had a discussion of "anticipatory schema" in thinking, and of "frames" as "a performance in outline, needing to be filled in" (1938, 798). If anything, the cognitive content was only increased in Osgood's *Method and Theory in Experimental Psychology* (1953), which in its discussions of learning, problem solving, and thinking introduced what was termed Tolman's "cognition theory," and freely discussed positing, to explain both animal and human performance, "representational mediation processes," described as "symbolic processes" (Osgood 1953, 382, 401, 663).

It is true that the rise of the computer, and the discussions of information processing in the 1950s, provided new models and analogies psychologists could use in framing theories of problem solving or other perceptual or cognitive tasks. The analogy of the computer was cited explicitly as providing grounds for thinking that the internal workings of complex information-handling devices *could* be understood at the "program level," and could be instantiated in a physical device whose operation was theoretically explicable (Green 1967). This comparison helped some psychologists overcome the behaviorist aversion to positing internal processes—though as we just saw, Osgood had already found the means for that in the work of Tolman and others.

In fact, early computer analogies in psychology did *not* yield computational theories of the sort described by Fodor (1975) and characteristic of cognitive science during the 1980s. Neisser's *Cognitive Psychology* (1967) is a case in point. It adopted a flow chart model for tracking information through the various processes by which it was received and transformed, and it compared the psychologist's task to that of discovering the "program" for human cognition. But it was skeptical about treating programs as models of actual psychological processes in which the computational steps in a computer are compared to fundamental psychological processes themselves. As Neisser put it, "the rest of the book can be considered as an extensive argument against models of this kind" (1967, 9). And in fact his book showed no sign of adopting a computational model of mind such as that described by Fodor (1975). My own impression is that the majority of American psychologists studying perception and cognition did not and has not fully joined the "cognitive science" movement. In the final section I explain this as a result of their distinctive approach to experimentation and theorizing about perception and cognition.

Cognitive science itself, in its "classical" formulation, was a mixture of artificial intelligence and linguistics, drawing on some areas of cognitive psychology, and sometimes attempting to make connections with neuroscience. Much of the history of this formulation has been told by Gardner (1985), though his chapter on psychology contains comparatively little on the *recent* contributions of psychology to cognitive science, focusing mainly on historical theories of perception and cognition, such as those of Wundt and the Gestaltists (Gardner 1985, ch. 5). The theoretical centerpiece of traditional cognitive science is the computer analogy, or, more accurately, the assertion that animal and human psychology occurs through computational processes in organisms involving physical symbol systems (Fodor 1975; Newell 1980). The idea is that psychological processes such as those studied in cognitive and perceptual psychology are realized, in animals and humans, by "subpersonal" (hence preconscious) innate symbol systems in which the programs of the mind are initially given and are subsequently modified (through experience). This conception offers a theory of how cognition really takes place in the organism: through the interaction of symbols that are processed by internal operations sensitive to their syntactic structure. In the end, this view holds that the mind actually runs like a computer. In the most updated versions, this computer is conceived as a massively parallel, modularized, naturally evolved device, but as a symbol-using computational machine nonetheless (Pinker 1997).

A prominent case of a *psychologist* adopting this sort of computer analogy was Stephen Kosslyn's (1980, 1983) original model of visual imagery. In this model, Kosslyn developed a Neisser-like decomposition of human imaging capacities, fitted together into a flow chart of processing activities. He then imagined these operations to be realized in digitally encoded data arrays (with color and lightness values assigned to "cells" organized into columns and rows, accessed through logical addresses and not as a physically real matrix of spatially contiguous locations). This theory fit so well the standard model of what a "classical" computational theory should be, while also engaging the experimental data of psychology, that Barbara Von Eckardt (1993) took it as a paradigm for work in cognitive science.

The problem is that the computer-analogy part of Kosslyn's original theory was like a free wheel spinning. The detailed flow charts and functional decomposition of imagery tasks into such operations as "lookfor," "scan," and "put" did real work and could be made to face the tribunal of experimental confirmation, for example, by studying the reaction times of subjects who performed imaging tasks. The hypothesis that these operations are instantiated in an underlying symbol system added nothing essential to the theory of imagery. It had the virtue of offering a precise characterization of how the operations are carried out, but as Anderson (1978) observed, any psychological process might be modeled by brute force using symbolic processing. Kosslyn at first considered dropping symbol systems (Kosslyn and Hatfield 1984). He subsequently (1994) altered his conception of the realization of images, to spatially organized arrays of "points," neurally instantiated in analog form (1994, 12–20). Curiously, he continued to call the points composing his depictive representations "symbols" (1994, 280–2). That label is misleading, since in his new model no operations are defined which respond to these points based on variation in their individual forms (as opposed to the depictive forms they collectively instantiate), as happens in classical symbol-processing models (Fodor 1975, ch. 2; Pylyshyn 1984, ch. 3).

Kosslyn's (1980) was a bold attempt to bring the new computational and symbolic theories of cognitive science into experimental psychology. Leaving aside his retention of the bare term "symbol," Kosslyn has moved away from the classical conception. Many of his colleagues in psychology never went there, or only flirted with the view and have now moved away.

Larry Barsalou (1999) has developed a line of thinking that promises to synthesize the perspectives of cognitive science with those of experimental psychology. However, unlike the early work of Kosslyn, which grafted a symbolist undercarriage onto a theory of imagery that could in fact stand on its own (or be joined to work in neuroscience), Barsalou is using psychological findings to criticize assumptions in classical cognitive science. He is turning the direction of purported influence around, and suggesting that cognitive science has proceeded too far without adequate input from perceptual and cognitive psychology. His target is in particular the "amodal" (i.e., represented in a manner independent of the various sensory modalities such as vision or hearing) symbols of Fodor (1975), Pylyshyn (1984), and others. In other words, he is going after the core of classical symbolist cognitive science.

Barsalou's point is that much of cognition relies on specifically perceptual modes of representation. He contends that concepts are typically stored in forms that represent the way things look, sound, feel, smell, and taste in perceptual (e.g., analog, as opposed to amodal symbolic) form. His argument draws on a large body of empirical work in psychology on memory and concepts. Some of this work tests the limitation of amodal theories by showing that concepts typically have a perceptual character. Work with neurological deficits reveals a connection between sensorimotor areas of the brain and conceptual abilities. Barsalou does not, of course, deny that humans have amodal symbolic abilities or that there is a psychology of such abilities. What he denies is the classical conception that amodal symbols are the coin of the realm of the psychological processes underlying perception and cognition, as classical cognitive science would have it (see also Ch. 2 and Hatfield 1991a).

The classical conception in cognitive science is under attack from many fronts, including the connectionist alternative to amodal symbolic processing. Connectionist models can themselves be conceived as realizing either amodal or perception-based representations. With the growth of subsymbolic connectionist models (Smolensky 1988), the notion that cognitive science is *defined* by symbolic computational processes is fading. But there is room for an alternative conception of cognitive science, one that does not demand that theorists use symbol-processing operations to instantiate all processing models. The mode of instantiation would remain open. Investigation could then proceed along the traditional lines of functionally decomposing psychological mechanisms, without yet adopting any particular micromodel of how psychological capacities are realized in the brain. Having dropped the imperialist demand for symbol-processing, cognitive science could now become a confederation of independent disciplines and perspectives—including psychology, philosophy, linguistics, computer science, and sometimes anthropology and neuroscience—each with its own methods and/or theories to contribute to the mix. This federational view of cognitive science has much to recommend over the symbolist-imperialist vision of Fodor and Pylyshyn. The proof of this brand of cognitive science is of course whether the various disciplines do have their own distinctive contributions to make. Focusing as we are on psychology, that brings us to our final question.

5. Will Psychology Go Away?

Gardner (1985) foresees that cognitive psychology will join forces with artificial intelligence and be absorbed into cognitive science. Gazzaniga (1998) contends that any part of psychology not going in that direction should be absorbed by neuroscience. By contrast, I think that psychology is here to stay for the foreseeable future.

Ernest Hilgard, a distinguished psychologist and historian of psychology with personal experience of much of twentieth-century American psychology (he was born in 1904), recently considered the question of what keeps psychology together as a unified discipline. He acknowledged the centrifugal forces that draw psychology into contact with other disciplines, including linguistics, artificial intelligence, biology, neuroscience, anthropology, and sociology. Yet, psychology retains its own identity. He explained:

What binds us together are agreement upon a preference for experimental approaches, the use of appropriate statistics in determining the reliability of such findings, and a preference for theories that integrate such findings. We have attained status as a legitimate social science and also a biological science, depending on the subfields under consideration. While we may expect changes, our role as a legitimate member of the scientific disciplines appears to be assured. (1997, xv)

Experiment and experimental design, characteristic use of statistical analysis, and development of theories that integrate empirical data gained through experiment. These are core values that distinguish psychological research from the sort of data collection and theorizing that go on in neuroscience, artificial intelligence, linguistics, and anthropology. Psychologists may indeed enter into cooperative arrangements with these other fields—testing a computational model against data, specifying or assessing normal and pathological psychological function for the neurologist, proposing psychological functions so that the neuroscientist can look for their neural realizations. But it seems unlikely that their distinctive contribution will be replicated in these other fields, without looking to psychologically trained specialists.

An appreciation of the basis of my prediction that psychology will retain its distinctive role can be gained by comparing three recent books in the interdisciplinary field of vision science. The books are Brian Wandell (1995), who integrates mathematical modeling with brain science, Hanspeter Mallot (2000), who takes a computer-vision approach, and Stephen Palmer, who adopts an information-processing approach, as seen from "a psychological perspective" (1999, xix). All three are good books, and they draw on some of the same literature. But the first two differ from the third in the nearly total lack of psychological models of perceptual processing, and nearly total lack of citation to psychological experiments. Let's see what this difference amounts to.

All three books discuss in detail the optical information available at the retina and the question of what is needed to extract information about the environment from that information. They all see the information available as in some respects ambiguous or underdetermining of the distal scene. They call upon cognitive or psychological operations to process the information so as to yield typically accurate perception and cognition of distal scenes. (We do typically succeed in discovering by vision many properties of surrounding objects.) All three invoke the notion of "information processing" in characterizing these operations. Mallot suggests that the observer draws on "prior knowledge or assumptions about the environment" to infer back from the image to the environment (2000, 14). Wandell proposes that the visual system uses statistical regularities to interpret the environment by drawing "accurate inferences about the physical cause of the image" (1995, 3). Palmer also sees the problem as one of making appropriate inferences on the information given.

The three books differ greatly in whether and how they characterize and discuss animal and human information processing. Mallot makes comparatively little reference to the literature of neuroscience or psychology, and includes almost no discussion of neurophysiology, postulated psychological processes, or behavioral tests of living systems. That is not the aim of his book. Rather, he has written a book that takes a "computational theory" approach (in the sense of that term defined in Marr 1982). As Mallot puts it, "the central issue is of what must be calculated in order to derive the desired information from the spatio-temporal stimulus distribution. ... On the level of computational theory, the brain and the computer are confronted with the same problems" (2000, 6). In other words, he is not interested in the problem of how biological perceivers actually carry out the information processing needed in order to perceive. Rather, he is interested in characterizing what mathematical relations hold between environment and senses, and what plausible assumptions about the structure of the environment would allow the recovery of information about the distal scene from the optical stimulus. As he puts it, this simply is "the problem of computer vision" (2000, 8). His various chapters then show in some detail how a mathematical reconstruction of the distal scene can be achieved using plausible assumptions. Such work provides highly useful information for building robots that can do visual tasks, or for characterizing tasks that *might be* carried out by biological systems. But it clearly does not directly engage the psychology of vision in living systems.

Wandell's basic approach shares Mallot's emphasis on computational analysis, but adds data from neuroscience. Mallot did not discuss even basic neuroanatomy or physiology. By contrast, Wandell covers the photoreceptors, neural pathways, and cortical physiology (more extensively than Marr 1982, who earlier sought to wed the computational approach with neural implementation). He distinguishes the job of "learning how we *might* see" by studying the inference rules needed to recover information from stimulation from the task of using "neural and behavioral measurements of our brains and our perceptions" in order to "learn how we *do* see" (1995, 402, my emphasis). He has an interest in neural and behavioral reality. At the same time, he admits that in our current state of knowledge we know more about the description of stimulation and photoreceptor response (the "encoding"), and the immediately subsequent neurophysiological representation, than we do about the "interpretation" stage that governs how we see. Consequently, in the third part of his book, on interpretation, he presents mainly three types of information: first, the sort of computational possibilities for interpretation emphasized by Mallot, to which he adds a more extensive discussion of linear models in color constancy; second, neurophysiological studies of the pathways and localization of the neural activity in vision; and third, evidence that certain neurons are sensitive to the sorts of information that his mathematical models describe in stimuli. But as Wandell himself contends, to understand how vision works we need not so much to know *where* the neural activity is, but *how* it serves vision (1995, 191, 336). The discussion of front-end edge or motion detectors ties his mathematical models to biological reality. But in preparing to discuss the interpretive, inferential processes he believes underlie vision, he concludes that the "neuron doctrine" of looking for ever more comprehensive single-cell "detectors" won't work, and that further behavioral and computational studies are needed (1995, 188–91). These studies will aim at correlating discriminative capacities with manipulations of the type of information described in his computational models. This would make for an elaborated psychophysics (and as such would bear resemblance to the psychologist James J. Gibson's theories of vision, 1950, 1966), but it leaves out the entire body of psychological literature that attempts to analyze experimentally the processing mechanisms themselves, by relating performance data, including reaction time, error rates, and phenomenal reports, to cleverly constructed perceptual tasks. Wandell's final chapter on "seeing" is an invitation to try to discover how we see. The only psychological theory discussed is Gregory's (1966) theory of the Müller-Lyer illusion, along with an experimental counterexample to its predictions.

Palmer's (1999) book is written as a contribution to the interdisciplinary field of vision science, considered as a subfield of cognitive science. It attempts to integrate findings from computer models, neuroscience, and experimental psychology. It differs from Wandell's book in three important respects. First, although Wandell's book examines computational theories in some detail, it generally avoids discussion of theories of organismic processes of information processing that result in vision itself (as opposed to those that code retinal information). Palmer devotes an entire chapter to such theories, including the classical theories of Helmholtz, the Gestaltists, and Gibson, computer theories, biological information-processing theories, Marr's hybrid computational and biological theory, and psychological information-processing theories. He also carries the discussion of the various theoretical perspectives into each of the subsequent subject areas, including color vision, spatial vision, motion and events, and visual awareness. Second, although Wandell mentions visual awareness, he has little to say about it. Palmer takes visual experience itself to be an important object of explanation in vision science. Third, Palmer exhaustively surveys the literature in perceptual psychology that bears on the problems of spatial, color, and motion perception. This means he includes theoretical issues that Wandell and Mallot, with their computational and neural focus, leave out (and only some of which Marr approached, with scant reference to the psychological literature). These include unconscious inference as opposed to relational theories of lightness constancy, experiments and theories on perceptual organization, theories and experiments on a variety of spatial constancies, and experimental and theoretical work on motion perception, apparent motion, and grouping by movement. These various lines of work attempt to analyze the actual psychological processes underlying perception.

In the end, Palmer contends that interdisciplinary vision science has advantages over isolated single-discipline work, because it combines the perspectives of the independent disciplines and recognizes that each has something to contribute. As he puts it:

Vision science may have made the boundaries between disciplines more transparent, but it has not eliminated them. Psychologists still perform experiments on sighted organisms, computer scientists still write programs that extract and transform optical information, and neuroscientists still study the structure and function of the nervous system. (1999, xix)

The use of experiments on organisms not simply to determine discriminative capacities and psychophysical correspondences, but to dissect internal processes, remains a fundamental contribution of the psychological study of vision.

Of course, one might believe that visual scientists can converge on these processes working from computations, discriminative capacity, and neuroscientific measurements alone. Wandell seems to think so. And yet neuroscientific treatments (e.g., as surveyed in Kandel *et al.* 2000), like Wandell's book, do not go beyond describing initial detector-like registration of features so as to examine theories of information processing in detail; they provide thorough discussions of anatomical localization but offer only summary descriptions of the processes to be localized. Moreover, it seems that to discover the neural instantiation of visual processes, one will need a characterization not only of what the processes accomplish (input–output relations), but of how it is accomplished (functional organization of the processes). At present, such functional-level processing in biologically real systems is primarily the responsibility of psychological investigations. But since one needs a functional-level theory in order to ask whether and how the brain realizes the processes described in the theory, it seems that brain science will remain dependent on psychological science for characterizations of global brain functioning in perception (see Ch. 15).

There is, of course, no real assurance that the discipline of psychology will retain its identity. Gazzaniga reports that his dean once told him that if the Psychology Department would rename itself the Department of Brain and Cognitive Science, "I could raise $25 million in a week" (1998, xii). That sort of consideration might settle the issue. But if the newly named department is to succeed in the study of perception and cognition, it will need to use the theories and methods of psychology. The study of those brain functions of interest to cognitive science *is* the study of the psychological processes of organisms. The structure of those processes is not read off single-cell recordings or images of brain activity. Rather, those recordings and images gain meaning by being related to a theory of what's being done functionally. Psychology is here to stay, even if disguised so as to fool the money lenders. There's no way around it.

15

What Can the Mind Tell Us about the Brain?

PSYCHOLOGY, NEUROPHYSIOLOGY, AND CONSTRAINT

1. Introduction

Philosophers have long speculated about the strong constraints that brain science will or should provide for any future possible psychological theories. Hempel (1935/1949) advocated replacing psychological language with physical language, which would be used to describe both behavior and brain states. Quine (1974) maintained that mentalistic talk could be tolerated in psychology only provisionally, as a means toward a full physiological or physical explanation of behavior. P. S. Churchland (1986) foresaw the replacement of "folk psychology" with neuroscientific descriptions. On the other side, Fodor (1974) has long plumped for the autonomy of psychology from neuroscience, by analogy with the (alleged) hardware-independence of computer programs.

These predictions of elimination or strong constraint were undertaken in virtually complete innocence of actual cases of interaction between scientific psychology and neurophysiology. Quine's discussions were simply so many promissory notes about the future course of science (Quine 1974, 33–4). Churchland's *Neurophilosophy* did not address genuine interactions between psychology and neuroscience, because the representative of psychology in that book was (philosophers') folk psychology, not the actual

First published as "The Brain's 'New' Science: Psychology, Neurophysiology, and Constraint," *Philosophy of Science* 67 (2000), S388–403, copyright © 2000 by the Philosophy of Science Association, except Sections 2.3 and 6, which are new. The whole has been revised. Portions reprinted with permission.

results of experimental psychology (see Corballis 1988; Hatfield 1988a). Further, Fodor's case for autonomy relied heavily on the computer metaphor (Fodor 1975, chs. 1–2), which turned out not to be the only game in town, and in any event he dismissed (1975, 17) the importance of physiology for psychology without engaging the living body of work in physiological psychology.

Contemporary philosophy of science seeks to understand the cognitive features of living science. Without aiming to be merely descriptive, it seeks to capture conceptual relations and explanatory structures that have a basis in actual scientific practice. In this chapter, I appeal to real cases in support of the argument that, typically, psychological theory has led the way toward neuroscientific understanding. Section 2 surveys some major results in sensory psychology. Section 3 examines the strongest alleged case for the neuroscientific revision of fundamental psychological theory, the neurological finding of selectively preserved memory in amnesiacs. In Section 4, I offer a simple and straightforward conceptual argument that psychology must lead the way toward a neuroscientific understanding of mental and psychological function and the brain's role therein. These reflections and arguments raise the question of how it could have seemed so obvious to some philosophers that neuroscience must strongly condition or even replace psychology. Section 5 examines this question and asks what it means to say instead that psychology conditions neuroscience. In Section 6, I develop the idea that the functional descriptions of psychology individuate and type-identify neurophysiological structures, taking sensory receptors (and their molecular structure) as an example. This case also exemplifies one way in which neurophysiological descriptions help advance psychological theory.

2. Sensory Physiology: Psychology Leads and Constrains Neurophysiology

Sensory physiology is an area of rich interaction between neuroscience and psychology, and one in which knowledge is well advanced in both domains. I consider the relation between psychology and neurophysiology in four cases that span the modern period. The earliest case serves as a reminder that a basic functional parsing of the body and nervous system is itself a fundamental achievement, and is by no means obvious. The four cases are: binocular single vision; stereopsis; the hypothesis of two functionally distinct visual streams; and opponent processes in color vision.

2.1. Newton and binocular single vision

We have two eyes with overlapping fields of vision, which receive slightly different impressions from objects in the area of overlap, and yet we usually see such objects singly. Since antiquity, these facts have led visual theorists to speculate about how single vision is achieved (Wade 1987). Early theorists, including Galen (discussed in Siegel 1970, 59–62), Alhazen (Ibn al-Haytham), and Witelo (discussed in Ch. 12), proposed a physiological unification of binocular stimulation in the optic chiasma (where the two optic nerves meet). But since the optic nerves separate at the chiasma and continue on to separate sides of the brain, a question remained about how the post-chiasmally separate optic nerves mediate single vision (see, e.g., the figure in Discourse 5 of Descartes' *Dioptrique*, 1637/1965, 99).

Various early modern solutions were proposed, including Descartes' unification of binocular stimulation at the pineal gland (Descartes 1664/1998, 148). In Query 15 to his *Opticks*, Newton speculatively advanced the anatomical scheme that in fact underlies single vision (1718, 320–1). He proposed that nerve fibers from the two eyes partially decussate—that is, partially cross—in the optic chiasma, so that fibers from each hemifield of the retina join in the chiasma and proceed to their respective side of the brain in a manner that preserves retinotopic order. His reasoning was based on some erroneous comparative anatomy (he mistakenly believed that fish and chameleons lack a chiasma), but his functional conjecture was sound and was confirmed by observations on brain-damaged patients during the eighteenth century (Finger 1994, 83). A prominent finding in sensory physiology in the mid twentieth century was the discovery, using single-cell recording techniques in cats and primates, of neurons in the visual cortex that are activated only by input from both eyes (Barlow *et al.* 1967; Poggio and Fischer 1977). Further, neurons receiving stimulation from one or both eyes are laid out retinotopically across the back of the brain (Barlow 1990*b*). So Newton's anatomical conjecture is largely confirmed (although the neurons from each eye merely cross and become contiguous in the chiasma, and actually unite only post-chiasmally, in the thalamus—more specifically, in the lateral geniculate nucleus, or LGN). Since only rudimentary anatomical knowledge of the brain was available in his time, with no techniques for examining neural microstructure, it is clear that Newton's understanding of the psychological function of single vision led the way to his neuroanatomical hypothesis.

2.2. Stereopsis

Our two eyes fixate the same objects from slightly different perspectives, with each eye receiving a slightly different image of those objects. The disparities between the two images are a powerful source of information for the relative depth of the parts of objects or among objects. (Convergence, or the angles formed by the optical axes, provides an independent source of information for absolute depth, via the geometry of angle–side–angle.) In the decades following the discovery of the stereoscope by Charles Wheatstone in the 1830s, P. L. Panum, A. W. Volkmann, W. Wundt, H. Helmholtz, and E. Hering, among others, investigated the psychophysics of the depth response (Turner 1994, 13–26), including acuity for disparity, the temporal course of the response, and the efficacy of crossed vs. uncrossed disparities (image elements reversed between the two eyes relative to the optic axis, or not). Although virtually nothing was known of the microphysiology of the brain, these investigators framed various speculative hypotheses about the anatomical and physiological basis of stereopsis.

When binocularly driven neurons were discovered in the 1960s, some of them showed sensitivity to particular degrees of disparity (finely or more coarsely tuned), and to crossed and uncrossed disparity. Investigators immediately conjectured that these "disparity detectors" serve the binocular depth response (Barlow *et al.* 1967). In this case, a newly confirmed anatomical structure and its physiological activity were interpreted in relation to a visual capacity whose properties had been discovered through psychophysical and psychological investigation alone. The precise psychological mechanism by which the detection of local retinal disparities produces a depth response remains unknown. But subsequent investigation has shown a deep interaction among neurophysiological work, computational simulation, neuropsychology, and psychophysical studies. Bishop and Pettigrew, leaders in the neurophysiological and psychological study of stereopsis, conclude in their 1986 review of the field that individual *neuro*physiological results continue to be interpreted largely on the basis of *psycho*physical findings.

In a 1992 review, Tychsen found work on stereopsis had recently undergone a conceptual shift which he related to the neuroanatomical division of visual neurophysiology into parvocellular and magnocellular pathways. The pathways are named for types of cells found in the retina which project to distinct layers of the lateral geniculate nucleus and on to the visual cortex. Parvocellular neurons are slow but finely tuned, magnocellular are fast and coarsely tuned. Tyler (1990) applied these findings to binocular vision, distinguishing a fine, slow, foveal system that is good for static targets from a coarse, fast, wide-scope system, with greater sensitivity to moving targets. Although Tyler acknowledged that neuroanatomical studies provided "the inspiration for the psychophysical partition of sensory processing into categories of specialized analysis" (Tyler 1990, 1877), he also noted that he himself had previously (Tyler 1983) postulated similar multiple systems of stereopsis "on the basis of psychophysical evidence alone." In now linking psychological theories of stereopsis with neurophysiological findings, he hoped to facilitate testing "of proposed associations between the separable processes in the two domains" (Tyler 1990, 1894). Here there is linkage between neuroscience and psychology, but no precedence of brain facts over psychological facts. Indeed, the psychological facts about stereopsis again led the way.

2.3. Two visual systems

In a widely cited article, Ungerleider and Mishkin (1982) described two cortical pathways or processing streams serving two distinct visual functions. They maintained that the *ventral* or occipitotemporal pathway subserves "object perception" by identifying *what* an object is, and that the *dorsal* or occipitoparietal pathway subserves "spatial perception" by analyzing *where* objects are. In support of their proposal, they cited neuropsychological studies in humans involving surgery or brain damage and comparative studies in monkeys involving behavioral experiments in connection with brain ablation, electrophysiological measurements, and brain mapping. They acknowledged that previous investigators (studying amphibians and mammals) had distinguished *what* and *where* systems (Schneider 1967) or had made related distinctions (Held 1968; Ingle 1967; Trevarthen 1968). But they observed that these investigators had ascribed the spatial system to a "tectofugal" pathway, which in mammals involves the superior colliculus rather than a pathway through the LGN into primary visual cortex.

Subsequently, Goodale and Milner (1992) argued that there are two systems, but that they are not object vs. spatial systems (what vs. where); rather, they are respectively specialized for (1) conscious visual perception that engages cognitive resources for object recognition and identification as well as short-term and long-term memory ("what"), and (2) on-the-fly visually guided action (now called the "how" system). Milner and Goodale (2006) reported a consensus among investigators that the ventral system receives both parvocellular and magnocellular inputs via the LGN, whereas the dorsal system receives magnocellular inputs from the LGN but also from the superior colliculus (reviving, as a secondary source of input, the tectofugal pathway that Ungerleider and Mishkin 1982 had displaced). In fact, the anatomy of the two systems is quite complex and is still under investigation.

Although Ungerleider and Mishkin (1982) cast their finding as an *anatomical* discovery that both systems are cortical (at least in primates), a further review of the history shows a long interaction between anatomical and *psychofunctional* hypotheses, with functional hypotheses leading the way and anatomical findings helping to confirm functional conjectures. As it happens, despite a common perception that the "where" term in "what vs. where" implies mere spatial localization (e.g., Lindsay and Norman 1972, 169–74; Palmer 1999, 38–9), the original studies of Held (1968), Ingle (1967), Schneider (1967), and Trevarthen (1968) emphasized from the start that the "where" system was a spatial orienting system for guiding action. All four of these authors were trained as psychologists, and they used behavioral tests to support psychofunctional hypotheses. As an early review of this literature suggested, work in this area depends on well-developed psychological theories of perceptual function (Bishop and Henry 1971, 120). This observation fits well with the detailed elaboration in the early literature of functional distinctions between mechanisms that identify and evaluate objects (such as predators or prey) and mechanisms that allow the organism to orient and act toward those objects.

Goodale and Milner (1992) did not introduce the idea of separate action-guiding and object-perceiving systems. But they did develop new theoretical directions. First, they elaborated the hypothesis that the ventral system underlies conscious perception, whereas the dorsal system nonconsciously guides motor action, including both eye-movements (as was previously known) and fairly complex reaching behaviors and other visually guided behaviors, such as walking (Goodale and Milner 2004, Milner and Goodale 2006). This hypothesis was suggested to them by study of a subject with neurological deficits that severely restricted her conscious perception but left intact the action-guiding system. Second, they emphasized that both systems must include spatial processing. They suggest that the dorsal system uses egocentric representations, whereas the ventral system is concerned with spatial relations among objects in the scene. Further, using a variety of techniques, including behavioral tests of brain-damaged subjects and functional brain imaging of normal and brain-damaged subjects, they have evaluated various functional and anatomical models of systems for conscious, cognitively engaged perception and nonconscious, in-the-moment action-guidance. This area of work shows how neurophysiological evidence can support and even suggest functional hypotheses; but it does not support the notion that neuroscientific evidence is in some way more primary than psychological ("behavioral") evidence (see also Goodale and Westwood 2004).

Finally, from the early days of the "two visual systems hypothesis" in the 1960s, psychological theorists have understood that the activity of the two systems must be integrated (Ingle 1967, 50; Trevarthen 1968, 331). If one system evaluates the significance of objects and the other system modulates actions toward those objects, then the latter system must be triggered and guided by the evaluations of the former system as regards a significant object in a location. In Milner and Goodale's terms, the conscious representations of the ventral system, which include perception of the affordances or functional characteristics of objects in a location, must guide the action system, which does not have cognitive (function-representing) resources of its own. Milner and Goodale (2006, ch. 8) acknowledge the role of conscious visual representations in setting targets for and ensuring the functional appropriateness of the motions regulated by the action system, even if the precise mechanisms of interaction between the two systems remain unknown (see also Wallhagen 2007).

2.4. Color vision and opponent pathways

The golden age of visual science in the latter nineteenth century saw two competing accounts of color vision (Turner 1994, chs. 6–7). Helmholtz revived and extended Thomas Young's proposal that there are only three types of color sensitive elements in the retina, each of which responds maximally to a particular wavelength (Helmholtz 1867/1924–5, 2:134–46). Perceived color results from combining the stimulation from the three types of element. In opposition to this simple trichromatic model, Hering argued that color vision results from three opponent processes in the central nervous system, one serving red–green perception, one blue–yellow, and one black–white (Hering 1875b; Turner 1994, 130–4). Neither position was based on detailed knowledge of retinal anatomy and microphysiology. Indeed, the photic properties of the cones, which are the retinal elements subserving color vision, were directly measured only in the latter twentieth century (Kaiser and Boynton 1996, ch. 5). Helmholtz's arguments relied on color matching experiments (on both normal and color deficient observers), in which lights of known spectral composition are adjusted until they look the same. Hering's arguments appealed to similar types of measurements and to phenomenal observations. On phenomenal grounds, Hering contended that there are four color primaries: red, yellow, blue, and green. He argued that afterimages reveal adaptation effects among the four primaries, thereby revealing linkage in the underlying physiology: yellow produces a blue afterimage, red a green one, and so on. He also observed that color deficient individuals are always "red and green blind" (or "blue and yellow blind"), but are never simply "red blind" or "green blind." On these grounds he speculatively postulated yoked physiological processes underlying red–green and blue–yellow perception, which operate in opponent fashion, so that a red sensation arises when the red–green channel is driven in one direction, and a green sensation when it is driven in the opposite, or opponent, direction.

Subsequently, some theorists proposed that three types of retinal receptor might feed into central opponent mechanisms (Turner 1994, 182–3). Initially, there was no real acceptance of this compromise. Helmholtz's trichromacy theory dominated the literature, although Hering's theory continued to garner mention. During the 1930s and 1940s, the American biophysicist Selig Hecht and the British physicist W. S. Stiles, working in the trichromacy tradition, advanced colorimetric standards and helped to determine the properties of retinal receptors. Hecht's work confirmed that rhodopsin is the photoreceptive element in rods and Stiles determined more precisely the spectral sensitivities of the cones. As a physicist, Stiles did not delve deeply into post-receptor processes (Alpern 1988). Hecht (1928; 1934, 815–16) sustained the Helmholtzian belief that the three retinal receptors are literally "color receptors" that produce distinctive sensations, which are combined in the brain, and he ridiculed Hering's idea of opponent neural processes (1934, 817). The philosopher-psychologist Christine Ladd-Franklin (1929, 80) also ridiculed this notion.

In the 1950s, psychologists Leo Hurvich and Dorothea Jameson (1951, 1957) revived the opponent-process theory, arguing from psychophysical and phenomenal data alone, including especially data from some color mixture experiments (cancellation experiments, reviewed in Hurvich 1981, chs. 5–6). Their revival met considerable resistance (Hurvich and Jameson 1989, 187). But neurophysiology came to the rescue. In the 1930s, physiologists had begun to record from single neurons. These techniques were applied to retinal cells. The Finnish physiologist Ragnar Granit, who was also trained in psychology, was able to record electrophysiologically retinal responses to various lights in fish, frog, snake, and mammals, thereby establishing spectral sensitivity functions for receptors (Granit 1947, ch. 19). He rightly considered these curves to provide data that were independent of whether the animals possessed color vision (and so, independent of the mechanism of color vision). In discussing color vision, he offered support for Hering's notion that brightness is achromatically detected independently of color, but he stuck with Helmholtzian trichromacy for color itself (Granit 1947, ch. 22). However, he subsequently remarked that retinal recordings of antagonistic responses to light coming "on" and going "off" had, in a general way, vindicated Hering's notion that "there are two fundamental processes of opposite character in the retina" (Granit 1955, 78), although of course he still did not accept opponent color channels. The alleged physiological implausibility of antagonistic or opponent processes had, in Hurvich's view (1969, 502), unjustifiedly trumped the psychophysical evidence in favor of opponent color processes. In any event, Gunnar Svaetichin (1956) subsequently measured opponent neural responses in the retina, which he interpreted as supporting Hering's theory, which he knew from the physiological literature (Linksz 1952, chs. 4–5; Tschermak-Seysenegg 1952, ch. 3). Within ten years, the physiological psychologist R. L. DeValois and his colleagues found opponent responses in the lateral geniculate nucleus (DeValois *et al.* 1966).

The theory that the three types of cones in normal human eyes are linked neurophysiologically into opponent processes is now widely accepted (Kaiser and Boynton 1996, ch. 7) and is presented as the standard theory of color vision within psychology (Palmer 1999, 110–12). In this case, neurophysiological findings were interpreted in light of functional psychological theories of color processing so as to provide an added source of evidence for such theories.

In the four cases reviewed, psychophysics, behavioral research, and phenomenal observations led the way to the postulation and subsequent confirmation of neural mechanisms. Of course, this is not to say that researchers do not work the other way around, using neurophysiological findings to generate new research questions. Ken Nakayama (1990) contended that findings about brain anatomy called for new psychological theorizing. Neurophysiologists had found that a larger portion of cerebral cortex is devoted to vision than had been thought, and that the areas are highly subdivided. He observed that, for once, "it is the physiologists who seem to be leading the way, at least as far as higher visual functions are concerned." In order to redress "this imbalance between psychology and neurophysiology," he offered a "speculative theory as to the overall functional organization of the visual system" (Nakayama 1990, 411). Physiology had shown the existence of apparently specialized areas, and psychology would now propose a functional organization for them, drawing on work from cognitive psychology, psychophysics, physiology, and artificial intelligence. Peter Kaiser and Robert Boynton, co-authors of the standard handbook on human color vision, allow that in work on color vision findings from anatomy, neurophysiology, and photochemistry have sometimes inspired new psychophysical experiments, but they maintain that "the data of the psychophysicist, together with theories developed from such data, provide a framework within which the electrophysiologist conducts his research" (1996, 26–7). Which suggests that while physiological facts and theories may inspire or confirm research and theory cast in psychological language, psychological language remains the primary vocabulary for describing the functions being investigated, including those investigated in neuroscientific research.

3. The Neuropsychology of Memory: H.M. Revisited

Standing in contrast to the findings of Section 2, Patricia Churchland (1986, 1996) has claimed that in some areas of work neurological results have led the way to a radical rethinking of basic theoretical categories in psychology. She makes the boldest claim for work in memory, declaring that "some data discovered by neuropsychologists are so remarkable, and so contrary to common assumptions, that they suggest that some basic assumptions about memory may be in need of radical revision" (Churchland 1986, 150). What are these basic assumptions? Are they merely the assumptions of "folk psychology," or does she mean the assumptions of scientific (experimental) psychology? Although "folk psychology" is her usual target, Churchland here addresses experimental psychology directly. She asserts that psychological theory on topics such as memory is in a "*statu nascendi,*" its current level of development being "pretheoretical" (1986, 149, 153). But she finds cause for hope. Studies of amnesiac patients led some neuropsychologists "to postulate two memory systems, each with its own physiological basis" (1986, 371). The two systems in question are the *descriptive* and *procedural* memories of Squire and Cohen (1984). As Churchland (1986, 372) tells it, their observations on amnesiac patients led them to posit distinct memory subsystems of a sort radically different from those on offer from psychologists who study memory in the intact human.

The issue in question is not whether neurological observations are germane to psychological research on memory, but whether in this case neurological observation led to the introduction of new theoretical categories, and specifically, to the introduction of a novel distinction between descriptive and procedural memory systems. As it happens, in Squire and Cohen's case (Cohen and Squire 1980; Squire and Cohen 1984; Cohen 1984) the theoretical framework they adopted was drawn from previous work in experimental psychology, cognitive science, and philosophy, as were the motivation for the empirical questions they asked and the experimental procedures they used.

The relevant part of Squire and Cohen's work concerned preserved learning and memory capacities in amnesiacs. The "preserved" capacities are those unaffected or only partially affected by the cause of the amnesia. It was well known that amnesiacs who suffer severe memory deficits may show no effects for perceptual-motor learning and memory (Milner *et al.* 1968). Squire and Cohen asked whether other sorts of skills are preserved. In Cohen and Squire (1980), they showed that amnesiac patients could perform well on a pattern-analyzing skill, which involved reading mirror-reversed words.

444   HISTORY AND PHILOSOPHY OF PSYCHOLOGY

Although the patients could not remember previous trials, even from day to day, their performance showed dramatic improvement over three consecutive days of testing and in a retest three months later. Cohen and Squire (1980) interpreted their results in relation to proposals made by Kolers (1975) and Winograd (1975). Kolers (1975) used psychological experiments to study memory in intact adult humans. He interpreted his findings on sentence-recognition tasks (including tasks with geometrically reversed stimuli) by distinguishing between "operational or procedural" and "semantic or substantive" memory. Kolers drew this distinction from a discussion of "knowing how" vs. "knowing that" in a book on the philosophy of education by Israel Scheffler (1965), who in turn drew upon Gilbert Ryle's (1949) analysis of intelligent behavior. Winograd (1975) characterized the distinction between "knowing how" and "knowing that" as dividing procedural (programmed) from declarative (database) knowledge. In a subsequent review and expansion of their results, Squire and Cohen (1984, 37) articulated their distinction, drawing directly on Ryle (1949), on work in psychology (Bruner 1969), and on artificial intelligence (including Winograd 1975). Finally, Cohen (1984) retested the much-studied amnesiac H.M. on a cognitive skill that had been well studied by experimental psychologists, the "Tower of Hanoi" problem, and he further articulated the procedural–declarative distinction, again drawing on Ryle, Bruner, Kolers, Winograd, and other work in artificial intelligence.

In this case, the methods of testing, the framework for posing empirical questions, and the theoretical concepts used are drawn from previous work at a psychological or philosophical level of analysis. Moreover, Squire and Cohen (1984, 4) did not present their work as requiring revision of *psychological* ideas about memory, but as a challenge to previous views on amnesia as a unitary phenomenon (an assumption they attributed to previous work in *neurology*). They presented themselves as developing and extending theoretical conceptions of memory and skilled performance extant in the psychological and philosophical literatures. Tests on various clinical populations provided a source of data about ways in which the normal functioning of human memory could be disrupted. Here, neurological results did not require a fundamental rethinking of the basic categories of psychological theory, but they inspired a refinement of those categories and allowed them to be mapped onto brain loci known to be damaged in the amnesiac patients. This is "co-evolution" of psychology and neuroscience as Churchland (1986) would have it, but with the leading theoretical contribution coming from extant psychological theory, a contribution that Churchland missed in her portrayal of psychology as in a "pretheoretical" state on these issues.

This case study does not show that reflection on neurological results, or on images or other recordings of brain activity, could not challenge the fundamental categories of psychological theory. Nonetheless, the image of neuroscience as arriving at its results independently of previous psychological theory invokes a naive Baconianism that is implausible. Experimental findings of the sort achieved by Squire and Cohen require posing questions to nature. This is true even if nature (or surgical procedures) have provided a "natural experiment" through a brain lesion. Subjects' performances are evaluated through systematic tests, not casual observation. Systematic experimental procedures are devised against a background of previous theory and previous experimental paradigms. Even casual observations are interpreted against a background of theory. In the case of psychological capacities such as learning and memory, it is natural to suppose that psychological theory will provide the background.

Again, this is not to say that neurological observation and neurophysiological measurement have not and will not continue to contribute to the advance of psychological theory. Indeed, subsequent work in memory has seen continuing interaction between psychological and neuroscientific research. The "memory systems" approach favored by Squire (1987) and by experimental psychologists such as Tulving (1983, 2002) has remained prominent (Schacter and Tulving 1994), and its proponents find support from neuroimaging (Schacter *et al.* 2000). Data from animal studies, clinical observations, brain imaging, and experiments on normal children and adults are used in testing theories about the psychological structure of memory and its neurophysiological substrate (Foster and Jelicic 1999; Jonides *et al.* 2008). Neuroscience has not provided an independent source of theory, but rather an additional source of data to test theories of function, along with evidence for localization. These are real contributions. But, as we shall see in Section 4, it is unclear that neuroscientific data provide any firmer constraint on psychological theory than do other kinds of data.

4. The Brain as a Mental and Psychological Organ

Review of some central cases from psychological science and neuroscience shows that psychology has led the way in the study of the brain, at least so far. At the same time, bottom-up studies of nervous systems and brains were revolutionized during the twentieth century, as a result of new staining, recording, and scanning techniques. The discovery of neuronal cell structure, the discovery and classification of neural transmitters, the ability to directly measure neural activity, and the advent of brain imagery stand as real and independent contributions of neuroscience.

Given the rapid advances in brain science during the twentieth century, one might conjecture that the leading role played by psychology in my case studies was the product of the different growth rates of psychological and specifically neuroscientific knowledge. Knowledge of the microstructure of brain tissue and measurement of neural activity required the development of microscopic techniques and technology for recording and, subsequently, imaging brain activity. The technology that made these results possible is less than a century old, and the more sophisticated techniques have arisen only in the past two decades. By contrast, psychology, at least at the beginning, could operate with less equipment. It could get started taxonomizing psychological function on the basis of data available through observation of everyday experience or behavior. One might think that its descriptions served well in an instrumentally simpler day, before the advent of techniques that made possible a direct assault on the brain. But in these auspicious times one might expect, with Quine and Churchland, that as science advances psychology will wither and neuroscientific concepts will replace its mentalistic descriptions.

While granting the great advances in the direct study of the brain's proper-ties, I reject this line of reasoning. I think an argument is available to show that psychology must (for all practical purposes) provide the functional vocabulary for describing much of the brain's activity. To understand the brain we must come to understand not only its microanatomy and microphysiology, but its global functioning. Some of its global functions serve to control vegetative functions, such as breathing or digestion. But the brain is most famous for its role in realizing mental functions, including sense perception, memory, emotions, and higher cognitive abilities. The description of these functions is mentalistic. This mentalism does not restrict itself to a statically traditional vocabulary—the "folk psychology" of neurophilosophical lore—but it avails itself of the devel-oping technical vocabulary of psychological science. For example, as sensory psychology progressed, the "sense of touch" was partitioned into numerous sensory systems (for haptic form, pressure, temperature, and more), altering the traditional notion of the "five senses" (Scheerer 1995, 825, 851–6). In this case, a traditional classification was overturned as psychology advanced. Still, as sensory psychology has developed into a mature science, its language has remained mentalistic, including talk of information, representation, com-binatorial processes, experienced qualities, perceived intensities, and so forth. Similarly, the language of attention research, while it has grown more precise, shows continuity with centuries of reflection on the phenomena of attention, mentalistically described (see Ch. 13). The mentalistic language of psychology should not be equated with outdated tradition. It is a living vocabulary. And it is the primary vocabulary for describing global brain function. The brain is (largely) a mental and psychological organ.

These considerations provide the basis for a relatively straightforward argument to the effect that psychology must provide the primary theoretical vocabulary for describing many brain functions. The argument goes as follows:

(1) The operations of the brain can be partitioned into various subsystems, study of which constitutes study of brain function.
(2) Some of the functions realized by the brain are mental functions (e.g., perception, attention, memory, emotions).
(3) Psychology is the experimental science that directly studies mental functions.
(4) Hence, psychology is the primary discipline covering a major subset of brain functions.
(5) Although it may be possible on occasion to reason from structure to function, in general knowledge or conjecture about function guides investigation of structure.
(6) And so psychology leads the way in behavioral brain science.

The premises have various bases, some tending toward the conceptual, some hinting at the empirical. But as in any conceptual argument about science, all of the premises have an empirical component. (1) records the fact that the brain is a complex system with identifiable subsystems, the operations of which can usefully be studied in relative independence of the other subsystems. (2) is a descriptive fact about the functions known to be realized by the brain. While it may seem bald and contentious, it is supported by reflection on the practice of behavioral brain science. Consult, for instance, the major and minor subdivisions of standard textbooks in neuroscience (e.g., Kandel *et al.* 2000). Neuroscientists use a psychological taxonomy to describe brain systems. They parse the brain's operations into sensory, motor, motivational, and memory systems (Kandel *et al.* 2000, pt. 4), which are further subdivided into sensation and perception; reflexive and voluntary movement; arousal, emotion, and motivation; and language, thought, mood, learning, and memory (pts. 5–7, 9). Item (3) comes as close to a conceptual truth as any. Psychology just is the science that studies mental functions in their own right. The only way to "eliminate" psychology from any foreseeable neuroscience would be simply to declare that theories of mental brain functions will from now on be called neuroscientific rather than psychological. That would be a merely terminological shuffle—unless, of course, neuroscience someday inspired the total replacement of the functional language of psychology (as Churchland 1986 predicts). But that seems unlikely; sensory psychology, for one, seems rightfully entrenched in its overall conception of sensory function as guiding thought and action by putting organisms into contact with distal objects. (4) follows from (1)–(3). (5) is supported by reflection on the history of biological science and by the cases reviewed in Sections 2–3. It records the fact that, typically, knowledge or conjecture about function guides the investigation of structure. Structure is hard to see in the absence of functional description. (5) blocks the supposition that a neuroscience devoid of psychological content could frequently provide a "bottom-up" route to discovering global brain function. (6) follows from (4) and (5).

5. Constraint

Suppose for the moment that this argument is correct. What implications does it have for the deeply held intuition that neuroscience is more basic than, and strongly conditions, psychology?

One could argue that psychology leads neuroscience only because of the epistemic limitations of the investigators. Because we start from a position of ignorance, we need to move from function to structure. But once we come to understand brain structure, we will see how it limits brain function. This position is intuitively plausible. But to understand its import we should consider further the notion of constraint.

How does knowledge of one science constrain another? Once one under-stands chemistry, it becomes apparent that you cannot make water from carbon and nitrogen. The constituents constrain what can be done, or made, with them. Perhaps adequate knowledge of the brain would constrain psychology in the same way.

This I think is the model of constraint implicit in the intuition that neuroscience must constrain psychology. At a very general level, we can suppose that some constraint of this sort is known to us. We perhaps can be said to know that the nervous system of an earthworm is incapable of supporting philosophical reflection. Given the worm's ganglia, we see that it is unable to do philosophy; there are not enough circuits to permit deep reflection. (In fact, our belief here is largely guided by knowledge of earthworm behavior in relation to its ganglia, but let us ignore this for the sake of argument.) Beyond extreme and very general instances such as this, so little is known about how brains realize psychological states and processes that this sort of direct constraint from constituent structure has no consequences for practice, now or in the foreseeable future. Where neuroscience provides constraining data for psychology, it usually does so in the context of choosing between psychological theories by finding neurophysiological data to support one theory rather than another (as in the discovery of opponent cells in color vision).

A related intuition behind the idea that neuroscience constrains psychology is that physics is the basic science of what there is, and neuroscience is closer to physics than is psychology. Because physics is basic, it sets boundaries on what is possible. As a practical matter, this argument falls prey to the observation that in the present state of knowledge we have little or no idea about how physical properties limit the psychological properties that material objects, and brains in particular, can realize.

Still, the basicality of physics might be expressed through the notion of nomic asymmetry. It may seem self-evident that psychology cannot postulate processes that violate the laws of physics, whereas physics is unconstrained by psychology. But in our present state of knowledge, this claim simply does not hold. Consider an example. Let us suppose that physics precludes psychology from positing processes in which information is transmitted from one location to another so that it arrives faster than the speed of light. We have been conditioned to nod assent to this. But should we treat this restriction as apodictic? Is it inconceivable that a psychological finding could cause us to question this statement? I think not. Conceive this. Under tightly controlled conditions, someone on earth is able to repeat what someone on the moon is thinking, and to do so with a time difference less than the time required for light to travel from the moon to earth. Teams of experts verify the empirical finding. Billionaires get interested in the phenomenon, and they hire the best scientists, physicists included, to monitor the test. It is concluded that the test is fair. What shall we do now? Posit the existence of extraphysical information transmission? Or consider revising the speed-of-light limitation on physical transfers? The latter option would seem to be open. So in this case, psychological facts might call physical theories into question. More generally, if facts are facts and truth is truth, it strikes me that physical facts, and true physical theories, cannot conflict with psychological facts and true psychological theories any more than the latter can conflict with the former.

The effective upshot of the basicality assumption is an abstract ontological asymmetry between physics and psychology. There can be physical things with no psychological properties, but many believe that nothing with psychological properties can fail to be realized in matter. Psychological properties cannot float free of physical realization. This abstract constraint is far removed from theorizing about the actual psychological capacities realized in the brain, and from determining their relations to brain structures.

There are two additional, closely related intuitions that may help to explain the widespread notion that neuroscience is privileged over, and does or will control, psychology. The first is publicity: the brain is a physical object in the public domain. But an important area of psychology, the psychology of perception, concerns private objects, in the form of sensory experiences. So psychology is methodologically suspect. "Objective" knowledge is only of what is public.

This argument is interesting in the abstract, but it runs afoul of actual scientific achievement. The first areas of psychology to be made objective, in the sense of achieving repeatable quantitative results, were sensory perception and psychophysics (Hearnshaw 1987, ch. 9). A plausible description of the subject matter of psychophysics is that it charts the relations between physical stimuli and perceptual experience, as in the case of the trichromacy matching-results achieved in the nineteenth century. The right-hand term of laws in psychophysics, then, is the content of a mental state, the content of perceptual experience (see Shapiro 1995). The much-touted "privacy" of psychological states, whatever interest it might have, has not blocked the scientific study of such states.

The second intuition concerns an alleged contrast in empirical rigor between physics and psychology. Allegedly, physics is hard and objective, psychology is soft and subjective. According to Quine (1974, 36), psychological notions thrive in darkness, and they will dissipate when physics, or neuroscience, turns on the light. This argument relies on an inaccurate portrayal of the achievements of psychology. Typically, it relies on the construal of psychology as "folk psychology," that is, as a codification of (allegedly) ordinary ascriptions of beliefs and desires to explain behavior. But, as suggested above, the mentalistic vocabulary of psychology is a living body of scientific description. If it is to be challenged, it must be challenged on its own terms, and not, as often happens, by surreptitiously changing the subject so as to substitute so-called "folk psychology" for the corpus of scientific psychology. (On this point see also Ch. 2; Wilkes 1980.)

Psychology conditions and constrains brain science by providing the basic functional description of numerous brain systems. This means that epistemically and methodologically psychology must lead the way in the study of global brain function. Ontologically, psychological functions may constrain and condition brain structure itself. Brain structures presumably have evolved so as to realize advantageous psychological functions. For example, trichromatic color systems allow finer discrimination of objects by color than do dichromatic systems.

The neural structures underlying trichromacy presumably exist in populations because of the psychological function they perform (Thompson 1995, ch. 4). If this is so, then the ontology of the brain is affected diachronically, through selection for advantageous psychological functions. In this way, psychological function constrains brain ontology. (See Chs. 1, 8 and Hatfield 1999 for further discussion.)

6. Function and Explanation without Reduction

Beyond the diachronic selection of brain mechanisms that serve psychological functions such as color vision, reflection on the interplay between ontology and functional context supports a further point about the ontology of physiological structures. This point concerns how we individuate and classify neurophysiological structures. By their biomolecular properties? Or by their functional properties as realized in these biomolecular properties? In investigating this matter, I turn again to the physiology of color vision.

As reviewed in Section 2.4, color vision occurs in normal human perceivers when the outputs of three types of visual photoreceptors are compared to yield color responses. These photoreceptors function as *transducers* that mediate between the characteristics of light energy and neural responses that can then be processed to yield color vision (Palmer 1999, 29).

The discovery of the molecular properties of the photopigments that serve mammalian and other forms of vision and their genetic basis is a triumph of twentieth-century vision science (Nathans and Hogness 1983; see Yokoyama 2000 for a review). The molecular characterization of the photosensitive substances (opsins and retinals) might be viewed as an apparently plausible case of the reduction of a psychologically relevant function to a molecular basis. In the human eye, the three types of daylight photoreceptors (or cones) differ in their sensitivity to light across the visible spectrum. The different sensitivities are explained by the fact that (to simplify) each type of cone contains one of three types of light-sensitive photopigment with a maximum sensitivity in the short, middle, or long-wavelength regions of the visible spectrum.

A great deal is known about the structure of the cones, the placement of the photopigments, and the events that cause a cone to produce a neural response. Has, then, the human cone been reduced to its molecular basis? It seems not. The identification of the various light-reactive substances as color-specialized visual photoreceptors already places them in a functional context that makes reference to the psychological function of color vision.

This functional context is not reducible to bare molecular talk, for such talk does not contain the needed theoretical concepts and vocabulary to describe the functions involved: sensitivity to light in a way that yields color vision, where the latter is fundamentally tied to the representation of object surfaces as having color in virtue of their being experienced with a specific hue. (In organisms deemed not to possess conscious color experience, the relevant psychological vocabulary would describe color-mechanisms that mediate color-dependent discriminatory behavior.)

Consider more closely what photopigments are and what they do. Photopigments consist of proteins called opsins bound to a vitamin-A related substance called retinal. The opsin (protein) component exhibits greater variety than the types of retinal, and the two together yield the differing light-reactive characteristics of the various photopigments. When light strikes a photopigment, the retinal changes shape (and chemical state, from one isomer to another), inducing changes in the opsin. In the biological context of the cone cell, these changes alter the electrical properties of the cell membrane. This change propagates to the portion of the cell that adjoins a neuron and, by causing the release of chemical transmitters, affects the electrical charge of the neuron.

Should the photopigments be described as inherently photoreceptive? The various photopigments are characterized by their reaction to distinct wavelength-distributions of light. If that makes them photoreceptive, then the discussion can end: they are what they are by their molecular basis. But many substances are differentially affected by light of differing wavelengths. We are interested in what makes the opsin-retinal complex into a photoreceptor in the vision science sense: a transducer of light energy into neural activity that serves vision. The identification of cones as transducers and of the photopigments as differentially light-sensitive materials that serve color vision depends on functional context. The chemical properties of the opsins and retinals can help explain *how* the function of visual transduction is carried out. But the chemical kinds cannot by themselves provide the basis for individuating the photopigment as a visual transducer. Only by placing the photopigments in the functional context of the visual system can they properly be described as components of sensory transducers.

One way of appreciating this conclusion is to consider the diversity of functions that the photopigments play in various organisms. Many of these functions do not serve vision. Photopigments (opsin-retinal complexes) may originally have arisen in ancient green algae (Deininger *et al.* 2000) as a way of detecting light and maximizing the light environment so as to provide energy to their chlorophyll. Photopigments also mediate chameleon-like pigment responses in the skin of frogs (Arnheiter 1998). Such color-adaptive responses may serve to camouflage the animal, implying sighted predators. But it need not have arisen for that reason. Arnheiter (1998, 633) suggests that "light-dependent intracellular pigment redistribution may have been invented not for colour adaptation but for thermoregulation and photoprotection." Leaving aside the metaphor of "invention," photoreceptive cells yoked to pigment redistribution may have arisen to serve the nonvisual functions of heat regulation (by changing the reflective/absorptive characteristics of the skin) or protection from the organically damaging effects of short-wavelength light.

Knowledge of the genetic basis of the diverse photopigments has allowed insight into the possible mechanisms of evolution of mammalian trichromacy (Jacobs and Rowe 2004). In the primate line, trichromacy arose from a polymorphism in the longer-wavelength-sensitive cone. This polymorphism involved a second opsin (and so a second cone type) with maximum sensitivity shifted toward the middle-wavelength region. Further, knowledge of the genetic basis and molecular structure of cone types has fostered insight into the complex color abilities of some new-world monkey species, in which the males are dichromatic and the females may be either dichromatic or trichromatic. In addition, genetic techniques that identify human polymorphisms in the middle-wavelength cone have helped find the physiological basis for psychophysical variations (in color matching experiments) exhibited by "anomalous" trichromats and by normal trichromats (Neitz *et al.* 1993). In these cases, functional descriptions provide a context for type-identifying molecular structures. Independent means of detecting and identifying those molecular structures then feed back into knowledge of the evolution and current distribution of photoreceptor variants, thereby allowing explanation of fine-grained psychophysical findings (subtle variations in color matching experiments) by appeal to its physiological basis.

Nonetheless, even within the visual context, there can be no equation of short, middle, or long-wavelength sensitive cones with color-vision receptors. As explained in Chapter 8.4, animals with two cone types possess color vision only if they have a nervous system that compares outputs from cones of each type. Distinct cone types with maximum sensitivities in the short and middle-wavelength ranges may have arisen to serve monochromatic vision by heightening sensitivity in differing aquatic contexts, such as seeing prey against light streaming down from above, where sensitivity that matches the wavelength of the most intense light serves best, by comparison with seeing light-reflecting objects horizontally, in which case a peak sensitivity of the most intense illumination creates contrast with the background (McFarland and Munz 1975).

The conclusion that neurophysiological structures such as retinal cones cannot be individuated and typed by their molecular properties alone does not require that their molecular constituents exhibit multiple biological functions, as in the cases reviewed here. These multiple realizations illustrate that molecular kinds can serve multiple functions. But the point can rest entirely on the sort of consideration brought out in Section 4 (and adumbrated in this section): molecular description, even dynamic descriptions of molecular responses to agents such as light energy, is not (bio/psycho-) functional description. It tells us how something reacts, but not what that reaction does for a system, or even what system the reaction occurs in. For vision, there is no way of describing the relevant functions without invoking the psychological vocabulary of combining or comparing information (e.g., from different cone types) in the service of discriminating objects by color. The very being of a retinal cone is the being of a functional component that enters into the psychological processes that yield a color response. Taken out of context, the cone constituents are just molecules with various properties. They are sensory transducers only in the context of visual function.

7. Conclusions

Reflection on neuroscience and psychology suggests that psychology has and must condition and constrain neuroscience. In the area of sensory perception, knowledge of psychological function has led the way in the individuation and investigation of visual neurophysiology. In neuropsychological investigation of memory, psychological theories of memory provided the framework within which questions were posed in the study of deficits caused by brain damage. More generally, the very identity of neural structures depends on their functional description. And for many sensory and brain functions, that description is irreducibly psychological.

These conclusions do not suggest (*pace* Fodor 1975, 17) that neurophysiology is irrelevant to psychology or that psychological theorists have nothing to learn from neuroscientific measurements and findings. We have seen cases of interaction between neuroscience and psychology in Sections 2 and 6. In Section 2.4, the opponent process theory of color vision received confirmation from electrophysiological recordings. In Section 6, subtle differences among photoreceptors were located using genetic methods, and these differences helped explain psychophysical findings. Such examples could be multiplied from the brain imaging literature (as in Sec. 2.3).

The matter in question is not the relevance of neuroscience for psychology, but the notion that neuroscience is in some way more basic than psychology and that its facts constrain psychology in a way that psychological facts cannot constrain neuroscience.

The idea that neuroscience can or should deeply constrain psychology is based on two sorts of arguments. First, there are abstract arguments concerning publicity, mushiness, nomic asymmetry, and ontological asymmetry. The first three of these are unconvincing. Ontological asymmetry provides a general constraint on solutions to the mind–body problem. But it does not offer real guidance for contemporary psychology.

The second sort of argument, from constituent structure, is based on the hope that future understanding of the brain will permit strong constraints on the range of possible psychological functions to be read directly off descriptions of neural structure and activity. At present, constraints of this sort are at best very general, such as that earthworms cannot do philosophy. We can hope that knowledge of the brain's properties will progress to the point where this sort of constraint from constituent elements becomes available. But most likely, the identification of constraints from brain structure will involve reasoning from structures that have already been type-identified on functional grounds, as in the case of the photopigments that underlie color vision. Prior experience and current reflection suggest that as brain science develops, it does so through interaction with functional descriptions, with psychology leading the way. For neuroscientists who have emerged from the behaviorist physicalism of the mid twentieth century, that shouldn't be a bad thing.

16

Introspective Evidence
in Psychology

Introspection was once the mainstay of psychological research, the primary source of psychological evidence. But, as history would have it (e.g., Lyons 1986, chs. 1–2), in the first part of the twentieth century it was discredited by behaviorists in psychology and by the likes of Wittgenstein and Ryle in philosophy. These critics purportedly showed that introspection was unscientific, conceptually impossible, or akin to believing in ghosts. As a result, introspection "disappeared" as a source of evidence in psychology and philosophy alike (Lyons 1986).

This standard account, as most, contains a grain of truth. Introspection, broadly conceived, was once the primary source of evidence in experimental psychology—although it was never, in any period of psychology's long past, considered to be the only source of evidence (Hatfield 2003*d*; Titchener 1912*a*). Even as one among several sources of evidence, introspection was in decline by the middle of the twentieth century, both in philosophy and psychology, largely but not exclusively because of attack from the behaviorists. Although the use of introspective evidence was not fully abandoned, criticisms from within psychology put an end to *analytical introspection*, narrowly defined to mean a specific method of seeking the "atomic" elements of experience.

Recently, interest has revived in introspection, in two contexts. In connection with questions about first-person knowledge, some authors have offered positive accounts of self-knowledge of some mental states, especially opinions and convictions (e.g., Moran 2001). In connection with theories of

First published in Peter Achinstein (ed.), *Scientific Evidence: Philosophical Theories and Applications* (Baltimore: Johns Hopkins University Press, 2005), 259–86, copyright © 2005 by Johns Hopkins University Press. Reprinted with permission.

consciousness, the question of introspective access to the self, or to private conscious states, has drawn considerable attention (e.g., Armstrong 1980; Lycan 1997). All the same, the notion of introspective awareness of specifically phenomenal aspects of perceptual states remains deeply suspect (Dretske 1995b, ch. 3; Jackson 1998, ch. 4; Tye 1995, ch. 5).

I am a friend of introspection. I introspect regularly. I think I find things out—though not everything there is to know, even about my own mind. I turn to introspection frequently in thinking about perceptual experience and in testing claims made by perceptual psychologists. More importantly, I believe that introspection maintains an ineliminable role in psychology itself, as a source of evidence. This is especially apparent in perceptual psychology, which will be my ultimate focus.

In preparation for examining the place of introspective evidence in scientific psychology, I begin by clarifying what introspection has been supposed to show and why some concluded that it couldn't deliver. This requires a brief excursus into the various uses to which introspection was supposed to have been put by philosophers and psychologists in the modern period, together with a summary of objections. I then reconstruct what I take to have been some of the actual uses of introspection (or related techniques, differently monikered) in the early days of experimental psychology. Here, I distinguish broader and narrower conceptions of introspection, and argue that recent critics have tended to misdescribe how introspection was supposed to work. Drawing upon the broader conception of introspection, I argue that introspective reports are ineliminable in perceptual psychology. I conclude with some examples of such ineliminable uses of introspective reports in both earlier and recent perceptual psychology.

1. Introspective Objectives

Introspection, broadly conceived, describes a mental state or activity in or through which persons are aware of properties or aspects of their own conscious experience. Being aware that one feels cold, is seeing red, or is worried, if mediated by awareness of conscious experiences that include feeling cold, seeing red, or feeling worried, are all instances of introspection. This broad description (which I refine below) is intended to cover the variety of uses ascribed to introspection in the history of philosophy and psychology.

Introspection has been undertaken with the aims of both self-knowledge and knowledge of self or mind. Self-knowledge, the use of introspection most typically discussed now by philosophers (e.g., Armstrong 1980; Moran 2001; Myers 1986; Shoemaker 1996), is knowledge of what is peculiar to a given person. This may include their beliefs and memories, and also may describe allegedly private states of consciousness (experiences of sense data were supposed to be such). By contrast, the search for knowledge of the self or mind is undertaken with the aim of attaining general, or intersubjectively common, descriptions of the self or mind. This general knowledge is to be achieved via introspective observations and their report. Psychophysics, in which subjects might match stimuli according to their appearances in specified circumstances, is an example. In such cases, introspection is supposed to serve as a basis for generalizations about all (or most) human selves or minds.

With this distinction between differing aims for introspection in place, let us consider the most important objectives for introspection, actual or purported, in the history of philosophy and psychology.

Explicit appeal to introspection is found in Augustine and Aquinas, and such appeals became widespread and prominent in the seventeenth century (Lyons 1986, ch. 1). Descartes especially is linked with the early history of introspection. His *Meditations* contain a studied turning away from the body, a "looking within" to find the foundations of knowledge. Purportedly, he discovered these foundations in incorrigibly known states of mind, from which he sought to infer the properties of a world beyond the mind.

What did Descartes claim to find when he turned inward? Opinions vary. Later philosophers, including Hume and Kant, argue as though Descartes or his rationalist descendants claimed to perceive the soul as a simple substance by a kind of direct inspection. Such perception of the soul or mind is our first purported objective for introspection:

(1) To perceive the mind as a simple substance.

Hume and Kant did not describe what they believed Descartes and other philosophers held this perception to be like: they merely asserted that *they* did not find a simple soul manifest in their own inner experience.[1] One

---

[1] Hume (1739–40), 252: "when I enter most intimately into what I call myself, I always stumble on some particular perception or other, of heat or cold, light or shade, love or hatred, pain or pleasure. I never can catch myself at any time without a perception, and never can observe any thing but the perception." Kant (1781/1787), A 355: "It is however obvious that through the *I* attached to thought the subject of inherence is designated only transcendentally, without noting any quality in it whatsoever, or in general being acquainted with or knowing anything from or of it"; also Kant (1781/1787), A 346/B 404, A 360, B 408, 420. As is usual, "A" and "B" refer to the original pagination of the first and second editions of Kant (1781/1787).

might assume that they believed Descartes and others had claimed to "see" a punctiform entity, a speck of immaterial substance.[2]

Although there was talk in the early modern period of whether the soul should be regarded as a point, Descartes refused to attribute to the soul any predicates derived from extension (1641/1984, 266). More importantly, he never claimed to perceive directly the soul itself as a simple substance. Rather, he claimed to perceive important features of the "nature of mind" via reflection.[3] According to Descartes, the mind manifests various characteristic types of experiences and various types of mental activity in relation to those experiences, which include perceiving through the senses, making judgments about such perceptions, imagining, remembering, understanding, or willing various things, feeling bodily sensations such as hunger and pain, and undergoing various passions or emotions—or at least seeming to do, feel, or undergo these acts and experiences (1641/1984, 19). From further reflection on and conceptualization of these mental activities, Descartes arrived at some conclusions about the nature of the human mind: that it is essentially an immaterial substance, that intellect and will are the two basic faculties of mind, and that mind is distinct from but interacts with the human body (1644/1985, 204, 208–19).

We thus have another objective for introspection:

(2) To discern the nature of mind.

Descartes claimed to meet this objective through an intellectual perception (or intuiting) of the essence of mind: not by "seeing" a speck, but by understanding an essence. Alternatively, the objective of knowing what a mind is might be met by describing what it does, that is, by cataloguing various mental activities. This more specific objective is:

(3) To discern the characteristic states and activities of mind.

---

[2] Neither philosopher ascribes this view directly to an opponent, but they do make clear that it would be inappropriate to view thoughts or the soul as mathematical points or as directly perceivable objects. Hume (1739–40), 235: "Neither ought a desire, tho' indivisible, to be consider'd as a mathematical point." Kant (1783/2004), 90: "to think of the soul as a simple substance already amounts to thinking of it as an object (the simple) the likes of which cannot at all be represented to the senses." A mathematical point is not visible, hence could not be seen; Kant might instead be alluding to the idea that "things in themselves" have no spatial properties at all, hence cannot even be described as points.

[3] In his correspondence, Descartes (1991, 306, 354–5, 356–7) distinguished between merely having a sensation and reflecting upon, or becoming aware of, the facts about and characteristics of the sensation (or other act of mind). Both sorts of mental state are "conscious," but the first sort may not happen to be remembered. Further, the reflective act is performed by the "pure intellect," and it is characterized as a "perception" that takes the sensation (or other act of mind) as its object. These reflective acts are akin to "introspection" considered as the perception of facts about a mental state. I discuss Descartes on consciousness in Hatfield (2003b), 122–5, 325–7.

An example of such a characterization is the claim (made prominent in the eighteenth century) that the three main divisions of mental life are perceiving, feeling, and desiring, rather than (as Descartes had it) perceiving and willing only.

Those investigating the mind by reflecting on their experience might observe that they can know more particular qualitative and temporal features of their mental states, or at least of those available in consciousness. Such features might include the division of sensory perceptions into various quality-groups, or *modalities*, such as vision, touch, hearing, taste, and smell. Such investigators might claim to compare the intensities or durations of various sensations, feelings, desires, and thoughts. This objective is:

(4) To ascertain the qualitative features and temporal relations of conscious states.

Such claims can be found in Descartes, but also in Hume, the mental geographer (1748/1999, 93). In the latter part of the nineteenth century, experimental psychology took as two of its principal aims (*a*) characterizing quality-groups through the experimental techniques of psychophysics, and (*b*) measuring temporal relations in mental processes.

One might hope, from observations of such qualitative features and temporal relations, to discover or infer the basic psychological processes or operations of the mind. We thus have a more specific version of (3), which is our fifth aim:

(5) To discover or infer the character of mental or psychological processes.

This aim was vigorously pursued in various theoretical contexts in the late nineteenth and early twentieth centuries. On the basis of observations, various psychologists claimed to discover of psychological processes:

(5.1) That they involve pure acts of intellect or imageless conceivings.
(5.2) That they are always imagistic.
(5.3) That such processes manifest genuine activity, as in attending or willing.
(5.4) That some processes are unconscious.

Findings (5.1) and (5.2) report the opposing views in the imageless-thought controversy that raged in the early twentieth century (on which, see Kusch 1999). Some psychologists claimed to discover a phenomenology of thought processes in the absence of any mental images. Others claimed that thought is always directed toward or involves images. During the same period, psychologists disagreed over whether instances of genuine psychological activity

are found introspectively (5.3), or whether in fact we have available only experiences that are not direct manifestations of activity even though the language
of "activity" is used to label them (see James 1912). Many psychologists in
the nineteenth century (and before) used introspective evidence as a basis
for positing unconscious (or perhaps "unnoticed") psychological processes
or operations (5.4) that yield conscious experience, while others sought to
rule out such processes (see Hatfield 1990b, chs. 2–5; 2003d). These various
areas of disagreement fueled the fires of behaviorists and other enemies of
introspection.

Uses (1) to (4) are found in earlier philosophical and psychological writings.
Uses collected under (5) were taken up by the new experimental psychology
in the nineteenth century. Use (4) and some parts of (5) are or should be of
interest in philosophy and psychology today.

Philosophers interested in epistemology also have made claims for the power
of introspection (or "immediate perception") of perceptual data. In the first
half of the twentieth century, sense data were said to be immediately perceived
objects of perception, perhaps incorrigibly known, and in any case the basis
for all other empirical knowledge. We thus have a sixth use:

(6) To perceive (incorrigibly known?) sense data, as the foundation for
    other knowledge.

Such data were supposed to provide an initial basis from which to construct or infer the external world and other minds, and sometimes they
were regarded as private. Bertrand Russell (1919) developed this talk of
"construction," which ultimately led him to a position of "neutral monism" that he shared with Ernst Mach and William James (Hatfield 2002c;
Ch. 10). On this view, only sense data (or rather "momentary particulars")
exist; external objects and minds (including one's self) are constructions from
such data. Adherents of a "representative" theory of perception treat private
sense data as the epistemic basis for knowledge of really existent external
objects and other minds (as in Russell 1912, 11–12 and ch. 2; Ayer 1958,
chs. 2–3, 5).

Finally, introspection has been taken to provide individual knowledge about
the self. To the extent that Augustine's *Confessions* are seen as the report of
a personal spiritual journey, they contain introspective reports of Augustine's
personal experiences and reactions. This gives us a seventh use:

(7) To know the particularities of one's self (hopes, aspirations, beliefs).

This is introspection as affording self-knowledge, that is, as providing privileged
access to specifically first-person facts. The extent to which this source of

knowledge can provide full insight into one's beliefs and desires has long been questioned. But the notion that at least some specifically first-person knowledge is available retains many advocates.

Of these uses, the first five purport to provide evidence for claims about mind, or mental states and processes, in general. They are not intended to provide special knowledge of an individual's own thoughts and beliefs, but are instead aimed at what I above termed "knowledge of self or mind": knowledge of the characteristics of the mind, or of mental processes, in general. In this context, individual introspective observations are taken to reveal characteristics common to all minds. The claims made on behalf of such uses range from knowledge of the nature of mind, as in (2), to knowledge of its states and processes, as in (3) to (5).

Uses (6) and (7) focus on knowledge specific to individuals. Use (7) in particular describes the sort of introspection (broadly conceived) that has been defended of late, under the title "first-person knowledge," by moral psychologists such as Moran (2001) and epistemologists such as Shoemaker (1996). They observe that, in many such cases, we attain self-knowledge by *deliberating* about what we hope or believe. Because they are *our* deliberations, we attain a specifically first-person knowledge of our beliefs, in the very act of deciding what they are. Moran (2001, 11–20) distinguishes this sort of first-person access from introspective knowledge of the phenomenal aspects of perceptual experience, which he thinks has been discredited. He associates the latter sort of "introspection" with a "perceptual model" of first-person knowledge that allegedly is directed toward a special inner object.

Although uses (6) and (7) fit the broad conception of introspection described above (since they involve conscious awareness of an allegedly private perceptual object, or of one's convictions), they are not my focus here. My primary concern is with reports or responses that serve as evidence for the characteristics of perceptual experience. Such reports or responses were conceived by earlier advocates—and should, I will argue, be so conceived today—as providing intersubjectively valid observational knowledge of (at least some of) the characteristics of perceptual states (and other sorts of mental states). The remainder of this chapter therefore leaves aside the specifically personal knowledge that has been the focus of some recent philosophers, and considers introspection as a source of evidence for general statements about mind, ultimately focusing on its use in providing scientific evidence in the study of perception. In considering objections to introspection in the next section, I therefore focus on uses (1) to (5); ultimately, I seek to vindicate aspects of uses (4) and (5).

2. Objections to Introspective Evidence

Many objections have been raised against actual or alleged uses of introspective evidence. Some of these objections are powerful and on target, while others have been based on a misdescription or caricature of introspective evidence or its objectives. I want to consider some telling objections, which limit the scope of introspective knowledge, and some misdirected objections, which I hope can be put aside.

Against use (1), which seeks direct introspective awareness of the soul or self as a simple substance, Hume's and Kant's reflections, as described above, are persuasive. However, alleged direct phenomenal acquaintance with the soul as a substance was not a mainstream position among metaphysicians of the soul (e.g., Descartes or Leibniz). Rather, they used arguments (which might include phenomenally based premises), rather than direct inspection, to arrive at their conclusions. In any case, it should be granted that introspection does not directly reveal the soul as a simple substance.

The more plausible claim of Descartes and others was that introspection revealed the nature of mind by revealing its characteristic states and activities as in use (2). In this use, Descartes and others could allow that the mind is only perceived through its properties (acts and states); perception of these properties allows one to grasp the mind's essence or nature. I suppose that few philosophers today believe that the "nature of mind" can be discerned in this way, in part because there are now few philosophical dualists who believe mind to be a separate substance with its own nature or essence. But even if we take "nature of mind" more broadly, to include functionally defined characteristics that have been popular of late (e.g., the mind is constituted of symbol-crunching processes), few to none would believe that this nature can be discovered directly through introspection.

Use (3) aims at discerning "the characteristic states and activities of mind." This objective supposes that such characteristic states are accessible to consciousness. Yet it is widely accepted today that many cognitive processes are not accessible to consciousness. One needn't endorse the Freudian unconscious to make this point. Cognitive psychology observes that many processes underlying perception and cognition—from simple visual capacities such as stereoscopic vision, in which minute spatial differences between the two retinal images are compared, to the recognition of a friend by her appearance—take place outside consciousness. While the *results* may be available to consciousness (in the experience of depth, or in the conscious recognition), the processes are not manifest. Acceptance of the point that some mental states and processes are not present to consciousness would not preclude introspection as a source of evidence, but it would limit its scope.

Three further objections have long been urged against uses (4) and (5). The first charges that introspection is unreliable; the second casts aspersion on its object; the third proclaims it to be conceptually impossible. The charge of unreliability was prominent in J. B. Watson's arguments against introspective psychology. He pointed to several examples, including the imageless-thought controversy, disagreements over the number of "degrees" of attention, and disagreements over the number of elemental sensations (Watson 1914, 6–7). These charges seek to undermine the use of introspection, as in (4) and (5), for determining the character of mental or psychological processes and the fundamental elements entering into them by observing the qualitative features and temporal relations of conscious states.

If the aim of psychological introspection is to find the "least elements" of mind, or to reveal fully the fundamental acts of mind (as in levels of attention), then Watson's charges stand. However, the problem may not be with introspection itself, but with the theoretical framework in which it was used. The notion that there are "least elements" of sensation to be discerned introspectively is, as James and the Gestalt psychologists (among others) observed, a theoretical construct. No one ever experiences a bare "least element" of sensation; such elements are posited by theory (see Hatfield 1990b, chs. 4–5). If the theory is wrong, then the sought-for least elements will not be discovered. As for the notion of "levels" of attention, it may have been an attempt to attribute overly fine phenomenological distinctions to the dynamics of attention. In a wider context, introspective techniques (broadly construed) are still used in studying attention, and to good effect (as discussed below). Finally, the imageless-thought controversy attempted to use introspection to discern facts about the content and structure of higher cognitive processes. The techniques were in many ways dissimilar from those used to elicit introspective reports in perception, because the object of experience was less restricted and defined. Such methods, which were sometimes called "systematic experimental introspection," came in for strong criticism from other introspective experimentalists (as reviewed by E. B. Titchener 1912b). Presumably, the adjective "systematic" was supposed to promote the legitimacy of the techniques in question, in which subjects might simply be asked to record observations on their thought processes after having carried out a given cognitive task. We may agree with Titchener's (1912b) conclusion that this form of introspection is of dubious reliability. However, the question of the reliability of introspective techniques in other contexts remains open.

The remaining two objections seek to rule out the possibility of introspection by casting aspersion on its objects or by claiming that it is conceptually impossible. These objections start from the assumption that to characterize introspection as "inner perception" or "inner observation" is to presuppose a special inner object. In the case of sense perception, which is my focus in this chapter, this object is supposed to be an existent thing that is distinct not only from external objects but also from perceptual experiences that are of external (as opposed to inner) objects. The existence or the knowability of such inner objects is then challenged on various metaphysical and epistemological grounds. I take up these two types of objection in turn.

Metaphysically, it has been suggested that experiential states containing their own mental or subjective content should not be countenanced, because to do so would be like believing in ghosts or other "unnatural" entities. Watson (1914, 20) and B. F. Skinner (1963) championed this sort of claim, and it can be found in many recent philosophers who would banish all mentalistic notions that cannot be "naturalized." Such philosophers may hold that notions such as "information" and "representation" *can* be naturalized by employing an engineering conception of "information" that rests on natural relations (such as conditional probabilities) among properties or states of affairs. Hence, the notion of representation may be retained, but, they argue, qualitative experiential states would be spooky entities that don't fit into a naturalistic outlook (e.g., Rey 1997, 255, 301).

This argument is directed against the alleged object of introspective awareness. It denies that introspection can provide a distinctive source of knowledge of the phenomenal, on the grounds that in order to do so, introspection would have to be directed upon a phenomenal object of dubious metaphysical status. It seeks to restrict the sort of evidence that psychologists should countenance, on the basis of a metaphysical assertion about what is natural and what is not. And yet the basis for the claim of what does or does not "belong to nature" is not spelled out. With the decline of philosophers' presumptions to have distinctive *a priori* insights into the fundamental elements of nature, such claims must in some way make contact with empirical knowledge. One typical way to decide on the range of natural states, processes, and objects is to look to the generalizations of the natural sciences. But if psychology is included among the natural sciences, the question of whether introspectible experiential states are found in nature reduces to the question of whether they are the object of generalizations (or other scientific assertions) in psychology. Philosophers' intuitions about what is natural and what is not would in this case give way to the question of what is being (or can be) studied in, and what is posited by, perceptual psychology (discussed in Sec. 3).

Turning to the epistemological objection, introspection is supposed to be conceptually impossible because it would require inward-looking descriptions of a sort that will not bear scrutiny. Wittgenstein's "private language argument" is supposed to tell against such descriptions. As the story goes,[4] the language in which we describe our perceptual experience is parasitic upon, and perhaps presupposes the existence of, external objects. As it was sometimes put, "is red" is more fundamental than "looks red." This means that our descriptions always start from attributions of properties to publicly perceivable things. From this, it is concluded that there is no conceptual space for knowledge or description of what is private or internal. Such descriptions would be forced to employ concepts proper to external objects, which is incompatible with the purportedly private status of their objects. Hence, the old idea that we start from awareness of inner states, so described, and work out to awareness, belief, or knowledge of an external world would be conceptually undermined. On this argument, uses (4) to (6) are ruled out.

Any reply to this argument must distinguish various purposes one might have in attempting to describe one's phenomenal experience. If one proceeds from the traditional philosophical aim of describing the foundation or basis for knowledge of the external world, then, if that foundation or basis is supposed to be conceptually independent of beliefs or knowledge about an external world, the "private language" argument could have some bite. But if the aim of describing or attending to phenomenal experience is simply to discover how things look, in the sense of how the world is perceptually presented to observers under specified conditions, then the matter is not so clear. In these circumstances, I might use the descriptive language applied to external objects in order to direct attention to aspects of how those objects are experienced. This is the case in contemporary perceptual psychology, which supposes that one can describe one's own experience using terms that are also used for describing the properties of external objects.

Let us take an example from color perception. In asking for reports on the colors of things, psychologists may instruct subjects to distinguish between the color they take an object actually to have, and the way in which the object looks or appears.[5] If, as I examine a piece of paper on my desk, I am asked

---

[4] I leave aside the question of whether Wittgenstein (1953) actually intended his "private language argument" to tell against introspective awareness; the matter is under dispute (Sluga 1996).

[5] This introduces a phenomenal-report sense of "looks," which is distinct from Austin's (1962) notion of "looks" as indicating doubt about the reality of things or the reliability of current perception. Mundle (1971, 15–20) admirably defends a phenomenal-description sense of "looks." (I confess to disagreeing with some of Mundle's phenomenal reports, as when he takes "perspectival shape" to indicate the "real" looks of things, 1971, 27–8.)

what color the paper looks to be, I may unhesitatingly say that it looks white. I perceive it to be white. An experimenter might then ask me to attend carefully to how the paper looks, and to respond to whether it appears with the same whiteness all over. Noting my uncertainty about the task, the experimenter may explain that I am to distinguish the question of whether I would judge or estimate the paper to be uniformly white (as opposed to being dyed or otherwise colored at any place), from my report on its current *appearance* as regards sameness or variation of color quality. Under such instructions, I report (let us imagine) that although I certainly judge the paper to be the same white everywhere, and I do so because of how it looks, nonetheless the paper appears darker and lighter in different areas across its surface, and it has a reddish tinge in one portion. Warming to the task, if I were next asked to go beyond simply describing the paper's appearance and to explain why it looks this way, I would say that because of its slight curvature and the direction of the light, the paper appears darker and lighter across its surface, and that it is next to a red ceramic cup that has reflected some reddish light onto it. I would still have no doubt that the paper *is the same white* across its entire surface. I would not say that it looks to me as if it is a piece of paper that is white in some areas but has been colored darker (or grey) in another area, and red in yet another. It looks to me as uniformly white paper does in many ordinary circumstances. All the same, I am able to use terms such as "white," "grey," and "red" to describe the varying appearance across the surface of the paper (even if I were myself unable to explain those appearances, but simply reported how the paper looked).[6]

In these circumstances, the experimenter has co-opted my ability to use color words to recognize the colors of objects by asking me to describe subtle variations in appearance. If I were claiming that the descriptions of the appearance were epistemically primary and provided the conceptual basis for constructing my knowledge of the external world, I might be in trouble. But if the aim is simply to describe in detail how the paper looks—where I've distinguished the attempt to describe the paper's appearance from what I would conclude about how the paper is physically constituted—then this problem about what is conceptually primary does not arise. I may develop and elaborate concepts of the phenomenal using whatever materials are available, including predicates normally used to describe external objects.

[6] In the technical literature of color perception, some theorists use the term "lightness" for the perceived object color of the paper itself (as white or grey), and "brightness" for the phenomenal variations of darker or lighter white (Rock 1975, 503–4). In this technical context, it is incorrect to say the paper looks "greyer" in a certain region, when this is not intended to ascribe an object color (pigmentation) to that region. But in nontechnical language, shadow may be described as "greying" a region of the paper.

Recently, another objection has been raised against "inner" description or describing the looks of things. It is a phenomenal objection, based upon a report of "how things look." According to this objection, phenomenally our experience seems to be "out there," not "in here." But introspection is supposed to be a "looking within" and is supposed to take as its object something besides the external object.

This objection has been stated by many authors (e.g., Dretske 1995b, 54, 62; Harman 1990; Tye 1995, 30). Georges Rey sums it up as follows: "as a number of writers (e.g. Harman 1990, Dretske 1995) have stressed, a great deal of what passes for introspection of one's 'inner' experience consists of reports about how the *outer* world seems: we don't so much report on the features of the 'inner movie' as upon what that movie *represents* (e.g. that *barns* seem red, *the sky* a dome)" (Rey 1997, 136–7). That is, we don't seem phenomenally to be attending to a special inner object. Rather, when asked to report, say, on the color of a piece of paper, it seems to us that all we see is a piece of paper.

Rey (1997, 136) describes this as a "problem" for introspection. How so? In fact, two points are compressed together here. Harman (1990), Dretske (1995b), and Tye (1995) all wish to reduce qualitative content in perception to the bare representation of properties of external objects. Hence, they deny that in perceptual experience we are presented with qualities that arise from how we subjectively represent objects (what Tye 2002 calls "qualities of experience"), such as is thought to be the case if we treat color as a subjective quality that serves as a mere "sign" for its cause in the object (Ch. 5). They don't want there to be features of our experience that depend on the subject's way of representing things, rather than on external-world content about objects. This sort of point cannot, of course, be decided just by reporting on the "diaphanous" or "transparent" character of our experience (names for the fact that in visual perception we seem to see the external world directly, without anything intervening, particularly not our own mental states); it depends on a substantive account of the metaphysics of perceptual qualities (such as color). But surely a decision on the metaphysics of qualities shouldn't be required before we can decide whether it is possible to describe phenomenal aspects of our perceptual experience. For even if these authors were right about the metaphysics, we could still ask how the external thing looks. Hence, this part of their "transparency" position is not relevant to my inquiry into the use of introspection as a source of evidence in psychology. The question of whether we can report on our experience does not require a prior solution to the metaphysical problem, even if such a solution might influence our view of what there is to report.

This brings us to the second point, which concerns what it is like to attend to our own experiences. The phenomenological point about transparency is supposed to undermine a notion of introspection as describing "inner" experience.[7] Our experiences seem "transparently" to be of external things; we don't seem to be aware of some inner object. But introspection is supposed to be "inner." Hence, at least in the case of sense perception, introspection does not find its intended object and so can be dismissed.

This objection is founded upon a misconstrual, or caricature, of how introspection has long been supposed to work. If we distinguish (a) the metaphysical question of whether introspection is directed upon objects that are distinct from external objects (as either "sense data" or "phenomenal qualities" might be), from (b) the phenomenal locating of the objects of introspection, we will find that very few authors in the history of psychology or philosophy held that the qualitative features of sense perceptions are experienced as phenomenally "inner" in a spatial sense. The early experimental psychologists who advocated introspection certainly did not. The relevant question, then, is not whether experienced qualities seem to be "in here" or "out there," but whether any relevant differences exist between simply observing external objects and observing characteristics of the experiences we have in doing so. Classical experimental psychology held that such differences exist. This point requires elaboration.

3. Actual Practices of Introspection in Psychology

The notion of introspection was refined over the course of the nineteenth century, partly in response to various charges that introspective observation is impossible. Comte (1830−42/1855, 33) argued that direct introspection of mental processes is not possible, because it would interrupt itself. The

---

[7] Our authors offer various views on introspection, but Rey (1997, 136−7) presents the "transparency" point as a problem for the phenomenology of introspection. Harman (1990) is directly negative about the possibility of introspection. Dretske (1995b, ch. 2) allows introspection in the form of beliefs about the content of perception, but thinks it can have no experiential content or phenomenology peculiar to it. Tye (1995, 2002) is the most liberal in his willingness to countenance introspective experiences, but he goes to heroic lengths to preserve the theory that their content is exhausted by external-world content; thus, in the case of things that look blurry (due to nearsightedness, let us say), he maintains that the content is as of a vague or blurred object in the world, thereby avoiding ascribing any specifically subjective content (Tye 2002). As stated in the text, my arguments in this chapter supporting introspection do not rely on any particular conception of the metaphysics of sensory qualities; elsewhere, I support the view that subject-dependent phenomenal qualities exist (Chs. 5, 10).

initial response to this charge was to grant that, although any attempt to observe our own thought processes directly would interrupt itself, we can "observe" by seeking to remember our thought processes just after they have taken place (J. S. Mill 1865, 64); introspection could operate via memory. Franz Brentano (1874/1995, 29–36) refined this response by allowing that introspective *observation* is possible only through memory, but he contended that there is also a kind of "incidental" perception of our mental states while we are having them. He called the fleeting awareness that we are having a certain sort of mental state an "inner perception," distinguishing it from introspection proper, which he called "inner observation."

These discussions took place before the widespread use of introspective techniques in experimental settings, which increased dramatically after 1880. At first, experimental psychologists such as Wilhelm Wundt agreed with Brentano's point that self-observation (*Selbstbeobachtung*) of mental states and processes is unreliable because it interrupts itself (Wundt 1882/1885, 136–7). But he soon reversed himself on this point and refined his position.

In a lengthy study on introspection, Wundt (1888) distinguished unaided inner perception from experimentally assisted self-observation (psychological introspection proper). He characterized self-observation as the "deliberate and immediate observation of inner processes" (1888, 297). The key terms all require explanation.

"Deliberate" implies that the subject directs his or her attention on the states or processes being observed. Although deliberate observation need not be previously planned (a botanist may observe with deliberateness a specimen that she has found serendipitously during a walk), it does suggest that the observer is paying careful attention to the object of observation. Wundt described "scientific observation" as the "deliberate direction of attention to the phenomena" (293). The observer is prepared to discriminate or discern characteristics of the observed phenomena, and to remember the results of such discrimination. The observer may direct his or her attention to selected aspects of the phenomena. Without this directing of attention, mere "inner perception" may allow us to be aware of the contents of our minds, but not in the deliberate manner of introspection. Introspection proper involves deliberate consideration with the intent of discriminating among psychological states or processes.

"Immediate" rules out the sort of memory-mediated introspection that Mill and Brentano allowed. According to Wundt, observation requires the presence of what is observed. Hence, retrospection does not count as introspection ("self-observation") of the remembered state or process; rather, it is observation (or introspection) of a present memory of the past state or process (1888, 294,

297–300). As such, it need not be wholly untrustworthy. But it introduces the usual limitations on memory as a source of evidence.

According to Wundt, experiment makes deliberate introspection possible (1888, 301–3). Experimental conditions allow the subject or observer to maintain an object of observation over a period of time, as when an observer is asked to match color samples. The samples can be examined for a preset period (two seconds, say), or subjects might simply be asked to declare the match only when they are sure. Also, an experimenter can elicit the same (or closely similar) psychological processes by arranging for an exact repetition of external conditions.[8] If higher thought processes were the object, the immediate results of techniques of directed attention would be suspect if considered to be observations of a constant object, for the directed attention of introspection might interrupt the thought process, and the thoughts themselves might alter from trial to trial as the result of learning or speculation by the observer. But in color matching, observation of properly arranged color stimuli for a few seconds introduces minimal change, and if proper precautions are taken, later observations will not be systematically altered by physiological or psychological after-effects from previous observations.

"Inner" is the main offending term, according to those who empha-size the "transparency" of perception (Dretske 1995b, Harman 1990). Many philosophers have supposed that this term must imply that the object of introspection seems to be "in the mind" or "in the head," rather than in the world—otherwise, the point about transparency would have no bite. They have also supposed that it implies an ontologically distinct entity, a "sense datum" or a subject-dependent "quale." Finally, they have supposed that, failing the existence of such an entity, there would be nothing to do in introspection except to report on the external object: there could be no "observation" of one's own experience.[9]

---

[8] Factors such as sensory adaptation and habituation limit the extent to which "the same" phenomena can be observed over time and in repeated trials. Such effects can be controlled for, and may be counted as experimental error, or they can be studied in their own right (Palmer 1999, 674).

[9] Dretske puts the point as follows: "If there is an inner sense, some quasi-perceptual faculty that enables one to know what experiences are like by 'scanning' them, this internal scanner, unlike the other senses, has a completely transparent phenomenology. It does not 'present' experiences of external objects in any guise other than the way the experiences present external objects. If one is aware of experiences in the way one is aware of external objects, the experiences look, for all the world, like external objects. This is very suspicious. It suggests that there is not really another sense in operation at all" (1995b, 62). However, the notion of an "inner sense," or of a "perceptual model" of introspection, is ambiguous. Dretske and others have interpreted the analogy between introspection and sensing or perceiving to mean that there must be a distinct object of sense, and that "perceiving" such objects introspectively must presuppose a perceiver–perceived relation distinct from that already extant in the perception of external objects. But one may interpret the notion of "perception" more broadly.

None of these assumptions applies to the classic notion of introspection as experimental psychologists such as Wundt developed it. In describing the objects of introspection, Wundt did not posit an "inner" location or require a specific metaphysical theory of qualia, but he nonetheless did allow an attitude of observation toward one's own experience. According to him, introspection takes the same (phenomenal) objects as ordinary perception, but approaches them with a different attitude or "point of view." Whatever may be the truth about the relation between the physical and the psychical (in sense perception, let us say), the phenomenal objects of observation are the same. Wundt rejected the definition of psychology as the "science of inner experience," for the reason that "it may give rise to the misunderstanding that psychology has to do with objects totally different from the objects of so-called 'outer experience'" (1901/1902, 2). Various perceptions, as of "a stone, a plant, a tone, a ray of light," can be viewed either as natural phenomena, or as "ideas" or presentations to a subject.

As a psychologist, Wundt was not concerned to determine the metaphysical status of perceptual experience. He regarded sense experience as presenting external objects (1901/1902, 4, 13). Methodologically, psychologists can study the same observational phenomena as do physicists, but they do so from a different point of view: "the expressions outer and inner experience do not indicate different objects, but *different points of view* from which we take up the consideration and scientific treatment of a unitary experience" (ibid., 3).[10] And again: "from this point of view, the question of the relation between psychical and physical objects disappears entirely. They are not different objects at all,

If we include cognitive aspects of perception (Palmer 1999, 13), such as classifying objects (seeing something *as a book*, rather than simply seeing its shape and color), as part of the perceptual act (and its phenomenology), then the "perceptual model" of introspection can be interpreted as the application of introspective concepts within everyday perceptual experience. To introspect would be to apply concepts in classifying one's immediate experience, for example, to conclude that the paper looks greyish here and reddish there, where this classifying is understood to be distinct from ascribing a surface-color property (a pigmentation) to the paper itself.

[10] In saying that a sensation is not a "different object" from external objects, Wundt may appear to be taking a metaphysical stance and adopting a form of monism. In fact, he preferred not to adopt a metaphysical "hypothesis" on the mind–body problem; in equating "inner" and "outer" sense perceptions as objects of experience, he was not making an assertion about their ontological status. Wundt himself subscribed to a form of psychological parallelism as a methodological principle, but he did not purport to refute materialism or idealism (spiritualism); rather, he characterized them as empirically sterile (1901/1902, 352–63). In this regard, he shared the position of Helmholtz (and others in the late nineteenth century) that the data of science are the materials of observation, and that these can be known independently of "metaphysical" notions such as material or mental substance. One might suspect that this position leads to the "neutral monism" common to Mach, James, and Russell, which itself may be thought to tend toward phenomenalism or even to idealism; but the view that perceptual experience can be investigated independently of a particular position on the mind–body problem can be defended without subscribing to neutral monism (see Ch. 10, and Sec. 4 below).

but one and the same content of experience" (11). In physics and chemistry, one seeks to describe objects by abstracting away from a subjective point of view as much as is possible (3, 357). Those sciences develop their own concepts, which describe objects in terms of stable physical and chemical properties (e.g., mass, force, acid, base, etc.). Psychology, by contrast, studies all aspects of experience, including those that are momentary, or that depend on momentary relations between the subject and an external object. Even though the objects in introspective studies of perception typically are existing external objects,[11] psychologists have developed special phenomenological concepts for describing them. These include notions such as "sensation," and, for a given sensory modality, the range of sensory qualities, such as hue, brightness, and saturation in the case of color. In a psychological investigation, one may ask subjects to describe the objects of perception phenomenally, in terms of how the objects look from moment to moment.

As an example of the two viewpoints, consider first a student in the chemistry lab who simply wants to know whether the litmus paper she has just dipped into a liquid has turned red or blue. She isn't interested in whether the appearance of those colors varies with the variations in lighting found in the chemistry classroom. Rather, the classification into *red* or *blue* (depending on whether the liquid was an acid or a base) is binary. In the psychology classroom down the hall, a student might simply report the classification into red and blue introspectively, as his awareness that the paper looked red or looked blue. But that bare classification into color classes need not exhaust the experimenter's interest in the look of the colored papers. In a study of color perception, a subject might be shown colored papers matching the red and blue of litmus paper under various conditions of illumination, and asked to compare how they look (their appearances). Far from simply declaring "red" or "blue," the student might note that (under ordinary illumination) the "red" sample would more accurately be described as pink, and the "blue" sample as bluish violet. He might also note that the samples take on differing phenomenal hues under variations in lighting, that the two swatches nonetheless continue to be distinguishable in color, and that under a wide range of illuminations he could still easily classify the samples as "red" or "blue," even though each sample doesn't look exactly the same under all those conditions. In describing how the litmus paper looks during the experiment, the psychology student employs concepts of phenomenal appearance rather than binary color classification. He never once need conceive of himself as accessing a special inner object that

---

[11] One can of course also study afterimages and other subjective phenomena, but let us stay focused on the primary case.

seems to be located within himself: he is always describing how the colored papers look.[12] Hence, whether the colors he reports are in fact subject- or perceiver-dependent (a metaphysical question we have, for now, put aside), the traditional object of introspection in the study of visual perception is characterized as *phenomenally* outer.

Wundtian experimentation took place in highly controlled conditions and used trained observers. When Wundt and others coupled this experimental practice with certain further theoretical assumptions, such as that sensory experience is constituted out of punctiform sensational "elements" or "atomic sensations," they evolved the introspective practices that are classed under the name of "analytical introspection."[13] In a broad sense, analytical introspection simply means introspection undertaken in order to discriminate and classify experiences (Titchener 1912b, 495–6). Here, "analytical" means classificatory, and the notion is unobjectionable. But in the narrow sense, it means introspection undertaken to uncover atomic sensations (1912b, 495). Here, "analytical" means resolution into least elements; in vision, these elements were (by hypothesis) punctiform sensations. In this latter guise, analytical introspection came in for heavy criticism from James (1890, ch. 6) and the Gestalt psychologists.[14]

Wolfgang Köhler devoted a chapter of his *Gestalt Psychology* (1947) to criticizing this form of introspection. He was especially concerned to question the notion that "hidden" elements, called "pure sensations," underlie phenomenal experience as we have it. The Gestalt psychologists emphasized that ordinary experience is of a world at a distance, experienced in three dimensions. They held that objects nearby are ordinarily experienced under conditions of spatial

[12] Some objects of introspective observation may be spatially "inner" in the sense of inside the skin, as a pain in the stomach is. Others, such as anger or joy, may be ascribed as feelings of the person, generally felt as localized in the region of the body. One wouldn't try to turn one's eyeballs around to see them; one would simply reflect on the character of one's emotions and feelings.

[13] Early on, Wundt (1862) adopted a "punctiform" analysis of perception (see Hatfield 1990b, ch. 5), and he retained sympathy for a "fusional" account of the origin of spatial structure from elemental or atomic sensations (1901/1902, 116–56) and of the development of tones from constituent sensations (100–13). Titchener (1910, 304–5) did not follow Wundt on the original nonspatiality of visual sensations.

[14] On "analytical introspection" vs. "phenomenological" or "naive" introspection, see Rock (1975, 11–12). Koffka (1935, 73) distinguished phenomenological introspection from the "American" version of introspection (i.e., analytical introspection). Palmer (1999, 48) attributes an "introspective" approach to the Gestaltists, owing to their appeal to "phenomenological observations of one's own conscious experience." He distinguishes this sort of introspection from that involved in the search for sensory atoms, which he (somewhat unhappily) calls "trained introspection" (1999, 50). Many psychologists still associate the term "introspection" with analytical introspection. I term this the "narrow" conception, and distinguish it from a broader notion (citing, if needed, the precedents just given, from past and present literature).

"constancy." This means that a dinner plate seen across the table (and so, at an angle of 45° to the line of sight) is nonetheless perceived as circular, rather than as an ellipse (its projective shape on the retina).[15] By contrast, an analytical introspectivist might hold that the "real" sensation conforms to the two-dimensional projection, while the fact (or—depending on the particularities of the theory—the report) that the plate looks round would be ascribed to learning.

The Gestalt psychologists held that an accurate phenomenal report of how the plate looks would say that it looks round. They would relegate the perception of it as an ellipse to circumstances in which the observer has adopted a special attitude, sometimes called the "painter's attitude," such as one might learn to adopt in drawing class when attempting to produce a perspectival picture of the plate. According to Köhler and his colleagues, such deliberately elicited experiences should not constitute the starting point in the psychology of perception. Perceptual psychology, or indeed any psychology, must start from the external world "as we have it": "There seems to be a single starting point for psychology, exactly as for all the other sciences: the world as we have it, naïvely and uncritically. The naïveté may be lost as we proceed" (1947, 3). He called the world as we have it the world of "direct experience." And he contended that such experience is "the raw material of both physics and psychology" (1947, 34).

Although rejecting analytical introspection, the Gestalt psychologists nonetheless relied on introspection, more broadly conceived. In their writings, they use demonstration drawings as a means of making readers become aware of aspects of their perceptual experience. The drawings illustrated figure/ground relations, grouping of phenomena, and other Gestalt principles. A familiar example is the Necker cube, which is like a drawing of a wire cube seen from one of its faces. The cube reverses in depth as one looks at it. One experiences this reversal, and can attend to it and report on it. Such reports, although not labeled introspective by Köhler (who limited that term to analytical introspection), are examples of the less restricted (or broader) practice of introspection, on which the Gestaltists relied heavily.

I classify the Gestalt approach, and the general Wundtian experimental approach (distinct from the assumptions of analytical introspection), as forms of introspection in a broad sense: forms of psychological investigation that are mediated by observers' or subjects' responses to their own experience.

---

[15] Here I adopt the usual description of shape constancy as yielding a Euclidean circle (for a round dinner plate); in fact, the space of visual constancy may be compressed with distance, so that the plate would be represented with a slight flattening of the front and rear edges—which would nonetheless be taken for the look that a true circle should have. On the compression of visual space, see Ch. 5.7.

This form of introspection has limits, as Wundt knew. He realized that many processes cannot be fully observed in consciousness. We should not expect introspection to directly reveal the nature of mind or the structure of psychological processes.[16] The development of cognitive and perceptual psychology has only confirmed this limitation. Nonetheless, the perceived qualities of objects, the temporal structure of experience, and the effects of experimental manipulations on experience can be investigated by techniques that rely on subjects' responses to what they experience, and can be used as evidence in investigating the structure of underlying psychological processes.

4. Introspective Reality

There are many examples of the use of introspection (broadly construed) in present-day psychology. Every textbook in perception employs demonstration drawings, sometimes similar to those used by the Gestaltists, to illustrate various perceptual phenomena. All of them depend upon the reader's being able to attend to the way the drawing looks, and to recognize appropriate aspects of how he or she experiences the drawings, including, in the case of figure/ground reversal, changes in phenomenal organization that occur while the physical object (the line drawing itself) remains the same on the printed page.

I want to examine some experiments in which subjects attend to or respond to aspects of their occurrent experience. I describe some psychological experiments on shape perception in some detail, and also mention some work on color perception and attention.

One phenomenon studied in perceptual psychology is *shape constancy*, the tendency of objects to appear to have a constant shape despite differences in viewing conditions (especially viewing angle, in the case of flat objects). Consider again a circular dinner plate. It appears circular when viewed at various angles from the frontal plane, say, from 0° (frontoparallel) through 45°. When it is perpendicular to the line of sight (0° slant), the plate projects a circular shape on the retina; at 45°, an ellipse (as at other angles, until the plate is seen edge-on, when it flattens to a long, thin shape with parallel edges, perhaps half-rounded at each end). A study of shape constancy might seek to distinguish the conditions in which full (or nearly full) constancy is obtained from those in which perception tends toward projective shape. One such set

---

[16] The Gestaltists thought it might, through an isomorphism relation, but in the form they held it this notion has been discredited (see Epstein and Hatfield 1994).

of conditions might include brief exposure to a set of stimuli that are generated as projectively equivalent shapes when viewed at predetermined angles (e.g., a circle viewed at 0°, and various ellipses that project a circle when rotated to various angles, say, 39°, 52°, and 65°). Experimenters may then elicit reports of perceived shape by, for example, asking subjects to pick out the one shape on a sheet of comparison shapes that most closely matches the perceived shape of an object they've just seen.

In studying shape constancy, experimenters have discovered that it is important to instruct observers concerning their attitude about what they are to report (Epstein *et al.* 1963). If observers believe that their job is to report the *perspective projection* of a shape, their reports will deviate from shape constancy (except at 0°). But such deviation may simply reflect their attitude about the task, not their perceptual experience of the shape. If subjects believe that they are to report what the actual or *objective shape* is, they may "correct" the appearance; under conditions of brief exposure, they may try to guess the objective shape. This could lead to reports closer to shape constancy than their perceptual experience would warrant. In consequence, subjects are typically instructed to report *phenomenal shape*, as opposed to *projective* or *objective* shape. Subjects are instructed to base their report on what the shape of the object looks to have, not what they would guess it to have nor what they think it should have.[17] Given such instructions, subjects have been found to report good shape constancy under conditions of binocular viewing (using both eyes, without moving the head), when viewing an object illuminated for less than one-fifth of a second, followed by darkness. When their viewing is interrupted by a visual "mask" (small, irregular white shapes on black) at very brief periods (from 0 to 50 milliseconds) after offset of the illumination on the object, they tend to report projective shape (Epstein *et al.* 1977). They also tend to report projective shape when viewing the shapes monocularly, that is, with one eye and no head movement (Epstein and Hatfield 1978).

---

[17] Epstein *et al.* (1977) instructed subjects as to the purpose of the experiment and about the kind of reports they were to make (how they should conceive the task). They were first told: "In this experiment we are trying to learn how the apparent shape, or the appearance of the shape, of an object is affected by variations in the time one is allowed to see the object." After a description of the experimental set up, and prior to explaining how responses were to be indicated, they were told: "I would like to make clear what it is that I am asking you to report. I want you to report the shape of the object directly as it appears to you, without any analysis or guessing on your part. The experiment will be spoiled if you base your response on a conscious attempt to figure out what the shape *ought* to be, instead of what it appears to be. Don't convert the situation into a guessing game or into an intellectual task. We are not trying to trick you in this experiment; we are really interested in the way things look to you." Similar instructions were given for trials on which slant (rather than shape) judgments were elicited.

We need not enter into the theoretical significance of these reports. What is interesting to note is that, under instructions to report the shape as it appears, subjects exhibited shape constancy when the stimulus object was illuminated for less than one-fifth of a second, and they tended toward projective shape when their viewing was interrupted after a very brief interval, or when binocular depth information was eliminated. These findings are consistent with the conclusion that the observer's experience of the same objective shape at the same slant changed under differing conditions of observation. The changes are in the direction expected by theory. Hence, the consistency of the data suggests that these techniques, which draw on subjects' responses as mediated by their attention to their phenomenal experience, allowed experimenters to study aspects of that experience.

Color perception has been studied in the laboratory for more than 150 years. The methods of study, called "psychophysics," have been highly refined. Palmer (1999, 665) defines psychophysics as "the behavioral study of quantitative relations between people's perceptual experiences and corresponding physical properties." The studies are behavioral because they rely on subjects' responses, whether verbal (saying "yes" or "no") or manual (pressing a button, adjusting a dial); they depend on perceptual experience because they concern color appearances. In studies of color matching (Kaiser and Boynton 1996, 124−5), subjects may look at a round area or disc that is illuminated by two different sources. On the left hemifield, a monochromatic light of known wavelength is projected. On the right, a mixture of two monochromatic lights is projected. The subject is asked to vary the mixture by turning a knob until the disc appears uniform (no border or difference between the two hemifields is apparent). The subjects' responses are mediated by the appearance of the disc: how it looks to them. The resulting color matches are among the fundamental data for color theory. The results are highly consistent (with very tight error bars) for normal human observers (normal trichromats).

Finally, work on attention has blossomed in the experimental literature in recent decades. Many techniques are used to measure the effects of attention, either directly or indirectly. Indirect measures may include subjects' abilities to report one sort of thing while attending to something else (say, to report on the shapes of objects they had recently seen, when they had only been told to look for a specific color).[18] One striking technique, which has been used to study

---

[18] In the terminology of this chapter, an experiment in which subjects are primed to look for color but then queried on shape is an example of both introspection (of the stimulus attribute they are directed to attend to) and inner perception (of the dimension they are subsequently asked to report). The first fits the notion that psychological introspection is a form of observation. The second presumably relies on memory of an undirected or "incidental" awareness of shape.

attentional processes, is called "pop out." It is based on the phenomenological observation that in a field of uniform objects, say, letters or shapes, even under brief exposure (too brief to allow eye movement or redirection of attention), a nonmatching shape (calibrated to be of similar size and color to surrounding shapes) will "pop out" or become phenomenally salient. If subjects are asked to detect the presence or absence of a diagonal line-segment among vertical line-segments of the same length, the time it takes them to do so is not affected by the number of vertical segments (ranging from 2 to 32). This finding led Triesman and Gelade (1980) to conclude that subjects process the identity of such shapes pre-attentively and in parallel (that is, all at once, as opposed to serially, one after another). Details of the studies aside, the important point is that subjects' responses are mediated by directed attention and phenomenal salience. Here again, experimental psychology uses introspectively mediated responses that exactly fit Wundt's broad conception of introspection.

5. Introspection as Evidence

When introspection is defined as deliberate and immediate attention to certain aspects of phenomenal experience, we see that it continues to be used as a source of evidence in perceptual and cognitive psychology. The psychologists who use it need not be, and often are not, committed to the existence of distinct entities that, like sense data, have phenomenal properties of their own, distinct from those involved in the direct perception of external objects. The key to introspection is not "looking within," but attending to relevant aspects of experience. Such relevant aspects include phenomenal variations in the looks of things. These variations may be at the coarse grain of object description ("the thing looks red"). For the purposes of perceptual psychology, however, the concepts involved will classify how things look at a finer grain of description than is used in ordinary typing of objects and their properties. Introspectively based responses may require persons to attend more closely to phenomenal shape than they normally do, or to inspect shades of color more closely than they usually do (except, perhaps, in the paint store).

Such responses are treated as scientific evidence in the literature of experimental psychology. The evidence purports to reveal facts about attention, or shape perception, or color perception in general. One person's introspectively based response is treated as yielding information about how others will respond as well—subject to known, or discovered, individual differences (as in color blindness).

This literature shows little or no concern with an epistemological worry raised by philosophers: that introspection is inherently "private" or "subjective." When philosophers make this objection, they may contrast the alleged privacy of introspection with the epistemologically more worthy perception of or response to "public" objects, such as tables and chairs. As philosophers often conceive these things, tables and chairs have properties that all of us can perceive and compare, by contrast with sense perceptions themselves, which are private to each subject. I can't have yours, you can't have mine, so we can't check or compare them.

This framing of the problem of privacy retains the earlier confusion about what the object of introspection is supposed to be in perceptual psychology. In the standard case, the focus of attention is how the distal object looks. In fact, knowledge of the "public" object depends on the same phenomenal experience. There are not two experiences: one of the table as public, one of the experience of the table as private.[19] The only difference between objective property reports and introspective reports are the concepts that are used to classify the experience. In the first case, the subject has learned to attribute determinate properties of color and shape that are counted as remaining the same under large variations in lighting and in viewing distance. We know to expect that the table's shape and color are stable. In the second case, we are interested in subtler variations in phenomenal color and shape. We may be describing the same table, looking exactly the same, in the two cases. But the concepts are of different grain and application. We classify a table we've just painted as "a uniform red across its surface" when we apply object-color concepts. But we may describe variations in the appearance of the uniformly red pigment (due to lighting variation, shadows, glare, etc.) when we adopt an attitude of phenomenal description.

It is true that two observers can't directly compare their phenomenal experiences in such cases. But they can't directly compare how they perceive the table as an external object, either. In both cases, we as observers coordinate our descriptions with repeated samplings of how the table looks, and we develop language for conveying those looks, with the stable table as the coordinating factor. There need be no mystery in this, as Köhler (1947, 19–33)

<hr />

[19] This does not deny that differences in attitude *can* (in some cases) cause the experience itself to differ, as when one takes what was described in the previous section as a "projectivist" attitude, or when one causes a figure/ground shift by redirecting attention. The point is that an introspective attitude need not change the spatial or chromatic character of experience. Nor need it be directed at a different experience of spatial and chromatic properties than that which occurs when one is observing an object without an introspective attitude. Moreover, introspecting may change the overall experience (by injecting a different conceptualization, one based on phenomenal concepts), without necessarily affecting spatial and chromatic characteristics.

has explained. The physical world itself is known to us directly only by our experiencing it—visually, according to how it looks, and tactually, according to how it feels.[20]

Introspection may be taken as a reliable source of data about objects of consciousness. In perception, introspectively based responses go to how things look. These responses provide data about phenomenal experience. Such data are legitimate objects of explanation in perceptual psychology. Introspectively based responses are no longer considered to provide direct access to the structure and functioning of the psychological processes that underlie visual perception. Rather, these processes must be inferred from, or hypotheses about them must be tested against, various patterns of data. The relevance of introspection for discovering fundamental psychological processes has been re-evaluated more than once during the past century. Introspection can yield data to mediate inferences or to test hypotheses. It is not and need not be seen as an oracle whose pronouncements can, by their immediacy, lay psychological processes bare. It provides evidence, and that's all. But that should be plenty.[21]

---

[20] I discuss epistemological worries more fully in Ch. 10.5.

[21] I am grateful to Yumiko Inukai, Jeffrey Scarborough, and Morgan Wallhagen for comments on an earlier version of this essay.

References

Abel, Jacob F. (1786). *Einleitung in die Seelenlehre*. Stuttgart: Metzler. Reprint, Hildesheim: Olms, 1985.

Achinstein, Peter (1983). *The Nature of Explanation*. New York: Oxford University Press.

Alhazen (or Alhacen). See Ibn al-Haytham.

Allen, Grant (1879). *The Colour-Sense: Its Origin and Development: An Essay in Comparative Psychology*. Trübner: London.

Alpern, Mathew (1988). Walter Stanley Stiles: 15 June 1901–15 December 1985. *Biographical Memoirs of Fellows of the Royal Society* 34:816–85.

Ames, Adelbert, Jr. (1961). The rotating trapezoid: Description of phenomena. In Franklin P. Kilpatrick (ed.), *Explorations in Transactional Psychology*, 222–37. New York: New York University Press.

Amundson, Ron (1983). E. C. Tolman and the intervening variable: A study in the epistemological history of psychology. *Philosophy of Science* 50:268–82.

—— (1986). The unknown epistemology of E. C. Tolman. *British Journal of Psychology* 77:525–31.

Amundson, Ron, and Laurence D. Smith (1984). Clark Hull, Robert Cummins, and functional analysis. *Philosophy of Science* 51:657–66.

Anderson, John. R. (1978). Arguments concerning representations for mental imagery. *Psychological Review* 85:249–77.

Arbib, Michael A., and Allen R. Hanson (1987). Vision, brain, and cooperative computation: An overview. In Michael A. Arbib and Allen R. Hanson (eds.), *Vision, Brain, and Cooperative Computation*, 1–83. Cambridge, Mass.: MIT Press.

Arend, Lawrence E., Jr., and Adam Reeves (1986). Simultaneous color constancy. *Journal of the Optical Society of America* A 3:1743–51.

Arend, Lawrence E., Jr., Adam Reeves, James Schirillo, and Robert Goldstein (1991). Simultaneous color constancy: Papers with divers Munsell values. *Journal of the Optical Society of America* A 8:661–72.

Ariew, André (2003). Natural selection doesn't work that way: Jerry Fodor vs. evolutionary psychology on gradualism and saltationism. *Mind and Language* 18:478–83.

Aristotle (1984a). *On the Soul*, trans. John I. Beare. In Jonathan Barnes (ed.), *Complete Works of Aristotle*, 2 vols., 1:641–92. Princeton: Princeton University Press. Cited, as is usual, with Bekker numbers.

—— (1984b). *Sense and Sensibilia*, trans. John I. Beare. In Jonathan Barnes (ed.), *Complete Works of Aristotle*, 2 vols., 1:693–720. Princeton: Princeton University Press. Cited, as is usual, with Bekker numbers.

Armstrong, David M. (1961). *Perception and the Physical World*. New York: Humanities Press.

_____ (1968). *Materialist Theory of Mind*. London: Routledge.

_____ (1980). What is consciousness? *Nature of Mind and Other Essays*, 55–67. St. Lucia: University of Queensland Press.

_____ (1999). *The Mind–Body Problem: An Opinionated Introduction*. Boulder: Westview Press.

Arnauld, Antoine, and Pierre Nicole (1683). *Logique, ou L'Art de penser*, 5th edn. Paris: Guillaume Desprez.

Arnheiter, Heinz (1998). Eyes viewed from the skin. *Nature* 391:632–3.

Atherton, Margaret (1990). *Berkeley's Revolution in Vision*. Ithaca: Cornell University Press.

Attneave, Fred (1954). Some informational aspects of visual perception. *Psychological Review* 61:183–93.

_____ (1982). Prägnanz and soap bubble systems: A theoretical exploration. In J. Beck (ed.), *Organization and Representation in Perception*, 11–29. Hillsdale, NJ: Erlbaum.

Augustine of Hippo (1969). *De musica*, ed. and trans. into Italian, G. Marzi. Florence: Sansoni. Cited by book, chapter, and section number.

_____ (1991). *Confessions*, trans. Henry Chadwick. Oxford: Oxford University Press. Cited by book, chapter, and section number.

_____ (1992). *Confessions*, ed. James J. O'Donnell. Oxford: Oxford University Press.

Austin, John L. (1962), *Sense and Sensibilia*. Oxford: Clarendon Press.

Autrum, Hansjochem (1979). Introduction. In H. Autrum (ed.), *Handbook of Sensory Physiology*, vol. 7, pt. 6A, *Comparative Physiology and Evolution of Vision in Invertebrates*, 1–22. Berlin: Springer.

Ayer, Alfred J. (1958). *The Problem of Knowledge*. London: Macmillan.

Ayers, Michael (1991). *Locke: Epistemology and Ontology*, 2 vols. London: Routledge.

_____ (2005). Ordinary objects, ordinary language, and identity. *Monist* 88:534–70.

Bach, Kent (1982). *De re* belief and methodological solipsism. In Andrew Woodfield (ed.), *Thought and Object: Essays on Intentionality*, 121–51. Oxford: Clarendon Press.

_____ (1987). *Thought and Reference*. Oxford: Clarendon Press.

Bacon, Roger (1962). *Opus majus*, trans. Robert Burke. New York: Russell and Russell.

_____ (1996). *Roger Bacon and the Origins of Perspectiva in the Middle Ages: Bacon's Perspectiva*, ed. and trans. David C. Lindberg. Oxford: Clarendon Press.

Ballard, Dana H., Geoffrey E. Hinton, and Terrence J. Sejnowski (1983). Parallel visual computation. *Nature* 306:21–6.

Barlow, Horace B. (1953). Summation and inhibition in the frog's retina. *Journal of Physiology* 119:69–88.

_____ (1961a). The coding of sensory messages. In W. H. Thorpe and O. L. Zangwill (eds.), *Current Problems in Animal Behavior*, 331–60. Cambridge: Cambridge University Press.

_____ (1961b). Possible principles underlying the transformations of sensory messages. In Walter A. Rosenblith (ed.), *Sensory Communication*, 217–34. New York: Wiley.

_____ (1974). Inductive inference, coding, perception, and language. *Perception* 3:123–34.

_____ (1982a). General principles: The senses considered as physical instruments. In Horace B. Barlow and John D. Mollon (eds.), *The Senses*, 1–33. Cambridge: Cambridge University Press.

_____ (1982b). Physiology of the retina. In Horace B. Barlow and John D. Mollon (eds.), *The Senses*, 102–113. Cambridge: Cambridge University Press.

_____ (1982c). What causes trichromacy? A theoretical analysis using comb-filtered spectra. *Vision Research* 22:635–44.

_____ (1990a). Conditions for versatile learning, Helmholtz's unconscious inference, and the task of perception. *Vision Research* 30:1561–71.

_____ (1990b). What does the brain see? How does it understand? In Horace B. Barlow, Colin Blakemore, and Miranda Weston-Smith (eds.), *Images and Understanding*, 5–25. Cambridge: Cambridge University Press.

Barlow, Horace B., Colin Blakemore, and J. D. Pettigrew (1967). The neural mechanism of binocular depth discrimination. *Journal of Physiology* 193:327–42.

Barsalou, Lawrence W. (1999). Perceptual symbol systems. *Behavioral and Brain Science* 22:577–660.

Barwise, Jon, and John Perry (1983). *Situations and Attitudes*. Cambridge, Mass.: MIT Press.

Bauer, Hans (1911). *Die Psychologie Alhazens*. Beiträge zur Geschichte der Philosophie des Mittelalters, vol. 10, pt. 5. Münster: Aschendorff.

Beck, Jacob (1972). *Surface Color Perception*. Ithaca: Cornell University Press.

Bennett, Bruce M., Donald D. Hoffman, and Chetan Prakash (1989). *Observer Mechanics: A Formal Theory of Perception*. San Diego: Academic Press.

Bergmann, Gustav, and Kenneth W. Spence (1941). Operationism and theory in psychology. *Psychological Review* 48:1–14.

Berkeley, George (1709). *An Essay Towards a New Theory of Vision*. Dublin: Rhames and Papyat.

_____ (1710). *A Treatise Concerning the Principles of Human Knowledge*. Dublin: Rhames and Papyat.

_____ (1733). *The Theory of Vision Vindicated and Explained*. London: J. Tonson.

_____ (1963). *Works on Vision*, ed. Colin Murray Turbayne. New York: Bobbs-Merrill.

Berlyne, Daniel E. (1974). Attention. In Edward C. Carterette and Morton P. Friedman (eds.), *Handbook of Perception*, vol. 1, *Historical and Philosophical Roots of Perception*, 123–47. New York: Academic Press.

Biederman, Irving (1987). Recognition-by-components: A theory of human image understanding. *Psychological Review* 94:115–47.

Bienenstock, Elie, and René Doursat (1991). Issues of representation in neural networks. In Andrei Gorea (ed.), *Representations of Vision: Trends and Tacit Assumptions in Vision Research*, 47–67. Cambridge: Cambridge University Press.

486 REFERENCES

Bishop, P. O., and G. H. Henry (1971). Spatial vision. *Annual Review of Psychology* 22:119–60.

Bishop, P. O., and J. D. Pettigrew (1986). Neural mechanisms of binocular vision. *Vision Research* 26:1587–1600.

Blackmore, Susan J., Gavin Brelstaff, Kay Nelson, and Tom Troscianko (1995). Is the richness of our visual world an illusion? Transsaccadic memory for complex scenes. *Perception* 24:1075–81.

Block, Ned (1980). Introduction: What is functionalism. In Ned Block (ed.), *Readings in the Philosophy of Psychology*, 2 vols., 1:171–84. Cambridge, Mass.: Harvard University Press.

Blumenfeld, Walter (1913). Untersuchungen über die scheinbare Grösse im Sehraume. *Zeitschrift für Psycholgie und Physiologie der Sinnesorgane* 65:241–404.

Boghossian, Paul A., and J. David Velleman (1989). Colour as a secondary quality. *Mind* 98:81–103.

—— (1991). Physicalist theories of color. *Philosophical Review* 100:67–106.

Bohr, Niels (1934). The atomic theory and the fundamental principles underlying the description of nature. *Atomic Theory and the Description of Nature*, 102–19. Cambridge: Cambridge University Press. Volume reprinted as *Philosophical Writings of Niels Bohr*, vol. 1. Woodbridge, Conn.: Oxbow Press, 1987. Lecture originally delivered in 1929.

—— (1935). Can quantum-mechanical description of physical reality be considered complete? *Physical Review* 48:696–702. Reprinted in *Philosophical Writings of Niels Bohr*, vol. 4, *Causality and Complementarity*, 73–82. Woodbridge, Conn.: Oxbow Press, 1998.

—— (1958). Atoms and human knowledge. *Atomic Physics and Human Knowledge*, 83–93. New York: Wiley. Volume reprinted as *Philosophical Writings of Niels Bohr*, vol. 2. Woodbridge, Conn.: Oxbow Press, 1987. Lecture originally delivered in Danish in 1955.

Boltzmann, Ludwig (1897). Über die Frage nach der objektiven Existenz der Vorgänge in der unbelebten Natur. *Sitzungsberichte der Akademie der Wissenschaften in Wien, Mathematisch-Naturwissenshaftliche Klasse* 106. As republished in Ludwig Boltzmann, *Populäre Schriften*, 162–87. Leipzig: Barth, 1905.

—— (1974). On the question of the objective existence of processes in inanimate nature. In Ludwig Boltzmann, *Theoretical Physics and Philosophical Problems*, ed. Brian McGuinness, trans. Paul Foulkes, 57–76. Dordrecht: Reidel.

Bonnet, Charles (1755). *Essai de psychologie; ou, considerations sur les operations de l'ame, sur l'habitude et sur l'education*. London: n.p.

—— (1769). *Essai analytique sur les facultés de l'ame*, 2nd edn., 2 vols. Copenhagen: Philibert.

Boring, Edwin G. (1929). *A History of Experimental Psychology*. New York: Century.

—— (1942). *Sensation and Perception in the History of Experimental Psychology*. New York: Appleton-Century-Crofts.

——(1950). *A History of Experimental Psychology*, 2nd edn. New York: Appleton-Century-Crofts.

——(1965). The perception of objects. In Herschel W. Leibowitz (ed.), *Visual Perception*, 67–85. New York: Macmillan.

Bowmaker, James K., and Herbert J. A. Dartnall (1980). Visual pigments of rods and cones in a human retina. *Journal of Physiology* 298:501–11.

Boyd, Robert, and Peter J. Richerson (1985). *Culture and the Evolutionary Process*. Chicago: University of Chicago Press.

Boynton, Robert M. (1979). *Human Color Vision*. New York: Holt, Rinehart and Winston.

——(1990). Human color perception. In K. Nicholas Leibovic (ed.), *Science of Vision*, 221–53. Berlin: Springer-Verlag.

Braunschweiger, David (1899). *Die Lehre von der Aufmerksamkeit in der Psychologie des 18. Jahrhunderts*. Leipzig: Haacke.

Brena, Carlo, Francesca Cima, and Paolo Burighel (2003). Alimentary tract of *Kowalevskiidae* (Appendicularia, Tunicata) and evolutionary implications. *Journal of Morphology* 258:225–38.

Brentano, Franz Clemens (1874). *Psychologie vom empirischen Standpunkt*. Leipzig: Duncker and Humblot.

——(1995). *Psychology from an Empirical Standpoint*, trans. Antos C. Rancurello, D. B. Terrell, and Linda L. McAlister. London: Routledge.

Brewer, Bill (2007). Perception and its objects. *Philosophical Studies* 132:87–97.

Bridgman, Percy W. (1927). *Logic of Modern Physics*. New York: Macmillan.

Broad, C. D. (1923). *Scientific Thought*. London: Kegan Paul, Trench, Trubner.

Brown, Christopher M., Dana H. Ballard, and O. A. Kimball (1982). Constraint interaction in shape-from-shading algorithms. *Proceedings of the DARPA Image Understanding Workshop*, 1–11. Springfield, Va.: National Technical Information Service.

Brown, Thomas (1824). *Lectures on the Philosophy of the Human Mind*, 2nd edn., 4 vols. Edinburgh: Tait.

Bruner, Jerome S. (1969). Modalities of memory. In G. A. Talland and N. C. Waugh (eds.), *The Pathology of Memory*, 253–9. New York: Academic Press.

Brunswik, Egon (1956). *Perception and the Representative Design of Psychological Experiments*, 2nd edn. Berkeley: University of California Press.

Buchsbaum, Gershon, and Allan Gottschalk (1983). Trichromacy, opponent colours coding and optimum colour information transmission in the retina. *Proceedings of the Royal Society of London* B 220:89–113.

Buffart, Hans, and Emanuel Leeuwenberg (1978). Introduction. In Emanuel Leeuwenberg and Hans Buffart (eds.), *Formal Theories of Visual Perception*, 3–6. New York: Wiley.

Burge, Tyler (1973). Reference and proper names. *Journal of Philosophy* 70:425–39.

——(1977). Belief *de re*. *Journal of Philosophy* 74:338–62.

Burge, Tyler (1986). Individualism and psychology. *Philosophical Review* 95:3−45.

Buridan, Jean (1518). *In librum Aristotelis De sensu et sensato*. In George Lockert (ed.), *Questiones et decisiones*. Paris: Ascensius and Resch.

Burtt, Edwin A. (1925). *Metaphysical Foundations of Modern Physical Science: A Historical and Critical Essay*. London: Kegan Paul.

Campbell, John (1993). A simple view of colour. In John Haldane and Crispin Wright (eds.), *Reality, Representation, and Projection*, 257−68. New York: Oxford University Press.

———(2002). *Reference and Consciousness*. Oxford: Clarendon Press.

———(2005). Transparency vs. revelation in color perception. *Philosophical Topics* 33:105−15.

Campbell, Keith (1990). *Abstract Particulars*. Oxford: Blackwell.

Caramazza, Alfonso, Gabriele Miceli, Gianpiero Villa, and Cristina Romani (1987). The role of the graphemic buffer in spelling: Evidence from a case of acquired dysgraphia. *Cognition* 26:59−85.

Carey, Susan, and Fei Xu (2001). Infants' knowledge of objects: Beyond object files and object tracking. *Cognition* 80:179−213.

Carlson, V. R. (1977). Instructions and perceptual constancy judgments. In William Epstein (ed.), *Stability and Constancy in Visual Perception: Mechanisms and Processes*, 217−54. New York: Wiley.

Carnap, Rudolf (1928). *Der logische Aufbau der Welt*. Berlin: Weltkreis-Verlag. Republished, with introduction from 1961, Hamburg: Meiner, 1998.

———(1932). Psychologie in physikalischer Sprache. *Erkenntnis* 3:107−42.

———(1938). Logical foundations of the unity of science. In Otto Neurath, Rudolf Carnap, and Charles Morris (eds.), *Encyclopedia and Unified Science*. Chicago: University of Chicago Press. Reprinted in Otto Neurath, Rudolf Carnap, and Charles Morris (eds.) *International Encyclopedia of Unified Science*, vol. 1, pt. 1:42−62. Chicago: University of Chicago Press, 1955.

———(1959). Psychology in physical language, trans. Frederic Schick. In Alfred Jules Ayer (ed.), *Logical Positivism*, 165−97. New York: Free Press.

———(1963). Intellectual autobiography. In Paul Arthur Schilpp (ed.), *Philosophy of Rudolf Carnap*, 3−84. La Salle, Ill.: Open Court.

———(1966). *Philosophical Foundations of Physics: An Introduction to the Philosophy of Science*. New York: Basic Books.

———(1967). *Logical Structure of the World*, trans. Rolf A. George. Berkeley: University of California Press.

Carruthers, Peter (2006). *The Architecture of the Mind*. Oxford: Clarendon Press.

Chalmers, David J. (1996). *The Conscious Mind: In Search of a Fundamental Theory*. Oxford: Oxford University Press.

Chambers, Ephraim (1738). *Cyclopaedia, or, An Universal Dictionary of Arts and Sciences*, 2nd edn., 2 vols. London: D. Midwinter and others.

Charniak, Eugene, and Drew McDermott (1985). *Introduction to Artificial Intelligence*. Reading, Mass.: Addison-Wesley.

Chomsky, Noam (1959). Review of B. F. Skinner's *Verbal Behavior*. *Language* 35:26–58.

_____ (1980). *Rules and Representations*. New York: Columbia University Press.

Churchland, Patricia Smith (1980). A perspective on mind-brain research. *Journal of Philosophy* 77:185–207

_____ (1986). *Neurophilosophy: Toward a Unified Science of the Mind-Brain*. Cambridge, Mass.: MIT Press.

_____ (1996). Toward a neurobiology of the mind. In R. Llinas and P. S. Churchland (eds.), *The Mind–Brain Continuum: Sensory Processes*, 281–303. Cambridge, Mass.: MIT Press.

Churchland, Patricia Smith, and Paul M. Churchland (1983). Stalking the wild epistemic engine. *Noûs* 17:5–18,

Churchland, Paul M. (1979). *Scientific Realism and the Plasticity of Mind*. Cambridge: Cambridge University Press.

_____ (1981). Eliminative materialism and the propositional attitudes. *Journal of Philosophy* 78:67–90.

Cicero (1968). *De oratione, Book III*, trans. H. Rackham. Cambridge, Mass.: Harvard University Press.

Clark, Austen (2000). *A Theory of Sentience*. Oxford: Oxford University Press.

_____ (2004). Feature-placing and proto-objects. *Philosophical Psychology* 17:443–69.

Cohen, Jonathan (2008). Colour constancy as counterfactual. *Australasian Journal of Philosophy* 86:61–92.

Cohen, Neal J. (1984). Preserved learning capacity in amnesia: Evidence for multiple memory systems. In Larry R. Squire and N. Butters (eds.), *Neuropsychology of Memory*, 83–103. New York: Guilford Press.

Cohen, Neal J., and Larry R. Squire (1980). Preserved learning and retention of pattern-analyzing skill in amnesia: Dissociation of knowing how and knowing that. *Science* 210:207–10.

Comte, Auguste (1830–42). *Cours de philosophie positive*. Paris: Rouen.

_____ (1855). *The Positive Philosophy*, ed. and trans. Harriet Martineau. New York: Blanchard.

Corballis, Michael C. (1988). Psychology's place in the science of the mind/brain? *Biology and Philosophy* 3:363–73.

Corcoran, D. W. J. (1971). *Pattern Recognition*. Harmondsworth: Penguin.

Cornman, James Welton (1971). *Materialism and Sensations*. New Haven: Yale University Press.

Crane, Tim (1992*a*). Introduction. In Tim Crane (ed.), *The Contents of Experience: Essays on Perception*, 1–17. Cambridge: Cambridge University Press.

_____ (1992*b*). The nonconceptual content of experience. In Tim Crane (ed.), *The Contents of Experience: Essays on Perception*, 136–57. Cambridge: Cambridge University Press.

_____ (2000). Introspection, intentionality, and the transparency of experience. *Philosophical Topics* 28:49–67.

_____ (2001). *Elements of Mind*. Oxford: Oxford University Press.

Crawford, M. L. J., R. S. Harwerth, E. L. Smith, and G. K. von Noorden (1993). Keeping an eye on the brain: The role of visual experience in monkeys and children. *Journal of General Psychology* 120:7–19.

Crombie, Alistair C. (1967). The mechanistic hypothesis and the scientific study of vision: Some optical ideas as a background to the invention of the microscope. In Savile Bradbury and Gerard L'Estrange Turner (eds.), *Historical Aspects of Microscopy*, 3–112. Cambridge: Royal Microscopical Society.

Cummins, Robert (1975). Functional analysis. *Journal of Philosophy* 72:741–64.

—— (1983). *The Nature of Psychological Explanation*. Cambridge, Mass.: MIT Press.

Cutting, James (1986). *Perception with an Eye for Motion*. Cambridge, Mass.: MIT Press.

Cutting, James, and Peter M. Vishton (1995). Perceiving layout and knowing distances: The integration, relative potency, and contextual use of different information about depth. In William Epstein and Sheena Rogers (eds.), *Perception of Space and Motion*, 69–117. San Diego, Calif.: Academic Press.

Danziger, Kurt (1980). The history of introspection reconsidered. *Journal of the History of the Behavioral Sciences* 16:241–62.

D'Arcy, Patrick (1765). Memoire sur la durée de la sensation de la vue. *Histoire de l'Académie Royale des Sciences avec les memoires de mathématique et de physique année,* Paris edn., 82:439–51.

Darwin, Charles (1859). *On the Origin of Species*. London: Murray.

—— (1872). *Expression of the Emotions in Man and Animals*. London: Murray.

Davidson, Donald (1973). The material mind. In Patrick Suppes *et al.* (eds.), *Logic, Methodology and Philosophy of Science IV*. Amsterdam: North-Holland Publishing Company. As republished in John Haugeland (ed.), *Mind Design*, 339–54. Cambridge, Mass.: MIT Press, 1981.

Davies, Martin (1995). Tacit knowledge and subdoxastic states. In Cynthia Macdonald and Graham Macdonald (eds.), *Debates on Psychological Explanation*, vol. 1, *Philosophy of Psychology*, 309–30. Oxford: Blackwell.

Deininger, Werner, Markus Fuhrmann, and Peter Hegemann (2000). Opsin evolution: Out of the wild green yonder? *Trends in Genetics* 16:158–9.

Dell, Gary S. (1985). Positive feedback in hierarchical connectionist models: Applications to language production. *Cognitive Science* 9:3–23.

Dennett, Daniel C. (1978). Two approaches to mental images. *Brainstorms: Philosophical Essays on Mind and Psychology*, 174–89. Montgomery, Vt.: Bradford Books.

—— (1983). Styles of mental representation. *Proceedings of the Aristotelian Society* 83:213–26.

—— (1988). Quining qualia. In Anthony J. Marcel and Edoardo Bisiach (eds.), *Consciousness in Contemporary Science*, 42–77. Oxford: Oxford University Press.

—— (1991). *Consciousness Explained*. Boston: Little, Brown and Company.

Descartes, René (1637). *Discours de la methode pour bien conduire sa raison et chercher la verité dans les sciences: plus la dioptrique, les meteores, et la geometrie, qui sont des essais de cete methode*. Leiden: Maire.

_____ (1641). *Meditationes de prima philosophia*. Paris: Soly. Trans. as *Meditations on First Philosophy*. In Descartes (1984–5), 2:1–397.

_____ (1642). *Meditationes de prima philosophia*, 2nd edn. Amsterdam: Elzevier.

_____ (1644). *Principia philosophiae*. Amsterdam: Elzevier. Trans. as *Principles of Philosophy*. In Descartes (1984–5), 1:179–291.

_____ (1664). *L'homme de René Descartes*, ed. Claude Clerselier. Paris: Charles Angot.

_____ (1955). *Philosophical Works of Descartes*, trans. Elizabeth S. Haldane and G. R. T. Ross, 2 vols. New York: Dover.

_____ (1965). *Discourse on Method, Optics, Geometry, and Meteorology*, trans. Paul J. Olscamp. New York: Bobbs-Merrill.

_____ (1969–75). *Oeuvres de Descartes*, ed. Charles Adam and Paul Tannery, new edn., 11 vols. Paris: Vrin. This edition of Descartes' works is referred to as AT.

_____ (1972). *Treatise of Man*, trans. Thomas S. Hall. Cambridge, Mass.: Harvard University Press.

_____ (1984–5). *Philosophical Writings of Descartes*, ed. John Cottingham, Robert Stoothoff, and Dugald Murdoch, 2 vols. Cambridge: Cambridge University Press.

_____ (1985). *Passions of the Soul*. In Descartes (1984–5), 1:325–404. Originally published in 1649. Cited by section number.

_____ (1991). *Philosophical Writings of Descartes*, vol. 3, *Correspondence*, ed. and trans. John Cottingham, Robert Stoothoff, Dugald Murdoch, and Anthony Kenny. Cambridge: Cambridge University Press.

_____ (1998). *Treatise on Man*. In *The World and Other Writings*, ed. and trans. Stephen Gaukroger, 99–169. Cambridge: Cambridge University Press.

DeValois, Russell L., I. Abramov, and Gerald H. Jacobs (1966). Analysis of response patterns of LGN cells. *Journal of the Optical Society of America* 56:966–77.

Donald, Merlin (1991). *Origins of the Modern Mind*. Cambridge, Mass.: Harvard University Press.

Drake, Durant (ed.) (1920). *Essays in Critical Realism: A Co-Operative Study of the Problem of Knowledge*. London: Macmillan.

Dretske, Fred (1969). *Seeing and Knowing*. Chicago: University of Chicago Press.

_____ (1981). *Knowledge and the Flow of Information*, Cambridge, Mass.: MIT Press.

_____ (1988). *Explaining Behavior: Reasons in a World of Causes*. Cambridge, Mass.: MIT Press.

_____ (1995a). Meaningful perception. In Stephen M. Kosslyn, and Daniel N. Osherson (eds.), *Invitation to Cognitive Science*, vol. 2, *Visual Cognition*, 2nd edn., 331–52. Cambridge, Mass.: MIT Press.

_____ (1995b). *Naturalizing the Mind*. Cambridge, Mass.: MIT Press.

Dummett, Michael (1993). *Origins of Analytical Philosophy*. Cambridge, Mass.: Harvard University Press.

Ebbinghaus, Hermann (1908). *Abriss der Psychologie*. Leipzig: Veit.

_____ (1911). *Psychology: An Elementary Textbook*, trans. M. Meyer. Boston: Heath.

Ebenholtz, Sheldon (1977). The constancies and object orientation: An algorithm processing approach. In William Epstein (ed.), *Stability and Constancy in Visual Perception: Mechanisms and Processes*, 71–90. New York: John Wiley.

Eckert, Michael P., Joel Brian Derrico, and Gershon Buchsbaum (unpublished). The Laplacian of images is a special case of predictive coding in the retina. Paper presented at the 1989 ARVO meeting.

Eddington, Arthur Stanley (1928). *Nature of the Physical World*. Cambridge: Cambridge University Press.

Edds, Mac V. (1951). The eye and seeing. In E. V. McLoughlin (ed.), *Book of Knowledge*, 20 vols., 11:3801–8. New York: Grolier.

Edelman, Shimon (1998). Representation is representation of similarities. *Behavioral and Brain Sciences* 21:449–98.

Elder, Crawford L. (1996). On the reality of medium-sized objects. *Philosophical Studies* 83:191–211.

Einstein, Albert (1934). *Mein Weltbild*. Amsterdam: Querido. Trans. Alan Harris, *The World as I See It*. New York: Covici-Friede, 1934.

Enç, Berent (1975). Numerical identity and objecthood. *Mind* 84:10–26.

Epstein, William (1963). Attitudes of judgment and the size-distance invariance hypothesis. *Journal of Experimental Psychology* 66:78–83.

—— (1967). *Varieties of Perceptual Learning*. New York: McGraw-Hill.

—— (1973). The process of "taking into account" in visual perception. *Perception* 11:75–83.

—— (1977a). Historical introduction to the constancies. In William Epstein (ed.), *Stability and Constancy in Visual Perception: Mechanisms and Processes*, 1–22. New York: John Wiley.

—— (1977b). What are the prospects for a higher-order stimulus theory of perception? *Scandinavian Journal of Psychology* 18:164–71.

—— (1993). On seeing that thinking is separate and thinking that seeing is the same. *Giornale Italiano di Psicologia* 20:731–47.

—— (1995). The metatheoretical context. In William Epstein and Sheena Rogers (eds.), *Perception of Space and Motion*, 1–22. San Diego, Calif.: Academic Press.

Epstein, William, Helen Bontrager, and John Park (1963). The induction of nonveridical slant and the perception of shape. *Journal of Experimental Psychology* 63:472–9.

Epstein, William, and Gary Hatfield (1978). Functional equivalence of masking and cue reduction in perception of shape at a slant. *Perception and Psychophysics* 23:137–44.

—— (1994). Gestalt psychology and the philosophy of mind. *Philosophical Psychology* 7:163–81.

Epstein, William, Gary Hatfield, and Gerard Muise (1977). Perceived shape at a slant as a function of processing time and processing load. *Journal of Experimental Psychology: Human Perception and Performance* 3:473–83.

Euclid (1945). The *Optics* of Euclid, trans. Harry Edwin Burton. *Journal of the Optical Society of America* 35:357–72. Originally written in the 4th c. BCE.

—— (1959). *L'optique el la catoptrique*, trans. Paul Ver Eecke. Paris: Albert Blanchard.

Evans, Gareth (1973). The causal theory of names. *Proceedings of the Aristotelian Society* 47 (supp.):187–208.

―――― (1982). *Varieties of Reference*. Oxford: Clarendon Press.

Farah, Martha J. (1984). The neurological basis of mental imagery: A componential analysis. *Cognition* 18:245–72.

Fechner, Gustav (1960). *Elements of Psychophysics*, trans. Helmut E. Adler. New York: Holt, Rinehart and Winston. Original German edition published in 1860.

Feldman, Jerome A. (1985a). Four frames suffice: A provisional model of vision and space. *Behavioral and Brain Sciences* 8:265–313.

―――― (1985b). Special issue: Connectionist models and their applications: Introduction. *Cognitive Science* 9:1–2.

Feldman, Jerome A., and Dana H. Ballard (1982). Connectionist models and their properties. *Cognitive Science* 6:205–54.

Finger, Stanley (1994). *Origins of Neuroscience*. New York: Oxford University Press.

Firth, Roderick (1965). Sense-data and the percept theory. In Robert J. Swartz (ed.), *Perceiving, Sensing and Knowing*, 204–70. Garden City: Doubleday.

Flanagan, Owen (1992). *Consciousness Reconsidered*. Cambridge, Mass.: MIT Press.

Fodor, Jerry A. (1968). *Psychological Explanation: An Introduction to the Philosophy of Psychology*. New York: Random House.

―――― (1974). Special sciences, or The disunity of science as a working hypothesis. *Synthese* 28:97–115.

―――― (1975). *Language of Thought*. New York: Crowell.

―――― (1980). Methodological solipsism considered as a research strategy in cognitive psychology. *Behavioral and Brain Sciences* 3:63–109.

―――― (1981). *Representations: Philosophical Essays on the Foundations of Cognitive Science*. Cambridge, Mass.: MIT Press.

―――― (1983). *Modularity of Mind: An Essay on Faculty Psychology*. Cambridge, Mass.: MIT Press.

―――― (1987). *Psychosemantics: The Problem of Meaning in the Philosophy of Mind*. Cambridge, Mass.: MIT Press.

―――― (1990). A theory of content, I: The problem. *A Theory of Content and Other Essays*, 51–87. Cambridge, Mass.: MIT Press.

―――― (1998). There are no recognitional concepts—not even RED. *In Critical Condition*, 35–47. Cambridge, Mass.: MIT Press.

―――― (2000). *The Mind Doesn't Work That Way: The Scope and Limits of Computational Psychology*. Cambridge, Mass.: MIT Press.

―――― (unpublished). On there not being an evolutionary theory of content, or, Why, if you've been waiting around for Darwin to pull Brentano's chestnuts out of the fire, my advice to you is: Forget it. Paper presented at the Columbia Conference on Representation, Realism, and Research, December, 1988.

Fodor, Jerry, and Zenon Pylyshyn (1981). How direct is visual perception? Some reflections on Gibson's "Ecological Approach." *Cognition* 9:139–96.

Fodor, Jerry, and Zenon Pylyshyn (1988). Connectionism and cognitive architecture: A critical analysis. *Cognition* 28:3−71.

Foster, Jonathan K., and Marko Jelicic (eds.) (1999). *Memory: Systems, Processes, or Function?* Oxford: Oxford University Press.

French, Robert E. (1987). *The Geometry of Vision and the Mind−Body Problem*. New York: Peter Lang.

Gallistel, Charles R. (1990). *The Organization of Learning*. Cambridge, Mass.: MIT Press.

—— (1998). Symbolic processes in the brain: The case of insect navigation. In Don Scarborough and Saul Sternberg (eds.), *Invitation to Cognitive Science*, vol. 4, *Methods, Models, and Conceptual Issues*, 1−51. Cambridge, Mass.: MIT Press.

Gallistel, Charles R., and John Gibbon (2002). *Symbolic Foundations of Conditioned Behavior*. Mahwah, N.J.: Erlbaum.

Gamble, Clive (1991). Raising the curtain on human origins. *Antiquity* 65:412−17.

Gardner, Howard E. (1985). *The Mind's New Science: A History of the Cognitive Revolution*. New York: Basic Books.

Gazzaniga, Michael S. (1998). *The Mind's Past*. Berkeley, Calif.: University of California Press.

Gehler, Johann Samuel Traugott (1787−96). *Physikalisches Wörterbuch, oder Versuch einer Erklärung der vornehmsten Begriffe und Kunstwörter der Naturlehre*, 6 vols. Leipzig: Schwickert.

Geiger, Roger L. (1986). *To Advance Knowledge: The Growth of American Research Universities, 1900−40*. Oxford: Oxford University Press.

Gibson, James J. (1950). *The Perception of the Visual World*. Boston: Houghton Mifflin.

—— (1966). *The Senses Considered as Perceptual Systems*. Boston: Houghton Mifflin.

—— (1971). The legacies of Koffka's *Principles*. *Journal of the History of the Behavioral Sciences* 7:3−9.

—— (1979). *The Ecological Approach to Visual Perception*. Boston: Houghton Mifflin.

—— (1982). *Reasons for Realism: Selected Essays of James J. Gibson*, ed. Edward S. Reed and Rebecca Jones. Hillsdale, N.J.: Erlbaum.

Gilchrist, Alan (1994). Introduction: Absolute versus relative theories of lightness perception. In Alan Gilchrist (ed.), *Lightness, Brightness, and Transparency*, 1−34. Hillsdale, N.J.: Erlbaum.

Glare, P. G. W. (1968). *Oxford Latin Dictionary*, combined edn., 8 vols. Oxford: Clarendon Press.

Gleitman, Henry (1986). *Psychology*, 2nd edn. New York: Norton.

Gluck, Mark A., and Gordon H. Bower (1988). Evaluating an adaptive network model of human learning. *Journal of Memory and Language* 27:166−95.

Godart, Guillaume-Lambert (1755). *La physique de l'ame*. Berlin: La Compagnie.

Gogel, Walter C. (1990). A theory of phenomenal geometry and its applications. *Perception and Psychophysics* 48:105−23.

Goldsmith, Timothy H. (1990). Optimization, constraint, and history in the evolution of eyes. *Quarterly Review of Biology* 65:281−322.

Goldstein, E. Bruce (1996). *Sensation and Perception*, 4th edn. Pacific Grove, Calif.: Brooks/Cole Publishing Company.

Goodale, Melvyn A., and A. David Milner (1992). Separate visual pathways for perception and action. *Trends in Neuroscience* 15:20–5.

———(2004). *Sight Unseen: An Exploration of Conscious and Unconscious Vision*. Oxford: Oxford University Press.

Goodale, Melvyn A., and David A. Westwood (2004). An evolving view of duplex vision: Separate but interacting cortical pathways for perception and action. *Current Opinion in Neurobiology* 14:203–11.

Goodman, Nelson (1968). *Languages of Art: An Approach to a Theory of Symbols*. Indianapolis: Bobbs-Merrill.

Gordon, Ian E. (1997). *Theories of Visual Perception*, 2nd edn. New York: Wiley.

Gould, Stephen Jay, and Richard C. Lewontin (1979). The Spandrels of San Marco and the Panglossian paradigm: A critique of the adaptationist programme. *Proceedings of the Royal Society* B 205:581–98.

Granit, Ragnar (1947). *Sensory Mechanisms of the Retina*. London: Oxford University Press.

———(1955). *Receptors and Sensory Perception*. New Haven, Conn.: Yale University Press.

Granrud, Carl E. (2004). Visual metacognition and the development of size constancy. In Daniel T. Levin (ed.), *Thinking and Seeing: Visual Metacognition in Adults and Children*, 75–95. Cambridge, Mass.: MIT Press.

Green, Bert F., Jr. (1967). The computer conquest of psychology. *Psychology Today* 1:56–61.

Gregory, Richard L. (1966). *Eye and Brain: The Psychology of Seeing*. London: Weidenfeld and Nicolson.

———(1974). Perceptions as hypotheses. In S. C. Brown (ed.), *Philosophy of Psychology*, 195–210. London: Macmillan.

———(1978). *Eye and Brain: The Psychology of Seeing*, 3rd edn. New York: McGraw-Hill.

———(1997). *Eye and Brain: The Psychology of Seeing*, 5th edn. Princeton: Princeton University Press.

Grice, Herbert Paul (1957). Meaning. *Philosophical Review* 66:377–88.

———(1974–5). Method in philosophical psychology (from the banal to the bizarre). *Proceedings and Addresses of the American Philosophical Association* 48:23–53.

Grünbaum, Adolf (1973). *Philosophical Problems of Space and Time*, 2nd edn. Dordrecht: Reidel.

Gurwitsch, Aron (1964). *The Field of Consciousness*. Pittsburgh, Pa.: Duquesne University Press.

Haber, Ralph N. (1986). Toward a theory of the perceived spatial layout of scenes. In A. Rosenfeld (ed.), *Human and Machine Vision II*, 109–48. Boston: Academic Press.

Haber, Ralph N., and Maurice Hershenson (1973). *Psychology of Visual Perception*. New York: Holt, Rinehart and Winston.

Haber, Ralph N., and Maurice Hershenson (1980). *Psychology of Visual Perception*, 2nd edn. New York: Holt, Rinehart and Winston.

Hacker, P. M. S. (1987). *Appearance and Reality: A Philosophical Investigation into Perception and Perceptual Qualities*. Oxford: Blackwell.

Hamilton, William (1859). *Lectures on Metaphysics*, ed. Henry L. Mansel and John Veitch. London: Blackwood.

——— (1895). Notes and supplementary dissertations. *Works of Thomas Reid*, ed. William Hamilton, 8th edn. Edinburgh: James Thin.

Hamlyn, D. W. (1957). *The Psychology of Perception: A Philosophical Examination of Gestalt Theory and Derivative Theories of Perception*. London: Routledge.

Hardin, Clyde L. (1988). *Color for Philosophers: Unweaving the Rainbow*. Indianapolis: Hackett Publishing Company.

Harman, Gilbert (1990). The intrinsic quality of experience. In James E. Tomberlin (ed.), *Philosophical Perspectives*, vol. 4, *Action Theory and Philosophy of Mind*, 31–52. Atascadero, Calif.: Ridgeview.

——— (1996). Explaining objective color in terms of subjective reactions. In Enrique Villanueva (ed.), *Philosophical Issues*, vol. 7, *Perception*, 1–17. Atascadero, Calif.: Ridgeview.

Hatfield, Gary (1979). Force (God) in Descartes' physics. *Studies in History and Philosophy of Science* 10:113–40.

——— (1986a). Perception. *Encyclopedia Americana*, 21:689–93. Danbury: Grolier.

——— (1986b). The senses and the fleshless eye: The *Meditations* as cognitive exercises. In Amélie Rorty (ed.), *Essays on Descartes' Meditations*, 45–79. Berkeley: University of California Press.

——— (1988a). Neuro-philosophy meets psychology: Reduction, autonomy, and physiological constraints. *Cognitive Neuropsychology* 5:723–46.

——— (1988b). Representation and content in some (actual) theories of perception. *Studies in History and Philosophy of Science* 19:175–214.

——— (1990a). Metaphysics and the new science. In David Lindberg and Robert S. Westman (eds.), *Reappraisals of the Scientific Revolution*, 93–166. Cambridge: Cambridge University Press.

——— (1990b). *The Natural and the Normative: Theories of Spatial Perception from Kant to Helmholtz*. Cambridge, Mass.: MIT Press.

——— (1991a). Representation and rule-instantiation in connectionist systems. In Terence Horgan and John Tienson (eds.), *Connectionism and the Philosophy of Mind*, 90–112. Boston: Kluwer.

——— (1991b). Representation in perception and cognition: Connectionist affordances. In William Ramsey, David E. Rumelhart, and Stephen P. Stich (eds.), *Philosophy and Connectionist Theory*, 163–95. Hillsdale, N.J.: Erlbaum.

——— (1992a). Color perception and neural encoding: Does metameric matching entail a loss of information? In David Hull and Micky Forbes (eds.), *PSA 1992*, vol. 1:492–504. East Lansing, Mich.: Philosophy of Science Association.

_____(1992*b*). Descartes's physiology and its relation to his psychology. In John Cottingham (ed.), *Cambridge Companion to Descartes*, 335–70. Cambridge: Cambridge University Press.

_____(1993). Commentary on Dennis Proffitt: A hierarchical approach to perception. In S. C. Masin (ed.), *Foundations of Perceptual Theory*, 93–8. Amsterdam: Elsevier.

_____(1994). Psychology as a natural science in the eighteenth century. *Revue de synthèse* 115:375–91.

_____(1995*a*). Philosophy of psychology as philosophy of science. In David Hull, Micky Forbes, and Richard M. Burian (eds.) *PSA 1994*, vol. 2:19–23. East Lansing, Mich.: Philosophy of Science Association.

_____(1995*b*). Remaking the science of mind: Psychology as a natural science. In Christopher Fox, Roy Porter, and Robert Wokler (eds.), *Inventing Human Science*, 184–231. Berkeley: University of California Press.

_____(1996). Was the scientific revolution really a revolution in science? In Jamil Ragep and Sally Ragep (eds.), *Tradition, Transmission, Transformation*, 489–525. Leiden: Brill.

_____(1997). Wundt and psychology as science: Disciplinary transformations. *Perspectives on Science* 5:349–82.

_____(1998). The cognitive faculties. In Michael Ayers and Daniel Garber (eds.), *Cambridge History of Seventeenth Century Philosophy*, 953–1002. Cambridge: Cambridge University Press.

_____(1999). Mental functions as constraints on neurophysiology: Biology and psychology of vision. In Valerie Gray Hardcastle (ed.), *Where Biology Meets Psychology: Philosophical Essays*, 251–71. Cambridge, Mass.: MIT Press.

_____(2000*a*). Descartes' naturalism about the mental. In Stephen Gaukroger, John Schuster, and John Sutton (eds.), *Descartes' Natural Philosophy*, 630–58. London: Routledge.

_____(2000*b*). The brain's "new" science: Psychology, neurophysiology, and constraint. *Philosophy of Science* 67:S388–403.

_____(2001). Epistemology and science in the image of modern philosophy: Rorty on Descartes and Locke. In Juliet Floyd and Sanford Shieh (eds.), *Future Pasts: Reflections on the History and Nature of Analytic Philosophy*, 393–413. New York: Oxford University Press.

_____(2002*a*). Perception as unconscious inference. In Dieter Heyer and Rainer Mausfeld (eds.), *Perception and the Physical World: Psychological and Philosophical Issue in Perception*, 115–43. New York: Wiley.

_____(2002*b*). Psychology, philosophy, and cognitive science: Reflections on the history and philosophy of experimental psychology. *Mind and Language* 17:207–32.

_____(2002*c*). Sense-data and the philosophy of mind. *Principia* 6:203–30.

_____(2003*a*). Behaviorism and psychology. In Thomas Baldwin (ed.), *Cambridge History of Philosophy, 1870–1945*, 640–8. Cambridge: Cambridge University Press.

_____(2003*b*). *Descartes and the Meditations*. London: Routledge.

Hatfield, Gary (2003c). Objectivity and subjectivity revisited: Colour as a psychobiological property. In Rainer Mausfeld and Dieter Heyer (eds.), *Colour Perception: Mind and the Physical World*, 187–202. Oxford: Oxford University Press.

——(2003d). Psychology old and new. In Thomas Baldwin (ed.), *Cambridge History of Philosophy, 1870–1945*, 93–106. Cambridge: Cambridge University Press.

——(2003e). Representation and constraints: The inverse problem and the structure of visual space. *Acta Psychologica* 114:355–78.

——(2004). Sense-data and the mind–body problem. In Ralph Schumacher (ed.), *Perception and Reality: From Descartes to the Present*, 305–31. Berlin: Mentis Verlag.

——(2005). Introspective evidence in psychology. In Peter Achinstein (ed.), *Scientific Evidence: Philosophical Theories and Applications*, 259–86. Baltimore: Johns Hopkins University Press.

——(2006). Psychology and philosophy. In Anthony Grayling, Andrew Pyle, and Naomi Goulder (eds.), *Continuum Encyclopedia of British Philosophy*, 4 vols., 3:2613–21. London: Thoemmes.

——(2008). Psychology in philosophy: Historical perspectives. In Sara Heinämaa and Martina Reuter (eds.), *Psychology and Philosophy: Inquiries into the Soul from Late Scholasticism to Contemporary Thought*, 1–25. Dordrecht: Springer.

——(ed.) (forthcoming-a). *Evolution of Mind, Brain, and Culture*. Philadelphia: University of Pennsylvania Museum of Anthropology and Archaeology.

——(forthcoming-b). Sense data and perception. In Michael Beaney (ed.), *Oxford Handbook of the History of Analytic Philosophy*. Oxford: Oxford University Press.

——(forthcoming-c). Transparency of mind: The contributions of Descartes, Leibniz, and Berkeley to the genesis of the modern subject. In Hubertus Busch (ed.), *Departure for Modern Europe: Philosophy between 1400 and 1700*. Hamburg: Meiner.

Hatfield, Gary, and William Epstein (1979). The sensory core and the medieval foundations of early modern perceptual theory. *Isis* 70:363–84.

——(1985). The status of the minimum principle in the theoretical analysis of vision. *Psychological Bulletin* 97:155–86.

Hatfield, Gary, and Edward N. Pugh (unpublished). Psychophysical laws, qualia, and psycho-neural linking hypotheses.

Haugeland, John (1978). The nature and plausibility of cognitivism. *Behaviorial and Brain Sciences* 1:215–26. As republished in John Haugeland (ed.), *Mind Design*. Cambridge, Mass.: MIT Press, 1981.

——(1985). *Artificial Intelligence: The Very Idea*. Cambridge, Mass.: MIT Press.

Hearnshaw, L. S. (1987). *The Shaping of Modern Psychology*. London: Routledge & Kegan Paul.

Hecht, Selig (1928). On the binocular fusion of colors and its relation to theories of color vision. *Proceedings of the National Academy of Sciences of the United States of America* 114:237–41.

——(1934). Vision II: The nature of the photoreceptor process. In Carl Murchison (ed.), *Handbook of General Experimental Psychology*, 504–828. Worcester, Mass.: Clark University Press.

Heelan, Patrick A. (1983). *Space-Perception and the Philosophy of Science*. Berkeley: University of California Press.

Heil, John (1983). *Perception and Cognition*. Berkeley: University of California Press.

——(2005). Real tables. *Monist* 88:493–509.

Heisenberg, Werner (1948). Die Einheit des naturwissenschaftlichen Weltbildes. In *Wandlungen in den Grundlagen der Naturwissenschaft: Acht Vorträge*, 8th edn. Zürich: Hirzel. Trans. F. C. Hayes, On the unity of the scientific outlook on nature. In F. C. Hayes (ed.), *Philosophic Problems of Nuclear Science*, 77–94. New York: Pantheon, 1952. Volume reprinted as *Philosophic Problems of Quantum Physics,* Woodbridge, Conn.: Ox Bow Press, 1979. Lecture originally given in 1941 at the University of Leipzig.

Held, Richard (1968). Dissociation of visual functions by deprivation and rearrangement. *Psychologische Forschung* 31:338–48.

Helm, Peter A. van der (2000). Simplicity versus likelihood in visual perception: From surprisals to precisals. *Psychological Bulletin* 126:770–800.

Helmholtz, Hermann (1867). *Handbuch der physiologischen Optik*. Leipzig: Voss. As republished in the 3rd German edn, 3 vols., Leipzig: Voss, 1910. The translations herein are the author's.

——(1868). Die neueren Fortschritte in der Theorie des Sehens. *Preussischen Jahrbücher*. Trans. as: Recent progress in the theory of vision. In Helmholtz (1995), 127–203.

——(1878). *Die Thatsachen in der Wahrnehmung*. Berlin: Hirschwald. Trans. as: The facts in perception. In Helmholtz (1995), 342–80.

——(1882–95). *Wissenschaftliche Abhandlungen*, 3 vols. Leipzig: Barth.

——(1894). Über den Ursprung der richtigen Deutung unserer Sinneseindrücke. *Zeitschrift für Psychologie und Physiologie der Sinnesorgane* 7:81–96. Trans. as: The origin and correct interpretation of our sense impressions. In *Selected Writings of Hermann von Helmholtz*, ed. Russell Kahl, 501–12. Middletown, Conn.: Wesleyan University Press, 1971.

——(1896). *Vorträge und Reden*, 4th edn., 2 vols. Braunschweig: Vieweg.

——(1924–5). *Helmholtz's Treatise on Physiological Optics*, ed. and trans. James P. C. Southall, 3 vols. Rochester, N.Y.: Optical Society of America. Trans. from 3rd German edn.

——(1995). *Science and Culture: Popular and Philosophical Essays by Hermann von Helmholtz*, ed. David Cahan. Chicago: University of Chicago Press.

Hempel, Carl G. (1935). Analyse logique de la psychologie. *Revue de synthèse* 10:27–42.

——(1949). Logical analysis of psychology, trans. Wilfrid Sellars. In Herbert Feigl and Wilfred Sellars (ed.), *Readings in Philosophical Analysis*, 373–84. New York: Appleton-Century-Crofts.

——(1963). The logic of functional analysis. *Aspects of Scientific Explanation and Other Essays in the Philosophy of Science*, 297–330. New York: Free Press.

Hering, Ewald (1875a). Zur Lehre von der Beziehung zwischen Leib und Seele. I. Mittheilung. Ueber Fechner's psychophysisches Gesetz. *Sitzungsberichte der Kaiserlichen Akademie der Wissenschaften zu Wien. Mathematisch-Naturwissenschaftliche Classe*, pt. 3, 72:310–48.

Hering, Ewald (1875b). Zur Lehre vom Lichtsinne, VI. Grundzüge einer Theorie des Farbensinnes. *Sitzungsberichte der Kaiserlichen Akademie der Wissenschaften in Wien. Mathematisch-naturwissenschaftliche Classe*, pt. 3, 70:169–204.

——(1905–20). *Grundzüge der Lehre vom Lichtsinn*. Leipzig: Engelmann.

——(1964). *Outlines of a Theory of the Light Sense*, trans. Leo M. Hurvich and Dorothea Jameson. Cambridge, Mass.: Harvard University Press.

Hershenson, Maurice (1999). *Visual Space Perception*. Cambridge, Mass.: MIT Press.

Hilbert, David R. (1987). *Color and Color Perception: A Study in Anthropocentric Realism*. Stanford, Calif.: Center for the Study of Language and Information.

——(1992). What is color vision? *Philosophical Studies* 68:351–70.

——(2005). Color constancy and the complexity of color. *Philosophical Topics* 33:141–58

Hilgard, Ernest R. (1987). *Psychology in America: A Historical Survey*. San Diego: Harcourt Brace Jovanovich.

——(1997). A personal view of 20th-century psychology: With an eye to the 21st century. In Robert L. Solso (ed.), *Mind and Brain Sciences in the 21st Century*, xi–xv. Cambridge, Mass.: MIT Press.

Hillebrand, Franz (1902). Theorie der scheinbaren Grösse beim binokularen Sehen. *Denkschrift der Kaiserlichen Akademie der Wissenschaften Wien, Mathematisch-Naturwissenschaftliche Classe* 72:255–307.

Hinton, Geoffrey E., James L. McClelland, and David E. Rumelhart (1986). Distributed representations. In David E. Rumelhart and James L. McClelland (eds.), *Parallel Distributed Processing: Explorations in the Microstructure of Cognition*, vol. 1, *Foundations*, 77–109. Cambridge, Mass.: MIT Press.

Hinton, Geoffrey E., and Terrence J. Sejnowski (1986). Learning and relearning in Boltzmann machines. In Rumelhart and McClelland (1986b), 1:282–317.

Hirsch, Eli (1982). *The Concept of Identity*. New York: Oxford University Press.

——(1997). Basic objects: A reply to Xu. *Mind and Language* 12:406–12.

Hochberg, Julian E. (1981). Levels of perceptual organization. In Michael Kubovy and James R. Pomeranz (eds.), *Perceptual Organization*, 255–278. Hillsdale, N.J.: Erlbaum.

Hodges, Wilfrid (1997). *A Shorter Model Theory*. Cambridge, Mass.: Cambridge University Press.

Hoorn, Willem van (1972). *As Images Unwind: Ancient and Modern Theories of Visual Perception*. Amsterdam: University Press.

Hopkins, Robert (1998). *Picture, Image, and Experience: A Philosophical Inquiry*. Cambridge, Mass.: Cambridge University Press.

Hornstein, Norbert (1984). *Logic as Grammar*. Cambridge, Mass.: MIT Press.

Hull, Clark L. (1943). *Principles of Behavior: An Introduction to Behavior Theory*. New York: Appleton-Century-Crofts.

Hume, David (1739–40), *Treatise of Human Nature*. London: John Noon.

——(1748), *Philosophical Essays Concerning Human Understanding*. London: Millar.

——(1999). *An Enquiry Concerning Human Understanding*, ed. Tom L. Beauchamp. Oxford: Oxford University Press.

Huntley-Fenner, Gavin, Susan Carey, and Andrea Solimando (2002). Objects are individuals but stuff doesn't count: Perceived rigidity and cohesiveness influence infants' representations of small groups of discrete entities. *Cognition* 83:203–21.

Hurlbert, Anya C. (1998). Computational models of color constancy. In Vincent Walsh and Janusz Kulikowski (eds.), *Perceptual Constancy: Why Things Look as They Do*, 283–322. Cambridge: Cambridge University Press.

Hurvich, Leo M. (1969). Hering and the scientific establishment. *American Psychologist* 24:497–514.

——(1981). *Color Vision*. Sunderland, Mass.: Sinauer.

Hurvich, Leo M., and Dorothea Jameson (1951). The binocular fusion of yellow in relation to color theories. *Science* 114:199–202.

——(1957). An opponent-process theory of color vision. *Psychological Review* 64:384–404.

——(1966). *Perception of Brightness and Darkness*. Boston: Allyn and Bacon.

——(1989). Leo M. Hurvich and Dorothea Jameson. In Gardner Lindzey (ed.), *A History of Psychology in Autobiography*, vol. 8:156–206. Stanford: Stanford University Press.

Hutchison, Keith (1991). Dormitive virtues, scholastic qualities, and the new philosophies. *History of Science* 29:245–78.

Ibn al-Haytham (1572). *De aspectibus*. In Friedrich Risner (ed.), *Opticae thesaurus: Alhazeni Arabis libri septem; De Crepusculis et nubium ascensionibus; Vitellonis Thuringopoloni libri X.* Basel: Episcopate. Reprint, New York: Johnson Reprint, 1972.

——(1989). *The Optics of Ibn al-Haytham: Books I–III, On Direct Vision*, vol. 1, *Translation*, ed. and trans. Abdelhamid I. Sabra. London: Warburg Institute. (Originally written c.1030.)

——(2001). *Alhacen's Theory of Visual Perception: A Critical Edition, with English Translation and Commentary, of the First Three Books of Alhacen's De aspectibus*, ed. and trans. A. Mark Smith. Philadelphia: American Philosophical Society.

Indow, Tarow (1982). An approach to geometry of visual space with no a priori mapping functions: Multidimensional mapping according to Riemannian metrics. *Journal of Mathematical Psychology* 26:204–36.

——(1991). A critical review of Luneburg's model with regard to global structure of visual space. *Psychological Review* 98:430–53.

——(1995). Psychophysical scaling: Scientific and practical applications. In Robert Duncan Luce, Michael D'Zmura, Donald Hoffman, Geoffrey J. Iverson, and A. Kimball Romney (eds.), *Geometric Representations of Perceptual Phenomena*, 1–34. Mahwah, N.J.: Erlbaum.

Indow, Tarow, Emiko Inoue, and Keiko Matsushima (1962). An experimental study of the Luneburg theory of binocular space (2). The alley experiments. *Japanese Psychological Research* 4:17–24.

Ingle, David (1967). Two visual mechanisms underlying the behavior of fish. *Psychologische Forschung* 31:44–51.

Jackson, Frank (1998). *From Metaphysics to Ethics: A Defence of Conceptual Analysis.* Oxford: Clarendon Press.

Jackson, Frank, and Robert Pargetter (1987). An objectivist's guide to subjectivism about colour. *Revue internationale de philosophie* 41:127–41.

Jacobs, Gerald H. (1981). *Comparative Color Vision.* New York: Academic Press.

—— (1993). The distribution and nature of colour vision among the mammals. *Biological Review* 68:413–71.

—— (1996). Primate photopigments and primate color vision. *Proceedings of the National Academy of Science USA* 93:577–81.

Jacobs, Gerald H., and Mickey P. Rowe (2004). Evolution of vertebrate colour vision. *Clinical and Experimental Optometry* 87:206–16.

James, William (1890). *Principles of Psychology*, 2 vols. New York: Henry Holt.

—— (1904). Does "consciousness" exist? *Journal of Philosophy, Psychology and Scientific Method* 1:477–91. As republished in James, *Essays in Radical Empiricism*, Lincoln, Nebr.: University of Nebraska Press, 1996 (reprint, with new introduction, of the original 1912 edition).

—— (1912). The experience of activity. *Essay in Radical Empiricism*, 155–89. New York: Longmans, Green, and Co.

Jameson, Dorothea, and Leo M. Hurvich (1989). Essay concerning color constancy. *Annual Review of Psychology* 40:1–22.

Jevons, W. Stanley (1871). Power of numerical discrimination. *Nature* 3:281–2.

Johansson, Gunnar, Claes von Hofsten, and Gunnar Jansson (1980). Direct perception and perceptual processes. *Behavioral and Brain Sciences* 3:388.

Johnston, Mark (1992). How to speak of the colors. *Philosophical Studies* 68:221–63.

Johnston, William A., and Veronica J. Dark (1987). Selective attention. *Annual Review of Psychology* 37:43–75.

Jonides, John, Richard L. Lewis, Derek Evan Nee, Cindy A. Lustig, Marc G. Berman, and Katherine Sledge Moore (2008). The mind and brain of short-term memory. *Annual Review of Psychology* 59:193–224.

Kaiser, Peter K., and Robert M. Boynton (1996). *Human Color Vision*, 2nd edn. Washington D.C.: Optical Society of America.

Kandel, Eric R., James H. Schwartz, and Thomas M. Jessell (2000). *Principles of Neural Science*, 4th edn. New York: McGraw-Hill.

Kanizsa, Gaetano (1979). *Organization in Vision: Essays on Gestalt Perception.* New York: Praeger.

—— (1985). Seeing and thinking. *Acta Psychologica* 59:23–33.

Kant, Immanuel (1781). *Kritik der reinen Vernunft.* Riga: Hartnoch. Translations in the text are by the author.

—— (1783). *Prolegomena zu einer jeden künftigen Metaphysik.* Riga: Hartnoch.

—— (1787). *Kritik der reinen Vernunft*, 2nd edn. Riga: Hartnoch. Translations in the text are by the author.

—— (1998). *Critique of Pure Reason,* ed. and trans. Paul Guyer and Allen Wood. Cambridge: Cambridge University Press.

_____ (2004). *Prolegomena to Any Future Metaphysics*, ed. and trans. Gary Hatfield, 2nd edn. Cambridge: Cambridge University Press.

Kaplan, David (1969). Quantifying in. In Donald Davidson and Jaakko Hintikka (eds.), *Words and Objections: Essays on the Work of W. V. Quine*, 206–42. Dordrecht: Reidel.

_____ (1989a). Demonstratives: An essay on the semantics, logic, metaphysics, and epistemology of demonstratives and other indexicals. In Joseph Almog, John Perry, and Howard Wettstein (eds.), *Themes from Kaplan*, 481–563. New York: Oxford University Press.

_____ (1989b). Afterthoughts. In Joseph Almog, John Perry, and Howard Wettstein (eds.), *Themes from Kaplan*, 565–614. New York: Oxford University Press.

Kaufman, E. L., M. W. Lord, T. W. Reese, and J. Volkmann (1949). The discrimination of visual number. *American Journal of Psychology* 62:498–525.

Kaufman, Lloyd (1974). *Sight and Mind: An Introduction to Visual Perception*. New York: Oxford University Press.

Kaukua, Jari, and Taneli Kukkonen (2007). Sense-perception and self-awareness: Before and after Avicenna. In Sara Heinämaa, Vili Lähteenmäki, and Pauliina Remes (eds.), *Consciousness: From Perception to Reflection in the History of Philosophy*, 95–119. Dordrecht: Springer.

Kellman, Philip J., and Elizabeth Spelke (1983). Perception of partly occluded objects in infancy. *Cognitive Psychology* 15:483–524.

Kepler, Johannes (1611). *Dioptrice*. Augsburg: David Franke. Reprint, Cambridge: Heffer, 1962.

_____ (1904). *Dioptrik*, trans. F. Plehn. Leipzig: Ostwald's Klassiker der exakten Wissenschaften.

_____ (1939). *Ad vitellionem paralipomena* (originally published in 1604). *Gesammelte Werke*, vol. 2. Munich: Beck.

_____ (1964). De modo visionis, trans. Alistair Cameron Crombie. In I. Bernard Cohen and René Taton (eds.), *Mélanges Alexandre Koyré*, 2 vols., 1:135–72. Paris: Hermann.

_____ (2000). *Optics: Paralipomena to Witelo and Optical Part of Astronomy*, ed. and trans. William H. Donahue. Santa Fe, N.M.: Green Lion Press.

Kienker, Paul K., Terrence J. Sejnowski, Geoffrey E. Hinton, and Lee E. Schumacher (1986). Separating figure from ground with a parallel network. *Perception* 15:197–215.

Kinchla, Ronald A. (1992). Attention. *Annual Review of Psychology* 43:711–42.

Kitcher, Patricia (1984). In defense of intentional psychology. *Journal of Philosophy*, 81:89–106.

_____ (1985). Narrow taxonomy and wide functionalism. *Philosophy of Science* 52:78–97.

Koch, Sigmund (1941). The logical character of the motivational concept. *Psychological Review* 48:15–38.

_____ (1964). Psychology and emerging conceptions of knowledge as unitary. In T. W. Wann (ed.), *Behaviorism and Phenomenology: Contrasting Bases for Modern Psychology*, 1–41. Chicago: University of Chicago Press.

Koenderink, Jan J., Andrea J. van Doorn, Astrid M. L. Kappers, and James. T. Todd (2002). Pappus in optical space. *Perception and Psychophysics* 64:380–91.

Koenderink, Jan J., Andrea J. van Doorn, and Joseph S. Lappin (2000). Direct measurement of the curvature of visual space. *Perception* 29:69–79.

Koffka, Kurt (1935). *Principles of Gestalt Psychology*. New York: Harcourt, Brace.

Köhler, Wolfgang (1929). *Gestalt Psychology*. New York: Liveright.

——(1947). *Gestalt Psychology: An Introduction to New Concepts in Modern Psychology*. New York: Liveright.

Kolers, Paul. A. (1975). Specificity of operations in sentence recognition. *Cognitive Psychology* 7:289–306.

Kosslyn, Stephen M. (1980). *Image and Mind*. Cambridge, Mass.: Harvard University Press.

——(1983). *Ghosts in the Mind's Machine: Creating and Using Images in the Brain*. New York: Norton.

——(1994) *Image and Brain: The Resolution of the Imagery Debate*. Cambridge, Mass.: MIT Press.

——(1995). Mental imagery. In Stephen M. Kosslyn and Daniel N. Osherson (eds.), *Invitation to Cognitive Science*, vol. 2, *Visual Cognition*, 2nd edn., 267–96. Cambridge, Mass.: MIT Press.

Kosslyn, Stephen M., and Gary Hatfield (1984). Representation without symbol systems. *Social Research* 51:1019–45.

Krantz, David H., R. Duncan Luce, Patrick Suppes, and Amos Tversky (1971). *Foundations of Measurement*, vol. 1, *Additive and Polynomial Representations*. New York: Academic Press.

Kriegel, Uriah (2002). Phenomenal content. *Erkenntnis* 57:175–98.

Kripke, Saul (1972). Naming and necessity. In Donald Davidson and Gilbert Harman (eds.), *The Semantics of Natural Language*, 254–355. Dordrecht: Reidel.

——(1981). *Wittgenstein on Rules and Private Language: An Elementary Exposition*. Oxford: Blackwell.

Krüger, Johann Gottlob (1756). *Versuch einer Experimental-Seelenlehre*. Halle: Hermerde.

Kubovy, Michael, and William Epstein (2001). Internalization: A metaphor we can live without. *Behavioral and Brain Sciences* 24:618–25.

Kusch, Martin (1995). *Psychologism: A Case Study in the Sociology of Philosophical Knowledge*. London: Routledge.

——(1999). *Psychological Knowledge: A Social History and Philosophy*. London: Routledge.

LaBerge, David (1995). *Attentional Processing: The Brain's Art of Mindfulness*. Cambridge, Mass.: Harvard University Press.

Ladd, George T. (1895). *Psychology: Descriptive and Explanatory*. New York: Charles Scribner's Sons.

Ladd-Franklin, Christine (1929). *Colour and Colour Theories*. London: Kegan Paul, Trench, Trubner.

Le Cat, Claude-Nicolas (1767). *Traité des sensations et des passions en général, et des sens en particulier*, 2 vols. Paris: Vallat-La-Chapelle.

Le Grand, Antoine (1694). *An Entire Body of Philosophy, According to the Principles of the Famous Renate des Cartes*, trans. Richard Blome. London: Samuel Roycroft and Richard Blome.

Leahey, Thomas H. (1980). *A History of Psychology*. Englewood Cliffs, N.J.: Prentice-Hall.

Leeuwenberg, Emanuel L. J. (1969). Quantitative specification of information in sequential patterns. *Psychological Review* 76:216–20.

Lehky, Sidney R., and Terrence J. Sejnowski (1988). Network model of shape-from-shading: Neural function arises from both receptive and projective fields. *Nature* 333:452–4.

Lehot, C. J. (1823). *Nouvelle theorie de la vision: premier mémoire, partie physiologique*. Paris: Huzard-Courcier.

Leibniz, Gottfried Wilhelm (1981). *New Essays on Human Understanding*, ed. and trans. Peter Remnant and Jonathan Bennett. Cambridge: Cambridge University Press. Cited by book, chapter, and section number.

Leijenhorst, Cees (2007). Attention, please! Theories of selective attention in late Aristotelian and early modern philosophy. In Paul J. J. M. Bakker and Johannes M. M. H. Thijssen (eds.), *Mind, Cognition and Representation: The Tradition of Commentaries on Aristotle's De anima*. Aldershot: Ashgate.

Lejeune, Albert (1948). *Euclide et Ptolémée, deux stades de l'optique géométrique grecque*. Louvain: Bibliothèque de l'Université.

Levine, Joseph (2001). *Purple Haze: The Puzzle of Consciousness*. Oxford: Oxford University Press.

Lewontin, Richard C. (1998). The evolution of cognition: Questions we will never answer. In Don Scarborough and Saul Sternberg (eds.), *An Invitation to Cognitive Science*, vol. 4, *Methods, Models, and Conceptual Issues*, 107–32. Cambridge, Mass.: MIT Press.

Lindberg, David C. (1976). *Theories of Vision from al-Kindi to Kepler*. Chicago: University of Chicago Press.

Lindemann, Bernd (2001). Receptors and transduction in taste. *Nature* 413:219–25.

Lindsay, Peter H., and Donald A. Norman (1972). *Human Information Processing: An Introduction to Psychology*. New York: Academic Press.

Linksz, Arthur (1952). *Physiology of the Eye*, vol. 2, *Vision*. New York: Grune & Stratton.

Lloyd, Dan (1989). *Simple Minds*. Cambridge, Mass.: MIT Press.

Locke, John (1690). *An Essay Concerning Human Understanding*. London: Bassett.

——— (1975). *An Essay Concerning Human Understanding*, ed. Peter H. Nidditch. Oxford: Clarendon Press. Cited by book, chapter, and section number.

Loeb, Jacques (1900). *Comparative Physiology of the Brain and Comparative Psychology*. New York: G. P. Putnam's Sons.

Loewy, Ariel G., and Philip Siekevitz (1969). *Cell Structure and Function*, 2nd edn. New York: Holt.

Lombardi, Olimpia (2005). Dretske, Shannon's theory and the interpretation of information. *Synthese* 144:23–39.

Lowe, E. Jonathan (1992). Experience and its objects. In Tim Crane (ed.), *The Contents of Experience*, 79–104. Cambridge: Cambridge University Press.

Lucretius (1965). *On Nature*, trans. Russel M. Geer. Indianapolis: Bobbs-Merrill. Cited by book and line number.

——(1967). *De rerum natura*, rev. edn. Oxford: Clarendon Press.

Ludwig, Kirk (1996). Explaining why things look the way they do. In Kathleen Akins (ed.), *Perception*, 18–60. New York: Oxford University Press.

Lumsden, Charles J., and Edward O. Wilson (1981). *Genes, Mind, and Culture*. Cambridge, Mass.: Harvard University Press.

Luneburg, Rudolf K. (1947). *Mathematical Analysis of Binocular Vision*. Princeton: Princeton University Press.

Lycan, William (1997). Consciousness as internal monitoring. In Ned Block, Owen Flanagan, and Guven Guzeldere (eds.), *Nature of Consciousness*, 755–71. Cambridge, Mass.: MIT Press.

Lyons, William (1986). *Disappearance of Introspection*. Cambridge, Mass.: MIT Press.

Lythgoe, John N. (1972). Adaptation of visual pigments to the photic environment. In Herbert J. A. Dartnall (ed), *Handbook of Sensory Physiology*, vol. 7, pt. 1, *Photochemistry of Vision*, 566–603. Berlin: Springer-Verlag.

——(1979). *The Ecology of Vision*. Oxford: Oxford University Press.

Lythgoe, John N., and Julian C. Partridge (1991). Modelling of optimal visual pigments of dichromatic teleosts in green coastal waters. *Vision Research* 31:361–71.

MacArthur, David J. (1982). Computer vision and perceptual psychology. *Psychological Bulletin* 92:283–309.

McBeath, Michael K., Dennis M. Shaffer, and Mary K. Kaiser (1996). On catching fly balls. *Science* 273:258–60.

McClelland, James L., David E. Rumelhart, and Geoffrey E. Hinton (1986). The appeal of parallel distributed processing. In David E. Rumelhart and James L. McClelland (eds.), *Parallel Distributed Processing: Explorations in the Microstructure of Cognition*, vol. 1, *Foundations*, 3–44. Cambridge, Mass.: MIT Press.

McDougall, William (1905). *Physiological Psychology*. London: Dent.

——(1912). *Psychology, The Study of Behaviour*. New York: Holt.

McDowell, John (1996). *Mind and World*. Cambridge, Mass.: Harvard University Press.

McFarland, William N., and Frederick W. Munz (1975). The evolution of photopic visual pigments in fishes. *Vision Research* 15:1071–80.

McLaughlin, Brian (2003). The place of colour in nature. In Rainer Mausfeld and Dieter Heyer (eds.), *Colour Perception: Mind and the Physical World*, 475–502. Oxford: Oxford University Press.

Mach, Ernst (1886). *Beiträge zur Analyse der Empfindungen*. Jena: Fischer.

——(1897). *Contributions to the Analysis of Sensations*, trans. C. M. Williams. La Salle, Ill.: Open Court.

Mackie, Roderick I. (2002). Mutualistic fermentative digestion in the gastrointestinal tract: Diversity and evolution. *Integrative and Comparative Biology* 42:319–26.

Malebranche, Nicolas (1980). *Search after Truth*, trans. Thomas M. Lennon and Paul J. Olscamp. Columbus: Ohio State University Press.

Mallot, Hanspeter A. (2000). *Computational Vision: Information Processing in Perception and Visual Behavior.* Cambridge, Mass.: MIT Press.

Maloney, Laurence T. (1986). Evaluation of linear models of surface spectral reflectance with small numbers of parameters. *Journal of the Optical Society of America* A 3:1673–83.

_____ (2003). Surface colour perception and environmental constraints. In Rainer Mausfeld and Dieter Heyer (eds.), *Colour Perception: Mind and the Physical World*, 279–300. Oxford: Oxford University Press.

Maloney, Laurence T. and Brian A. Wandell (1986). Color constancy: A method for recovering surface spectral reflectance. *Journal of the Optical Society of America* A 3:29–33.

Marcel, Anthony J. (1983). Conscious and unconscious perceptions: An approach to the relations between phenomenal experience and perceptual processes. *Cognitive Psychology* 15:197–237.

Marr, David (1982). *Vision: Computational Investigation into the Human Representation and Processing of Visual Information.* San Francisco: Freeman.

Massaro, Dominic W. (1989). *Experimental Psychology: An Information Processing Approach.* San Diego: Harcourt Brace Jovanovich.

Matthen, Mohan (1988). Biological functions and perceptual content. *Journal of Philosophy* 85:5–27.

_____ (2005). *Seeing, Doing, and Knowing: A Philosophical Theory of Sense Perception.* Oxford: Clarendon Press.

Mausfeld, Rainer (1998). Color perception: From Grassman codes to a dual code for object and illumination colors. In W. G. K. Braukhaus, R. Kiegl, and J. S. Werner (eds.), *Color Vision: Perspectives From Different Disciplines*, 381–430. Berlin: de Gruyter.

_____ (2003). "Colour" as part of the format of different perceptual primitives: The dual coding of colour. In Rainer Mausfeld and Dieter Heyer (eds.), *Colour Perception: Mind and the Physical World*, 475–502. Oxford: Oxford University Press.

Maynard Smith, John (1978). Optimization theory in evolution. *Annual Review of Ecology and Systematics* 9:31–56.

Mayr, Ernst (1970). *Populations, Species, and Evolution.* Cambridge, Mass.: Harvard University Press.

Mehler, Jacques, John Morton, and Peter W. Jusczyk (1984). On reducing language to biology. *Cognitive Neuropsychology* 1:83–116.

Mellars, Paul (1989). Major issues in the emergence of modern humans. *Current Anthropology* 30:349–85.

Michaels, Claire F., and Claudia Carello (1981). *Direct Perception.* Englewood Cliffs, N.J.: Prentice-Hall.

Mill, John Stuart (1865). *Auguste Comte and Positivism.* London: Trübner.

Mill, John Stuart (1974). *System of Logic, Ratiocinative and Inductive*, 2 vols. London: Routledge & Kegan Paul.

Millikan, Ruth G. (1984). *Language, Thought, and Other Biological Categories: New Foundations for Realism*. Cambridge, Mass.: MIT Press.

——— (1986). Thoughts without laws: Cognitive science with content. *Philosophical Review* 95:47–80.

Milner, A. David, and Melvyn A. Goodale (2006). *The Visual Brain in Action*, 2nd edn. Oxford: Oxford University Press.

Milner, Brenda, Suzanne Corkin, and H.-L. Teubner (1968). Further analysis of the hippocampal amnesic syndrome: 14-year follow-up study of H.M. *Neuropsychologia* 6:215–34.

Mithen, Steven (1990). *Thoughtful Foragers: A Study of Prehistoric Decision Making*. Cambridge: Cambridge University Press.

——— (1996). *The Prehistory of the Mind: A Search for the Origin of Art, Science and Religion*. London: Thames and Hudson.

Molière, Jean Baptiste (1965). *Le Malade imaginaire*, ed. Peter H. Nurse. Oxford: Oxford University Press. Originally published in 1673.

Mollon, John D. (1989). "'Tho' she kneel'd in that place where they grew…'" The uses and origins of primate colour vision. *Journal of Experimental Biology* 146:21–38.

Moran, Richard (2001). *Authority and Estrangement: An Essay on Self-Knowledge*. Princeton: Princeton University Press.

Mundle, Clement W. K. (1971). *Perception: Facts and Theories*. Oxford: Oxford University Press.

Myers, Gerald E. (1986). Introspection and self-knowledge. *American Philosophical Quarterly* 23:199–207.

Nagel, Ernst (1979). Teleology revisited. *Teleology Revisited and Other Essays in the Philosophy and History of Science*, 275–316. New York: Columbia University Press.

Nakayama, Ken (1990). The iconic bottleneck and the tenuous link between early visual processing and perception. In Colin Blakemore (ed.), *Vision: Coding and Efficiency*, 411–22. Cambridge: Cambridge University Press.

Nakayama, Ken, Zijiang J. He, and Shinsuke Shimojo (1995). Visual surface recognition: A critical link between lower-level and higher-level vision. In Stephen M. Kosslyn and Daniel N. Osherson (eds.), *Invitation to Cognitive Science*, vol. 2, *Visual Cognition*, 2nd edn., 1–70. Cambridge, Mass.: MIT Press.

Nathans, Jeremy, and David S. Hogness (1983). Isolation, sequence analysis, and intron-exon arrangement of the gene encoding bovine rhodopsin. *Cell* 34:807–14.

Natsoulas, Thomas (1991). "Why do things look as they do?": Some Gibsonian answers to Koffka's question. *Philosophical Psychology* 4:183–202.

Neisser, Ulric (1967). *Cognitive Psychology*. New York: Appleton-Century-Crofts.

——— (1976). *Cognition and Reality: Principles and Implications of Cognitive Psychology*. San Francisco: Freeman.

Neitz, Jay, Maureen Neitz, and Gerald H. Jacobs (1993). More than three different cone pigments among people with normal color vision. *Vision Research* 33:117–22.

Neumann, Odmar (1971). Aufmerksamkeit. In Joachim Ritter (ed.), *Historisches Wörterbuch der Philosophie*, vol. 1:635−45. Darmstadt: Wissenschaftliche Buchgesellschaft.

Newell, Allen (1980). Physical symbol systems. *Cognitive Science* 4:135−83.

Newell, Allen, Paul S. Rosenbloom, and John E. Laird (1989). Symbolic architectures for cognition. In Michael I. Posner (ed.), *Foundations of Cognitive Science*, 93−131. Cambridge, Mass.: MIT Press.

Newell, Allen, and Herbert A. Simon (1976). Computer science as empirical inquiry: Symbols and search. *Communications of the Association for Computing Machinery*, 19:113−26. As republished in John Haugeland (ed.), *Mind Design*, 35−66. Cambridge, Mass.: MIT Press, 1981.

Newton, Isaac (1718). *Opticks: or, A Treatise of the Reflections, Refractions, Inflections and Colours of Light*, 2nd edn. London: Innys.

Noë, Alva (2004). *Action in Perception*. Cambridge, Mass.: MIT Press.

O'Donnell, John M. (1979). The crisis in experimentalism in the 1920s: E. G. Boring and his uses of history. *American Psychologist* 34:289−95.

O'Neil, William M. (1982). *Beginnings of Modern Psychology*, 2nd edn. Sydney: Sydney University Press.

Osgood, Charles Egerton (1953). *Method and Theory in Experimental Psychology*. New York: Oxford University Press.

Palmer, Stephen E. (1978). Fundamental aspects of cognitive representation. In Eleanor Rosch and Barbara B. Lloyd (eds.), *Cognition and Categorization*. Hillsdale, N.J.: Erlbaum.

_____ (1999). *Vision Science: Photons to Phenomenology*. Cambridge, Mass.: MIT Press.

Palmer, Stephen E., and Ruth Kimchi (1986). The information processing approach to cognition. In Terry J. Knapp and Lynn C. Robertson (eds.), *Approaches to Cognition: Contrasts and Controversies*. Hillsdale, N.J.: Erlbaum.

Parasuraman, Raja and D. R. Davies (1984). Preface. In Raja Parasuraman and D. R. Davies (ed.), *Varieties of Attention*, xi−xvi. Orlando: Academic Press.

Pasnau, Robert (1997). *Theories of Cognition in the Later Middle Ages*. Cambridge: Cambridge University Press.

_____ (2002). *Thomas Aquinas on Human Nature: A Philosophical Study of Summa theologiae 1a 75−89*. Cambridge: Cambridge University Press.

Pastore, Nicholas (1971) *Selective History of Theories of Visual Perception*. New York: Oxford University Press.

Pastore, Nicholas, and Hélène Klibbe (1969). The orientation of the cerebral image in Descartes' theory of visual perception. *Journal of the History of the Behavioral Sciences* 5:385−9.

Peacocke, Christopher (1983). *Sense and Content: Experience, Thought, and Their Relations*. Oxford: Clarendon Press.

_____ (1984). Colour concepts and colour experience. *Synthese* 58:365−82.

_____ (1992). Scenarios, concepts and perception. In Tim Crane (ed.), *The Contents of Experience: Essays on Perception*, 105−35. Cambridge: Cambridge University Press.

Pecham, John (1970). *John Pecham and the Science of Optics: Perspectiva Communis*, ed. and trans. David C. Lindberg. Madison: University of Wisconsin Press.

Perry, John (2000). What are indexicals? *The Problem of the Essential Indexical and Other Essays*, 313–23. Stanford: CSLI Publications.

Peterson, Mary A. (2001). Object perception. In E. Bruce Goldstein (ed.), *Blackwell Handbook of Perception*, 168–203. Oxford: Blackwell.

Pettigrew, John D., and Masakazu Konishi (1976). Neurons selective for orientation and binocular disparity in the visual Wulst of the barn owl (*Tyto alba*). *Science* 193:675–8.

Piaget, Jean (1971). *Psychology and Epistemology*, trans. Arnold Rosin. New York: Grossman.

Pillsbury, Walter Bowers (1911). *Essentials of Psychology*. New York: Macmillan.

Pinker, Steven (1997). *How the Mind Works*. New York: Norton.

Pinker, Steven, and Paul Bloom (1990). Natural language and natural selection. *Behavioral and Brain Science* 13:707–84.

Pinker, Steven, and Alan Prince (1988). On language and connectionism: Analysis of a parallel distributed processing model of language acquisition. *Cognition* 28:73–193.

Pitcher, George (1977). *Berkeley*. London: Routledge and Kegan Paul.

Place, Ullin T. (1956). Is consciousness a brain process? *British Journal of Psychology* 47:44–50.

Planck, Max (1932). *Where Is Science Going?* trans. James Murphy. New York: Norton.

Poggio, G. F., and B. Fischer (1977). Binocular interaction and depth sensitivity in striate and prestriate cortex of behaving rhesus monkey. *Journal of Neurophysiology* 40:1392–1405.

Polyak, Stephen (1957). *The Vertebrate Visual System*. Chicago: University of Chicago Press.

Porterfield, William (1759). *A Treatise on the Eye: The Manner and Phenomena of Vision*, 2 vols. Edinburgh: Balfour.

Proffitt, Dennis R. (1993). A hierarchical approach to perception. In S. C. Masin (ed.), *Foundations of Perceptual Theory*, 75–93, 103–11. Amsterdam: Elsevier.

Proffitt, Dennis R., and Mary K. Kaiser (1995). Perceiving events. In William Epstein and Sheena Rogers (eds.), *Perception of Space and Motion*, 227–61. San Diego, Calif.: Academic Press.

—— (1998). The internalization of perceptual processing constraints. In Julian Hochberg (ed.), *Perception and Cognition at Century's End*, 169–97. San Diego, Calif.: Academic Press.

Ptolemy, Claudius (1956). *L'Optique de Claude Ptolémée, dans la version latine d'après l'arabe de l'émir Eugène de Sicile*, ed. Albert Lejeune. Louvain: Publications Universitaires.

—— (1989). *L'Optique de Claude Ptolémée, dans la version latine d'après l'arabe de l'émir Eugène de Sicile*, ed. and trans. Albert Lejeune. Leiden: Brill.

—— (1996). *Ptolemy's Theory of Visual Perception: An English Translation of the Optics*, ed. A. Mark Smith. Philadelphia: American Philosophical Society.

Putnam, Hilary (1967). The mental life of some machines. In Hector-Neri Castanñeda (ed.), *Intentionality, Minds, and Perception*. Detroit: Wayne State University Press. As republished in Putnam 1975*a*, 408–28.

——(1973*a*). Explanation and reference. In Glenn Pearce and Patrick Maynard (eds.), *Conceptual Change*, 199–221. Dordrecht: Reidel. As republished in Putnam 1975*a*, 196–214.

——(1973*b*). The meaning of "meaning." In Keith Gunderson (ed.), *Language, Mind and Knowledge*, 131–93. Minneapolis: University of Minnesota Press. As republished in Putnam 1975*a*, 215–71.

——(1975*a*). *Philosophical Papers*, vol. 2, *Mind, Language and Reality*. Cambridge: Cambridge University Press.

——(1975*b*). Philosophy and our mental life. In Putnam 1975*a*, 291–303.

——(1981). *Reason, Truth, and History*. Cambridge: Cambridge University Press.

——(1988). *Representation and Reality*. Cambridge, Mass.: MIT Press.

Pylyshyn, Zenon (1980). Computation and cognition: Issues in the foundation of cognitive science. *Behavioral and Brain Sciences* 3:111–69.

——(1984). *Computation and Cognition: Toward a Foundation for Cognitive Science*. Cambridge, Mass.: MIT Press.

——(1989). Computing in cognitive science. In Michael I. Posner (ed.), *Foundations of Cognitive Science*, 49–92. Cambridge, Mass.: MIT Press.

——(2003). *Seeing and Visualizing: It's Not What You Think*. Cambridge, Mass.: MIT Press.

——(2007). *Things and Places: How the Mind Connects with the World*. Cambridge, Mass.: MIT Press.

Quine, W. V. (1953). Two dogmas of empiricism. In *From a Logical Point of View: 9 Logico-Philosophical Essays*, 20–46. Cambridge, Mass.: Harvard University Press.

——(1960). *Word and Object*. Cambridge, Mass.: MIT Press.

——(1974). *The Roots of Reference*. La Salle, Ill.: Open Court.

Quinlan, Philip T. (1991). *Connectionism and Psychology: A Psychological Perspective on New Connectionist Research*. Chicago: University of Chicago Press.

Raphael, Bertram (1976). *The Thinking Computer: Mind Inside Matter*. San Francisco: Freeman.

Ratliff, Floyd (1965). *Mach Bands: Quantitative Studies on Neural Networks in the Retina*. San Francisco: Holden-Day.

Recanati, François (1993). *Direct Reference: From Language to Thought*. Oxford: Blackwell.

Reed, Edward S. (1986). James J. Gibson's revolution in perceptual psychology: A case study in the transformation of ideas. *Studies in History and Philosophy of Science* 17:65–98.

Regis, Pierre-Sylvain (1691). *Systeme de philosophie*, 7 vols. Lyon: Anisson, Posuel et Rigaud.

Reid, Thomas (1785). *An Inquiry into the Human Mind*, 4th edn. Edinburgh: Bell and Creech.

Reid, Thomas (1863). *Works of Thomas Reid*, ed. William Hamilton, 2 vols. Edinburgh: MacLachlan and Stewart.

Rey, Georges (1997). *Contemporary Philosophy of Mind: A Contentiously Classical Approach*. Cambridge, Mass.: Blackwell.

Richardson, Alan W. (1998). *Carnap's Construction of the World: The Aufbau and the Emergence of Logical Empiricism*. Cambridge: Cambridge University Press.

Roback, Abraham Aaron (1923). *Behaviorism and Psychology*. Cambridge, Mass.: University Book Store.

Robinson, Howard (1994). *Perception*. London: Routledge.

Rock, Irvin (1954). The perception of the egocentric orientation of a line. *Journal of Experimental Psychology* 48:367–74.

—— (1975). *Introduction to Perception*. New York: Macmillan Publishing Co.

—— (1977). In defense of unconscious inference. In William Epstein (ed.), *Stability and Constancy in Visual Perception: Mechanisms and Processes*, 321–73. New York: John Wiley.

—— (1983). *The Logic of Perception*. Cambridge, Mass.: MIT Press.

Rock, Irvin, and Sheldon Ebenholtz (1959). The relational determination of perceived size. *Psychological Review* 66:387–401.

Rohault, Jacques (1735). *System of Natural Philosophy*, trans. Samuel Clarke, 3rd edn., 2 vols. London: Knapton. Original version published in 1671.

Rosenberg, Alexander (1985). *Structure of Biological Science*. Cambridge: Cambridge University Press.

Rosenfeld, Azriel (1990). Pyramid algorithms for efficient vision. In Colin Blakemore (ed.), *Vision: Coding and Efficiency*, 423–30. Cambridge: Cambridge University Press.

Rubin, Edgar (1921). *Visuell wahrgenommene Figuren*. Copenhagen: Gyldendals.

Ruckmich, Christian A. (1912). History and status of psychology in the United States. *American Journal of Psychology* 23:517–31.

Rumelhart, David E. (1989). The architecture of mind: A connectionist approach. In Michael I. Posner (ed.), *Foundations of Cognitive Science*, 133–60. Cambridge, Mass.: MIT Press.

Rumelhart, David E., and James L. McClelland (1986a). On learning the past tense of English verbs. In James L. McClelland and David E. Rumelhart (eds.), *Parallel Distributed Processing: Explorations in the Microstructure of Cognition*, vol. 2, *Psychological and Biological Models*, 216–71. Cambridge, Mass.: MIT Press.

—— (eds.) (1986b). *Parallel Distributed Processing: Explorations in the Microstructure of Cognition*, 2 vols. Cambridge, Mass.: MIT Press.

Runeson, Sverker (1977). On the possibility of smart perceptual mechanisms. *Scandinavian Journal of Psychology* 18:172–9.

Russell, Bertrand (1912). *The Problems of Philosophy*. New York: Henry Holt.

—— (1914a). On the nature of acquaintance. *Monist* 24:1–16, 161–87, 435–53. As republished in Russell (1956), 125–74.

_____ (1914*b*). *Our Knowledge of the External World as a Field for Scientific Method in Philosophy*. Chicago: Open Court.

_____ (1914*c*). Relation of sense-data to physics. *Scientia* 16:1–27.

_____ (1915). The ultimate constituents of matter. *Monist* 25:399–417.

_____ (1919). On propositions: What they are and how they mean. *Proceedings of the Aristotelian Society*, suppl. vol. 2, *Problems of Science and Philosophy*, 1–43. As republished in Russell (1956), 285–320.

_____ (1921). *The Analysis of Mind*. London: Allen and Unwin.

_____ (1945). *History of Western Philosophy*. New York: Simon and Schuster.

_____ (1953). The cult of common usage. *British Journal for the Philosophy of Science* 3:303–7.

_____ (1956). *Logic and Knowledge: Essays, 1901–1950*, ed. Robert C. Marsh. New York: Macmillan.

Ryle, Gilbert (1949). *The Concept of Mind*. London: Hutchinson.

Sabbah, Daniel (1985). Computing with connections in visual recognition of origami objects. *Cognitive Science* 9:25–50.

Sabra, Abdelhamid I. (1978). Sensation and inference in Alhazen's theory of visual perception. In Peter Machamer and Robert Turnbull (eds.), *Studies in Perception*, 160–85. Columbus: Ohio State University Press.

_____ (1989). *The Optics of Ibn al-Haytham: Books I–III, On Direct Vision*, vol 2, *Introduction, Commentary, Glossaries, Concordance, Indices*. London: Warburg Institute.

Saltzman, Irving J., and Wendell Garner (1948). Reaction time as a measure of span of attention. *Journal of Psychology* 25:227–41.

Schacter, Daniel L., and Endel Tulving (1994). What are the memory systems of 1994? In Daniel L. Schacter and Endel Tulving (eds.), *Memory Systems*, 1–38. Cambridge, Mass.: MIT Press.

Schacter, Daniel L., A. D. Wagner, and R. Buckner (2000). Memory systems of 1999. In Endel Tulving and Fergus I. M. Craik (eds.), *Oxford Handbook of Memory*, 627–43. Oxford: Oxford University Press.

Scheerer, Eckart (1994). Psychoneural isomorphism: Historical background and current relevance. *Philosophical Psychology* 7:183–210.

_____ (1995), Die Sinne. In J. Ritter and K. Gründer (eds.), *Historisches Wörterbuch der Philosophie*, vol. 9, *Se–Sp*, 824–69. Basel: Schwabe.

Scheffler, Israel (1965). *Conditions of Knowledge*. Chicago: Scott, Foresman.

Schiffer, Stephen (1978). The basis of reference. *Erkenntnis* 13:171–206.

Schmid, Carl C. E. (1796). *Empirische Psychologie*, 2nd edn. Jena: Cröker.

Schmidt-Nielsen, Knut (1990). *Animal Physiology: Adaptation and Environment*, 4th edn. Cambridge: Cambridge University Press.

Schnaitter, Roger (1986). A coordination of differences: Behaviorism, mentalism, and the foundations of psychology. In Terry J. Knapp and Lynn C. Robertson (eds.), *Approaches to Cognition: Contrasts and Controversies*, 291–315. Hillsdale, N.J.: Erlbaum.

Schneider, Gerald E. (1967). Contrasting visuomotor functions of tectum and cortex in the golden hamster. *Psychologische Forschung* 31:52–62.

Schoumans, Nicole, Astrid M. Kappers, and Jan Koenderink (2002). Scale invariance in near space: Pointing under influence of context. *Acta Psychologica* 110:63–81.

Schrödinger, Erwin (1958). *Mind and Matter*, Cambridge: Cambridge University Press. As republished in Schrödinger, *What Is Life?* and *Mind and Matter*, Cambridge: Cambridge University Press, 1967.

——(1961). *Meine Weltansicht*. Hamburg: Zsolnay. Trans. C. Hastings, *My View of the World*, Cambridge: Cambridge University Press, 1964.

Schultz, Duane P., and Sydney E. Schultz (1987). *A History of Modern Psychology*, 4th edn. San Diego: Harcourt Brace Jovanovich.

Schwartz, Peter (2002). The continuing usefulness account of proper function. In André Ariew, Robert Cummins, and Mark Perlman (eds.), *Functions: New Essays in the Philosophy of Psychology and Biology*, 244–60. Oxford: Oxford University Press.

Schwartz, Robert (1994). *Vision: Variations on Some Berkeleian Themes*. Oxford: Basil Blackwell.

——(2006). *Visual Versions*. Cambridge, Mass.: MIT Press.

Searle, John R. (1983). *Intentionality: An Essay in the Philosophy of Mind*. Cambridge: Cambridge University Press.

——(1995). *The Construction of Social Reality*. New York: Free Press.

Sejnowski, Terrence J., and Geoffrey E. Hinton (1989). Separating figure from ground with a Boltzmann machine. In M. A. Arbib and A. R. Hanson (eds.), *Vision, Brain, and Cooperative Computation*, 703–24. Cambridge, Mass.: MIT Press.

Sellars, Roy Wood (1916). *Critical Realism*. Chicago: Rand McNally.

Shannon, Claude E. (1948). A mathematical theory of communication. *Bell System Technical Journal* 27:379–423, 623–56.

Shapere, Dudley (1969). Notes toward a post-positivistic interpretation of science. In Peter Achinstein and Stephen F. Barker (eds.), *The Legacy of Logical Positivism*, 115–60. Baltimore: Johns Hopkins Press.

Shapiro, Lawrence (1992). Darwin and disjunction: Foraging theory and univocal assignments of content. *PSA: Proceedings of the Biennial Meeting of the Philosophy of Science Association*, vol. 1:469–80.

——(1994). Behavior, ISO functionalism, and psychology. *Studies in History and Philosophy of Science* 25:191–209.

——(1995). What is psychophysics? In D. Hull, M. Forbes, and R. M. Burian (eds.), *PSA 1994*, vol. 2, *Symposia and Invited Papers*, 47–57. East Lansing, Mich.: Philosophy of Science Association.

——(1996). Representation from bottom and top. *Canadian Journal of Philosophy*, 26:523–42.

——(1997). The nature of nature: Rethinking naturalistic theories of intentionality. *Philosophical Psychology* 10:309–22.

——(1998). Do's and don'ts for Darwinizing psychology. In Colin Allen and Denise Cummins (eds.), *Evolution of Mind*, 243–59. New York: Oxford University Press.

Shastri, Lokendra (1988). A connectionist approach to knowledge representation and limited inference. *Cognitive Science* 12:331–92.

_____ (1990). Connectionism and the computational effectiveness of reasoning. *Theoretical Linguistics* 16:65–87.

Shastri, Lokendra, and Venkat Ajjanagadde (1993). From simple associations to systematic reasoning: A connectionist representation of rules, variables and dynamic bindings using temporal synchrony. *Behavioral and Brain Sciences* 16:417–94.

Shaw, Robert, and Michael T. Turvey (1981). Coalitions as models for ecosystems: A realist perspective on perceptual organization. In Michael Kubovy and James R. Pomeranz (eds.), *Perceptual Organization*, 343–415. Hillsdale, N.J.: Erlbaum.

Shebilske, Wayne L., and Aaron L. Peters (1995). Perceptual constancies: Analysis and synthesis. In Wolfgang Prinz and Bruce Bridgeman (eds.), *Handbook of Perception and Action*, vol. 1, *Perception*, 227–51. London: Academic Press.

Shepard, Roger (1975). Form, formation, and transformation of internal representations. In Robert L. Solso (ed.), *Information Processing and Cognition*, 87–122. New York: Wiley.

_____ (1981). Psychophysical complementarity. In Michael Kubovy and James R. Pomeranz (eds.), *Perceptual Organization*, 279–341. Hillsdale, N.J.: Erlbaum.

_____ (1984). Ecological constraints on internal representation: Resonant kinematics of perceiving, imagining, thinking, and dreaming. *Psychological Review* 91:417–47.

_____ (1992). The perceptual organization of colors: An adaptation to regularities of the terrestrial world? In Jerome H. Barkow, Leda Cosmides, and John Tooby (eds.), *The Adapted Mind: Evolutionary Psychology and the Generation of Culture*, 495–532. New York: Oxford University Press.

_____ (1994). Perceptual-cognitive universals as reflections of the world. *Psychonomic Bulletin and Review* 1:2–28.

Shepard, Roger, and Susan Chipman (1970). Second-order isomorphism of internal representations: Shapes of states. *Cognitive Psychology* 1:1–17.

Sherrington, Charles Scott, Sir (1940). *Man on His Nature*. Cambridge: Cambridge University Press.

_____ (1951). *Man on His Nature*, 2nd edn. Cambridge: Cambridge University Press.

Shoemaker, Sydney (1996). *The First-Person Perspective and Other Essays*. Cambridge: Cambridge University Press.

Siegel, R. E. (1970). *Galen on Sense Perception*. Basel: Karger.

Simmons, Alison (1994). Explaining sense perception: A scholastic challenge. *Philosophical Studies* 73:257–75.

Singer, Edgar A. (1911). Mind as an observable object. *Journal of Philosophy, Psychology and Scientific Methods* 8:180–6.

Skinner, B. F. (1938). *Behavior of Organisms: An Experimental Analysis*. New York: Appleton-Century.

_____ (1945). Operational analysis of psychological terms. *Psychological Review* 52:270–7, 291–4.

_____ (1957). *Verbal Behavior*. New York: Appleton-Century-Crofts.

_____ (1963). Behaviorism at fifty. *Science* 140:951–8.

Slomann, Aage (1968). Perception of size: Some remarks on size as a primary quality and "size constancy." *Inquiry* 11:101–13.

Sluga, Hans (1996). "Whose house is that?" Wittgenstein on the self. In Hans Sluga and David G. Stern (eds.), *Cambridge Companion to Wittgenstein*, 320–53. Cambridge: Cambridge University Press.

Smart, J. J. C. (1959). Sensations and brain processes. *Philosophical Review* 68:141–56.

——(1961). Colours. *Philosophy* 36:128–42.

——(1962). Sensations and brain processes. In Vere C. Chappell (ed.), *Philosophy of Mind*, 160–72. Englewood Cliffs, N.J.: Prentice-Hall.

Smith, Edward E. (1995). Concepts and categorization. In Edward E. Smith and Daniel N. Osherson (eds.), *Invitation to Cognitive Science*, vol. 3, *Thinking*, 2nd edn., 3–33. Cambridge, Mass.: MIT Press.

Smith, Edward E., and Douglas L. Medin (1981). *Categories and Concepts*. Cambridge, Mass.: Harvard University Press.

Smith, Laurence D. (1981). Psychology and philosophy: Toward a realignment, 1905–1935. *Journal of the History of the Behavioral Sciences* 17:28–37.

——(1986). *Behaviorism and Logical Positivism: A Reassessment of the Alliance*. Stanford: Stanford University Press.

Smith, Robert (1738). *A Compleat System of Opticks*, 2 vols. Cambridge: printed for the author.

Smolensky, Paul (1988). On the proper treatment of connectionism. *Behavioral and Brain Sciences* 11:1–74.

Snodderly, D. Max (1979). Visual discriminations encountered in food foraging by a neotropical primate: Implications for the evolution of color vision. In Edward H. Burtt, Jr. (ed.), *Behavioral Significance of Color*, 237–79. New York: Garland.

Spelke, Elizabeth S. (1990). Principles of object perception. *Cognitive Science* 14:29–56.

Spelke, Elizabeth S., and Richard Kestenbaum (1986). Les origins du concept d'object. *Psychologie française* 31:67–72.

Spelke, Elizabeth S., Grant Gutheil, and Gretchen Van de Walle (1995). The development of object perception. In Stephen M. Kosslyn and Daniel N. Osherson (eds.), *Visual Cognition*, 297–330. Cambridge, Mass.: MIT Press.

Sperling, George (1960). The information available in brief visual presentations. *Psychological Monographs* 74 (11, Whole No. 498).

Squire, Larry R. (1987). *Memory and Brain*. New York: Oxford University Press.

Squire, Larry R., and Neal J. Cohen (1984). Human memory and amnesia. In G. Lynch, J. L. McGaugh, and N. M. Weinberger (eds.), *Neurobiology of Memory*, 3–64. New York: Guilford Press.

Stabler, Edward P. (1983). How are grammars represented? *Behavioral and Brain Sciences* 6:391–421.

——(1987). Kripke on functionalism and automata. *Synthese* 70:1–22.

Steinbuch, Johann Georg (1811). *Beytrag zur Physiologie der Sinne*. Nurnberg: J. L. Schragg.

Steneck, Nicholas (1974). Albert the Great on the classification and localization of the internal senses. *Isis* 65:193–211.

Sterling, Peter (1990). Retina. In G. M. Shepherd (ed.), *The Synaptic Organization of the Brain*, 3rd edn., 170–213. New York: Oxford University Press.

Stewart, Dugald (1793). *Elements of the Philosophy of the Human Mind*. Philadelphia: William Young.

Stich, Stephen (1983). *From Folk Psychology to Cognitive Science: The Case Against Belief*. Cambridge, Mass.: MIT Press.

Stout, George F. (1923). Are the characteristic of things universal or particular? *Proceedings of the Aristotelian Society* 3 (supp.):114–22.

Strawson, Galen (1989). Red and "red." *Synthese* 78:193–232.

——(1994). *Mental Reality*. Cambridge, Mass.: MIT Press.

Strawson, Peter F. (1959). *Individuals: An Essay in Descriptive Metaphysics*. London: Methuen.

Stroud, Barry (2000). *The Quest for Reality: Subjectivism and the Metaphysics of Color*. New York: Oxford University Press.

Sturdee, David (1997). The semantic shuffle: Shifting emphasis in Dretske's account of representational content. *Erkenntnis* 47:89–103.

Suppes, Patrick (1977). Is visual space Euclidean? *Synthese* 35:397–421.

Suppes, Patrick, and Joseph L. Zinnes (1963). Basic measurement theory. In R. Duncan Luce, Robert R. Bush, and Eugene Galanter (eds.), *Handbook of Mathematical Psychology*, 2 vols., 1:1–76. New York: Wiley.

Svaetichin, Gunnar (1956). Spectral response curves from single cones. *Acta Physiologica Scandinavica* 39 (supp. 134), 17–46.

Swets, John A., Wilson P. Tanner, and Theodore G. Birdsall (1961). Decision processes in perception. *Psychological Review* 68:301–40.

Teller, Davida Y., and Edward N. Pugh (1983). Linking propositions in color vision. In John D. Mollon and Lindsey T. Sharpe (eds.), *Colour Vision: Physiology and Psychophysics*, 577–89. London: Academic Press.

Theophrastus (1917). *On the Senses*, trans. George M. Stratton. In Stratton, *Theophrastus and the Greek Physiological Psychology before Aristotle*. New York: Macmillan.

Thomasson, Amie L. (2007). *Ordinary Objects*. New York: Oxford University Press.

Thompson, Evan (1995). *Colour Vision: A Study in Cognitive Science and the Philosophy of Perception*. London: Routledge.

Thorndyke, Perry W. (1981). Distance estimation from cognitive maps. *Cognitive Psychology* 13:526–50.

Thouless, Robert H. (1931). Phenomenal regression to the real object. I. *British Journal of Psychology* 21:339–59.

——(1932). Phenomenal regression to the "real" object. II. *British Journal of Psychology* 22:1–30.

Thrane, Gary (1977). Berkeley's "proper object of vision." *Journal of the History of Ideas* 38:243–60.

Titchener, Edward B. (1908). *Lectures on the Elementary Psychology of Feeling and Attention.* New York: Macmillan.

—— (1910). *A Text-Book of Psychology.* New York: Macmillan.

—— (1912*a*). Prolegomena to a study of introspection. *American Journal of Psychology* 23:427–48.

—— (1912*b*). The schema of introspection. *American Journal of Psychology* 23:485–508.

Todd, James T. (1981). Visual information about moving objects. *Journal of Experimental Psychology: Human Perception and Performance* 7:795–810.

Todd, James T., Augustinus H. J. Oomes, Jan J. Koenderink, and Astrid M. L. Kappers (2001). On the affine structure of perceptual space. *Psychological Science* 12:191–6.

Tokuda, Gaku, Nathan Lo, Hirofumi Watanabe, Gaku Arakawa, Tadao Matsumotos, and Hiroaki Noda (2004). Major alteration of the expression site of endogenous cellulases in members of an apical termite lineage. *Molecular Ecology* 13:3219–28.

Tolman, Edward C. (1926). A behavioristic theory of ideas. *Psychological Review* 33:352–69.

—— (1927). A behaviorist's definition of consciousness. *Psychological Review* 34:433–9.

—— (1932). *Purposive Behavior in Animals and Men.* New York: Century.

—— (1936). Operational behaviorism and current trends in psychology. In H. W. Hill (ed.), *Proceedings of the Twenty-Fifth Anniversary Celebration of the Inauguration of Graduate Studies.* Los Angeles: University of Southern California Press.

—— (1951). *Collected Papers in Psychology.* Berkeley: University of California Press.

Tomasello, Michael (1999). *Cultural Origins of Human Cognition.* Cambridge, Mass.: Harvard University Press.

Tourtual, Caspar T. (1827). *Die Sinne des Menschen in den wechselseitigen Beziehungen ihres psychischen und organischen Lebens: Ein Beitrag zur physiologischen Aesthetick.* Münster: Coppenrath.

Toye, Richard C. (1986). The effect of viewing position on the perceived layout of space. *Perception and Psychophysics* 40:85–92.

Travis, Joseph (1989). The role of optimizing selection in natural populations. *Annual Review of Ecology and Systematics* 20:279–96.

Tremoulet, Patrice D., Alan M. Leslie, and G. Hall (2001). Infant attention to the shape and color of objects: Individuation and identification. *Cognitive Development* 15:499–522.

Trevarthen, Colwyn B. (1968). Two mechanisms of vision in primates. *Psychologische Forschung* 31:299–337.

Triesman, Anne M., and Garry Gelade (1980). A feature integration theory of attention. *Cognitive Psychology* 12:97–136.

Tschermak-Seysenegg, Armin von (1952). *Introduction to Physiological Optics*, trans. Paul Boeder. Springfield, Ill.: Thomas.

Tulving, Endel (1983). *Elements of Episodic Memory.* Oxford: Oxford University Press.

—— (2002). Episodic memory: From mind to brain. *Annual Review of Psychology* 53: 1–25.

Turner, R. Steven (1994). *In the Eye's Mind: Vision and the Helmholtz–Hering Controversy.* Princeton: Princeton University Press.

Turvey, Michael T., Robert E. Shaw, Edward S. Reed, and William M. Mace (1981). Ecological laws of perceiving and acting: In reply to Fodor and Pylyshyn. *Cognition* 9:237–304.

Tychsen, L. (1992). Binocular vision. In W. M. Hart (ed.), *Adler's Physiology of the Eye*, 773–853. St. Louis: Mosby.

Tye, Michael (1991). *The Imagery Debate.* Cambridge, Mass.: MIT Press.

_____ (1995). *Ten Problems of Consciousness: A Representational Theory of the Phenomenal Mind.* Cambridge, Mass.: MIT Press.

_____ (2000). *Consciousness, Color, and Content.* Cambridge, Mass.: MIT Press.

_____ (2002). Representationalism and the transparency of experience. *Noûs* 36:137–51.

_____ (2003). *Consciousness and Persons: Unity and Identity.* Cambridge, Mass.: MIT Press.

Tyler, C. W. (1983). Sensory processing of binocular disparity. In C. M. Schor and K. J. Ciuffreda (eds.), *Vergence Eye Movements: Basic and Clinical Aspects*, 199–295. Boston: Butterworths.

_____ (1990). A stereoscopic view of visual processing streams. *Vision Research* 30:1877–95.

Ullman, Shimon (1979). *The Interpretation of Visual Motion.* Cambridge, Mass.: MIT Press.

_____ (1980). Against direct perception. *Behavioral and Brain Sciences* 3:373–415.

Ungerleider, Leslie G., and Mortimer Mishkin (1982). Two cortical visual systems. In David J. Ingle, Melvyn A. Goodale, and Richard J. W. Mansfield (eds.), *Analysis of Visual Behavior*, 549–86. Cambridge, Mass.: MIT Press.

University of Pennsylvania (1938). The college. *Bulletin* 38 (no. 24).

Van de Walle, Gretchen, Susan Carey, and Meredith Prevor (2000). Bases for object individuation in infancy: Evidence from manual search. *Journal of Cognition and Development* 1:249–80.

Veysey, Laurence R. (1965). *Emergence of the American University.* Chicago: University of Chicago Press.

Vogel, Erin, Maureen Neitz, and Nathaniel J. Dominy (2007). Effect of color vision phenotype on the foraging of wild white-faced capuchins, Cebus capucinus. *Behavioral Ecology* 18:292–7.

Von Eckardt, Barbara (1984). Cognitive psychology and principled skepticism. *Journal of Philosophy* 81:67–88.

_____ (1993). *What Is Cognitive Science?* Cambridge, Mass.: MIT Press.

Wade, Nicholas J. (1987). On the late invention of the stereoscope. *Perception* 16:785–818.

Wagner, Mark (1985). The metric of visual space. *Perception and Psychophysics* 38:483–95.

_____ (2006). *Geometries of Visual Space.* Mahwah, N.J.: Erlbaum.

Wallhagen, Morgan (2007). Consciousness and action: Does cognitive science support (mild) epiphenomenalism? *British Journal for the Philosophy of Science* 58:539–61.

Walls, Gordon L. (1942). *The Vertebrate Eye and its Adaptive Radiation*. Bloomfield Hills, Mich.: Cranbrook Institute of Science.

Walsh, Denis M. (1996). Fitness and function. *British Journal for the Philosophy of Science* 47:553−74.

———(2002). Brentano's chestnuts. In André Ariew, Robert Cummins, and Mark Perlman (eds.), *Functions: New Essays in the Philosophy of Psychology and Biology*, 314−37. Oxford: Oxford University Press.

Wandell, Brian A. (1995). *Foundations of Vision*. Sunderland, Mass.: Sinauer Associates.

Watson, John B. (1913). Psychology as the behaviorist views it. *Psychological Review* 20:158−77.

———(1914). *Behavior: An Introduction to Comparative Psychology*. New York: Holt.

———(1919). *Psychology from the Standpoint of a Behaviorist*. Philadelphia: Lippincott.

———(1925). *Behaviorism*. New York: Norton.

Weiskrantz, Lawrence (1986). *Blindsight: A Case Study and Implications*. Oxford: Clarendon Press.

Weizenbaum, Joseph (1976). *Computer Power and Human Reason*. San Francisco: Freeman.

Wilkes, Kathleen V. (1978). *Physicalism*. London: Routledge and Kegan Paul.

———(1980). More brain lesions. *Philosophy* 55:455−70.

Williams, Donald C. (1953). On the elements of being. *Review of Metaphysics* 7:3−18, 171−92.

Williams, George C. (1966). *Adaptation and Natural Selection: A Critique of Some Current Evolutionary Thought*. Princeton: Princeton University Press.

Wilson, Daniel J. (1990). *Science, Community, and the Transformation of American Philosophy, 1860−1930*. Chicago: University of Chicago Press.

Winograd, Terry (1975). Frame representations and the declarative−procedural controversy. In D. G. Bobrow and A. Collins (eds.), *Representation and Understanding: Studies in Cognitive Science*, 185−210. New York: Academic Press.

Witelo (1572). *Perspectiva*. In Friedrich Risner (ed.), *Opticae thesaurus: Alhazeni Arabis libri septem; De Crepusculis et nubium ascensionibus; Vitellonis Thuringopoloni libri X*. Basel: Episcopate. Reprint, New York: Johnson Reprint, 1972.

———(1991). *Witelonis perspectivae liber secundus et liber tertius = Books II and III of Witelo's Perspectiva*, ed. and trans. Sabetai Unguru. Wroclaw: Ossolineum.

Wittgenstein, Ludwig (1953). *Philosophische Untersuchungen, Philosophical Investigations*, ed. and trans. G. E. M. Anscombe. New York, Macmillan.

Wolff, Christian (1738). *Psychologia empirica*. Frankfurt and Leipzig: Renger.

———(1740). *Psychologia rationalis*. Frankfurt and Leipzig: Renger.

Woodger, Joseph Henry (1938). *The Axiomatic Method in Biology*. Cambridge, Mass.: Cambridge University Press.

Woodhouse, J. Margaret, and Horace Basil Barlow (1982). Spatial and temporal resolution and analysis. In Horace Basil Barlow and John D. Mollon (eds.), *The Senses*, 133−64. Cambridge: Cambridge University Press.

Woodworth, Robert (1938). *Experimental Psychology*. New York: Henry Holt.

Woodworth, Robert, and Harold Schlossberg (1954). *Experimental Psychology*, rev. edn. New York: Henry Holt.

Wright, Larry (1973). Functions. *Philosophical Review* 82:139–68.

Wundt, Wilhelm (1862). *Beiträge zur Theorie der Sinneswahrnehmung*. Leipzig: Winter.

_____(1874). *Grundzüge der physiologischen Psychologie*. Leipzig: Engelmann.

_____(1882). Die Aufgaben der experimentellen Psychologie. *Unsere Zeit* 3:389–406. As republished in Wundt (1885), 127–53.

_____(1885). *Essays*. Leipzig: Engelmann.

_____(1888). Selbstbeobachtung und innere Wahrnehmung. *Philosophische Studien* 4:292–309.

_____(1901). *Grundriss der Psychologie*, 4th edn. Leipzig: Engelmann.

_____(1902). *Outlines of Psychology*, trans. Charles H. Judd. Leipzig: Engelmann.

_____(1902–3). *Grundzüge der physiologischen Psychologie*, 5th edn., 3 vols. Leipzig: Engelmann.

Xu, Fei (1997). From Lot's wife to a pillar of salt: Evidence that physical object is a sortal concept. *Mind and Language* 12:365–92.

Xu, Fei, and Susan Carey (1996). Infants' metaphysics: The case of numerical identity. *Cognitive Psychology* 30:111–53.

Yaglom, Isaak M. (1962–75). *Geometric Transformations*, trans. A. Shields, 3 vols. New York: Random House.

Yokoyama, Shozo (2000). Molecular evolution of vertebrate visual pigments. *Progress in Retinal and Eye Research* 19:385–419.

Yolton, John W. (1984). *Perceptual Acquaintance from Descartes to Reid*. Minneapolis: University of Minnesota Press.

Young, Thomas (1807). *Course of Lectures on Natural Philosophy and the Mechanical Arts*, 2 vols. London: Joseph Johnson.

Yrjönsuuri, Mikko (2008). Perceiving one's own body. In Simo Knuuttila and Pekka Kärkkäinen (eds.), *Theories of Perception in Medieval and Early Modern Philosophy*, 101–16. Dordrecht: Springer.

Yue, Xiaomin, Bosco S. Tjan, and Irving Biederman (2006). What makes faces special? *Vision Research* 46:3801–11.

Index

recognitional 21, 190, 214
see also under introspection; perceptual processes; visual experience
cones (receptors) 191–2, 272, 327, 331–2
  evolution of 192–4, 277–9, 288–90, 326, 330, 453
  molecular constituents of 452–4
  ontology of 451–4
connectionism 28–9, 71–4, 104–13, 151–2, 428
consciousness 4–6, 8, 18, 160, 178 n.
constancy, perceptual 9, 178–82
  Ptolemy and 126–7, 362
  Ibn al-Haytham and 128, 139, 145
  Descartes and 179, 374
  Helmholtz and 129 n.
  Hering and 129 n.
  of color 128–9, 167, 184, 185–6, 193–4, 283, 287, 289–91
  instructions and 183–4, 186, 190, 197, 477–8
  inverse-inference view of 129, 168, 171, 184–5, 189 n. 8, 193, 195
  of shape 118, 178–9, 182–4, 186–7, 190, 203–6, 359, 474–5, 476–8
  of size 128, 171, 181–5, 187–90, 195–8
constraints, see under perceptual processes
constructivism viii, 26
  cognitive 45, 51–2, 55–6, 60–1, 70
  noncognitive 7, 26–7, 46, 52–3, 63–7
content 17–19, 50–3, 74–86, 95, 97–101, 107–8, 122
  conceptual 5, 13–14, 60, 83–5, 122–3, 139–40, 180
  nonconceptual 7, 17–18, 33–4, 180 n., 221–2, 253, 275–6, 334 n. 9
  phenomenal 17–18, 144, 159–61, 220, 226, 322, 334, 350
  semantic 80, 85, 113–14, 234
contracted visual space, see space, contracted
convergence (of eyes) 132 n., 134–5, 374 n. 44, 437
convergence (of parallels) 168, 171–4, 187–9, 201–3
Copernicus, and "sunrise" 300 n., 342–3
Crane, Tim 138, 264
Cummins, Robert 8, 15, 44, 89
Cutting, James 196

Darwin, Charles 14
demonstratives 230, 234, 249–50, 254
Dennett, Daniel C. 31, 130 n., 316
Descartes, René 372–8, 383–4, 412–13
  on attention 392, 396, 398

on distance perception 132–3, 140, 374
and instrospection 458–60, 463
and mental faculties 133–4
and mind as natural 295, 390
and "no resemblance" 373 n. 43
and phenomenality of sensation 145
and pineal gland 372–4, 436
and post-retinal transmission 372–3, 377, 436
and secondary qualities 285
on size perception 128, 132–3, 374, 413
on three grades of sense 374–8
on unnoticed judgments 133–4, 140, 375–8
DeValois, Russell L. 442
Dewey, John 420, 421
direct realism, see under realism, perceptual
direct theory of visual perception, see under theories of visual perception
distance perception 126–8, 132–5, 366
Drake, Durant 350 n.
Dretske, Fred viii
  on indicator content 22–3, 98
  on information 22–3, 39, 334 n.
  on intensionality of explanation 24
  on introspection 468–9
  his naturalism 25, 39, 98, 222–3, 309 n. 9
  on object reference 214, 216 n., 217, 222–3, 227, 234–5
  on pictures 221–2
  on phenomenal content 264, 298, 316, 318–19, 323, 328–9, 332–3
  on representation 22–3, 39, 98–101, 122
  on "seeing" 224–8

early vision, see vision, early
Ebbinghaus, Hermann 388
Ebenholz, Sheldon 63 n., 196
ecological factors 16–17, 58–9, 78–81, 262, 273–5, 279, 332–3
Enç, Berent 237
epistemology 33, 96–7, 337–40, 461
  and intersubjectivity 286, 294–6, 299 n., 305, 307, 316–18, 458, 462
  and privacy 161, 294–5, 297–8, 317–18, 450, 461, 466, 480–1
  and subjectivity 161, 294–6, 297–8, 318–19, 468, 480–1
Epstein, William viii, 27, 63–4, 155–6, 185, 424, 477
Euclid 126, 361–2
Evans, Gareth 217, 218, 221–3, 229, 231, 234–5